W9-BJZ-605

The following points should be considered when reviewing Chapters 7, 11, 13 and 14 which relate to studies conducted with NORMODYNE® (labetalol HCl):

■ NORMODYNE is not approved for the treatment of angina pectoris.

■ Drug has not been studied for antianginal efficacy and safety in normotensive patients with angina.

■ Patients with coronary artery disease should be advised to consult their physician before discontinuing therapy.

■ NORMODYNE is contraindicated in hypertensive patients with overt cardiac failure.

■ Patients with non-allergic bronchospasm should, in general, not receive beta blockers. NORMODYNE may be used, with caution however, in patients who do not respond to, or cannot tolerate, other antihypertensive agents.

NOR-288/13246700

Clinical Pharmacology
of the
β-Adrenoceptor
Blocking Drugs

Clinical Pharmacology of the β-Adrenoceptor Blocking Drugs

Second Edition

William H. Frishman, M.D.
Associate Professor of Medicine
Albert Einstein College of Medicine
Chief of Medicine
Hospital of the Albert Einstein
College of Medicine
Bronx, New York

APPLETON-CENTURY-CROFTS/Norwalk, Connecticut

0-8385-1155-4

Notice: Our knowledge in the clinical sciences is constantly changing. As new information becomes available, changes in treatment and in the use of drugs become necessary. The author(s) and the publisher of this volume have taken care to make certain that the doses of drugs and schedules of treatment are correct and compatible with the standards generally accepted at the time of publication. The reader is advised to consult carefully the instruction and information material included in the package insert of each drug or therapeutic agent before administration. This advice is especially important when using new or infrequently used drugs.

First Edition, 1980
Second Edition, 1984

Copyright © 1984 by Appleton-Century-Crofts
A Publishing Division of Prentice-Hall, Inc.
Except for pages 257–272 from Circulation; 273–298 from Excerpta Medica; 341–366 from American Journal of Cardiology; 393–442 and 459–477 from American Journal of Medicine.

All rights reserved. This book, or any parts thereof, may not be used or reproduced in any manner without written permission. For information, address Appleton-Century-Crofts, 25 Van Zant Street, East Norwalk, Connecticut 06855.

84 85 86 87 88 89 / 10 9 8 7 6 5 4 3 2 1

Prentice-Hall International, Inc., London
Prentice-Hall of Australia, Pty. Ltd., Sydney
Prentice-Hall Canada, Inc.
Prentice-Hall of India Private Limited, New Delhi
Prentice-Hall of Japan, Inc., Tokyo
Prentice-Hall of Southeast Asia (Pte.) Ltd., Singapore
Whitehall Books Ltd., Wellington, New Zealand
Editora Prentice-Hall do Brasil Ltda., Rio de Janeiro

Library of Congress Cataloging in Publication Data

Frishman, William H., 1946-
  Clinical pharmacology of the beta-adrenoceptor blocking drugs.

  Bibliography: p.
  Includes index.
  1. Adrenergic beta receptor blockaders. 2. Cardiovascular system—Diseases—Chemotherapy. I. Title.
  [DNLM: 1. Adrenergic beta receptor blockaders.
  2. Cardiovascular diseases—Drug therapy. QV 132 F917c]
  RM323.5.F74 1984   615'.71   83-22349
  ISBN 0-8385-1155-4

Design: Jean M. Sabato

PRINTED IN THE UNITED STATES OF AMERICA

To my wife Esther Rose
and our children
Sheryl, Amy, and Michael Aaron

CONTRIBUTORS

Deborah Aronson, M.D.
Department of Medicine, Montefiore Hospital and Medical Center,
Bronx, New York

Ronald M. Becker, M.D.
Associate Professor of Medicine, Division of Cardiothoracic Surgery,
Albert Einstein College of Medicine, Bronx, New York

Jeffrey Bernstein, B.A.
Albert Einstein College of Medicine, Bronx, New York

Saul S. Bloomfield, M.D.
Professor of Medicine and Clinical Pharmacology, University of
Cincinnati School of Medicine, Cincinnati, Ohio

Lawrence J. Brandt, M.D.
Associate Director, Division of Gastroenterology, Montefiore Hospital
and Medical Center, Associate Professor of Medicine, Albert Einstein
College of Medicine, Bronx, New York

Shlomo Charlap, M.D.
Division of Cardiology, Albert Einstein College of Medicine, Bronx,
New York

Winston T. Edwards, M.D.
Clinical Assistant Professor of Medicine, University of Alabama
School of Medicine, Baptist Medical Center, Montgomery, Alabama

Edward S. Eisenberg, M.D.
Associate Chief of Medicine, Hospital of the Albert Einstein College of
Medicine, Bronx, New York

Uri Elkayam, M.D.
Director of In-Patient Cardiology, Los Angeles County—USC Medical Center, Los Angeles, California

Paul Farkas, M.D.
Associate Clinical Professor of Medicine, Tufts University School of Medicine, Bay State Medical Center, Springfield and Mercy Hospitals, Springfield, Massachusetts

Frank A. Finnerty, M.D.
Clinical Professor of Medicine, George Washington University School of Medicine, Medical Director, Washington Center for Clinical Studies, Washington, D.C.

William J. Flanigan, M.D.
Professor of Medicine, Director of Transplantation, University of Arkansas for Medical Sciences, Little Rock, Arkansas

Robert W. B. Frater, M.B., Ch.B., M.S.
Professor of Surgery and Chief, Division of Cardiothoracic Surgery, Albert Einstein College of Medicine, Bronx, New York

Edward D. Freis, M.D.
Senior Medical Investigator, Veterans Administration Medical Center, Professor of Medicine, Georgetown University Medical Center, Washington, D.C.

William H. Frishman, M.D.
Associate Professor of Medicine, Albert Einstein College of Medicine, Chief of Medicine, Hospital of the Albert Einstein College of Medicine, Bronx, New York

Curt D. Furberg, M.D.
Chief, Clinical Trials Branch, Division of Heart and Vascular Diseases, National Heart Lung and Blood Institute, Bethesda, Maryland

Harold Jacob, M.D.
Attending Physician, Division of Gastroenterology, Department of Medicine, Brooklyn Veterans Hospital, Brooklyn, New York

Brian F. Johnson, M.D.
Professor of Medicine and Pharmacology, Director of Clinical Pharmacology, University of Massachusetts College of Medicine, Worcester, Massachusetts

Bruce Kimmel, M.D.
Division of Cardiology, Albert Einstein College of Medicine, Bronx, New York

Benjamin Kirschenbaum, M.D.
Department of Medicine, Albert Einstein College of Medicine, Bronx New York

Marc Kirschner, M.D.
Division of Cardiology, Albert Einstein College of Medicine, Bronx, New York

Neal Klein, M.D.
Assistant Director, Coronary Care Unit, St. Joseph's Hospital, Phoenix, Arizona

Eliot Lazar, M.D.
Department of Medicine, Albert Einstein College of Medicine, Bronx, New York

James E. Lewis, M.D.
Associate Clinical Professor of Medicine, Stanford University School of Medicine, Sunnyvale Medical Center, Sunnyvale, California

Charles Lucas, M.D.
Professor of Medicine, Wayne State University School of Medicine, Detroit, Michigan

E. Paul MacCarthy, M.B., B.Ch.
Director of Hypertension Program, University of Cincinnati Medical Center, Cincinnati, Ohio

Eric L. Michelson, M.D.
Chief, Clinical Research Unit, The Lankenau Medical Research Center, Philadelphia, Pennsylvania

Yasu Oka, M.D.
Professor of Anesthesiology, Albert Einstein College of Medicine, Chief of Cardiac Anesthesiology, Hospital of the Albert Einstein College of Medicine, Bronx, New York

Heschi H. Rotmensch, M.D.
Assistant Professor of Medicine and Pharmacology, Assistant Director, Division of Clinical Pharmacology, Jefferson Medical College, Philadelphia, Pennsylvania

Henry S. Sawin, M.D.
Clinical Research Unit
The Lankenau Medical Research Center
Philadelphia, Pennsylvania

Ralph Silverman, M.D.
Assistant Clinical Professor of Medicine, Albert Einstein College of
Medicine, Bronx, New York

Edmund H. Sonnenblick, M.D.
Professor of Medicine, Chief, Division of Cardiology, Albert Einstein
College of Medicine, Bronx, New York

Carl R. Spivack, M.D.
Department of Medicine, Misericordia Hospital, Bronx, New York

Joel A. Strom, M.D.
Associate Professor of Medicine and Radiology, Albert Einstein
College of Medicine, Bronx, New York

Babette B. Weksler, M.D.
Professor of Medicine, Cornell University Medical College, New York
New York

CONTENTS

PREFACE TO THE SECOND EDITION

Twenty-five years ago the first β-adrenergic blocking drug, dichloroiso-prenaline (DCI), was synthesized. The discovery of DCI corroborated the dual adrenoceptor hypothesis, which stated that there were two distinct types of adrenergic receptors, classified as α and β. The finding that DCI selectively blocked pharmacologic responses that were mediated by β-receptors has proven to be one of the most significant advances in human pharmacotherapy.

The β-blocking drugs developed after DCI were initially utilized for the treatment of patients with angina pectoris, supraventricular arrhythmias, and systemic hypertension. It soon became clear that these drugs had much to offer in other cardiovascular and noncardiovascular disorders. Today there is no group of synthetic drugs that have had such widespread utility in human therapeutics.

The application of these agents has been accelerated by the development of β-blocking compounds possessing partial agonist activity, α-adrenergic blocking actions, and a degree of selectivity for various subgroups of the β-receptor population. β-Blocking drugs with widely different pharmacokinetic properties have been synthesized and new drug delivery systems for β-blockers have also been developed.

There are close to 20 β-blockers being marketed worldwide, and perhaps 9 of them will be available for clinical use in the United States by 1984. Tens of thousands of original scientific articles have been written about these drugs. Because of the need to synthesize this knowledge for easy reference and my career-long interest in β-blockers, my colleagues and I at the Albert Einstein College of Medicine prepared 13 consecutive monthly articles for *The American Heart Journal* (May 1979 to May 1980), based on our own original research and critical reviews of the literature. In late 1980, these articles were compiled and reproduced in the original edition of this book, the first comprehensive text dealing in its entirety with the β-blocking drugs.

Since 1980 this area has grown tremendously, both in the basic science and clinical spheres. The purpose of this second edition is to highlight the advances and update the information base on β-blockade, including our own research with these drugs. Much of this volume contains chapters based on journal articles written by my colleagues and myself since 1980, as well as completely revised updates of many chapters from the first edition. The text includes contributions from *The American Heart Journal, The American Journal of Cardiology, The American Journal of Medicine, The Annals of Internal Medicine, Cardiovascular Reviews and Reports, Circulation, Hospital Practice, The International Journal of Cardiology, The New England Journal of Medicine,* and *Pharmacotherapy.*

The first seven chapters of the book discuss the clinical and molecular pharmacology of β-blockers. The first chapter reviews the molecular pharmacology of α and β-blockade and the recent advances in adrenergic receptor research. The next two chapters deal with the pharmacodynamic and pharmacokinetic properties of the different β-blocking drugs and their physiologic and metabolic effects. Chapter 4 is an encyclopedic review of the major clinical studies of β-blockers in angina pectoris, systemic hypertension, and arrhythmia, and also details the other cardiovascular and noncardiovascular uses of the drugs. Chapter 5 discusses the adverse reaction profiles of the β-blockers, drug interactions, and how the clinician should choose a specific β-blocker for a given patient. The sixth chapter reviews our own experience and the world experience with β-blocker overdose, and the approach to treatment. Chapter 7 is a comprehensive review of the clinical pharmacology of labetalol, the first combined α- and β-adrenergic blocker. Drugs in this subclass will provide an innovative approach to patients with cardiovascular diseases.

β-Blockers are important drugs in the management of patients with ischemic heart disease—unstable and stable angina pectoris, acute myocardial infarction, and now for prolonging life in survivors of an acute myocardial infarction. They may also prolong life in patients at risk for a first myocardial infarction. The next five chapters in the book deal with the use of β-blockers in myocardial ischemia. Chapter 8 is a critical appraisal of how β-blockers might alter the pathophysiology of myocardial ischemia. Chapter 9 deals specifically with one of the possible antiischemic actions of β-blockers—their role as inhibitors of platelet aggregation. The chapter includes our own laboratory and clinical investigations in support of this concept. Chapter 10 is a comprehensive review of β-blocker use in experimental and clinical myocardial infarction. The chapter discusses how the drugs may alter the natural history of patients with preinfarction angina and hyperacute myocardial infarction, and how the drugs may reduce the long-term risk of mortality and reinfarction in survivors of a myocardial infarction and other high-risk patients. Chapter 11 reports on the results of the first North American Study using oral labetalol in patients with both hypertension and angina pectoris. The last chapter in Part II is an original study of ours that provides conclusive evidence for continued β-blocker therapy in patients undergoing coronary artery bypass surgery.

The next two chapters describe two multicenter trials that involved our group, using labetalol in patients with mild to moderate systemic hypertension. The first trial compares labetalol to metoprolol using a double-blind study design. The second evaluates the long-term efficacy and safety of labetalol used alone and in combination with a diuretic.

The final three chapters of the book discuss special topics—the use of β-blockers during pregnancy, the effects of β-blockade on the gastrointestinal system, and the neuropsychiatric actions of β-blockers.

The book does not cover every aspect of β-blockade since it reflects, in part, my own personal experience with these drugs. However, over 2000 published references through November 1983 are cited for the reader who wishes to research a specific area in more detail. This edition, as was the first, is directed to the teachers, researchers, and students of adrenergic pharmacology on the undergraduate and postgraduate levels, whether they be in general medicine, cardiology, anesthesiology, surgery, pediatrics, psychiatry, pharmacology, pharmacy, toxicology, or epidemiology, and particularly to all clinicians who prescribe β-blockers in daily medical practice.

As with the first edition, this book is largely the result of many individual efforts. It is impossible to acknowledge the names of the many medical students, house officers, and cardiology fellows from The Albert Einstein College of Medicine and its affiliated hospitals from whom I absorbed many ideas and who have served indispensable roles as research collaborators, coauthors, critics, supporters, and constant sources of stimulation. I am grateful to my devoted and loyal secretaries in the Cardiology Division and the Department of Medicine—Joanne Cioffi, Anne Paladino, Eve Ponzio (Administrative Secretary), Nina Scotti,

Mary Senatore, and Mary Jo Soreca—for their valuable help in preparing the manuscript. To Joanne Cioffi, a special tribute—it was on her capable shoulders that an immense amount of this work fell. I also wish to acknowledge Barry Shapiro and Linval Monfreis for their excellent artwork. I wish to thank my professional colleagues from The Albert Einstein College of Medicine and from other academic institutions, who were my collaborators in research and in preparation of this book. I will always be indebted to The American Heart Association and The National Institutes of Health, who have supported and continue to support my efforts in medical education. The education of my colleagues was always the primary motivation for writing this book. I wish to acknowledge Richard Lampert and the production staff of Appleton–Century–Crofts for their expert guidance in the preparation of this edition. Finally, my most important collaborators were my wife Esther Rose and our three children, Sheryl, Amy, and Michael Aaron, on whose constant love, patience, devotion and forbearance I have always relied, and whose confidence in the outcome of my academic efforts was always greater than mine.

This book commemorates the first 25 years of the β-blocker legacy. There is little doubt that in the next 25 years β-blockers will have achieved an even more prominent place in the annals of medical pharmacotherapy.

William H. Frishman
Bronx, New York
October, 1983

PREFACE TO THE FIRST EDITION

The introduction of β-adrenoceptor blocking drugs to clinical medicine has provided the most significant advance in the medical management of cardiovascular diseases during the past 20 years. While the original investigators envisioned these agents for the treatment of patients with angina pectoris, hypertension, and arrhythmias, their therapeutic benefits have extended well beyond the cardiovascular sphere. For instance, the β-blockers have been utilized in the treatment of porphyria, acne vulgaris, and a host of neuropsychiatric conditions. No group of synthetic drugs have had such widespread applicability in human pharmacotherapy.

Although the competitive inhibition of a β-adrenoceptor is a simple pharmacologic concept, there are many unsettled issues regarding the molecular and clinical pharmacology of these drugs. There are a host of β-adrenergic blocking agents that are now being marketed worldwide. These agents have similarities and differences that have clinical relevance. Thousands of scientific articles have been written about these drugs. This bulk of knowledge has never been synthesized for the clinician's easy reference. This book was conceived to organize this plethora of knowledge.

The controversies and questions involving the β-blocking drugs and their pharmacodynamic and pharmacokinetic differences are discussed. The clinical applications of these agents and their adverse reactions are reviewed in detail. Special chapters deal with the problems of overdose, and the use of these drugs in surgery and pre- and postmyocardial infarction. Specific drugs are discussed in detail based on the author's personal experiences in order to illustrate how chemical and pharmacokinetic differences can influence the therapeutic applications of these agents. The final chapter concludes with the changing concepts in adrenergic molecular pharmacology and extrapolates this new knowledge to disease and pharmacotherapy.

This book is directed to the teachers and students of adrenergic pharmacology (undergraduate and postgraduate), whether they be in general medicine, basic science, research cardiology, anesthesiology, surgery, pediatrics, psychology, pharmacy, toxicology, and epidemiology, and particularly to all clinicians who use β-blockers in daily medical practice.

The list of people and organizations to whom I am indebted directly or indirectly for helping me complete my work would easily fill an entire page. I want to start with my mother and father. The memory of my father who died from premature coronary artery disease inspired my interest in cardiovascular medicine and pharmacology.

It is hardly possible to acknowledge the many medical students, house officers, and cardiac fellows from whom I absorbed many ideas and who have served indispensable roles as collaborators, critics, supporters, and constant sources of stimulation.

To my devoted and loyal secretary, Nina Scotti, a special tribute: it was on her very capable shoulders that an immense amount of work fell. Her patience, good humor, skill, and unremitting labors deserve more thanks than I can ever provide.

On the medical side, I should like to begin with Dr. Thomas Killip, III, who gave me the opportunity to work in adult cardiology and encouraged my early research endeavors in cardiovascular pharmacology. I wish to express my sincere thanks to Dr. Edmund Sonnenblick for his critical review of the manuscript and the constant support and encouragement he has given me.

I wish to thank my professional colleagues at the Albert Einstein College of Medicine and the New York Hospital-Cornell Medical Center who were my collaborators in research and in preparation of this book.

I will always be grateful to the American Heart Association who chose me as their "Teaching Scholar" enabling me to pursue my interests in medical education. Education of my colleagues and students was the primary motivation for writing this book. I also wish to thank the National Heart-Lung Institute (HL-00653-1) who have supported my efforts in preventive cardiology, of which β-adrenoceptor blockade has and will play an important role.

I wish to acknowledge my appreciation for the efforts of Albert Nitzburg and Marcia Poland for their editorial reviews. I am particularly grateful to my editor, Robert E. McGrath of Appleton-Century-Crofts, for his expert guidance in the preparation of this volume.

In many ways, my most important collaborators were my wife, Esther, and my two daughters, Sheryl and Amy, whose patience, devotion, and forebearance were commendable and whose confidence in the outcome of my efforts was far greater than mine.

Bronx, New York
March 1980

Clinical Pharmacology of the β-Adrenoceptor Blocking Drugs

PART ONE

Basic and Clinical Pharmacology

CHAPTER 1

The β-Adrenergic Receptors: Current Concepts

William H. Frishman

The introduction of β-adrenoceptor blocking drugs to clinical medicine has provided one of the major pharmacotherapeutic advances of the twentieth century. These drugs are now being utilized for a wide variety of cardiovascular and noncardiovascular disorders.[1,2] The versatility of the β-blockers in medical practice demonstrates the importance of the sympathetic nervous system and the β-receptors in disease states and drug therapy. In this chapter, the recent advances in knowledge about β-adrenergic receptors will be reviewed.

ADRENERGIC RECEPTORS AND THEIR FUNCTION

Catecholamines are neurohumoral substances that mediate a variety of physiologic and metabolic responses in human beings. The effects of the catecholamines ultimately depend on their physiochemical interactions with receptors, discrete macromolecular components located on the plasma membranes themselves. The catecholamine–receptor complex activates the enzyme adenyl cyclase, located on the internal surface of the plasma membrane. The activated adenyl cyclase accelerates the intracellular formation of cyclic adenosine monophosphate (cyclic AMP), which then stimulates or inhibits various metabolic or physiologic processes.[3,4]

Adrenergic receptors are, therefore, recognition sites on cell membranes that translate the interaction of catecholamines with the cell into

3

a physiologic response. Agonist drugs are agents that interact with a receptor to elicit a full physiologic response. A partial agonist drug is an agent that causes a response that is qualitatively similar to an agonist but of lesser intensity. An antagonist agent interacts with the receptor, but causes no response, and, at the same time, prevents the action of agonists.

Previously, most research in hormonal or drug–receptor interactions bypassed the initial binding step on the plasma membrane and examined either the accumulation of cyclic AMP or the end result, the physiologic or metabolic effect. In recent years, new biochemical research techniques have become available to study the initial binding to the receptor. These new techniques involve the use of radioactively labeled hormone and drug derivatives called radioligands that attach to and label receptors.[3-6] The basis of a radioligand-binding assay for studying receptors involves first incubating a radioligand with a tissue, then removing the unbound radioactivity by filtration or centrifugation and measuring the radioactivity remaining within the tissue.[4,5] In these experiments it must be proven that the tissue-bound radioactivity represents radioligand bound to receptors and not to nonspecific binding sites.[5]

A great deal of new information regarding the molecular pharmacology of receptors has been obtained with radioligand-binding assay, which has increased our understanding of human disease and its drug therapy.

CLASSIFICATION OF ADRENERGIC RECEPTORS

As previously mentioned, the catecholamines norepinephrine and epinephrine are important regulators of many physiologic and metabolic actions in human beings. Norepinephrine acts primarily as a neurotransmitter released from sympathetic nerve terminals; epinephrine functions as a circulating hormone released from chromaffin tissue in the adrenal medulla. Thirty-five years ago Ahlquist sought to characterize the receptors by which the natural catecholamines (norepinephrine and epinephrine) and the synthetic catecholamine (isoproterenol) mediated their physiologic effects. In his detailed studies, Ahlquist used the differences in the ability of various catecholamines to stimulate a number of physiologic processes as criteria to separate adrenergic receptors into two distinct types, which he termed α-adrenergic and β-adrenergic receptors.[7]

For α-receptors, epinephrine has a greater affinity than norepinephrine and isoproterenol. For β-receptors, isoproterenol has a greater affinity than epinephrine or norepinephrine.[4] In addition, α- and β-adrenergic receptors may be identified further by the fact that certain antagonist drugs have greater affinity for α-receptors, whereas other antagonists, such as propranolol, have a greater affinity for β-receptors.[6]

A third type of adrenergic response stimulated by the norepinephrine precursor, dopamine, has also been defined.[8] These receptors are found in certain areas of the brain and in renal vessels where they cause vasodilation.

Subsequent studies by Lands and others, using indirect pharmacologic research methods, suggested that β-adrenergic receptors existed as two discrete subtypes called β_1 and β_2.[9] These β-subtypes mediate different physiologic and metabolic responses. Radioligand-binding techniques have recently demonstrated that the pharmacologic properties of β_1 and β_2 receptors truly differ, and that the receptors are distinct molecular entities.[10–12] Specific drugs have been synthesized that will selectively inhibit or block β_1 and β_2 receptors.[13]

The α-receptors are also subdivided.[6] α_1-Receptors are, for the most part, postsynaptic receptors which mediate smooth-muscle contraction.[6] The α_2- receptors are presynaptic autoregulatory receptors that, when stimulated, will inhibit norepinephrine release from the nerve terminal (Figure 1). α_2-Receptors are also found on platelet membranes.[6] Special

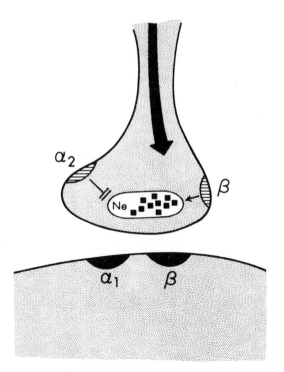

Figure 1. Schematic representation of the sympathetic neuroneffector cell synapse showing pre- and postsynaptic receptors. Stimulation of the presynaptic α_2 receptor inhibits further norepinephrine (Ne) release; stimulation of the presynaptic β-receptor facilitates norepinephrine release.

agonist and antagonist drugs have been developed that will selectively stimulate (clonidine α-$_2$) or block (prazosin α-$_1$) these α-receptor subtypes.[6]

Recently, β-receptors have also been identified in the sympathetic nerve terminal as presynaptic autoregulators. In contrast to the effects of stimulating presynaptic α_2 receptors, when the presynaptic β-receptor is stimulated, norepinephrine release from the nerve terminal will be augmented (Fig. 1).[14]

Some of the known physiologic effects of α- and β-adrenergic stimulation are shown in Table 1.[15]

ALTERATIONS OF β-ADRENERGIC DENSITY AND SENSITIVITY

Using radioligand assay techniques, it appears that the classical concept of adrenoreceptors as static entities on cell membranes that simply serve to initiate the chain of events leading to catecholamine activity is no longer tenable.[3,5,13] Considerable evidence indicates that adrenoreceptors (both α and β) are subject to a wide variety of controlling influences

TABLE 1. SOME EFFECTS OF ADRENERGIC RECEPTOR STIMULATION[15]

Organ System	α-Adrenergic Receptors	β-Adrenergic Receptors
Heart		Increase heart rate (β_1) Increase contractility (β_1) Increase conduction velocity (β_1) Shorten refractory period at atrioventricular node (β_1)
Blood vessels	Constrict	Dilate (β_1)
Bronchi		Dilate (β_2)
Stomach	Contract sphincter	Decrease motility and tone
Intestinal musculature	Relax	Relax
Uterine smooth muscle	Contract	Relax
Urinary bladder	Contract sphincter	Relax
Platelets	Increase aggregation (α_2)	
Eye	Dilation of pupil	
Renin release	Decrease ?	Increase (β_1)
Lipolysis		Increase (β_2?)
Glycogenolysis	Liver-increase	Cardiac and skeletal muscle-increase (β_2)

that dynamically regulate the number of adrenoceptors in tissues.[4,5,13] It is likely that these changes in the tissue concentrations of receptors are involved in mediating important fluctuations in tissue sensitivity to drugs (Tables 2 and 3).[4,5,13]

The density of β-adrenergic receptors in tissues appears to be inversely related to the magnitude of stimulation of these receptors by catecholamine agonists. When sympathetic nervous system activity is high, the density of β-adrenergic receptors will be low (down-regulation).[4] Conversely, when sympathetic activity is low, β-adrenergic receptor density will be high (up-regulation).[4] Similar changes appear to take place in α-receptor density and sensitivity (Table 3).[5]

The concentration of β-adrenoceptors in the membrane of mononuclear cells (a radioligand model for studying receptor numbers in man) significantly decreases with age.[4,13] This might explain the progressive resistance of β-adrenoceptor blocker therapy reported with increasing age of the hypertensive population. As shown in a study of Buhler et al., a good response to β-adrenoceptor blocker therapy occurred in 90 percent of hypertensive patients in their twenties, but the percentage of responders fell progressively with increasing age.[16]

An apparent increase in the number of β-adrenoceptors, and thereby a supersensitivity to β-agonists, may be induced by chronic exposure to β-antagonists.[17,18] This phenomenon was described by Glaubiger and Lefkowitz[19] and may explain the "β-blocker withdrawal phenomenon" seen in some patients with ischemic heart disease upon sudden discontinuation of β-adrenoceptor blocking therapy. With pro-

TABLE 2. FACTORS ASSOCIATED WITH ALTERATIONS IN β-ADRENERGIC RECEPTOR BINDING SITES[5]

Regulatory Agent or Condition	Effect on β-Receptors*
Beta-adrenergic agonists[21,25–29]	↓
Propranolol (antagonist)[19,30]	↑
Pindolol (partial agonist)[31]	↔
Denervation[32–34]	↑
Hyperthyroidism[23,35–37]	↑
Hypothyroidism[36,38]	↓
Cortisone[39,40]	↓
Alcohol withdrawal[24]	↑
Aging[41,42]	↓

* ↑ Increase
↔ No change
↓ Decrease

TABLE 3. FACTORS ASSOCIATED WITH ALTERATIONS IN α-ADRENERGIC RECEPTOR BINDING SITES[5]

Regulatory Agent or Condition	Effect on α-Receptors
Alpha-adrenergic agonists[43,44]	↓
Denervation[45]	↑
Hyperthyroidism[35,46,47]	↓
Estrogen[48,49]	↑
Thrombocytosis[50]	↓

↑ Increase
↔ No change
↓ Decrease

longed β-adrenoceptor blocker therapy, receptor occupancy of cate-cholamines would be diminished and the number of available receptors increased. When the β-adrenoceptor blocker is suddenly withdrawn, an increased pool of sensitive receptors would be open to endogenous cate-cholamine stimulation. The resultant adrenergic stimulation could then precipitate angina pectoris or a myocardial infarction (see Chapter 5).[18]

Using radioligand assay techniques, a decrease in β-adrenoceptor sites in the myocardium has been demonstrated in transplanted hearts from patients with chronic congestive heart failure.[20] An apparent reduc-tion in β-adrenoceptors has also been associated with the development of refractoriness or desensitization to endogenous and exogenous cate-cholamines in patients with heart failure, a phenomenon caused by the prolonged exposure of these adrenoceptors to high levels of catechol-amines.[21] This desensitization phenomenon is not caused by changes in receptor formation or degradation, but rather by catecholamine-induced changes in the conformation of the receptor sites, thus rendering them ineffective.[3,5] In vitro, these changes are reversible over a period of hours.[5] β-Adrenoceptor blocking drugs do not induce desensitization or changes in the conformation of receptors. They do, however, block the ability of catecholamines to desensitize receptors, and this may explain their suggested use in patients with chronic congestive heart failure.

The effects of thyroid hormone on adrenoceptor numbers in exper-imental studies may provide at least a partial explanation for the thera-peutic efficacy of β-adrenergic blockers in the treatment of patients with thyrotoxicosis.[22] β-Receptor-binding sites increase in hyperthyroidism[5,23] and decrease in hypothyroidism.[5] The number of β-adrenoceptors also increases with acute alcohol[24] and narcotic withdrawal in chronic users,[5] which may explain the reported beneficial effects of β-blockers in these situations (see Chapter 4).

CONCLUSION

Radioligand assay techniques are providing new information regarding adrenoreceptors and leading to a better understanding of the physiologic and pharmacologic mechanisms that regulate β-receptor function. These new biochemical concepts concerning adrenoreceptor function and regulation have also increased our knowledge of how adrenergic receptors and changes in sympathoadrenal activity influence human disease and its drug treatment.

REFERENCES

1. Frishman WH: β-Adrenoceptor antagonists: new drugs and new indications. N Engl J Med 305:500, 1981.
2. Frishman WH: The beta-adrenoceptor blocking drugs. Int J Cardiol 2:165, 1982.
3. Lefkowitz RJ, Michel T: Plasma membrane receptors. J Clin Invest 72:185, 1983.
4. Motulsky HJ, Insel PA: Adrenergic receptors in man: direct identification, physiologic regulation and clinical alterations. N Engl J Med 307:18, 1982.
5. Lefkowitz R: Direct binding studies of adrenergic receptors: biochemical, physiologic, and clinical implications. Ann Intern Med 91:450, 1979.
6. Hoffman BB, Lefkowitz RJ: Alpha-adrenergic receptor subtypes. N Engl J Med 302:1390, 1982.
7. Ahlquist RP: A study of adrenotropic receptors. Am J Physiol 53:586, 1948.
8. Goldberg LI: Comparison of putative dopamine receptors in blood vessels and the CNS. Adv Neurol 9:53, 1975.
9. Lands AM, Arnold A, McAuliff JP, et al: Differentiation of receptor systems activated by sympathomimetic amines. Nature 214:597, 1967.
10. Minneman KP, Hegstrand LR, Molinoff PB: The pharmacological specificity of beta₁ and beta₂ adrenergic receptors in rat heart and lung in vitro. Mol Pharmacol 16:21, 1979.
11. Hancock AA, DeLean AL, Lefkowitz RJ: Quantitative resolution of beta-adrenergic receptor subtypes by selective ligand binding: application of a computerized model fitting technique. Mol Pharmacol 16:1, 1979.
12. Lavin T, Nambi T, Heald SL, et al: [125](I)paraazidobenzyl carazolol, a photoaffinity label for the beta-adrenergic receptor: Characterization of the ligand and photoaffinity labelling of the beta₁ and beta₂ adrenergic receptor. J Biol Chem 257:1232, 1982.
13. Watanabe AM: Recent advances in knowledge about beta-adrenergic receptors: application to clinical cardiology. J Am Coll Cardiol 1:82, 1983.
14. Starne L, Brundin J: Dual adrenoceptor-mediated control of noradrenaline secretion from vasoconstrictor nerves. Facilitation by β-receptors and inhibition by α-receptors. Acta Physiol Scand 94:139, 1982.

15. Lefkowitz RJ: β-Adrenergic receptors: recognition and regulation. N Engl J Med 295:323, 1976.
16. Buhler FR, Bukart F, Benno LE, et al: Antihypertensive β-blocking action as related to renin and age. A pharmacological tool to identify pathogenic mechanisms in essential hypertension. Am J Cardiol 36:653, 1975.
17. Shand DG, Wood AJJ: Propranolol withdrawal syndrome—why? Circulation 58:202, 1978.
18. Prichard BNC, Walden RJ: The syndrome associated with the withdrawal of β-adrenergic receptor blocking drugs. Br J Clin Pharmac 13:337s, 1982.
19. Glaubiger G, Lefkowitz RJ: Elevated β-receptor number after chronic propranolol treatment. Biochem Biophys Res Commun 78:720, 1977.
20. Bristow MR, Ginsberg R, Minobe W, et al: Decreased catecholamine sensitivity and β-adrenergic receptor density in failing human hearts. N Engl J Med 307:205, 1982.
21. Colucci WS, Alexander RW, Williams GH, et al: Decreased lymphocyte β-adrenergic receptor density in patients with heart failure and tolerance to the β-adrenergic agonist perbuterol. N Engl J Med 305:185, 1981.
22. Ingbar SH: The role of anti-adrenergic agents in the management of thyrotoxicosis. Card Rev Rep 2:683, 1981.
23. Williams LT, Lefkowitz RJ, Watanabe AM, et al: Thyroid hormone regulation of β-adrenergic receptor number. J Biol Chem 252:2787, 1977.
24. Banerjee SP, Sharma VK, Khanna JM: Alterations in β-adrenergic receptor binding during ethanol withdrawal. Nature 276:407, 1978.
25. Lefkowitz RJ, Mukherjee C, Limbird LE, et al: Regulation of adenylate cyclase coupled β-adrenergic receptors. Recent Prog Horm Res 32:597, 1976.
26. Mickey JV, Tate R, Mullikin D, Lefkowitz RJ: Regulation of adenylate cyclase-coupled beta-adrenergic receptor binding sites by beta adrenergic catecholamines in vitro. Mol Pharmacol 12:409, 1976.
27. Mukherjee C, Caron MG, Lefkowitz RJ: Regulation of adenylate cyclase coupled β-adrenergic receptors by β-adrenergic catecholamines. Endocrinology 99:347, 1976.
28. Shear M, Insel PA, Melmon KL, Coffino P: Agonist specific refractoriness induced by isoproterenol: Studies with mutant cells. J Biol Chem 251:7572, 1976.
29. Su Y-F, Harden TK, Perkins JP: Isoproterenol-induced desensitization of adenylate cyclase in human astrocytoma cells: relation of loss of hormonal responsiveness and decrement in β-adrenergic receptors. J Biol Chem 254:38, 1979.
30. Dolphin A, Adrien J, Hamon M, Bockaert J: Identity of (^{3}H)-Dihydroalprenolol binding sites and β-adrenergic receptors coupled with adenylate cyclase in the central nervous system: pharmacological properties, distribution and adaptive responsiveness. Mol Pharmacol 15:1, 1979.
31. Molinoff PB, Aarons RD, Nies AS, et al: Effects of pindolol and propranolol on β-adrenergic receptors on human lymphocytes. Br J Clin Pharmacol 13:365s, 1982.
32. Glaubiger G, Tsai BS, Lefkowitz RJ, et al: Chronic guanethidine treatment increases cardiac β-adrenergic receptors. Nature 273:240, 1978.

33. Sporn JR, Harden TK, Wolfe BB, Molinoff PB: β-Adrenergic receptor involvement in 6-hydroxydopamine-induced sensitivity in rat cerebral cortex. Science 194:624, 1976.

34. Banerjee SP, Sharma VK, Kung LS: β-Adrenergic receptors in innervated and denervated skeletal muscle. Biochem Biophy Acta 470:123, 1977.

35. Ciaraldi T, Marinetti GV: Thyroxin and propylthiouracil effects in vivo or alpha and beta-adrenergic receptors in rat heart. Biochem Biophys Res Commun 74:984, 1977.

36. Banerjee SP, Kung LS: β-Adrenergic receptors in the rat heart: Effects of thyroidectomy. Eur J Pharmacol 43:207, 1977.

37. Tsai JS, Chen A: L-Triiodothyronine increases the level of β-adrenergic receptor in cultured myocardial cells. (Abstr) Clin Res 25:303a, 1977.

38. Stiles GL, Stadel JM, DeLean A, Lefkowitz RJ: Hypothyroidism modulates beta-adrenergic receptor-adenylate cyclase interactions in rat reticulocytes. J Clin Invest 68:1450, 1981.

39. Wolfe BB, Harden TK, Molinoff PB: β-Adrenergic receptors in rat liver: Effects of adrenalectomy. Proc Natl Acad Sci USA 73:1343, 1976.

40. Davies AO, Lefkowitz R: Corticosteroid-induced differential regulation of β-adrenergic receptors in circulating polymorphonuclear leukocytes and mononuclear leukocytes. J Clin Endocrin Metab 51:599, 1981.

41. Schocken DD, Roth GS: Reduced β-adrenergic receptor concentrations in aging man. Nature 267:856, 1977.

42. Vestal RE, Wood AJJ, Shand DG: Reduced beta-adrenoceptor sensitivity in the elderly. Clin Pharmacol Ther 26:181, 1979.

43. Strittmatter WJ, Davis JN, Lefkowitz RJ: α-Adrenergic receptors in rat parotid cells: II. Desensitization of receptor binding sites and potassium release. J Biol Chem 252:5478, 1977.

44. Cooper B, Handin RI, Young LH, Alexander RW: Agonist regulation of the human platelet α-adrenergic receptor. Nature 274:703, 1978.

45. Pointon SE, Banerjee SP: Alpha- and beta-adrenergic receptors of the rat salivary gland: elevation after chemical sympathectomy. Biochem Biophys Acta 584:231, 1979.

46. Sharma VK, Banerjee SP: α-Adrenergic receptor in rat heart: Effects of thyroidectomy. J Biol Chem 253:5277, 1978

47. Williams RS, Lefkowitz RJ: Thyroid hormone regulation of alpha-adrenergic receptors: studies in rat myocardium. J Cardiovasc Pharmacol 1:181, 1979.

48. Williams LT, Lefkowitz RJ: Regulation of rabbit myometrial alpha-adrenergic receptors by estrogen and progesterone. J Clin Invest 60:815, 1977.

49. Roberts JM, Insel PA, Goldfien RD, Goldfien A: α-Adrenoreceptors but not β-adrenoreceptors increase in rabbit uterus with oestrogen. Nature 270:624, 1977.

50. Kaywin P, McDonough M, Insel PA, Shattel SJ: Platelet function in essential thrombocythemia: decreased epinephrine responsiveness associated with a deficiency of platelet α-adrenergic receptors. N Engl J Med 299:505, 1978.

CHAPTER 2

Pharmacodynamic and Pharmacokinetic Properties

William H. Frishman

The introduction of β-adrenoceptor blocking drugs to the armamentarium of clinical medicine has provided one of the major therapeutic advances in this century. Although β-blockers were intended initially for the treatment of patients with angina pectoris, it soon became clear that they had much to offer for a diversity of clinical disorders: hypertension, arrhythmia, thyrotoxicosis, hypertrophic cardiomyopathy, migraine, glaucoma, myocardial infarction, and gastrointestinal hemorrhage.[1-4] As a class, the β-adrenoceptor blocking drugs have been so successful that many of them have been synthesized, and over 20 are available on the world market.

The application of these agents has been accelerated by the development of drugs possessing a degree of selectivity for two subgroups of the β-adrenoceptor population: β_1-receptors in the heart and β_2-receptors in the peripheral circulation and bronchi.[5,6] More controversial has been the introduction of β-blocking drugs with α-adrenergic blocking properties, varying amounts of intrinsic sympathomimetic activity (partial agonist action) and nonspecific membrane stabilizing effects.[3,7-11] There are also major pharmacokinetic differences between β-blocking drugs that may be of clinical importance.[1,7,8,12]

Based on an article that appeared in the International Journal of Cardiology, Volume 2, August 1982, pp 165–178, with permission.

Six β-adrenergic blockers are now marketed in the United States: propranolol, for angina pectoris, arrhythmia, systemic hypertension, migraine headache prophylaxis, and for reducing the risk of mortality in survivors of an acute myocardial infarction; nadolol, for angina pectoris and hypertension; timolol, for open angle glaucoma and for reducing the risk of mortality and reinfarction in survivors of an acute myocardial infarction; and metoprolol, atenolol, and pindolol, for hypertension. Labetalol will be marketed shortly. Acebutolol, oxprenolol, and penbutolol are now under consideration by the FDA.

Despite the extensive experience with β-blockers in clinical practice, there are no studies suggesting that one of these agents has major advantages or disadvantages in relation to another for therapy of cardiovascular disease.[1-3,9] When any available β-blocker is titrated to the proper dose, it can be effective in patients with arrhythmia, hypertension or angina pectoris.[1,3,5,9,13]

One agent, however, may be more effective than another in reducing adverse reactions in certain patients and for specific clinical situations.[7,9,10] To assess the value of different β-adrenoceptor blockers, one must compare those pharmacodynamic and pharmacokinetic properties of each drug that may provide an added margin of safety for the patient, alter any tendency toward undesirable side effects, reduce the incidence of drug interactions, or influence the ease of effective dosing.[5,9,14-16]

In this chapter the comparative pharmacodynamics and pharmacokinetics of β-blockers are discussed.

BASIC PHARMACOLOGIC DIFFERENCES

Potency
β-Adrenoceptor blocking drugs are competitive inhibitors of catecholamine binding at β-adrenoceptor sites. They reduce the effect of any concentration of catecholamine agonist on a sensitive tissue. The dose–response curve of the agonist is shifted to the right; a given tissue response requires a higher concentration of agonist in the presence of β-blocking drugs.[1,3,7] $β_1$-Blocking potency can be assessed by the inhibition of tachycardia produced by isoproterenol or exercise; potency varies from compound to compound (Table 1).[1,7]

These differences in potency are of no therapeutic relevance. However, they do explain the different drug dosages needed to achieve effective β-adrenergic blockade when initiating therapy in patients or when switching from one agent to another.

TABLE 1. PHARMACODYNAMIC PROPERTIES OF β-ADRENOCEPTOR BLOCKING DRUGS

Drug	β_1-Blockade Potency Ratio (Propranolol = 1.0)	Relative β_1 Selectivity	Intrinsic Sympathomimetic Activity	Membrane-Stabilizing Activity
Acebutolol	0.3	+	+	+
Atenolol	1.0	+ +	0	0
Esmolol (ASL-8052)	0.01	+ +	0	0
Labetalol*	0.3	0	+ ?	0
Metoprolol	1.0	+ +	0	0
Nadolol	1.0	0	0	0
Oxprenolol	0.5–1.0	0	+	+
Pindolol	6.0	0	+ +	+
Propranolol	1.0	0	0	+ +
Sotalol	0.3	0	0	0
Timolol	6.0	0	0	0
Isomer: D-Propranolol				+ +

*Labetalol has additional α-adrenergic blocking activity and direct vasodilatory actions.

Structure–Activity Relationships

The chemical structures of most β-adrenergic blockers have several features in common with the agonist isoproterenol (Fig. 1), an aromatic ring with a substituted ethanolamine side chain linked to it by an $-OCH_2$ group.[3] The β-blocker timolol has a catecholamine-mimicking side chain, but it is attached to a five-membered heterocyclic ring containing nitrogen and sulfur (a thiadiazole), which is in turn attached to another heterocyclic ring containing nitrogen and oxygen (a morpholino compound). It is possible that the thiadiazole–morpholino structure may confer on timolol properties not possessed by other β-blockers, but these are as yet unidentified.

Most β-blocking drugs exist as pairs of optical isomers and are marketed as racemic mixtures.[1,3,7] Almost all the β-blocking activity is found in the negative (−) levorotatory stereoisomer. The two stereoisomers of β-adrenergic blockers are useful for differentiating between the pharmacologic effects of β-blockade and membrane stabilizing activity (possessed by both optical forms). The (+) dextrorotatory stereoisomers of β-blocking agents have no recognized clinical value.[3,7]

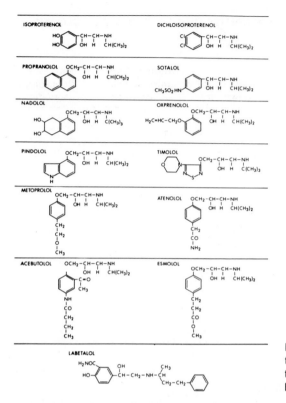

Figure 1. Molecular structure of the β-adrenergic agonist isoproterenol and some β-adrenergic blocking drugs.

Membrane Stabilizing Activity

In high concentrations well above therapeutic levels, certain β-blockers have a quinidine-like or "local anesthetic" membrane stabilizing effect on the cardiac action potential.[1,3,7] This property is exhibited equally by the two stereoisomers of the drug and is unrelated to β-adrenergic blockade and to major therapeutic antiarrhythmic effects.[17]

There is no evidence that membrane-stabilizing activity is responsible for any direct negative inotropic effects of β-blocking drugs since both drugs with and without this property equally depress left ventricular function.[1,9] Membrane-stabilizing activity can manifest itself clinically during massive β-blocker intoxications.[18]

Selectivity

The β-adrenoceptor blockers may be classified as selective or nonselective according to their relative abilities to antagonize the actions of sympathomimetic amines in some tissues at lower doses than those required in other tissues.[5,19] When used in low doses, β_1-selective blocking agents such as atenolol and metoprolol inhibit cardiac β_1-receptors but have less influence on bronchial and vascular β-adrenoceptors (β_2).[5,6] In higher doses, however, β_1-selective blocking agents will also block β_2-receptors.[5,6]

Because selective β_1-blockers have less of an inhibitory effect on the β_2-receptors, they have two theoretical advantages. The first is that β_1-selective agents may be safer than nonselective ones in patients with obstructive pulmonary disease because β_2-receptors remain available to mediate adrenergic bronchodilatation.[1,3 5–7] In some clinical trials on patients with asthma, relatively low doses of β_1-selective agents caused a lower incidence of side effects than did similar doses of propranolol.[6] However, even selective β-blockers may aggravate bronchospasm in certain patients, so that these drugs should generally not be used in patients with bronchospastic disease.[5–7]

The second theoretical advantage is that unlike nonselective β-blockers, β_1-selective blockers in low doses may not block the β_2-receptors that mediate dilation of arterioles.[1] This property might be an advantage in treatment of hypertension with relatively low doses of β_1-adrenergic drugs, but this possibility has not been demonstrated. During infusion of epinephrine, nonselective β-blockers can cause a pressor response by blocking β_2-receptor mediated vasodilation, since α-adrenergic vasoconstrictor receptors are still operative. Selective β_1-antagonists may not induce this pressor effect in the presence of epinephrine and may lessen the impairment of peripheral blood flow.[1,5]

It is possible that leaving the β_2-receptors unblocked and responsive to epinephrine may be functionally important in some patients with asthma, hypoglycemia, hypertension, or peripheral vascular disease treated with β-adrenergic blocking drugs.[1]

Intrinsic Sympathomimetic Activity (Partial Agonist Activity)
Certain β-adrenoceptor blockers (acebutolol, alprenolol, oxprenolol, and pindolol) possess partial agonist activity.[20] These drugs cause a slight to moderate activation of the β-receptor,[1,21] in addition to preventing the access of natural or synthetic catecholamines to the receptor sites (Fig. 2). Dichloroisoproterenol, the first β-adrenoceptor blocking drug, exerted such marked partial agonist activity that it caused tachycardia in patients and was unsuitable for clinical use.[22] However, compounds with less partial agonist activity, such as pindolol, are effective β-blocking drugs.[2]

A quantitative assessment of the partial agonist activity in a β-blocker can be made in animals whose resting sympathetic tone has been abolished by adrenalectomy and pretreatment with reserpine or syringoserpine.[23,24] If in such animals a β-blocker increases the heart rate or force of myocardial contraction, the drug has partial agonist activity.[24] The increases in heart rate and contractility are mediated through β-adrenergic stimulation because they can be antagonized by propranolol.[24] The partial agonist effects of β-adrenoceptor blocking drugs differ from those of such agonists as epinephrine and isoproterenol in that the maximum pharmacologic effect is less, although the affinity for the receptor is high.[1,21] In laboratory animals, pindolol has up to 50 percent of the agonist activity of isoproterenol[21]; however, this activity is probably lower in human beings.[25] Unlike the relative selectivity of atenolol and metoprolol for β_1-adrenoceptors, which is attenuated as higher therapeutic doses are used,[1,5,6] the partial agonist activity of pindolol is not lost when higher doses are given.[11] The partial agonist effect of pindolol appears with low doses and has a flat dose–response curve, since the effect on the resting heart rate remains unchanged within a wide range of therapeutic doses.[26,27]

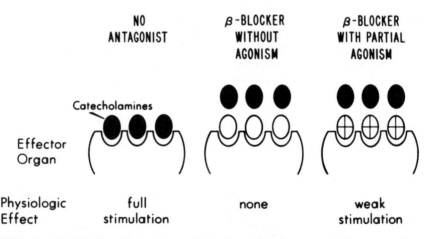

Figure 2. Physiologic effects of β-adrenergic blocking drugs with and without partial agonist activity in the presence of circulating catecholamines. When circulating catecholamines (●) combine with β-adrenergic receptors, they produce a full physiologic response. When these receptors are occupied by a β-blocker lacking partial agonist activity (○) no physiologic effects from catecholamine stimulation can occur. A β-blocking drug with partial agonist activity (⊕) also blocks the binding of catecholamines to β-adrenergic receptors, but in addition the drug also causes a relatively weak stimulation of the receptor. *(Reprinted from the New England Journal of Medicine 308:941, 1983, with permission).*

The evaluation of the partial agonist activity of β-blockers administered to human beings is complicated by the necessity to study the intact subject. However, the presence, extent, and clinical relevance of partial agonist activity can be assessed if equivalent pharmacologic doses of β-blocking drugs with and without this property are compared. Drugs with partial agonist activity, such as pindolol, cause less slowing of the resting heart rate than drugs without this activity, such as propranolol, atenolol, or metoprolol.[28-31] On the other hand, the increments in heart rate with exercise[28] or isoproterenol are decreased similarly by both types of β-blockers. An explanation for these findings is that the relative importance of the partial agonist effect of pindolol, as compared with its β-blocking action, is greatest when sympathetic tone is low and therefore is appreciated only in resting subjects.[31] Since the drug's chronotropic effect is weak relative to endogenous catecholamines, the net effect of pindolol in resting subjects is not a positive chronotropic action; it can cause either no change in heart rate or a smaller decrease than that caused by β-blockers lacking partial agonist activity. During exercise, when sympathetic activity is high, the β-blocking effect of pindolol predominates over its partial agonist activity. Thus, all β-blockers, with or without partial agonist activity, are equally effective in reducing the increases in heart rate and blood pressure that occur with exercise[31]— a finding that has been verified in many clinical studies.[26,28,32]

It is still debated whether the presence of partial agonist activity in a β-blocker constitutes an overall advantage or disadvantage in cardiac therapy.[1] It may reduce peripheral vascular resistance and may also depress atrioventricular conduction less than would agents lacking this property.[1,19] It has been claimed by some investigators that partial agonist activity in a β-blocker protects against myocardial depression, bronchial asthma, and peripheral vascular complications.[14,33] The evidence supporting these claims is not definite, and more definitive clinical trials are necessary to resolve these questions.

α-Adrenergic Activity

Labetalol is a β-blocker with antagonistic properties at both α- and β-adrenoceptors.[10] The drug is reviewed in detail in Chapter 7. Before labetalol, only antagonists acting at α- or β-adrenoceptors, but not at both, were available. Labetalol has been shown to be 6 to 10 times less potent than phentolamine at α-adrenoceptors, 1.5 to 4 times less potent than propranolol at β-adrenoceptors, and is itself 4 to 16 times less potent at α- than at β-adrenoceptors.[10]

Labetalol, like other β-blockers, has been shown to be a useful agent in the treatment of arrhythmias, hypertension, and angina pectoris (see Chapter 13).[34] However, unlike most β-blocking drugs, the additional α-adrenergic blocking actions of labetalol lead to a reduction in peripheral vascular resistance that may maintain cardiac output in patients.[10] Whether concomitant α-adrenergic activity is actually advantageous in a β-blocker remains to be determined.

Pharmacokinetics

Although the β-adrenergic blocking drugs as a group have similar pharmacologic effects in cardiovascular disease, their pharmacokinetics are markedly different (Tables 2, 3).[7-9,35] Their varied aromatic ring structures lead to differences in completeness of gastrointestinal absorption, amount of first-pass hepatic metabolism, lipid solubility, protein binding, extent of distribution in the body, penetration into the brain, concentration in the heart, rate of hepatic biotransformation, pharmacologic activity of metabolites, and renal clearance of a drug and its metabolites that may influence the clinical usefulness of these drugs in some patients.[1,7,9] The desirable pharmacokinetic characteristics of this group of compounds are a lack of major individual differences in bioavailability and in metabolic clearance of the drug, and a rate of removal from the active tissue sites that is slow enough to allow longer dosing intervals.[1]

The β-adrenergic blocking drugs can be divided by their pharmacokinetic properties into two broad categories: those eliminated by hepatic metabolism, which tend to have relatively short plasma half-lives, and those eliminated unchanged by the kidney, which tend to have longer half-lives.[1] Propranolol and metoprolol are both lipid soluble, are almost completely absorbed from the small intestine, and are largely metabolized by the liver. They tend to have highly variable bioavailability and relatively short plasma half-lives.[1,5,7] A lack of correlation between the duration of clinical pharmacologic effect and plasma half-life may still allow these drugs to be administered once or twice daily.[1]

In contrast, agents like atenolol and nadolol are more water soluble, are incompletely absorbed through the gut, and are eliminated unchanged by the kidney.[6,12] They tend to have less variable bioavailability in patients with normal renal function, in addition to longer half-lives, allowing one dose a day.[6,12] The longer half-lives may be useful in those patients who find compliance with β-blocker therapy a problem.[6]

Recently, a long-acting preparation of propranolol was approved for marketing (Tables 2,3). The propranolol is part of a soluble matrix inside tiny spheroids made up of an insoluble membrane. Gastrointestinal fluid

TABLE 2. PHARMACOKINETIC PROPERTIES OF β-ADRENOCEPTOR BLOCKING DRUGS

Drug	Extent of Absorption (% of dose)	Extent of Bioavailability (% of dose)	Dose-Dependent Bioavailability (Major First-Pass Hepatic Metabolism)	Interpatient Variations in Plasma Levels	β-Blocking Plasma Concentrations	Protein Binding (%)	Lipid Solubility*
Acebutolol	≈70	≈50	No	7-fold	0.2–2.0 μg/ml	30–40	Weak
Atenolol	≈50	≈40	No	4-fold	0.2–5.0 μg/ml	<5	Weak
Esmolol†	NA‡	NA	NA		0.3–1.0 μg/ml		
Labetalol	>90	≈33	Yes	10-fold	0.7–3.0 μg/ml	≈50	Weak
Metoprolol	>90	≈50	No	7-fold	50–100 ng/ml	12	Moderate
Nadolol	≈30	≈30	No	7-fold	50–100 ng/ml	≈30	Weak
Oxprenolol	≈90	≈40	No	5-fold	80–100 ng/ml	80	Moderate
Pindolol	>90	≈90	No	4-fold	5–15 ng/ml	57	Moderate
Propranolol	>90	≈30	Yes	20-fold	50–100 ng/ml	93	High
LA Propranolol (long-acting)	>90	≈20	Yes	10–20-fold	20–100 ng/ml	93	High
Sotalol	≈70	≈60	No	4-fold	0.5–4.0 μg/ml	0	Weak
Timolol	>90	≈75	No	7-fold	5–10 ng/ml	≈10	Weak

*Determined by the distribution ratio between octanol and water.
†Ultrashort acting β-blocker, only available in intravenous form.
‡NA = Not applicable.

TABLE 3. ELIMINATION CHARACTERISTICS OF ORALLY ACTIVE β-ADRENOCEPTOR BLOCKING DRUGS

Drug	Elimination Half-Life (hr)	Total Body Clearance (ml/min)	Urinary Recovery of Unchanged Drug (% of dose)	Total Urinary Recovery (% of dose)	Predominant Route of Elimination*	Active Metabolites	Drug Accumulation in Renal Disease
Acebutolol	3–4	6–15	≈40	>90	RE	Yes	No
Atenolol	6–9	130	≈40	>95	RE	No	Yes
Esmolol†	≈10 min	285	< 1	>70	HM‡	No	No
Labetalol	3–4	2700	< 1	>90	HM	No	No
Metoprolol	3–4	1100	≈3	>95	HM	No	No
Nadolol	14–24	200	70	70	RE	No	Yes
Oxprenolol	2–3	380	2–5	70–95	HM	No	No
Pindolol	3–4	400	≈40	>90	RE (≈40% unchanged) and HM	No	No
Propranolol	3–4	1000	< 1	>90	HM	Yes	No
LA Propranolol (Long-acting)	10	1000	< 1	>90	HM	Yes	No
Sotalol	8–10	150	≈60	>90	RE	No	Yes
Timolol	4–5	660	≈20	65	RE (≈20% unchanged) and HM	No	No

*RE denotes renal execretion and HM hepatic metabolism.
†Ultrashort acting β-blocker, only available in intravenous form.
‡Metabolized by blood, tissue and hepatic esterases.

enters the spheroids and propranolol exits via a concentration gradient into the gut lumen and then the bloodstream.[36] Long-acting propranolol absorption is not dependent on gastric acidity or enzymatic action, and the drug is metabolized by the liver in its first pass, an effect similar to conventional propranolol.[36] Studies have shown that long-acting propranolol provides a much smoother curve of daily plasma levels than comparable divided doses of conventional propranolol, which tends to yield high plasma level peaks. As expected, long-acting propranolol has been shown to have fewer side effects than conventional propranolol and provides sustained β-blockade for 24 hours.[37,38]

Ultra-short-acting β-blockers are now in the early stages of clinical testing. These drugs are designed for use in the hospital setting when β-blockade is required, and a short duration or action is desired (in patients with questionable congestive heart failure). One of these compounds, esmolol (ASL-8052), a β_1-selective drug (Tables 1–3), has been shown to be useful in the treatment of supraventricular tachyarrhythmias. The short half-life (approximately 10 minutes) relates to the rapid metabolism of the drug by blood, tissue, and hepatic esterases. Metabolism does not seem to be altered by disease states.[39-41]

Specific pharmacokinetic properties of individual β-adrenergic blockers (first-pass metabolism, active metabolites, lipid solubility, and protein binding) may be important to the clinician. When drugs with extensive first-pass metabolism are taken by mouth, they undergo so much hepatic biotransformation that relatively little drug reaches the systemic circulation.[1,7,8] Depending on the extent of the first-pass effect, an oral dose of β-blocker must be larger than an intravenous dose to produce the same clinical effects.[5,7,8] Some β-adrenergic blockers are transformed into pharmacologically active compounds rather than inactive metabolites. The total pharmacologic effect, therefore, depends on the amounts of both the drug administered and its active metabolites.[1,35]

Characteristics of lipid solubility in a β-blocker have been associated with the ability of the drug to concentrate in the brain.[1] Many side effects of these drugs, which have not been clearly related to β-blockade, seem to result from their actions on the central nervous system (lethargy, mental depression, and hallucinations).[1,12] It is still not clear, however, whether drugs that are less lipid-soluble cause fewer of these adverse reactions.[6,12]

Relationship Between Dose, Plasma Level, and Efficacy
Attempts have been made to establish a relationship between the oral dose, plasma level measured by gas chromotography, and pharmacologic effect of each β-blocking drug. After administration of a certain

oral dose, β-blocking drugs that are largely metabolized in the liver show large interindividual variation in circulating plasma levels.[1] Wide individual differences also exist in the relation between plasma concentrations of β-blockers and any associated therapeutic effect. Many explanations have been proposed to explain this observation. First of all, patients may have different levels of "sympathetic tone" (circulating catecholamines and active β-adrenoceptor binding sites), and may thus require different drug concentrations to achieve adequate β-blockade.[7] Secondly, many β-blockers have flat plasma–drug-level response curves.[35] Thirdly, the active drug isomer and active metabolites are not specifically measured by many plasma assays. Fourthly, the clinical effect of a drug may last longer than the period suggested by the drug's half-life in plasma.[7] Despite the lack of correlation between plasma levels and therapeutic effect, there is some evidence that a relation does exist between the logarithm of the plasma level and the β-blocking effect (blockade of exercise or isoproterenol-induced tachycardia).[5,7,35]

When using different β-blockers in clinical practice, plasma levels have little to offer as therapeutic guides, except for ensuring compliance. Pharmacodynamic characteristics and clinical response should be used as guides in determining the optimal β-blocking damage for each patient.

REFERENCES

1. Frishman WH: β-Adrenoceptor antagonists: new drugs and new indications. N Engl J Med 305:500, 1981.
2. Frishman W, Silverman R: Clinical pharmacology of the new beta-adrenergic blocking drugs. Part 3. Comparative clinical experience and new therapeutic applications. Am Heart J 98:119, 1979.
3. Conolly ME, Kersting F, Dollery CT: The clinical pharmacology of beta-adrenoceptor blocking drugs. Prog Cardiovasc Dis 19:203, 1976.
4. Lebrec D, Poynard T, Hillon, P, Benhamou JP: Propranolol for prevention of recurrent gastrointestinal bleeding in patients with cirrhosis: a controlled study. N Engl J Med 305:1371, 1981.
5. Koch-Weser J: Metoprolol. N Engl J Med 301:698, 1979.
6. Frishman WH: Atenolol and timolol, two new systemic β-adrenoceptor antagonists. N Engl J Med 306:1456, 1982.
7. Frishman W: Clinical pharmacology of the new beta-adrenergic blocking drugs. Part 1. Pharmacodynamic and pharmacokinetic properties. Am Heart J 97:663, 1979.
8. Waal-Manning HJ: Hypertension: which beta-blocker? Drugs 12:412, 1976.
9. Opie LH: Drugs and the heart. 1. Beta-blocking agents. Lancet 1:693, 1980.
10. Frishman W, Halprin S: Clinical pharmacology of the new beta-adrenergic

blocking drugs. Part 7. New horizons in beta-adrenoceptor blockade therapy: labetalol. Am Heart J 98:660, 1979.

11. Frishman WH: Pindolol: A new β-adrenoceptor antagonist with partial agonist activity. N Engl J Med 308:940, 1983.

12. Frishman WH: Nadolol: a new β-adrenoceptor antagonist. N Engl J Med 305:678, 1982.

13. Thadani U, Davidson C, Singleton W, Taylor SH: Comparison of the immediate effects of five β-adrenoceptor blocking drugs with different ancillary properties in angina pectoris. N Engl J Med 300:750, 1979.

14. Frishman W, Silverman R, Strom J, et al: Clinical pharmacology of the new beta-adrenergic blocking drugs. Part 4. Adverse effects. Choosing a β-adrenoceptor blocker. Am Heart J 98:256, 1979.

15. Frishman WH: Clinical Pharmacology of the Beta-adrenoceptor Blocking Drugs, New York, Appleton-Century-Crofts, 1980.

16. Frishman WH: Beta-adrenergic blockade in clinical practice. Hosp Practice 17:57, 1982.

17. Singh BN, Jewitt DE: β-Adrenergic receptor blocking drugs in cardiac arrhythmias. Drugs 7:426, 1974.

18. Frishman W, Jacob H, Eisenberg E, Ribner H: Clinical pharmacology of the new beta-adrenergic blocking drugs. 8. Self-poisoning with beta-adrenoceptor blocking agents: Recognition and management. Am Heart J 98:798, 1979.

19. Cruickshank JM: The clinical importance of cardioselectivity and lipophilicity in beta-blockers. Am Heart J 100:160, 1980.

20. Frishman W, Silverman R: Clinical pharmacology of the new beta-adrenergic blocking drugs, 2. Physiologic and metabolic effects. Am Heart J 97:797, 1979.

21. Clark BJ, Menninger K, Bertholet A: Pindolol—the pharmacology of a partial agonist. Br J Clin Pharmacol 13 (Suppl 2):149s, 1982.

22. Glover WE, Greenfield ADM, Shanks RG: Effects of dichloroisoprenaline on the peripheral vascular responses to adrenaline in man. Br J Pharmacol Chemother 19:235, 1962.

23. Barrett AM, Carter J: Comparative chronotropic activity of β-adrenoceptive antagonists. Br J Pharmacol 40:373, 1970.

24. Cocco G, Burkart F, Chu D, Follath F: Intrinsic sympathomimetic activity of β-adrenoceptor blocking agents. Eur J Clin Pharmacol 13:1, 1978.

25. Man in't Veld AJ, Schalekamp MADH: Pindolol acts as a beta-adrenoceptor agonist in orthostatic hypotension: Therapeutic implications. Br Med J 282:929, 1981.

26. Carruthers SG, Twum-Barima Y: Measurements of partial agonist activity of pindolol. Clin Pharmacol Ther 30:581, 1981.

27. Carruthers SG: Cardiac dose-response relationships of oral and intravenous pindolol. Br J Clin Pharmacol 13 (Suppl 2):193s, 1982.

28. Kostis JB, Frishman W, Hosler MH, et al: Treatment of angina pectoris with pindolol: The significance of intrinsic sympathomimetic activity of beta-blockers. Am Heart J 104:496, 1982.

29. McNeil JJ, Louis WJ: A double-blind crossover comparison of pindolol, metoprolol, atenolol and labetalol in mild to moderate hypertension. Br J Clin Pharmacol 8 (Suppl 2):163s, 1979.
30. Gonasun LM: Antihypertensive effects of pindolol. Am Heart J 104:374, 1982.
31. Frishman WH, Kostis J: The significance of intrinsic sympathomimetic activity in beta-adrenoceptor blocking drugs. Cardiovasc Rev Rep 3:503, 1982.
32. Aellig WH: Pindolol—a β-adrenoceptor blocking drug with partial agonist activity: Clinical pharmacological considerations. Br J Clin Pharmacol 13 (Suppl 2):187s, 1982.
33. Taylor SH, Silke B, Lee PS: Intravenous beta-blockade in coronary heart disease: is cardioselectivity or intrinsic sympathomimetic activity hemodynamically useful? N Engl J Med 306:631, 1982.
34. Frishman WH, Strom J, Kirschner M, et al: Labetalol therapy in patients with systemic hypertension and angina pectoris: Effects of combined alpha- and beta-adrenoceptor blockade. Am J Cardiol 48:917, 1981.
35. Johnsson G, Regardh CG: Clinical pharmacokinetics of β-adrenoceptor blocking drugs. Clin Pharmacokinet 1:233, 1976.
36. Frishman WH, Teicher M: Long-acting propranolol. Card Rev Rep 4:1100, 1983.
37. Halkin H, Vered I, Saginer A, Rabinowitz B: Once daily administration of sustained release propranolol capsules in the treatment of angina pectoris. Eur J Clin Pharmacol 16:387, 1979.
38. Parker JO, Porter A, Parker JD: Propranolol in angina pectoris: comparison of long-acting and standard formulation propranolol. Circulation 65:1351, 1982.
39. Zaroslinski J, Borgman RJ, O'Donnel JP, et al: Ultra-short acting beta-blockers: a proposal for the treatment of the critically ill patient. Life Sci 31:899, 1982.
40. Gorczyski RJ, Shaffer JE, Lee RJ, Vuong A: Pharmacology of ASL-8052, a novel beta-adrenergic receptor antagonist with an ultra-short duration of action. J Cardiovasc Pharmacol 5:668, 1983.
41. Murthy VS, Hwang T-F, Zagar ME, et al: Cardiovascular pharmacology of ASL-8052. An ultra-short acting beta-blocker. Eur J Pharmacol in press, 1983.

CHAPTER 3

Physiologic and Metabolic Effects

William H. Frishman and Ralph Silverman

Twenty-five years after their discovery, the therapeutic efficacy and safety of β-adrenoceptor blocking drugs has been well established in patients with angina pectoris, cardiac arrhythmias, hypertension, and in survivors of acute myocardial infarction. β-Blockers are also being used now for a growing number of new clinical indications (see Chapter 4). The basic pharmacodynamic and pharmacokinetic properties of β-blocking agents are discussed in Chapter 2. The main emphasis in this chapter is directed toward the physiologic and metabolic effects of these drugs in human beings.

CARDIOVASCULAR EFFECTS

Blood Pressure (Tables 1 and 2)
It is now well recognized that β-adrenergic blockers are effective in reducing the blood pressure of many patients with systemic hypertension. At the present time, there is no consensus of opinion as to the mechanism(s) whereby these drugs lower blood pressure. It is probable that some, or all, of the mechanisms proposed in the following sections play a part.

Negative Chronotropic and Inotropic Effects. Slowing of the heart rate and some decrease in myocardial contractility with β-blockers lead to a decrease in cardiac output, which in both the short and long term may lead

27

TABLE 1. PROPOSED MECHANISMS TO EXPLAIN THE ANTIHYPERTENSIVE ACTIONS OF β-BLOCKERS

1. Reduction in cardiac output
2. Inhibition of renin
3. Reduction in plasma volume
4. Central nervous system effects
5. Reduction in peripheral vascular resistance
6. Resetting of baroreceptor levels
7. Reduction in venomotor tone
8. Effects on prejunctional β-receptors—reductions in norepinephrine release

Most important effect of β-Blockers—Prevents the pressor response to catecholamines with exercise and stress

to a reduction in blood pressure.[1] It might be expected that these factors would be of particular importance in treatment of hypertension related to high cardiac output,[2] and increased sympathetic tone.

A Central Nervous System Effect. There is now good clinical and experimental evidence to suggest that most β-blockers cross the blood-brain barrier and enter the central nervous system.[3] The occurrence of dreams, insomnia, hallucinations, and depression during therapy with many β-blockers support this conjecture.[4]

Infusion of *l*- and *d,l*-propranolol into the cerebral ventricles of conscious rabbits was reported to cause a marked antihypertensive effect, whereas *d*-propranolol alone caused the blood pressure to rise.[5] By injecting drugs into the vertebral arteries of anesthetized dogs, other investigators found a central antihypertensive action for alprenolol, but not for propranolol.[6] Although there is little doubt that β-blockers with high lipophilicity (e.g., metoprolol, propranolol) enter the central nervous system in high concentrations, a direct antihypertensive effect mediated by this property is not well defined. Also, β-blockers that are less lipid soluble, and less likely to concentrate in the brain, appear to be as effective in lowering blood pressure as propranolol.[7,8]

Differences in Effects on Plasma Renin. The relationship between the hypotensive action of β-blocking drugs and their ability to reduce plasma renin activity remains one of the more controversial areas in hypertension research. There is no doubt that some β-blocking drugs can antagonize sympathetically mediated renin release.[9] Adrenergic activity is not the only mechanism whereby renin release is mediated, however. Other major determinants are sodium balance, posture, and renal perfusion pressure.

Laragh et al.[9] have suggested that a decrease in renin output by the kidney is the major factor contributing to the antihypertensive effects of β-blockers. Propranolol lowers plasma renin activity in normal[10] and hypertensive subjects[11] and blocks the orthostatic rise in plasma renin activity with standing.[12] The dextroisomer of propranolol has no effect on renin release,[13] unlike the inhibitory action of racemic propranolol in the same patients.[12] The suppressant effect of racemic propranolol is therefore dependent on the β-blocking action of the levoisomer.

The effect of different β-blockers on resting and orthostatic renin release is variable. Among the nonselective β-blockers, propranolol causes the greatest reduction of both resting and orthostatic renin release,[14] timolol causes significant reduction,[15] oxprenolol has less effect (especially on orthostatic renin release),[16] and pindolol has the least effect.[13,17] Weber et al.[13] found that in the rabbit, pindolol causes a rise in plasma renin activity; Stokes et al.[18] found that when patients were switched from propranolol to pindolol, they continued to have good control of their blood pressure despite a rise in plasma renin activity. It has been suggested that oxprenolol and pindolol have a lesser effect on renin than propranolol because of their partial agonist properties.[18]

β$_1$-Selective blockers show similar variation in their effects on renin; practolol has no effect on renin[19]; metoprolol lowers resting and furosemide induced renin release[20,21]; and with atenolol, the reports are conflicting (Amery et al.[22] showed no effect, whereas Aberg[23] demonstrated a significant decrease in resting renin). The lack of a renin-lowering effect with practolol may be related to its partial agonist activity. The effectiveness of some β$_1$-selective adrenergic blockers in reducing renin suggests that, in humans, renin release is mediated by a β$_1$-receptor-mediated mechanism.

The important question remains whether there is a clinical correlation between the β-blocker effect on plasma renin activity and the lowering of blood pressure. Laragh and associates[9] found that "high renin" patients respond well to propranolol, "low renin" patients do not respond or may even show a rise in blood pressure, and "normal renin" patients have less predictable responses. Other investigators have been unable to confirm this relationship with either propranolol or with other β-blockers.[7,8,17,18,24] In the "high renin" hypertensive patient, it has been suggested that renin may not be the only factor responsible for the high blood pressure. At present, the exact role of renin reduction in blood pressure control is not well defined.

Venous Tone. Reduced plasma volume and venous return may play a role in the control of blood pressure by β-blockers. A few studies have demonstrated these actions of β-blockers when heart failure was not present in both acute and long-term clinical trials. Since one would expect an impaired cardiac output with β-blockade to cause a reflex increase in plasma volume, these observations, though not yet fully substantiated, are of interest.

Peripheral Resistance. Nonselective β-blockers have no primary action in lowering peripheral resistance and, indeed, may cause it to rise by unopposed α-stimulatory mechanisms.[26] The vasodilating effect of catecholamines on skeletal muscle blood vessels is $β_2$-mediated, suggesting a positive therapeutic advantage of $β_1$-selective blockers, agents with partial agonist activity, and drugs with α-blocking activity. Since $β_1$-selectivity diminishes as the drug dosage is raised, and since hypertensive patients generally have to be given far larger doses than are required simply to block the $β_1$-receptors alone, $β_1$-selectivity[27] offers little, if any, real specific advantage in antihypertensive treatment.[27,28]

"Quinidine Effect" (Membrane-Stabilizing Activity). Some early clinical investigations[29] indicated that the antihypertensive effect of propranolol paralleled the antihypertensive effect of quinidine, suggesting that the "membrane-stabilizing" effect in the β-blocker might be important. Subsequent studies refuted these early findings.[30] All β-blockers appear to reduce blood pressure, regardless of the presence or absence of "membrane" effects.[21] D-Propranolol, with predominant "membrane" effects, does not affect blood pressure.

Resetting of Baroreceptors. It has been suggested that the baroreceptors in long-standing hypertension react less strongly to a reduction in blood pressure than in normal subjects, and that baroreceptor sensitivity can be increased by β-blockade.[31] The clinical significance of this proposed mechanism remains unknown.

Effects on Prejunctional β-Receptors. Apart from their effects on postjunctional tissue β-receptors, it is believed that blockade of prejunctional β-receptors may be involved in the hemodynamic actions of β-blocking drugs. The stimulation of prejunctional $α_2$-receptors leads to a reduction in the quantity of norepinephrine released by the postganglionic sympathetic fibers.[32,33] Conversely, stimulation of prejunctional β-receptors is followed by an increase in the quantity of noradrenaline released by postganglionic sympathetic fibers.[34-36] Blockade of the prejunctional β-receptors should, therefore, diminish the amount of norepinephrine released, leading to a weaker stimulation of postjunctional α-receptors, an effect that would produce less vasoconstriction. Opinions differ, however, on the contributions of presynaptic β-blockade to both a reduction in the peripheral vascular resistance and the antihypertensive effects of β-blocking drugs.

In summary, β-blockers have been found to be useful in treating systemic hypertension, although their precise mechanism of action remains unclear. Whether β-blockers with β_1-selectivity, partial agonist activity, or α-adrenergic blocking activity will ultimately prove more advantageous than nonselective β-blocking drugs for treating hypertension must still be determined.

Effects on Heart Rate, Effects in Angina Pectoris (Table 2)
In 1948 Ahlquist[37] demonstrated that sympathetic innervation of the heart causes the release of norepinephrine activating β-adrenoreceptors in myocardial cells. This adrenergic stimulation causes an increment in heart rate, isometric contractile force, and maximal velocity of muscle fiber shortening, leading to an increase in cardiac work and myocardial oxygen consumption.[38] The decrease in intraventricular pressure and volume caused by the sympathetic mediated enhancement of cardiac contractility, tends, on the other hand, to reduce myocardial oxygen consumption by reducing myocardial wall tension (Law of LaPlace).[39] Although there is a net increase in myocardial oxygen demand, this is normally balanced by an increase in coronary blood flow. Angina pectoris is felt to occur when oxygen demand exceeds supply, i.e., when coronary blood flow is restricted by coronary atherosclerosis. Since the conditions that precipitate anginal attacks (exercise, emotional stress, food, etc.) cause an increase in cardiac sympathetic activity, it might be expected that blockade of cardiac β-adrenoreceptors would relieve the symptoms of the anginal syndrome. It is on this basis that the early clinical studies with β-blocking drugs in angina were initiated,[40] leading to one of the major important therapeutic discoveries of this century. The antiischemic actions of β-blockers are discussed more extensively in Chapter 8.

Four main factors—heart rate, ventricular systolic pressure, rate of rise of left ventricular pressure, and the size of the left ventricle—contribute to the myocardial oxygen requirements of the left ventricle. Of these, heart rate and systolic pressure appear to be the most important (heart rate times systolic blood pressure product is a reliable index for predicting the precipitation of angina in a given patient).[41]

The reduction in heart rate affected by β-blockade has two favorable consequences: (1) decrease in cardiac work, thereby reducing myocardial oxygen needs, and (2) a longer diastolic filling time associated

TABLE 2. PHARMACODYNAMIC PROPERTIES AND CARDIAC EFFECTS OF β-ADRENOCEPTOR BLOCKERS

Drug	Relative β₁-Selectivity*	Partial Agonist Activity	Membrane Stabilizing Activity	Resting Heart Rate
Acebutolol	+ +	+	+	↓
Atenolol	+ +	0	0	↓
Esmololol	+ +	0	0	↓
Labetalol‡	0	+ ?	0	↔
Metoprolol	+ +	0	0	↓
Nadolol	0	0	0	↓
Oxprenolol	0	+	+	↓ ↔
Pindolol	0	+ +	0	↓ ↔
Propranolol	0	0	+ +	↓
Sotalol	0	0	0	↓
Timolol	0	0	0	↓
Isomer d-propranolol	0	0	+ +	↔

*β₁-Selectivity is only seen with low therapeutic drug concentrations. With higher concentrations, β₁-selectivity is not seen.
† + + = strong effect; + = modest effect; 0 = absent effect.
↑ = elevation; ↓ = reduction; ↔ = no change
‡Labetalol has additional α-adrenergic blocking properties and direct vasodilatory activity.
¶Effects of d-propranolol occur with doses in humans well above the therapeutic level. The isomer also lacks β-blocking activity.

with a slower heart rate, allowing for increased coronary perfusion. β-Blockade also reduces exercise-induced blood pressure increments, the velocity of cardiac contraction, and myocardial oxygen consumption at any patient workload.[42]

Studies in dogs have shown propranolol to cause a decrease in coronary blood flow.[43] However, subsequent experimental animal studies demonstrated β-blocking-induced shunting to occur in the coronary circulation, maintaining blood flow to ischemic areas, especially in the subendocardial region.[44] In humans, concomitant with the decrease in myocardial oxygen consumption, β-blockers can cause a reduction in coronary blood flow and a rise in coronary vascular resistance.[42] The overall reduction in myocardial oxygen needs as a whole with β-blockers, however, may be sufficient cause for this decrease in coronary blood flow.

Virtually all β-blockers, whether or not they have partial agonist activity, α-blocking effects, membrane-stabilizing activity, or general or

Exercise Heart Rate	Resting Myocardial Contractility	Resting Blood Pressure	Exercise Blood Pressure	Resting Atrio-ventricular Conduction	Anti-arrhythmic Effect
↓	↓	↓	↓	↓	+
↓	↓	↓	↓	↓	+
?	↓	↓	?	?	+
↓	↓ ↔	↓	↓ ↓	↓ ↔	+
↓	↓	↓	↓	↓	+
↓	↓	↓	↓	↓	+
↓	↓ ↔	↓	↓	↓ ↔	+
↓	↓ ↔	↓	↓	↓ ↔	+
↓	↓	↓	↓	↓	+
↓	↓	↓	↓	↓	+
↓	↓	↓	↓	↓	+
↔	↔ ↓ ¶	↔	↔	↔ ↓ ¶	+ ¶

selective β-blocking properties, produce some degree of increased work capacity without pain in patients with angina pectoris. Therefore, it must be concluded that this results from their common property: blockade of cardiac β-receptors.[45] Both d- and l-propranolol have membrane-stabilizing activity, but only l-propranolol has significant β-blocking activity. The racemic mixture (d- and l-propranolol) causes a decrease in both heart rate and force of contraction in dogs, while the d- isomer has hardly any effect.[46] In humans, d-propranolol, which has "membrane" activity but no β-blocking properties, has been found to be ineffective in relieving angina pectoris even with very high doses.[47]

Although exercise tolerance improves with β-blockade, the increments in heart rate and blood pressure with exercise are blunted, the rate–pressure product (systolic blood pressure times heart rate) achieved when pain occurs is less than that reached during a control run.[48] The depressed pressure-rate product at the onset of pain (about 20 percent reduction from control) is reported to occur with various β-blocking drugs: propranolol (membrane-stabilizing activity), oxprenolol (membrane-stabilizing and intrinsic sympathomimetic activity), practolol (β_1-selective blocker with intrinsic sympathomimetic activity), and sotalol (minimal membrane-stabilizing activity).[49] Thus, although there is increased exercise tolerance with β-blockade, patients exercise less than might be expected. This probably relates to the action of β-blockers to increase left ventricular size, causing increased left ventricular wall tension and an increase in oxygen consumption at a given blood pressure.[50]

All β-blockers will limit the heart rate increment with exercise; however, they have differing effects on the resting heart rate. Propranolol and metoprolol slow the resting pulse more than do oxprenolol, pindolol, and labetalol; *d*-propranolol has very little resting pulse slowing activity. Morgan et al.[51] also found differences in pulse slowing activity among four β-blockers they tested: propranolol and timolol reduced pulse rate more than pindolol and alprenolol. It would appear that β-blockers lacking partial agonist activity slow the resting pulse rate more than β-blockers with partial agonist activity or α-adrenergic blocking actions.

The therapeutic benefit of β-blockers in angina pectoris is now established beyond question. Many double-blind studies of β-blockers have demonstrated a significant reduction in the frequency of anginal attacks. Observed improvement is dose-related and dosage must be titrated for each individual patient.

Electrophysiologic Effects (Tables 2 and 3)

Although β-blocking drugs have been used for treating cardiac arrhythmias for 15 years, their precise mode of action remains unclear. Two main effects of these drugs in arrhythmia have been identified—β-blockade and membrane-stabilizing activity.

β-Blockade. By blocking adrenergic stimulation of cardiac pacemaker potentials, β-blocking drugs are useful in controlling arrhythmias that are caused by enhanced automaticity and reentry. In concentrations that cause significant inhibition of cardiac adrenergic receptors, the slope of the pacemaker action potential (either sinus or ectopic) is reduced, particularly in the presence of catecholamines or ouabain.[52,53] Thus, ar-

TABLE 3. ANTIARRHYTHMIC MECHANISMS FOR β-BLOCKERS

1. β-Blockade
   Electrophysiology: depress excitability; depress conduction
   Prevention of ischemia: decrease automaticity; inhibit re-entrant mechanisms
2. Membrane-stabilizing effects
   Local anesthetic, "quinidine-like" properties: depress excitability;
      prolong refractory period; delay conduction
   Clinically—probably not significant
3. Special pharmacologic properties (β₁-selectivity, intrinsic sympathomimetic activity,
      α-blocking activity) do not appear to contribute to antiarrhythmic effectiveness.

rhythmias related to sympathetic hyperactivity would be expected to respond to β-blockade. Similarly, in myocardial infarction, where there is heightened sympathetic nervous activity causing enhanced automaticity, β-blockers are likely to be useful.[54] This is not to say, however, that β-blockers will only be effective in arrhythmias directly related to catecholamines (e.g., pheochromocytoma, halothane anesthesia). Clinically, their usefulness has been demonstrated in many other conditions associated with arrhythmia. Their beneficial effect in these situations probably derives from removal of normal adrenergic stimulatory effects that may be unfavorably added to the major arrhythmia-causing stimulus. One such example would be arrhythmias related to digitalis toxicity.[55]

Membrane Stabilizing Action. The second possible mechanism to explain the antiarrhythmic effect of β-blocking drugs involves their membrane-stabilizing or depressant action, often referred to as the "quinidine-like" or "local anesthetic" action. This property is unrelated to catecholamine inhibitory actions and is manifested to an equal extent by both the *d* and *l* isomers of these drugs (*d* isomers have virtually no β-blocking activity).[56] It is characterized by a reduction in the rate of rise of the intracardiac action potential without affecting the duration of the spike or the resting potential.[57] The effect has been explained by an inhibition of the depolarizing inward sodium current.

It should be noted, however, that in in vitro experiments with human ventricular muscle, the concentration of propranolol required to produce this effect is 50 to 100 times the concentration generally associated with inhibition of exercise-induced tachycardia.[58] The concentrations of propranolol needed to produce this effect are in the millimolar range, whereas therapeutic doses produce micromolar concentrations, at which level only β-blocking effects occur.

It seems probable, therefore, that in usual therapeutic doses, the main factor in the antiarrhythmic effect of these drugs is β-blockade. Coltart et al.[59] and Shand[60] have shown that arrhythmias are suppressed by plasma propranolol concentrations 1 to 2 percent of the level needed for membrane stabilizing action. Jewitt and Singh[61] observed that *d*-propranolol, which possesses membrane stabilizing properties but no β-blocking actions, is a weak antiarrhythmic drug even in very high doses. Metropolol, on the other hand, is a clinically effective antiarrhythmic drug, although it lacks membrane-stabilizing characteristics.[62]

If β-blockade is, indeed, the major mechanism for antiarrhythmic action, and the clinical relevance of membrane stabilizing properties is negligible, then we would expect all β-blockers to have similar antiarrhythmic effects for a comparable degree of β-blockade. This, in fact,

TABLE 4. PHARMACODYNAMIC PROPERTIES AND NONCARDIAC EFFECTS OF β-ADRENOCEPTOR BLOCKERS

Drug	Relative β₁-Selectivity*	Partial Agonist Activity	Membrane Stabilizing Activity	Bronchial Tone	Platelet Aggreg-ability
Acebutolol	+ ‡	+	+	↑ ↔ ↓	
Atenolol	+ +	0	0	↑ ↔ ↓	
Labetalol¶	0	+ ?	0	↑ ↔ ↓	↔
Metoprolol	+ +	+ +	0	↑ ↔ ↓	
Nadolol	0	0	0	↔ ↓	
Oxprenolol	0	+	+	↑ ↔ ↓	↓
Pindolol	0	+ +	+	↑ ↔ ↓	↓
Propranolol	0	0	+ +	↔ ↓	↓
Sotalol	0	0	0	↔ ↓	
Timolol	0	0	0	↔ ↓	↓
Isomer d-propranolol	0	0	+ +	↔	↓

*β₁-Selectivity is only seen with low therapeutic drug concentrations. With higher concentrations, β₁-selectivity is not seen.
†RBF = renal blood flow; GFR = glomerular filtration rate; HDL-CHOL = high-density lipoprotein cholesterol; LDL-Chol = low-density lipoprotein cholesterol; VLDL-TRI = very low density lipoprotein triglycerides
‡+ + = Strong effect; + = modest effect; 0 = absent effect; ↑ = elevation; ↓ = reduction; ↔ = no change.
¶Labetalol has additional α-adrenergic blocking properties and direct vasodilatory activity.

appears to be the case. No clinical superiority of one β-blocking agent over another for the treatment of arrhythmias has ever been demonstrated.

Effects on the Sinus Node and Atrioventricular Conduction (Tables 2 and 3)

In animals and in humans, β-blockers slow the rate of discharge of the sinus and ectopic pacemakers and increase the functional refractory period of the atrioventricular (AV) node. They also slow both antegrade and retrograde conduction in anomalous conduction pathways.[63]

Since all β-blockers studied to date cause some increase in atrioventricular conduction time, advancing AV block is a potential complication when β-blockers are used in managing arrhythmias. From both animal and human studies, it is apparent that β-blockers that do not possess intrinsic sympathomimetic activity, but have potent membrane stabilizing properties (e.g., propranolol), cause the greatest increment in atrioventricular conduction time. In contrast, Giudicelli et al.[64] showed

Plasma Renin Activity	Peripheral Vascular Resistance	RBF†	GFR	HDL-Chol	LDL-Chol	VLDL-TRI
↔↓	↔↑	↔↔	↔↔	?	?	?
↓↔	↑↔	↓↔	↓↔	↔	↔	↔
↓↔	↓	↔	↔	↔	↔	↔
↓↔	↑↔	↓↔	↓↔	↔↓	↔	↑↔
↓↔	↑	↑	↔	?	?	?
↓↔	↑↔	↓↔	↓↔	?	?	?
↓↔↑	↔↓	↓↔	↓↔	↔	↔	↔
↓	↑	↓	↓	↓	↔	↑
↓	↑	↓	↓	?	?	?
↓	↑	↓	↓	?	?	?
↔	↔	↔	↔	?	?	?

that the partial agonist activity of pindolol provided some protection against the AV conduction impairment induced by β-blockade.

It should be noted that β-blocking drugs can, in large doses, induce sinus node dysfunction that may lead to sinus arrest or sinoatrial block. β-Blocking drugs, therefore, are best avoided in patients with "sick sinus syndrome" a condition that could be aggravated by β-blockade.

Vascular Resistance and Peripheral Blood Flow (Table 4)

Isoproterenol mediates its effects on cardiac contractility through the β_1-receptor and its peripheral vasodilatory effects through the β_2-receptor. Propranolol, by blocking both receptors, leaves uninhibited the α-adrenergic tone in the periphery. This would tend to increase peripheral vascular resistance with catecholamine stimulation, an effect that has been clearly demonstrated with propranolol.[65] This increase in peripheral resistance might potentiate the rate-slowing effects of propranolol and negate some of its antihypertensive effects.[27] The increase in peripheral resistance can also affect blood flow in the limbs, coronary arteries,[42] renal circulation,[66] splanchnic vessels,[67] and in the brain.[68] Drugs with β_1-selectivity (e.g., metoprolol) have little or no effect on peripheral vessels (in doses where the drugs are β_1-selective) and tend therefore not to increase peripheral resistance.[27,28] Drugs with intrinsic sympathomimetic activity (e.g., pindolol) or α-adrenergic blocking properties (e.g., labetalol) may tend to lower peripheral vascular resistance.[17,69]

Inhibition of peripheral vasodilatation is probably one mechanism to explain the beneficial effect of nadolol and propranolol in migraine.[70,71] Pindolol, perhaps because of its partial agonist activity, has shown little or no effect in the treatment of patients with migraine.

Renovascular Hemodynamics and Renal Function (Table 4)

There is a paucity of information on the acute effects of β-adrenoceptor blockers on renal blood flow and renal function. Of all the β-blockers, only nadolol (nonselective) has been shown to maintain renal blood flow while, at the same time, decreasing cardiac output.[72] Propranolol (nonselective) use in hypertension is characteristically associated with decrements in renal blood flow and glomerular filtration rate of about 10 to 20 percent.[73] β-Blockers with partial agonist activity, $β_1$-selectivity, or α-blocking activity may cause a lesser reduction in renal blood flow than propranolol and may preserve renal perfusion.[73,74] The unique renovascular effect of nadolol compared to other β-blockers may reflect a dopaminergic effect of the drug on the renal vasculature.[72]

There is no evidence that β-blockers are directly nephrotoxic. The mechanism by which they alter renal plasma flow and glomerular filtration rate is probably hemodynamic.[73] Reductions in renal blood flow with certain β-blockers probably relates to diminished cardiac output and, by reflex mechanisms, increased renovascular resistance.[73] It is also possible that β-blockers may inhibit natural vasodilation by the kallikrein-kinin system.[75]

With long-term β-blocker use, there is some evidence that the short-term effects on renal blood flow persist, and may even progress.[73] However, the clinical importance of β-blocker induced renal changes is unknown. These drugs appear to have no adverse effects in patients with normal pretreatment renal function, nor is there evidence that patients with impaired renal function are harmed by these agents.[73] Some serum creatinine and blood urea levels should be periodically monitored. If renal function does deteriorate on a specific β-blocker, the clinician can switch therapy to nadolol, labetalol, or to an entirely different class of antihypertensive medication—prazosin, hydralazine, methyldopa, captopril.

NONCARDIOVASCULAR EFFECTS

Oxygen Transport (Effects on the Oxyhemoglobin Dissociation Curve)

Altered oxyhemoglobin dissociation could facilitate oxygen availability to poorly perfused zones of myocardium in patients with ischemic heart disease. It was suggested that the oxyhemoglobin dissociation curve could be affected by administration of β-blocking drugs. Oski and Miller[76] showed that propranolol produced a favorable alteration of the curve to the right in normal subjects, probably by a release of membrane bound 2,3 diphosphoglycerate (2,3 DPG). These results were not confirmed by Brain, who found no significant change in P_{50} (Po$_2$ at 50 percent hemoglobin saturation) using a higher oral dose of propranolol, and no alteration in erythrocyte 2,3 DPG was seen.[77] We also were not able to corroborate the findings of Oski regarding changes in P_{50} and 2,3 DPG (during rest and with exercise) in patients with angina pectoris treated with propranolol.[78,79]

Although the effects on P_{50} with other β-blockers has not yet been well investigated, it would appear that the direct effects of β-blockers on the oxyhemoglobin dissociation curve and on O_2 delivery are negligible.

Effects on the Bronchial Tree (Table 4)

Bronchodilation is mediated in part through catecholamine stimulation of β$_2$-receptors in the lung. Propranolol, which blocks β-receptors (β$_1$ and β$_2$) can precipitate bronchospasm in some patients.

All β-blocking drugs, including those with β$_1$-selectivity, partial agonist activity and α-blocking effects, can induce bronchoconstriction in patients with asthma and asthmatic bronchitis. Comparative studies have shown, however, that compounds with partial agonist activity (pindolol),[80,81] β$_1$-selectivity (metoprolol),[8,28,82] and α-blocking activity (labetalol)[83] are less likely to increase airways resistance [as measured by forced expiratory volume in one second (FEV$_1$)] in asthmatic patients than propranolol. Patients who develop asthma while taking a β$_1$-selective blocker will respond readily with bronchodilation from standard doses of β$_2$-stimulant drugs such as albuterol, whereas patients taking a nonselective β-blocker like propranolol will not.[84]

Effects of β-Adrenergic Blocking Agents on Metabolism

Blood Glucose. Hypoglycemia has been reported as a side effect of nonselective β-blockade in diabetics receiving insulin.[85] The severity of this insulin-induced hypoglycemia may be lessened with β$_1$-selective blockers.[28,86] The symptoms of hypoglycemia are also attenuated by propranolol, but sweating is enhanced.

In humans, epinephrine stimulates glycolysis in skeletal muscle predominantly via β-adrenoceptors, and in the liver predominantly via α-adrenoceptors.[87] In normal subjects, abolition of glucose mobilization requires simultaneous blockade of α-adrenergic receptors in the liver and β-adrenergic receptors in skeletal muscle, with phenoxybenzamine and propranolol, respectively.[88] Resting plasma glucose and insulin concentrations in normal individuals are not affected by propranolol. The fall of plasma glucose levels after administration of insulin is also unaffected. The rate of return of blood glucose levels to normal, however, after insulin-induced hypoglycemia, is reduced and the increase of plasma glycerol is prevented. These effects depend, in part, on the β-adrenergic effect of catecholamines released in response to hypoglycemia. For this reason, in diabetic patients treated with insulin, and in some other situations (e.g., fasting), β-blockade with propranolol may be associated with hypoglycemia.[89]

In some patients, propranolol has been reported to precipitate hyperglycemia and hyperosmolar nonketotic coma, and to prevent recurrent hypoglycemia in a patient with insulinoma.[90,91] These contrasting effects in diabetic patients result from an interplay of several factors: gluconeogenesis, liver and skeletal muscle glycogenolysis, peripheral glucose utilization, and growth hormone, glucagon, and insulin secretion. β-Blockers inhibit glucose–sulfonylurea-stimulated insulin secretion. There is good evidence that the β-receptor for insulin secretion is of the β_2-type.[92]

Although the metabolic effects of β-blockade are not nearly as prominent as their hemodynamic effects, and the incidence of metabolic side effects is low, β-adrenergic blocking agents should be used with caution in patients prone to hypoglycemia, particularly insulin-treated diabetic patients. β_1-Selective blockers (e.g., metoprolol, atenolol)[93,94] or drugs with intrinsic sympathomimetic activity (e.g., pindolol) may not interfere as much with metabolic compensations for insulin-induced hypoglycemia.

Free Fatty Acids. Administration of propranolol has been shown to reduce plasma free fatty acid levels at rest, after prolonged fasting and during exercise, emotion, or insulin-induced hypoglycemia.[95,96] Also, propranolol, but not practolol (β_1-selective) blocks the lipolytic activity of isoproterenol.[97,98] The increase in free fatty acids occurring during epinephrine infusion is blocked by propranolol, but accentuated by phentolamine, suggesting the presence of an additional inhibitory α-adrenergic control.[99] Lipolytic activity of epinephrine can also be blocked by practolol, but only at doses significantly higher than those affecting its cardiovascular manifestations.[100] Thus, although the receptor sites associated with adrenergic stimulation of lipolysis fulfill many of the characteristics of a β-receptor, the presence of an inhibitory effect that can be reversed by phentolamine, and a reduced sensitivity to practolol, show that they are not identical with those affecting heart rate and force of contraction.

Plasma Lipids and Lipoproteins (Table 4). Certain β-adrenoceptor blocking agents were recently reported to alter plasma lipids and lipoproteins.[101,102] Propranolol has been shown, in multiple studies, to modestly raise plasma triglycerides and reduce levels of high-density lipoprotein cholesterol.[102,103] Low-density lipoprotein-cholesterol levels do not seem to be altered.[103] These observations with propranolol (nonselective), do not represent a class action of β-blockers since $β_1$-selective agents, partial agonist β-blockers, and labetalol do not appear to alter plasma lipids to any extent.[101,104,105] The mechanism by which propranolol affects plasma lipids and the clinical significance of these changes in humans has yet to be determined.

Effects on Serum Calcium and Parathormone Secretion. The release of parathormone from the parathyroid glands is mediated in part by catecholamine stimulation.[106] In experimental studies, it was demonstrated that propranolol could reduce parathormone secretion through its β-blocking effects.[107] Some reports have described a beneficial action of propranolol in patients having primary hyperparathyroidism, with a reduction in both serum calcium and parathormone secretion.[108] In normal individuals, however, β-blockers, in therapeutic doses, appear to have no effect on calcium, phosphate, or parathormone secretion.[109]

Effects on Blood Coagulation (Table 4). Adrenergic stimuli may interact with the hemostatic processes at several points. Exercise or epinephrine administration causes a rapid rise in Factor VIII (antihemophilic globulin) levels, which can reach two to four times control level.[110] This increase can be totally blocked by propranolol or alprenolol, but not by phenoxybenzamine or practolol.[111,112]

Propranolol has been shown to interfere with exercise-induced increments in fibrinolytic activity whereas practolol has been shown to have no effect.[113]

In contrast to this potential detrimental effect on fibrinolysis, some β-blockers have a potential beneficial effect on platelet activity (see Chapter 9). Excessive reactivity of blood platelets may contribute to arteriosclerotic vascular disease and its complications. The platelets of patients with thrombotic vascular disease show increased turnover rates and augmented responses to a variety of aggregating agents.[113-115] We have observed that the platelets of patients with angina pectoris have exaggerated aggregation responses that become normal during propranolol therapy.[116]

From in vitro experiments (see Chapter 9), propranolol (in concentrations similar to those safely achieved in vivo) both abolished the second wave of human platelet aggregation induced by adenosine diphosphate (ADP) and epinephrine and inhibited aggregation induced by collagen and thrombin.[116] Propranolol blocked the release of C-serotonin from platelets, inhibited platelet adhesion to collagen, interfered with clot retraction, and inhibited platelet thrombaxane release. Inhibition of platelet aggregation appeared unrelated to β-adrenergic blockade as (+) d-propranolol (which lacks β-blocking activity) was equipotent with (−) l-propranolol. Moreover, practolol, a β-blocking drug that is not membrane active (nonlipophilic), did not inhibit platelet function. These studies suggested that propranolol, like local anesthetics, decreases platelet responsiveness by a direct action on the platelet membrane. Modulation of platelet function by propranolol may occur at concentrations achieved with usual clinical doses of the drug.[116,117]

Oxprenolol[118] and pindolol, drugs with membrane activity, have also been shown to reduce platelet aggregability, though to a lesser degree than propranolol. If platelet hyperaggregability contributes to atherosclerosis and its complications, then β-blockers, with effects on platelet membranes, may provide an extra protective effect in patients.

Heightened platelet aggregability has been described in patients with angina pectoris who were withdrawn abruptly from chronic propranolol treatment. Whether or not platelet hyperresponsiveness contributes to the "rebound phenomenon" described with β-blocker withdrawal is provocative and warrants further investigation.[119,120]

REFERENCES

1. Hansson L, Zweifler AJ, Julius S, Hunyor SN: Hemodynamic effects of acute and prolonged β-adrenergic blockade in essential hypertension. Acta Med Scand 196:27, 1974.
2. Frohlich ED: Hyperdynamic circulation and hypertension. Postgrad Med 52:64, 1972.
3. Myers MG, Lewis PJ, Reid JL, Dollery CT: Brain concentration of propranolol in relation to hypotension effects in the rabbit with observations on brain propranolol levels in man. J Pharmacol Exp Ther 192:327, 1975.
4. Frishman WH, Razin A, Swencionis C, Sonnenblick EH: Beta-adrenergic blockade in anxiety states: A new approach to therapy? Card Rev Rep 2:447, 1981.

5. Reid JL, Lewis PJ, Myers MG, Dollery CT: Cardiovascular effects of intracerebroventricular *d*-, *l*-, and *dl*-propranolol in the conscious rabbit. J Pharmacol Exp Ther 188:394, 1974.
6. Offerhaus L, Van Zweiten PA: Comparative studies on central factors contributing to the hypotensive action of propranolol, alprenolol and their enantiomers. Cardiovasc Res 8:488, 1974.
7. Frishman WH: Nadolol: A new β-adrenoceptor antagonist. N Engl J Med 305:678, 1982.
8. Frishman WH: Atenolol and timolol, two new systemic β-adrenoceptor antagonists. N Engl J Med 306:1456, 1982.
9. Laragh JH: Vasoconstriction-volume analysis for understanding and treating hypertension: the use of renin and aldosterone profiles. Am J Med 55:261, 1973.
10. Winer N, Chekshi DS, Yoon MS, Freedman AD: Adrenergic receptor mediation of renin secretion. J Clin Endocrinol Metab 29:1168, 1969.
11. Michelakis AM, McAllister RG: The effect of chronic adrenergic receptor blockade on plasma renin activity in man. J Clin Endocrinol Metab 34:386, 1972.
12. Tobert JA, Slater JDH, Fugelman F, et al: The effect in man of (+) propranolol and racemic propranolol on renin secretion stimulated by orthostatic stress. Clin Sci 44:291, 1973.
13. Weber MA, Stokes GS, Gain JM: Comparison of the effects of renin release of beta-adrenergic antagonists with differing properties. J Clin Invest 54:1413, 1974.
14. Leonetti G, Mayer G, Morganti A, et al: Hypotensive and renin suppressing activities of propranolol in hypertensive patients. Clin Sci Mol Med 48:491, 1975.
15. Lydtin H, Schuchard J, Wober W, et al: The effect of timolol on renin, angiotensin II, plasma catecholamines, and blood pressure in the human, in Magnani B (ed), Beta-Adrenergic Blocking Agents in the Management of Hypertension and Angina Pectoris. New York, Raven, 1974, p. 81.
16. Kuramoto K, Kurihara H, Murata K, et al: Haemodynamic effects and variations in plasma activity after oral administration of oxprenolol. J Intern Med Res 2:448, 1973.
17. Frishman WH: Pindolol: A new β-adrenoceptor antagonist with partial agonist activity. N Engl J Med 308:940, 1983.
18. Stokes GS, Weber MS, Thornell IR: β-Blockers and plasma renin activity in hypertension. Br Med J 1:60, 1974.
19. Esler MD: Effect of practolol on blood pressure and renin release in man. Clin Pharmacol Ther 15:484, 1970.
20. Waal-Manning HJ: Metabolic effects of β-adrenoceptor blockade, in Simpson FO (ed), Proceedings Queenstown Symposium. Drugs II:121, 1976.
21. Waal-Manning HJ: Hypertension: Which beta blocker? Drugs 12:412, 1976.

22. Amery A, Billiet L, Fagard R: Beta receptors and renin release. N Engl J Med 290:284, 1974.
23. Aberg H: Beta receptors and renin release. N Engl J Med 290:1025, 1974.
24. Morgan TO, Roberts R, Carney SL, et al: β-Adrenergic receptor blocking drugs, hypertension and plasma renin. Br J Clin Pharmacol 2:159, 1975.
25. Krauss XH, Schalekamp MADH, Kolsters G, et al: Effects of beta-adrenergic blockade on systemic and renal haemodynamic responses to hyper osmotic saline in hypertensive patients. Clin Sci 43:385, 1972.
26. Prichard BNC: Propranolol as an antihypertensive agent. Am Heart J 79:128, 1970.
27. Imhof PR: Characterization of beta-blockers as antihypertensive agents in the light of human pharmacology studies, in Schweizer W (ed), Beta-Blockers—Present Status and Future Prospects. Bern, Huber, 1974, pp 40–50.
28. Koch-Weser J: Metoprolol. N Engl J Med 301:698, 1979.
29. Waal HJ: Hypotensive action of propranolol. Clin Pharmacol Ther 7:588, 1966.
30. Rahn KH, Hawlina A, Kersting F, Planz G: Studies on the antihypertensive action of the optical isomers of propranolol in man. Naunyn Schmiedebergs Arch Pharmacol 286:319, 1974.
31. Pickering TG, Gribbin B, Petersen ES, et al: Effects of autonomic blockade on the baroreflex in man at rest and during exercise. Circ Res 30:177, 1972.
32. Langer SZ: Presynaptic receptors and their role in the regulation of transmitter release. Br J Pharmacol 60:481, 1977.
33. Berthelsen S, Pettinger, WA: A functional basis for classification of α-adrenergic receptors. Life Sci 21:77, 1977.
34. Yamaguchi N, de Champlain J, Nadeau RL: Regulation of norepinephrine release from cardiac sympathetic fibers in the dog by presynaptic α- and β-receptors. Circ Res 41:108, 1977.
35. Stjärne L, Brundin J: β-Adrenoceptors facilitate noradrenaline secretion from human vasoconstrictor nerves. Acta Physiol Scand 97:88, 1976.
36. Majewski HJ, McCulloch MW, Rand MJ, Story DF: Adrenaline activation of pre-junctional β-adrenoceptors in guinea pig atria. Br J Pharmacol 71:435, 1980.
37. Ahlquist RP: A study of the adrenotropic receptors. Am J Physiol 153:586, 1948.
38. Sonnenblick EH, Ross J Jr., Braunwald E: Oxygen consumption of the heart. Newer concepts of its multifactorial determination. Am J Cardiol 22:328, 1968.
39. Sonnenblick EH, Shelton CL: Myocardial energetics: Basic principles and clinical implications. N Engl J Med 285:668, 1971.
40. Black JW, Stephenson JS: Pharmacology of a new adrenergic beta-receptor blocking compound (Nethalide). Lancet 2:311, 1962.
41. Robinson BF: Relation of heart rate and systolic blood pressure to the on-

set of pain in angina pectoris. Circulation 35:1073, 1967.

42. Wolfson S, Gorlin R: Cardiovascular pharmacology of propranolol in man. Circulation 40:501, 1969.

43. Parratt JR, Grayson J: Myocardial vascular reactivity after β-adrenergic blockade. Lancet 1:388, 1966.

44. Becker LC, Fortuin NJ, Pitt B: Effects of ischemia and antianginal drugs on the distribution of radioactive microspheres in the canine left ventricle. Circ Res 28:263, 1971.

45. Boakes AJ, Prichard BNC: The effects of AH 5158, pindolol, propranolol, and d-propranolol on acute exercise tolerance in angina pectoris. J Pharm Pharmacol 47:673, 1973.

46. Barrett AM: A comparison of the effect of (±) propranolol and (+) propranolol in anesthetized dogs; β-receptor blocking and hemodynamic action. J Pharm Pharmacol 21:241, 1969.

47. Bjorntorp P: Treatment of angina pectoris with beta-adrenergic blockade, mode of action. Acta Med Scand 184:259, 1968.

48. Gianelly RS, Goldman RH, Treister B, Harrison DC: Propranolol in patients with angina pectoris. Ann Intern Med 57:1216, 1967.

49. Prichard BNC: β-Receptor antagonists in angina pectoris. Ann Clin Res 3:344, 1971.

50. Robinson BF: The mode of action of beta-antagonists in angina pectoris. Postgrad Med J 47 (Suppl 2):41, 1971.

51. Morgan TO, Sabto J, Anavekar SM, et al: A comparison of beta-adrenergic blocking drugs in the treatment of hypertension. Postgrad Med J 50:253, 1974.

52. Hoffman BF, Singer DH: Appraisal of the effects of catecholamines on cardiac electrical activity. Ann NY Acad Sci 139:914, 1967.

53. Carmeliet E, Verdanok F: Interaction between ouabain and butridine, a beta-adrenergic blocking substance on the heart. Eur J Pharmacol 1:269, 1967.

54. Opie LH, Lubbe WF: Catecholamine-mediated arrhythmias in acute myocardial infarction: experimental evidence and role of beta-adrenoceptor blockade. S Afr Med J 56:871, 1979.

55. Singh BN, Jewitt DE: β-Adrenoceptor blocking drugs in cardiac arrhythmias, in Avery G (ed); Cardiovascular Drugs. Baltimore, University Park Press 1977, vol 2, pp 141–142.

56. Levy JV, Richards V: Inotropic and chronotropic effects of a series of β-adrenergic blocking drugs: Some structure activity relationships. Proc Soc Exp Biol Med 122:373, 1966.

57. Vaughan Williams EM, Papp J: The effect of oxprenolol on cardiac intracellular potentials in relation to its antiarrhythmia local anesthetic and other properties. Postgrad Med J 46:22, 1970.

58. Coltart DJ, Shand DG: Plasma propranolol levels in the quantitative assessment of β-adrenergic blockade in man. Br Med J 3:731, 1970.

59. Coltart DJ, Gibson DG, Shand DG: Plasma propranolol levels associated

with suppression of ventricular ectopic beats. Br Med J 1:490, 1971.

60. Shand DG: Pharmacokinetic properties of beta-adrenergic blocking drugs. Drugs 7:39, 1974.
61. Jewitt DE, Singh BN: The role of beta-adrenergic blockade in myocardial infarction. Prog Cardiovasc Dis 16:421, 1974.
62. Rydén L, Ariniego R, Arnman K, et al: A double-blind trial of metoprolol in acute myocardial infarction—effects on ventricular tachyarrhythmias. N Engl J Med 308:614, 1983.
63. Singh BN, Jewitt DE: Beta-adrenergic receptor blocking drugs in cardiac arrhythmias. Drugs 7:426, 1974.
64. Giudicelli JF, Lhoste F, Bossier JR: β-Adrenergic blockade and atrioventricular conduction impairment. Eur J Pharmacol 31:216, 1975.
65. Achong MR, Piafsky KM, Ogilvie RI: The effects of timolol (MK 950) and propranolol on peripheral vessels in man. Clin Pharmacol Ther 17:228, 1975.
66. Nies AS, McNeil JS, Schrier R: Mechanisms of increased sodium reabsorption during propranolol administration. Circulation 44:596, 1976.
67. Price HL, Coopereman LH, Warden JC: Control of the splanchnic circulation in man. Circ Res 21:333, 1967.
68. Meyer JS, Okamoto S, Shimazu K, et al: Cerebral metabolic changes during treatment of subacute cerebral infarction by alpha and beta adrenergic blockade with phenoxybenzamine and propranolol. Stroke 5:180, 1974.
69. Frishman W, Halprin S: Clinical pharmacology of the new beta-adrenoceptor blocking drugs. Part 7. New horizons in beta-adrenoceptor blocking therapy: labetalol. Am Heart J 98:660, 1979.
70. Packard RC: Uses of propranolol. N Engl J Med 293:1205, 1975.
71. Frishman WH: β-Adrenoceptor antagonists: New drugs and new indications. N Engl J Med 305:500, 1981.
72. Textor SC, Fouad FM, Bravo EL, et al: Redistribution of cardiac output to the kidneys during oral nadolol administration. N Engl J Med 307:601, 1982.
73. Epstein M, Oster JR: Beta-blockers and the kidney. Mineral Electrolyte Metab 8:237, 1982.
74. Thompson FD, Joekes AM, Hussein MM: Monotherapy with labetalol for hypertensive patients with normal and impaired renal function. Br J Clin Pharmacol 8 (Suppl 2):129s, 1979.
75. Warren SE, O'Connor DT, Cohen IM, Mitas JA: Renal hemodynamic changes during long-term antihypertensive therapy. Clin Pharmacol Ther 29:310, 1981.
76. Oski FA, Miller LD, Delivoria-Papadopoulous M, et al: Oxygen affinity in red cell changes induced in vivo by propranolol. Science 175:1372, 1972.
77. Brain MC, Card RT, Kane J, et al: Acute effects of varying doses of propranolol upon oxygen haemoglobin effects in man. Br J Clin Pharm 1:67, 1974.
78. Frishman W, Smithen C, Christodoulou J, et al: Medical management of

angina pectoris: Multifactorial action of propranolol, in Norman J, Cooley D (eds), Coronary Artery Medicine and Surgery. New York, Appleton, 1975, pp 285–295.

79. Frishman W, Wilner G, Smithen C, et al: Effects of exercise and propranolol on hemoglobin oxygen affinity in patients with angina pectoris. Clin Res 24:614, 1976.

80. Beumer HM, Hardonk HJ: Effects of beta-adrenergic blocking drugs on ventilatory function in asthmatics. Eur J Clin Pharmacol 5:77, 1972.

81. Frishman WH, Davis R, Strom J, et al: Clinical pharmacology of the new beta-adrenoceptor blocking drugs. Part 5. Pindolol (LB-46) therapy for supraventricular arrhythmia: a viable alternative to propranolol in patients with bronchospasm. Am Heart J 98:393, 1979.

82. Skinner C, Gaddie J, Palmer KNV: Comparison of effects of metoprolol and propranolol on asthmatic airway obstruction. Br Med J 1:504, 1976.

83. Skinner C, Gaddie J, Palmer KNV: Comparison of intravenous AH 5158 (labetalol) and propranolol on asthma. Br Med J 2:59, 1975.

84. Johnson G, Svedmyr M, Thirnger G: Effects of intravenous propranolol and metoprolol and their interaction with isoprenaline on pulmonary function, heart rate and blood pressure in asthmatics. Eur J Clin Pharmacol 8:175, 1975.

85. Kotler MN, Berinda L, Rubenstein AH: Hypoglycemia precipitated by propranolol. Lancet 2:1389, 1966.

86. Deacon SP, Barnett D: Comparison of atenolol and propranolol during insulin-induced hypoglycemia. Br Med J 2:272, 1976.

87. Porte D: Sympathetic regulation of insulin secretion. Its relation to diabetes mellitus. Arch Intern Med 123:252, 1969.

88. Antonis A, Clark MI, Hodge RL, et al: Receptor mechanisms in the hyperglycemic response to adrenaline in man. Lancet 1:1135, 1967.

89. Wray R, Sutcliffe SBJ: Propranolol-induced hypoglycaemia and myocardial infarction. Br Med J 2:592, 1972.

90. Podolsky S, Pattavina CG: Hyperosmolar non-ketotic diabetic coma: a complication of propranolol therapy. Metabolism 22:685, 1973.

91. Blum I, Duren M, Laron Z, et al: Prevention of hypoglycemic attacks by propranolol in a patient suffering from insomnia. Diabetes 24:535, 1975.

92. Loubatiere A, Mariani MM, Sorel G, Savi L: The action of β-adrenergic blocking drugs and stimulating agents on insulin secretion. Characteristics of the type of beta-receptor. Diabetologica 7:127, 1971.

93. Deacon SP, Karunanuyake A, Barnett D: Acebutolol, atenolol and propranolol and metabolic responses to acute hypoglycemia in man. Br Med J 2:1255, 1977.

94. Smith U: Effect of beta-adrenoceptor blocking agents on the reaction to hypoglycemia and the physical working capacity. Card Rev Rep 2:563, 1981.

95. Allison SP, Chamberlain MJ, Miller JE, et al: Effects of propranolol on blood sugar, insulin and free fatty acids. Diabetologica 5:339, 1969.

96. Abramson EA, Arky RA, Woeber KA: Effects of propranolol on the hormonal and metabolic responses to insulin-induced hypoglycaemia. Lancet 2:1386, 1966.
97. Harrison DC, Griffin JR: Metabolic and circulatory responses to selective adrenergic stimulation and blockade. Circulation 34:218, 1974.
98. Miller DW, Allen DO: Antilipolytic activity of 4- (2 hydroxy 3 isopropylaminopropoxy) acetanilide (practolol). Proc Soc Exp Biol Med 136:715, 1971.
99. Mohs JM, Langley PE, Chase GR, Burns TW: In vivo observations on the rule of alpha and beta adrenergic receptor sites in human lipolysis. (Abstr). Clin Res 20:57, 1972.
100. Sirtori CR, Azarnoff DL, Shoeman DW: Dissociation of the metabolic and cardiovascular effects of the beta-adrenergic blocker practolol. Pharmaceut Res Commun 4:123, 1972.
101. Johnson BF: The emerging problem of plasma lipid changes during antihypertensive therapy. J Cardiovasc Pharmacol 4 (Suppl 2):213s, 1982.
102. Leren P, Helgeland A, Holme I, et al: Effect of propranolol and prazosin on blood lipids. The Oslo Study. Lancet 2:4, 1980.
103. Shulman RS, Herbert PN, Capone RJ, et al: Effects of propranolol on blood lipids and lipoproteins in myocardial infarction. Circulation 67 (Suppl 1):19, 1983.
104. Leren P, Eide I, Foss OP: Antihypertensive drugs and blood lipids: The Oslo Study. Br J Clin Pharmac 13:441s, 1982.
105. Frishman WH, Michelson EL, Johnson BF, Poland MP: Multiclinic comparison of labetalol to metoprolol in treatment of mild-to-moderate systemic hypertension. Am J Med 75(4A):54, 1983.
106. Hanley DA, Takatsuki K, Birnbaumer ME, et al: In vitro perfusion for the study of parathyroid hormone secretion: Effects of extracellular calcium concentration and beta-adrenergic regulation on bovine parathyroid hormone secretion in vitro. Calcif Tiss Int 32:19, 1980.
107. Fischer JA, Blum JW, Binswanger U: Acute parathyroid response to epinephrine in vivo. J Clin Invest 52:2434, 1973.
108. Caro JF, Castro JH, Glennon JA: Effect of long-term propranolol administration on parathyroid hormone and calcium concentration in primary hyperthyroidism. Ann Intern Med 9:740, 1979.
109. Frishman WH, Klein N, Charlap S, et al: Comparative effects of verapamil and propranolol on parathyroid hormone and serum calcium concentrations. In Packer M, Frishman WH (eds), Calcium Channel Antagonists in Cardiovascular Disease. Norwalk, Appleton-Century-Crofts, 1983, p 343.
110. Cohn RJ, Epstein SE, Cohen LS, Dennis LH: Alterations of fibrinolysis and blood coagulation induced by exercise and the role of beta-adrenergic blockade. Lancet 2:1264, 1968.
111. Ingram GIC, Vaughan Jones R: The rise in clotting factor 8 induced in man by adrenaline. Effect of alpha- and beta-blockers. Physiol 187:447, 1966.
112. Gader AMA, da Costa J, Cash JD: The effect of propranolol, alprenolol

and practolol on the fibrinolytic and factor 8 responses to adrenaline and salbutamol in man. Thromb Res 2:9, 1973.

113. Steele PP, Weily HS, Davies H, Genton E: Platelet function in coronary artery disease. Circulation 48:1194, 1973.

114. Harker LA, Slichter S: Platelet and fibrinogen consumption in man. N Engl J Med 287:999, 1972.

115. Frishman WH, Weksler B, Christodoulou JP, et al: Reversal of abnormal platelet aggregability and change in exercise tolerance in patients with angina pectoris following oral propranolol. Circulation 50:887, 1974.

116. Weksler BB, Gillick M, Pink J: Effect of propranolol on platelet function. Blood 49:185, 1977.

117. Campbell WB, Callahan KS, Johnson AR, Graham RM: Anti-platelet activity of beta-adrenergic antagonists: inhibition of thrombaxane synthesis and platelet aggregation in patients receiving long-term propranolol treatment. Lancet 2:1382, 1981.

118. Rubegni M, Provedi D, Bellini PG, et al: Propranolol and platelet aggregation. Circulation 52:964, 1975.

119. Frishman WH, Christodoulou J, Weksler B, et al: Abrupt propranolol withdrawal in angina pectoris. Effects on platelet aggregation and exercise tolerance. Am Heart J 95:169, 1978.

120. Frishman W, Weksler BB: Effects of beta-adrenoceptor blocking agents on platelet function in normal subjects and patients with angina pectoris, in Roskamm DH, Graefe K-H (eds), Advances in β-Blocker Therapy. Proceedings of an International Symposium. Amsterdam, Excerpta Medica, pp 164–190.

CHAPTER 4

Comparative Clinical Experiences and New Therapeutic Applications

William H. Frishman, Jeffrey Bernstein, Deborah Aronson, and Benjamin Kirschenbaum

β-Blockers have been available for 20 years in clinical practice, but the list of their recognized and potential indications continues to grow.[1,2] In addition to angina pectoris, for which they were originally intended, prominent cardiovascular applications of β-blockers include arrhythmias, hypertension, myocardial infarction, hypertrophic cardiomyopathy, dissecting aneurysm, tetralogy of Fallot, and mitral valve prolapse (Table 1).[1,2] Noncardiovascular applications include migraine headache prophylaxis, open-angle glaucoma, thyrotoxicosis, some anxiety states, essential tremor, and gastrointestinal hemorrhage (Table 2).[1,2] No other class of synthetic compounds has been put to so many different clinical uses.

What accounts for this versatility? As discussed in Chapter 3, there are still many unanswered questions regarding how β-blockers influence disease, despite a host of studies delineating their pharmacologic properties and physiologic effects. Yet innumerable observations confirming the clinical efficacy of β-blockers in a wide variety of pathologic states support the concept that the sympathetic nervous system is critically important in health and disease.

There have been thousands of reports of clinical trials in tens of thousands of patients, examining the safety and efficacy of different β-

Adapted in part from Clinical Essays on the Heart. New York: McGraw-Hill, vol II, pp 25–63, with permission.

TABLE 1. REPORTED CARDIOVASCULAR INDICATIONS FOR β-ADRENOCEPTOR BLOCKING DRUGS[1,2]

1. Hypertension[187,275]
2. Angina Pectoris[95,96]
3. Supraventricular Arrhythmias[334]
4. Ventricular Arrhythmias[347]
5. Reducing the risk of mortality and reinfarction in survivors of acute myocardial infarction[302–304]
6. Hyperacute phase of myocardial infarction[302,317]
7. Dissection of the aorta[5,6]
8. Hypertrophic cardiomyopathy[358]
9. Digitalis intoxication[7]
10. Mitral valve prolapse[366]
11. "QT interval" prolongation syndrome[8]
12. Tetralogy of Fallot[9]
13. Mitral stenosis[10,11]
14. Congestive cardiomyopathy[12]
15. Fetal tachycardia[13]
16. Neurocirculatory asthenia[14]
17. Pulmonary stenosis and atresia[15,16]
18. Erythromelalgia[17]
19. Hypertensive response with endotracheal intubation[18]
20. Hypertensive response with human coitus[19]

blockers. However, no two studies were performed under the same conditions, or with the same experimental design, and the ability to compare results is often difficult. Additionally, because so many physiologic and metabolic variables are affected by the β-adrenergic system, and, hence, its blockade, the exact nature of the β-blocking effect in different clinical entities is nearly impossible to define precisely. However, an overall impression of these agents in clinical disease can be derived from the results of clinical trials, and in this chapter the results from many of these studies in different pathophysiologic states are summarized. Some of the newer applications and potential uses for β-blockers are also discussed.

ANGINA PECTORIS

The therapeutic benefit of β-blockade in angina pectoris is now established beyond question. There are many double-blind studies with various protocol designs demonstrating a significant reduction in the fre-

**TABLE 2. REPORTED NONCARDIOVASCULAR INDICATIONS FOR
β-ADRENOCEPTOR BLOCKING DRUGS[1,2]**

Neuropsychiatric	Other
1. Migraine[395]	18. Glaucoma[401,420]
2. Parkinson's disease[20]	19. Tetanus[33]
3. Essential tremor[403]	20. Acne vulgaris[34]
4. Anxiety[407]	21. Acute prophyria[35]
5. "Exam nerves"[21]	22. Endotoxin shock[36]
6. Alcohol withdrawal (delirium) tremens)[22]	23. Hemorrhagic shock[37]
7. Narcotic withdrawal[23]	24. Ureteral colic[38]
8. Cocaine toxicity[24]	25. Urinary incontinence[39]
9. LSD-induced anxiety states[25]	26. Phantom limb[40]
10. Schizophrenia[409,410]	27. Bile acid-induced diarrhea[41]
11. Lithium-induced tremor[26]	28. Spastic colon[42]
12. Narcolepsy[27]	29. Dysfunctional labor[43]
Endocrine	30. Hypothermia and hypoxia[44]
13. Thyrotoxicosis[373,385]	31. Disseminated intravascular coagulation[45]
14. Hyperparathyroidism[28,29]	32. Oleander poisoning[46]
15. Insulinoma[30]	33. Portal hypertension[423]
16. Unstable juvenile diabetes mellitus[31]	34. Gastrointestinal bleeding[424]
17. Renal osteodystrophy[32]	

quency of anginal attacks and an improvement in exercise tolerance.[3] Observed improvement is dose-related, and dosage must be titrated for each individual patient. Although the drugs were studied using different trial designs, all the various β-blocker compounds, despite their differing pharmacologic characteristics and activities, appear to have similar effects in the relief of effort angina.[3,4,47]

It should be borne in mind, however, that variations in study designs, run-in periods, fixed versus variable dosage schedules, duration of assessment, acute versus chronic administration, and other variables may be responsible for some differences in the results obtained.

Acebutolol

Acebutolol (Sectral) is a β_1-selective blocker with weak intrinsic sympathomimetic and membrane-stabilizing activities. The drug is not approved for clinical use in the United States.

Trials Versus Placebo. Fiserova et al. demonstrated a considerable reduction in anginal attacks and increased exercise tolerance in a study involving 14 patients who received a fixed daily dose of acebutolol (600 mg daily) for a 6-week period.[48]

Twenty-three patients with documented coronary artery disease were placed in a double-blind study by Rod et al.[49] to assess the antianginal efficacy of acebutolol (200 mg three times daily and 400 mg three times daily). Both dosages were found to be therapeutically effective. With the larger daily dose (1200 mg), heart rate decreased further compared to the lower dose, and there was a greater improvement in exercise tolerance.

Substantial support for the efficacy of acebutolol in angina pectoris is provided in a multicentric study by DiBianco et al.,[50] where 44 patients with chronic stable angina were entered in a double-blind, placebo-controlled, randomized, crossover trial. Compared to placebo, acebutolol was found to significantly reduce spontaneous anginal frequency, decrease nitroglycerin consumption, and increase exercise capacity.

Further support for the efficacy of acebutolol was provided from the results of a double-blind crossover trial by Steele and Gold in which 20 men with angiographically documented coronary artery disease were treated with acebutolol (400 mg three times daily in 19 patients; 300 mg three times daily in one patient).[51] Their findings demonstrated that acebutolol increases exercise performance and decreases the occurrence of angina symptoms when compared to placebo treatment in male patients with coronary artery disease.

Comparative Studies. A 28-week, multicenter, placebo-controlled, randomized, double-blind, crossover study comparing the antianginal efficacy of acebutolol versus propranolol in 46 male patients was conducted by DiBianco et al.[52] Dosages of acebutolol and propranolol were 1650 ± 375 mg/day and 219 ± 50 mg/day, respectively. When compared to placebo, acebutolol produced a greater reduction in mean systolic and diastolic blood pressures, and a smaller reduction in resting heart rate than propranolol. This difference between β-blockers may relate to the partial agonist property of acebutolol. Both agents produced a similar improvement in exercise duration and exercise work. Anginal frequency and nitroglycerin use were decreased significantly by both acebutolol and propranolol.

DePonti et al. investigated the comparative antianginal efficacies of nifedipine alone, acebutolol alone and nifedipine plus acebutolol in a randomized, double-blind, placebo-controlled study of 16 patients with documented coronary artery disease.[53] When used alone, both agents improved exercise tolerance. At the doses used, nifedipine was found to be more efficacious than acebutolol. The drug combination was more effective than any of the single-drug treatments.

Atenolol

Atenolol (Tenormin) has relative β_1-selectivity and no intrinsic sympathomimetic activity or membrane-stabilizing activity. It is not approved for use in angina pectoris in the United States.

Open Studies. Daltro and Lion conducted an open study in which ten chronic angina patients were treated with a single daily dose of atenolol 100 mg for a minimum period of 30 days.[54] Atenolol, was effective in reducing anginal frequency, nitroglycerin consumption, heart rate, systolic blood pressure, ECG ST-segment deviations, and it prolonged exercise time. It also prolonged exercise time. Langbehn et al. treated 125 patients with coronary artery disease and previous myocardial infarction with 50 mg of atenolol twice daily for 4 weeks.[55] In their study, the number and severity of anginal attacks were also reduced.

The comparative efficacies of atenolol at three dose levels (100 mg once daily, 100 mg twice daily, and 200 mg once daily) were investigated by Backman et al.[56] Five patients were given atenolol at each dose level for a period of 4 weeks. The three doses were determined to be equally effective in reducing resting and exercise heart rates and in increasing maximum work time.

Investigations Versus Placebo. In a trial of 11 patients with severe angina, Roy et al. found that atenolol, in doses of 50, 100, and 200 mg administered twice daily, produced a significant reduction in anginal attacks and nitroglycerin consumption when compared to placebo.[57] A dose–response relationship was also suggested by their results. There was an insignificant improvement in exercise tolerance with the drug. The efficacy of atenolol as compared to placebo was further demonstrated in a randomized, double-blind investigation of 19 patients by Erikssen et al.[58] In this study, doses of 50 mg twice daily and 100 mg twice daily caused significant drops in resting heart rate, exercise heart rate, blood pressure, and double-product in all patients. A 44 percent increase in bicycle exercise performance was observed at the different dose levels. Van der Vijgh et al. evaluated the therapeutic effectiveness of a single daily oral dose of atenolol 100 mg and 200 mg in a double-blind, crossover, randomized study of ten patients.[59] Compared to placebo, significant reductions in resting and exercise heart rates were observed with both doses. Maximal effects were obtained 3 to 6 hours after administration of the dose, with persistent effects throughout the 24-hour period following the dose. Reductions in systolic and diastolic blood pressure, an attenuation of ST-segment changes, a decrease in anginal frequency, and an improvement in exercise tolerance were reported with both doses. Jackson et al., in a definitive, single-blind dose-ranging trial of ten patients, reported that once daily dosing with 25, 50, 100, and 200 mg of atenolol significantly decreased the frequency of anginal attacks and nitroglycerin consumption.[60] The best results were obtained with the 100- and 200-mg doses. The 24-hour ambulatory electrocardiographic recordings showed a decrease in mean hourly heart rate throughout the dosing period, with preservation of diurnal variation. Maximal, symptom-limited, treadmill exercise tests performed 3 hours after drug ingestion showed significant increases in exercise time and a decrease in double-product and heart rate for all doses, especially with 100 and 200 mg. Exercise time 24 hours after drug ingestion was still improved with a decrease in maximum heart rate and double-product, the doses of 100 and 200 mg again being the most effective. Atenolol serum levels correlated with the percent reduction in exercise heart rate and increased exercise time. These investigators concluded that the 100 mg once daily dose of atenolol was preferable for relief of angina and for increasing exercise tolerance.

The long-term efficacy of once daily atenolol was investigated by Schwartz et al. in a placebo-controlled, single-blind, dose-finding trial involving nine patients with chronic stable exercise-induced angina.[61] Two-week drug dosing periods using 25, 50, 100, and 200 mg of oral atenolol were followed by daily treatments of 100 or 200 mg for a period of 1 year. Throughout the study, angina frequency and nitroglycerin use were decreased compared to placebo baseline. The 24-hour ambulatory electrocardiographic monitor studies and treadmill exercise tests demonstrated a sustained heart rate decrease. Exercise duration until angina onset was prolonged during all periods of atenolol administration. Maximal improvement in exercise tolerance and angina relief was not observed until after 3 months of atenolol therapy, despite stable serum drug concentrations.

Comparative Studies. In a double-blind, randomized comparison trial of oral atenolol and oral propranolol, Jackson et al. demonstrated that twice daily doses of 25, 50, and 100 mg of atenolol were as effective as propranolol 80 mg three times daily.[62] All dose levels were found to decrease anginal attacks, consumption of nitroglycerin, resting and exercise heart rate, resting and exercise systolic blood pressure, and to prolong exercise duration. Of the 14 patients, 9 continued in a trial comparing the effects of atenolol 200 mg once daily versus 100 mg twice daily. Both regimens were found to be equally effective in reducing anginal attacks, nitroglycerin consumption, systolic blood pressure, and heart rate. Ambulatory electrocardiographic monitoring demonstrated that atenolol consistently reduced heart rate throughout the 24-hour period whether given once or twice daily.

In a double-blind crossover study, Haghfelt et al. demonstrated that equipotent doses of atenolol and propranolol comparably decreased the frequency of anginal attacks and improved working capacity.[63] A greater reduction in the exercise double-product was noted with atenolol. The employment of a once-daily 100 mg dose of atenolol produced similar antianginal effects as propranolol used in doses up to 320 mg daily.

Labetalol

Labetalol (Trandate, Normodyne) is a nonselective β-blocker with α-blocking direct vasodilatory and intrinsic sympathomimetic activities. The drug has no membrane-stabilizing action. Labetalol is not approved for treatment of angina pectoris in the United States. The effects of this drug in patients with angina pectoris and hypertension are described in Chapter 11.

Metoprolol

Metoprolol (Betaloc, Lopressor), has relative β_1-selectivity and no intrinsic sympathomimetic or membrane activity. It is not approved for clinical use in angina in the United States.

Dose-Finding Trial. Uusitalo et al. assessed the antianginal efficacy of metoprolol using single oral doses of 50, 100, and 200 mg in a dose-finding trial involving 23 patients.[64] The effects were assessed 1½ hours following ingestion of the dose. Resting systolic blood pressures were similar with all three doses but resting heart rates were lower with 200 mg than with 50 mg. The mean exercise heart rate at the highest comparable work load was lowest with the 200-mg dose, followed by the 100- and 50-mg doses. Systolic blood pressure during exercise did not differ significantly. The total work capacity and the time until the onset of anginal pain was significantly greater with metoprolol 200 mg than with the other two dosage regimens.

Comparative Studies. Using equipotent doses of metoprolol and propranolol, Comerford and Besterman compared the antianginal effects of the drugs in a double-blind, crossover study in 14 patients, with long-term follow-up for 72 weeks.[65] Metoprolol was noted to cause a greater increase in total work and exercise tolerance to ST-segment depression than propranolol. Borer et al. performed a comparative, crossover, placebo-controlled study using equipotent doses of metoprolol (150 and 300 mg daily) and propranolol (120 and 240 mg daily) in 10 patients with angina pectoris.[66] A comparable reduction in anginal frequency and nitroglycerin consumption was observed and an improvement in total work performance was demonstrated with both agents. Resting and exercise heart rates were decreased by both metoprolol and propranolol. Conversely, arterial pressure was unchanged at rest but was decreased with exercise. The maximum dose of both medications was preferred by most patients. Finally, Frick and Luurila performed a double-blind investigation in 20 patients to compare equipment doses of metoprolol (450 mg/day) and propranolol (360 mg/day) with respect to their antianginal effects.[67] Both agents were equally effective in improving exercise tolerance and relieving angina pectoris.

In a randomized, double-blind, crossover, placebo-controlled trial in 16 patients, Thadani et al. compared propranolol, practolol, oxprenolol, metoprolol, and tolamolol with respect to their antianginal effects.[68] All five agents caused a significant improvement in exercise tolerance, a reduction in ST-segment depression, resting heart rate, blood pressure, and double-product. The optimal dose for metoprolol was 200 mg/day.

Thadani et al. conducted a follow-up double-blind, placebo-controlled, randomized, crossover investigation to assess the comparative antianginal effect of these five agents on a long-term basis.[69] Twenty-three patients participated in this 6-month study. Equipotent doses of practolol (100 mg), oxprenolol (40 mg), propranolol (40 mg), metoprolol (50 mg), and tolamolol (50 mg) were provided for the patients on a twice daily basis. Anginal frequency and nitroglycerin consumption were comparably reduced by all five drugs in comparison to placebo, and exercise tolerance was improved. In addition, significant reductions in ST-segment depression, exercising heart rate, systolic blood pressure, and double-product were noted with each of the five drugs—effects markedly different from those obtained with placebo. The investigators concluded that all five drugs were equally effective antianginal agents with sustained use.

Twenty patients participated in a placebo-controlled, double-blind, crossover study comparing the antianginal efficacy of the calcium-entry blocker verapamil (360 mg/day) and metoprolol (200 mg twice daily).[70] Subjective parameters (mean daily rate of anginal episodes and nitroglycerin consumption) decreased with both agents. Although both verapamil and metoprolol significantly increased exercise capacity, the former had a significantly greater effect. On the other hand, the rest and exercise double-products were reduced only by metoprolol.

Nadolol

Nadolol (Corgard) is a long-acting nonselective β-blocker that lacks intrinsic sympathomimetic activity and membrane-stabilizing activity. It is approved for once daily use in the treatment of angina pectoris.

Trials Versus Placebo. Multiple studies performed in patients with stable angina have demonstrated the once daily use of nadolol to be superior to placebo for reducing the frequency of anginal attacks, for decreasing nitroglycerin consumption, and for increasing the capability for exercise.[71] Shapiro et al. confirmed these results with nadolol in a double-blind, randomized, placebo-controlled study involving 37 patients.[72] Compared to placebo, the drug (in a fixed dose of 240 mg once daily) significantly decreased the number of angina attacks, nitroglycerin consumption, resting and peak heart rates, and peak rate–pressure products 24 hours postdose; exercise time and work were significantly prolonged.

Comparative Trials. Multiple studies have been conducted to assess the relative efficacies of nadolol used once daily and propranolol used four times a day.[71] Ling and Groel showed that nadolol given once daily is as effective an antianginal agent as propranolol four times a day.[73] Prager, in a trial involving 29 patients comparing nadolol once daily to propranolol four times daily, noted that both drugs had similar effects regarding the number of anginal attacks and nitroglycerin consumed.[74] These investigators observed, however, that nadolol produced a better performance in exercise time. Conversely, Furberg et al. observed that optimal daily dosages of nadolol (100 mg) and propranolol (112 mg) were equally effective in prolonging exercise time in patients with angina.[75] These investigators also noted the continued antianginal effectiveness of nadolol when used on a long-term basis (23 months).

In a more extensive study, Jones and Mir compared the antianginal efficacies of conventional propranolol, long-acting propranolol, sustained-release oxprenolol, and nadolol in a randomized, double-blind, crossover trial in 12 patients.[76] A fixed dose regimen of 160 mg once daily was used for all four medications. Observations were made 24 hours following a single 160-mg dose. All the drugs were found to cause a reduction in anginal attack rate and nitroglycerin use. Exercise tolerance was prolonged more by propranolol, long-acting propranolol, and nadolol than with sustained-release oxprenolol. Subjectively, patients preferred nadolol and long-acting propranolol over the other two preparations.

Oxprenolol

Oxprenolol (Trasicor, Iset) is nonselective β-blocker with membrane-stabilizing and intrinsic sympathomimetic activities. It is not approved for clinical use in the United States.

Open Trials. In a simple, noncomparative study assessing the antianginal efficacy of oxprenolol in general practice, Watt found complete or substantial relief of symptoms in 80 percent of the patients studied.[77] Monitored release studies were performed in Great Britain by Burley to assess the antianginal efficacy of oxprenolol in 5492 patients with angina of effort.[78] Of the patients, 5238 were followed in general practice. Of these, 4403 were treated with oxprenolol alone. Oxprenolol was added to long-acting nitrates in the remaining patients. The favorable response rate was found to be 85 to 90 percent, with the optimal oxprenolol dose being 120 to 200 mg/day.

Studies Versus Placebo. Using a fixed dosage regimen (80 mg three times daily) of oxprenolol in 13 patients with angina, Sandler and Pistevos failed to show a significant beneficial effect of the drug on angina or exercise performance.[79] Bianchi et al., using a fixed dose of oxprenolol, 40 mg four times per day in 62 patients, demonstrated a decrease in frequency of angina attacks and in nitroglycerin consumption.[80] Both these studies used 2-week assessment periods and lacked appropriate run-in periods (the run-in period prior to a trial provides an opportunity for patients to become familiar with the experimental protocol and for adjustment of drug dosage). Wilson et al., performing a 2-week trial using a variable dose schedule (60 to 400 mg oxprenolol per day) that was preceded by a run-in period, demonstrated a significant antianginal benefit in oxprenolol in 17 of 18 patients.[81] These results were confirmed in a double-blind, placebo-controlled study performed by Taylor and Thadani.[82] A single oral dose of 160 mg was effective in improving exercise tolerance, in attenuating exercise tachycardia and decreasing systolic blood pressure. Maximal effects were noted 1-hour postdose and declined slowly over 8 hours.

Forrest utilized a placebo-controlled, randomized, double-blind design to assess the comparative antianginal efficicies of oxprenolol (40 mg) and practolol (100 mg).[83] Both agents were equally effective in decreasing the frequency of anginal attacks and nitroglycerin consumption.

Other studies comparing oxprenolol with other β-blockers were described earlier in this chapter.[68,69]

Trials with Sustained-Release Oxprenolol. Forrest conducted a study in which 102 patients were treated in an open-protocol study using once daily sustained-release oxprenolol (160 mg per tablet).[83,84] Eighty-eight patients were successfully managed on once daily oxprenolol, and 70 percent achieved significant benefit with a single morning dose of 160 mg. The mean number of anginal attacks and mean nitroglycerin consumption were both reduced. Majid et al. compared the antianginal efficacy of sustained-release oxprenolol (160 mg/day) and conventional propranolol (40 mg three times daily) in a double-blind, randomized, placebo-controlled, crossover study of 18 patients.[85] Relative to placebo values, both agents comparably reduced the frequency and severity of anginal attacks, prolonged exercise tolerance, and decreased the exercise heart rate.

More recently Olowoyeye et al. compared sustained-release oxprenolol (160 mg/day) to propranolol (40 mg four times daily).[86] Twenty-three patients participated in this randomized, double-blind, crossover trial. The overall antianginal efficacy of the two drugs did not differ significantly. Resting heart rate was significantly higher 7½ and 24 hours after a propranolol dose. Exercise tolerance 24 hours after oxprenolol was significantly less than 7½ hours after oxprenolol and less than 4 and 12 hours after propranolol.

Pindolol

Pindolol (Visken) is a nonselective β-blocker with intrinsic sympathomimetic activity and no membrane stabilizing effect or β_1-selectivity. Pindolol is not approved for angina pectoris in the United States.

Trials Versus Placebo. Leary and Asmal assessed the antianginal efficacy of 15 to 25 mg of pindolol daily in 15 patients with chronic angina and coexistent moderate hypertension.[87] The investigators used a single-blind, randomized design. In this study, pindolol was found to be effective in decreasing supine and erect blood pressure, the frequency of anginal episodes, and nitroglycerin consumption.

In a randomized, double-blind, crossover study of 20 patients, Storstein investigated the effects of IV (0.4 mg) pindolol and oral pindolol (5 mg three times daily) on exercise tolerance and electrocardiographic ST-segment changes.[88] Pindolol significantly decreased heart rate at rest and during exercise. The time intervals before the appearance of ST-segment depression were significantly increased, and exercise tolerance was enhanced.

In two recent studies, pindolol was demonstrated to have, at best, a modest beneficial effect in patients with angina pectoris.[89,90] Each of these trials employed a double-blind, crossover protocol design and studied 12 patients with chronic stable angina and documented coronary artery disease. Dwyer et al. found that pindolol (15 and 30 mg/day) slightly decreased the number of anginal episodes and nitroglycerin tablets consumed while showing evidence of β-blockade during exercise.[89] However, they could not demonstrate any effect on exercise endurance with either dose. Harston and Friesinger demonstrated that a dosage of 5 mg four times daily of pindolol did not significantly reduce nitroglycerin consumption and anginal episodes.[90] Also, treadmill exercise tolerance and ST-segment depression with exercise were not significantly altered. However, there was a statistically significant reduction in myocardial oxygen demand as measured by the double-product of blood pressure and heart rate during exercise. The investigators concluded that pindolol significantly reduced myocardial oxygen demands, but clinical ischemia was not significantly reduced. They suggested possible mechanisms to explain the disparity between reduction in estimated myocardial oxygen demand (double-product) and objective improvement in ischemia.[91] These include coronary spasm and altered regional flow resulting from β-blockade. Alternative explanations proposed were the relatively small fixed dose of pindolol and the small number of patients studied in their trial.[90,91]

Comparative Trials. Frishman et al., in a large, placebo-controlled clinical study of 41 patients with classical angina pectoris, observed that pindolol (10 to 40 mg/day in four divided doses) reduced angina attacks and nitroglycerin consumption and increased exercise tolerance at least as effectively as propranolol (40 to 160 mg/day in four divided doses).[4,92] Both drugs effectively blunted increments in blood pressure and heart rate with exercise. However, unlike propranolol, pindolol with partial agonist activity did not affect the resting heart rate. The investigators concluded that although β-blocking drugs are effective in patients with angina pectoris of effort, in patients with angina pectoris at rest or with low heart rates, propranolol and other β-blockers without partial agonist activity would probably have a distinct advantage over pindolol.

In a single-blind, randomized, parallel study protocol, Cocco et al. assessed the comparative antianginal efficacies of pindolol (10 mg three times daily) and nifedipine (10 mg three times daily) in 42 patients with stable angina.[93,94] Pindolol and nifedipine were found to cause equal reductions in angina attacks and nitroglycerin consumption while improving exercise tolerance. Exercise heart rate was slightly decreased with pindolol and slightly increased with nifedipine. Nifedipine was found to be more effective in relieving asymptomatic myocardial ischemia than pindolol.

Propranolol

Propranolol (Inderal, Inderal-LA) is a nonselective β-blocker with membrane-stabilizing activity and no intrinsic sympathomimetric activity. There have been many clinical trials with propranolol using different daily dosages that have demonstrated its clinical effectiveness in angina.[95,96] Propranolol is approved for clinical use in angina in the United States as a conventional tablet and as a long-acting sustained-release capsule.

Trials Versus Placebo. A dose-dependent reduction of anginal attacks with propranolol was well demonstrated in an early study by Prichard and Gillam.[97] Sixteen patients were administered four different dose levels of propranolol and placebo in a double-blind fashion. The average doses ranged from 0 (placebo) to 417 mg/day. As the dosage increased, there was a progressive decrease in the number of anginal attacks and in the amount of nitroglycerin used, giving a linear dose-response curve, whose slope did not flatten even at the 417-mg dosage level (suggesting that maximum effect had not yet been obtained).

Alderman et al. conducted a double-blind, placebo-controlled, randomized, crossover study in 17 patients assessing the comparative efficacy of doses of 80, 160, and 320 mg of propranolol.[98] Significant decreases in the frequency of anginal episodes and nitroglycerin consumption were noted with 160 and 320 mg. A significant improvement in exercise tolerance was only achieved with 320 mg. Resting heart rate was significantly decreased by all three doses. Although standing systolic blood pressure was significantly decreased by all three doses, standing diastolic blood pressure and supine diastolic and systolic blood pressures were not. The investigators also confirmed the prominent linear relationship between clinical response and the log of the propranolol dosage that had been noted previously by Prichard and Gillam.[97]

Thadani and Parker assessed the comparative duration of effect of single oral doses of 80 and 160 mg of propranolol during acute and sustained therapy in nine patients.[99,100] Treadmill walking time to onset of angina, total duration of exercise, and total external work performed were significantly increased 1, 8, and 12 hours postdose with both acute and sustained therapy. Similar effects were observed with 80 and 160 mg. The improvement in exercise tolerance was accompanied by a significant decrease in the magnitude of ST-segment depression. Rest and exercise heart rates, systolic blood pressure, and double-product were significantly reduced with propranolol. These effects were noted 12 and 24 hours postdose.

In a more recent trial involving 25 patients, Thadani and Parker investigated the comparative efficacies of propranolol given twice a day or four times a day.[101] The same total daily dose of 160 or 320 mg was administered with each dosing regimen. A double-blind, crossover, randomized design was used in this trial. Similar results were obtained in the frequency of anginal episodes, prolongation of exercise time, reduction in ST-segment depression, and decrease in heart rate, systolic blood pressure, and double-product with both dosage regimens. The investigators concluded that for the treatment of stable angina, propranolol given twice daily is as effective as the same dose given four times daily.

Trials with Sustained-Release Propranolol. The comparative antianginal efficacies of standard formulation propranolol (40 mg four times daily) and sustained-release propranolol (160 mg once daily) was assessed in a double-blind, placebo-controlled, crossover, randomized trial in eight patients.[102] The frequencies of anginal episodes and nitroglycerin consumption were decreased by both formulations. The peak heart rate increment was reduced by both long-acting and standard propranolol, as was the maximal double-product and the degree of ST-segment depression.

The equivalent antianginal efficacy of long-acting propranolol (160 mg once daily) and standard propranolol (40 mg four times daily) was further supported in a trial by Parker et al.[103] Twenty patients participated in this double-blind, crossover, placebo-controlled, randomized study. A similar reduction in anginal episodes and nitroglycerin consumption was observed with both formulations. Resting values for heart rate, systolic blood pressure, and rate–pressure product were similar when determined 25.4 hours after a dose of long-acting propranolol and 10.7 hours after standard propranolol. When the patients exercised at these times, patients on long-acting propranolol and standard propranolol had similar walking times to the onset of angina and to the development of moderate angina. The values for heart rate, systolic blood pressure, and rate–pressure product were similar at rest and during exercise with these two treatment programs. Sustained-release propranolol has recently received FDA approval for once daily use in patients with angina pectoris.

Comparative Studies. See previous acebutolol, atenolol, metoprolol, nadolol, oxprenolol, and pindolol sections.

Eleven patients participated in a short-term, single-blind, randomized, crossover trial by Leon et al. to assess the comparative antianginal efficacies of propranolol (160 to 320 mg/day), verapamil (480 mg/day), and a combination of these two drugs (propranolol optimal dose, verapamil 160 to 480 mg).[104] Each of the regimens significantly increased exercise time, with propranolol having the least effect and the combination the greatest.

The comparative efficacies of propranolol and verapamil were further investigated by Johnson et al. in a double-blind, randomized, placebo-controlled, crossover study involving 18 patients.[105] Doses of propranolol, 40 and 80 mg every 6 hours, and verapamil, 80 and 120 mg every 6 hours, were administered to the participants. Low- and high-dose propranolol, as well as high-dose verapamil, significantly reduced the frequency of angina episodes, whereas nitroglycerin consumption was only significantly reduced by high-dose verapamil. Episodes of ST-segment deviations noted on 24-hour ambulatory ECG monitoring were decreased only with high-dose verapamil. Propranolol alone produced a significant reduction in resting heart rate. Peak heart rate with exercise was significantly blunted with both agents, but significantly more with propranolol. Verapamil significantly decreased resting systolic blood pressure, while propranolol significantly reduced exercise systolic blood pressure. Both agents produced a significant and comparable reduction in exercise-induced ST-segment deviation.

In addition, a study conducted by Subramanian et al.[106] compared the antianginal effects of propranolol and verapamil used alone and as combination therapy. Twenty-two patients participated in this double-blind, placebo-controlled, crossover study (verapamil 360 mg/day; propranolol 240 mg/day; and verapamil 360 mg/day plus propranolol 120 mg/day). A significant increase in exercise time was observed with all three regimens. The combination had a significantly greater effect than verapamil alone, which in turn was significantly better than propranolol.

In another double-blind, randomized, crossover trial, Frishman et al. further demonstrated the comparable effectiveness of verapamil and propranolol in patients with stable angina.[107]

Lynch et al. conducted a double-blind, placebo-controlled, randomized, crossover study to assess the comparative antianginal efficacies of propranolol (240 and 480 mg/day), nifedipine (30 and 60 mg/day), and a combination of both drugs.[108] The incidence of anginal pain and nitroglycerin consumption was significantly decreased with both drugs when compared with placebo, but propranolol produced significantly greater reductions than nifedipine for both clinical end points. Although there was no difference in antianginal efficacy with the two propranolol doses, the higher dose of nifedipine produced a significantly greater reduction in angina attack frequency and nitroglycerin consumption than did the lower dose. When the higher doses of these two drugs were combined, an additional decrease in anginal frequency and nitroglycerin consumption was observed. In addition, the number of episodes of ST-segment depression observed on an ambulatory 24-hour Holter electrocardiogram significantly decreased from placebo baseline with both agents used alone, with a significantly greater effect noted with combination therapy.

In a double-blind, placebo-controlled, randomized, crossover trial, Kenmure and Scruton further assessed the comparative efficacies of nifedipine (10 mg three times daily), propranolol (80 mg three times daily), and a combination (nifedipine 10 mg three times daily and propranolol 40 mg three times daily).[109] Twenty-one patients participated in the study. Both agents used alone significantly reduced the frequency of anginal episodes, with propranolol having a greater effect (not statistically significant) than nifedipine. The drug combination had the greatest effect. Comparable results were seen regarding nitroglycerin consumption. Nifedipine produced no change in heart rate but did cause a significant fall in systolic and diastolic blood pressures. Propranolol caused a significant decrease in both heart rate and blood pressure. The combination produced a lesser reduction in heart rate than with propranolol alone, but a greater fall in both systolic and diastolic blood pressures.

These results were supported by a double-blind, placebo-controlled, randomized, crossover trial conducted by Dargie et al.[110] Sixteen patients participated in this study, which utilized 30 and 60 mg/day of nifedipine and 240 and 280 mg/day of propranolol. The frequency of angina and consumption of nitroglycerin tablets were significantly decreased by all active treatments. The effect of propranolol was slightly greater than that of nifedipine. Although the high dose of propranolol provided no additional benefit, nifedipine at 60 mg/day was significantly more effective than nifedipine at 30 mg/day. An additional reduction in both angina and nitroglycerin consumption was observed with the high-dose combination of propranolol and nifedipine. Both propranolol and nifedipine used alone significantly reduced exercise-induced ECG ST-segment depressions, with the combination producing an additional reduction. The combination and propranolol alone produced a significant and comparable reduction in the double-product. All three treatment regimens significantly reduced the episodes of ST-segment depression assessed on a 24-hour ambulatory ECG monitor with a greater reduction observed with combination treatment. Resting systolic and diastolic blood pressures were decreased with the higher doses of nifedipine and propranolol when used alone and by both doses of the combination. Propranolol and combination therapy significantly decreased exercise systolic blood pressure and the resting heart rate.

In two additional studies, the antianginal efficacy and safety of combined nifedipine–propranolol treatment was confirmed.[111,112]

Sotalol

Sotalol (Betacordone, Sotacor) has no intrinsic sympathomimetic activity, no membrane-stabilizing activity, and no cardioselectivity. Sotalol is not available for clinical use in the United States.

Trials Versus Placebo. In a fixed, multidose level (80, 160, 320, 640, 1,280 mg sotalol per day) trial in nine patients, Toubes et al. demonstrated a significant decrease in the frequency and severity of anginal attacks and a reduction in nitroglycerin consumption at all dose levels.[113] Contrasting results were obtained in a double-blind crossover trial of 15 patients performed by Kentala et al.[114] A fixed daily dose of 160 mg was utilized in this study. Sotalol was observed to significantly decrease resting heart rate and systolic blood pressure, with a significant increase in heart volume. The frequency of anginal attacks and nitroglycerin consumption were not significantly altered; however, a relatively low drug dose was utilized. Sotalol was found to decrease the number and intensity of anginal attacks in a double-blind crossover study of 69 patients conducted by Milei and Fortunato.[115] The antianginal efficacy of the drug was further substantiated by the results of a double-blind, crossover study in 17 patients conducted by Slome, who determined that 320 mg of sotalol (160 mg twice daily) was effective in decreasing the mean number of angina attacks, nitroglycerin consumption, and heart rate at rest and during exercise.[116] This dosage regimen also improved exercise tolerance.

Timolol

Timolol (Blocadren) is a drug that has no β_1-selectivity, intrinsic sympathomimetic activity, or membrane-stabilizing activity. This drug is not approved for use in the United States for the treatment of angina pectoris.

Trials Versus Placebo. Brailovsky, using an average dose of 30 mg of timolol in a large multinational, multicenter trial in 390 patients, found a highly significant reduction in the frequency of anginal attacks and nitroglycerin consumption compared with placebo.[117]

In a 2-day double-blind, randomized, crossover investigation of 16 patients, Villa et al. demonstrated that timolol, compared to placebo, significantly increased exercise duration, decreased resting and exercise double-product, and delayed the onset of ischemic ST-segment depression during exercise.[118]

The beneficial effects of timolol were also demonstrated by Aronow et al. in a double-blind, randomized, crossover study of 23 patients with chronic angina.[119] Utilizing the optimal timolol dose for each patient (10 to 30 mg twice daily), these investigators found that compared to placebo, timolol significantly reduced anginal attack frequency, nitroglycerin consumption, resting and exercise heart rate and blood pressure (systolic and diastolic), and double-product. Timolol also prolonged exercise duration and reduced electrocardiographic manifestations of myocardial ischemia.

In a single-blind, controlled study of 20 stable angina patients, DiSegni et al. assessed the efficacy of timolol in doses of 10 to 30 mg/day.[120] They determined that timolol caused a significant decrease in the number of anginal attacks and amount of nitroglycerin consumption. Significant reductions in resting heart rate and blood pressure and exercising blood pressure were also noted. Work capacity was found to improve significantly.

Aronow et al., in the most recent of these trials, investigated the effect of timolol on exercise duration at 2 and 12 hours after drug ingestion.[121] Doses of 10 to 30 mg of timolol twice daily were used in this double-blind, randomized, crossover study of seven patients. Exercise duration to angina or marked fatigue was prolonged in 100 percent of patients 2 hours after drug ingestion and in 43 percent of patients 12 hours postdose. The mean exercise duration was significantly increased at both testing intervals.

COMBINED USE OF β-BLOCKERS WITH OTHER ANTIANGINAL THERAPIES IN STABLE ANGINA

Nitrates

Combined therapy with nitrates and β-blockers may be more efficacious for treatment of angina pectoris than either drug alone (Table 3).[122] The primary effects of β-blockers are to cause a reduction in both resting heart rate and the heart rate response to exercise. Since nitrates produce a reflex increase in heart rate, owing to a reduction in arterial pressure, concomitant β-blocker therapy will be extremely effective because it will block this reflex heart rate increment. Similarly, the preservation of diastolic coronary flow with a reduced heart rate will also be benefi-

TABLE 3. HEMODYNAMIC EFFECTS OF NITRATES, β-BLOCKERS AND COMBINATION TREATMENT[122]

	Nitrates	β-Blockers	Combination
1. Heart rate	↑ (reflex)	↓	↓ ↔
2. Contractility	↑ (reflex)	↓	↔
3. Wall tension:	↓	↔	↓
a. Systemic blood pressure	↓	↓	↓
b. Left ventricular volume	↓	↑	↔ ↑
4. Coronary resistance	↓	↑ ↔	↓ ↔

cial.[123] In patients with a propensity for myocardial failure who might have a slight increase in heart size with the β-blockers, the nitrates will counteract this tendency by reducing heart size due to its peripheral venodilatory effects. During the administration of nitrates, the reflex increase in contractility that is mediated through the sympathetic nervous system will be checked by the presence of β-blockers. Similarly, the increase in coronary resistance associated with β-blocker administration can be ameliorated by the administration of nitrates.[122]

Calcium-Entry Blockers

Calcium-entry blockers are a new group of antianginal drugs that block transmembrane calcium currents in vascular smooth muscle to cause arterial vasodilation. Some calcium-entry blockers also will slow the heart rate and reduce atrioventricular conduction. Combined therapy with β-adrenergic and calcium-entry blockers can provide substantial clinical benefits for patients with angina pectoris who remain symptomatic with either agent used alone (Table 4).[106,108–110] Because adverse effects can

TABLE 4. HEMODYNAMIC EFFECTS OF CALCIUM-ENTRY BLOCKERS, β-BLOCKERS, AND COMBINATION TREATMENT

	Ca^{2+} Blockers	β-Blockers	Combination
1. Heart rate	↓ ↔ ↑ (reflex)	↓	↓ ↔
2. Contractility	↓ ↔ (reflex)	↓	↓ ↔
3. Wall tension:	↓	↔	↓
a. Systolic blood pressure	↓	↓	↓
b. Left ventricular volume	↓ ↔	↑	↑ ↔
4. Coronary resistance	↓	↑ ↔	↓ ↔

occur, however, patients being considered for such treatment need to be carefully selected and observed.[124]

ANGINA AT REST AND VASOSPASTIC ANGINA

Although β-blockers are effective in the treatment of patients with angina of effort, clinical studies in patients with angina at rest have been based largely on uncontrolled observations and have not been conclusive. The rationale for therapy with β-blockers was based on an approach that considered the pathogenesis of chest pain at rest to be similar to that in patients with exertional symptoms. Recent studies, however, have emphasized that angina pectoris can be caused by multiple mechanisms and that coronary vasospasm is responsible for ischemia in a significant proportion of patients with angina at rest.[125,126] Therefore, drugs such as propranolol and other β-blockers that primarily reduce myocardial oxygen consumption, but fail to exert vasodilating effects on the coronary vasculature, may not be as effective in patients in whom angina is caused by dynamic alterations in coronary luminal diameter.[127,128] Despite their theoretical dangers in rest and vasospastic angina, β-blockers have been successfully used alone and in combination with vasodilating agents in many patients.[129]

β-ADRENOCEPTOR BLOCKER WITHDRAWAL

Following the abrupt cessation of β-blocker therapy after chronic administration, exacerbation of angina pectoris and, in some cases, acute myocardial infarction have been reported (see Chapter 5).[130,131] Two early double-blind randomized trials confirmed the reality of a propranolol withdrawal syndrome.[132,133] The mechanism for the propranolol withdrawal effect is unclear and may be related to the multifactorial actions of the drugs.[134] Reduced exercise tolerance following abrupt withdrawal of chronic propranolol therapy in patients with angina pectoris may be due to loss of sympathetic blockade of cardiovascular function, resulting in an acute increase in myocardial oxygen demands. Our group demonstrated that abrupt propranolol withdrawal can possibly harm some patients with angina pectoris by causing rebound platelet hyperaggregability associated with increased anginal frequency, decreased exercise tolerance, and possible compromise of coronary blood flow.[135]

A "rebound" effect has not been well-defined with the other β-blocking agents. When necessary, it would appear prudent to discontinue β-blocker therapy gradually and cautiously in patients with ischemic heart disease.

HYPERTENSION

There are several points to be noted when evaluating β-blocker trials in patients with hypertension:

1. Patients may vary in their individual dose requirements and rapidity of response. Hence, trials using small (or fixed) doses and short treatment periods may fail to show much effect.
2. In double-blind studies in which placebo follows active therapy, the duration of placebo therapy must be long enough to allow blood pressure to return to pretreatment levels. If this is not done, then the therapeutic benefit of active drug will appear to be modest.
3. The best results of β-blockers in hypertension are achieved when the drugs are used in combination with other antihypertensive agents, especially diuretics.

The β-blockers differ in terms of the presence or absence of intrinsic sympathomimetic activity, membrane-stabilizing effects, β_1-selectivity, α-blocking properties, and relative potencies and durations of action. It is unclear whether these differences have any practical relevance in the clinical treatment of hypertension: all β-blockers to date appear to have blood pressure–lowering effects.

Three points, however, can be made:

1. β-Blocking drugs with intrinsic sympathomimetic activity (partial agonist activity) or α-blocking activity will cause less bradycardia.
2. The presence or absence of membrane-stabilizing effect seems to be irrelevant.
3. If a β-blocker has to be given to a potential asthmatic patient, it is best to use a β_1-selective blocker, one with ISA, or one having α-blocking effects.[3]

Acebutolol

Acebutolol (Sectral) is not approved for the treatment of systemic hypertension.

Acebutolol Versus Diuretics and Combination Treatment. Nadeau compared acebutolol to hydrochlorothiazide in 24 patients with essential hypertension using a double-blind, randomized, crossover study design.[136] The average daily dose of acebutolol was 621 mg, which resulted in a reduction in blood pressure from 151/97 to 140/87 mm Hg, and in heart rate from 73 to 67 beats per minute. The average daily dose of hydrochlorothiazide was 168 mg, which resulted in a comparable reduction in blood pressure of 153/98 to 143/92 mm Hg, with an increase in heart rate from 74 to 77 beats per minute.

In a randomized, double-blind study of 24 patients with hypertension, Franz compared the antihypertensive effects of acebutolol alone to the diuretic combination of hydrochlorothiazide and amiloride. Patients were assessed at rest and with exercise.[137] At rest, both regimens, acebutolol 500 mg and hydrochlorothiazide 50 mg plus amiloride 5 mg, produced similar reductions in blood pressure. However, with exercise, the blood pressure response of the acebutolol-treated group was significantly greater than that seen in the diuretic treatment group. Acebutolol significantly decreased heart rate at rest and during exercise.

Gorkin et al. added acebutolol to diuretics in 15 hypertensive patients who failed to respond to diuretics alone for treatment of their hypertension (hydrochlorothiazide 50 mg, two times daily or chlorthalidone 100 mg/day).[138] Blood pressure, heart rate, and plasma renin activity responses were monitored. Patients were randomized in a double-blind study and nine patients continuing on diuretics were treated with acebutolol 200 to 600 mg two times daily, with the other six given placebo. Six of the nine treated patients responded with a diastolic blood pressure of under 90 mm Hg. There was an average diastolic blood pressure reduction in the acebutolol group of 11 ± 3 mm Hg, compared to 1 ± 3 mm Hg in the placebo group. The average heart rate of the patients treated with acebutolol was reduced 16 ± 5 beats per minute and the plasma renin activity was also lowered. This study suggested an antihypertensive effect for acebutolol in some patients found refractory to diuretic treatment alone.

Acebutolol Versus Other Antihypertensive Drugs. Chatterji compared the antihypertensive effects of acebutolol and methyldopa in a double-blind, crossover study.[139] In the patients who completed the trial, a significant reduction in blood pressure was seen in 27 subjects treated with acebutolol, and in 25 subjects treated with methyldopa. However, the methyldopa treated group complained of more side effects, such as drowsiness and impotence.

Studies comparing acebutolol to other β-blockers are described later in this chapter.

Atenolol

Atenolol (Tenormin) is approved for clinical use in the therapy of systemic hypertension as a once daily drug.

Open Studies. In a series of 43 patients receiving 100 mg of atenolol twice daily, Hansson et al.[140,141] were able to demonstrate excellent blood pressure responses with few side effects.

In a second open, multicenter trial, the same investigators[141,142] treated 117 patients with an average atenolol dose of 211 mg/day (range 50 to 800 mg/day) over a 2-year period. A significant decrease in average supine and standing blood pressure was noted for all 117 patients.

Hansson et al.[142] further assessed the efficacy of atenolol (up to 200 mg/day) over a 1-week treatment period in a third multicenter open trial of 20 hospitalized patients. Both supine and standing blood pressures were significantly reduced.

The antihypertensive efficacy of atenolol was assessed by Hansson et al.[143] in another open, multicenter trial in 262 patients. An average daily dose of 174 mg (12.5 to 600 mg) administered twice daily, but occasionally once daily, was given over an average period of 23 months. In several patients atenolol was combined with a diuretic and/or hydralazine. The investigators reported that there was a significant reduction in supine and erect blood pressures with atenolol used alone and in combination.

In an open trial by Gudbrandsson and Hansson,[144] atenolol (100 mg/day) was added to diuretics in 14 patients. These investigators noted a significant reduction in standing and supine blood pressure once atenolol was added.

Zacharias[145] carried out a 3-year open study evaluating the antihypertensive efficacy of atenolol in 422 patients. Patients were divided into three groups by age, and the mean atenolol doses used ranged from 355 to 420 mg/day. A significant decrease in systolic and diastolic blood pressure was noted for each age group. Many of the patients were concurrently receiving other antihypertensive medications.

Trials versus Placebo. Hansson et al.[146] confirmed the antihypertensive efficacy of atenolol noted earlier in a double-blind, randomized study of 45 patients. Atenolol caused a significant reduction in blood pressure when compared to placebo. The optimum daily dose for moderate hypertension was found to be 200 mg/day.

Myers et al.[147] conducted a two-part investigation involving 14 patients to further assess the antihypertensive efficacy of atenolol compared to placebo. The first part was an initial run-in stage during which the maximum effective dose of atenolol was determined for each patient. The atenolol dose ranged from 75 to 900 mg/day. Once the maximum effective dose was determined, the patients entered a 16-week randomized, double-blind, crossover phase. A significantly greater decrease in supine, erect, and exercising blood pressure was noted with atenolol than with placebo.

The antihypertensive efficacy of atenolol was compared to placebo in a two-part, multicenter, randomized, double-blind, crossover study carried out by Cilliers.[148] In the first part, 50 previously untreated patients received atenolol 100 mg once daily and placebo once daily, each for a 4-week period, using the study design mentioned above. They then received atenolol 100 mg once daily for an additional 8-week period. The second group consisted of 60 patients who were previously treated with a non-β-blocker antihypertensive agent. This medication was continued throughout the 16-week study. The patients received atenolol and placebo in the manner mentioned above. A significant reduction in systolic and diastolic blood pressures was observed in both groups with atenolol as compared to placebo.

Dose-Finding Studies. DeTollenaere and Verdonk[149] determined in a 16-week single-blind, placebo-controlled study of 31 patients that atenolol in doses of 100, 200, and 400 mg once daily gave comparable reductions in blood pressure.

In a placebo-controlled study in 18 patients, Lehtonen[150] obtained a significant reduction in systolic and diastolic blood pressure with atenolol in doses ranging from 50 mg twice daily to 300 mg twice daily. They determined 100 to 200 mg/day to be the optimal therapeutic dose range for atenolol in hypertension.

The antihypertensive efficacy of atenolol twice daily was compared to that of a once-daily regimen in a study conducted by Harris et al.[151] Atenolol, in doses of 50 to 200 mg twice daily and 100 to 400 mg once daily were found to cause significant and comparable reductions in blood pressure.

In a double-blind, placebo-controlled, randomized, crossover trial conducted by Douglas-Jones and Cruickshank,[152] the antihypertensive efficacy of atenolol in dosages of 25, 50, and 100 mg once daily was assessed. A significant reduction in supine and standing systolic and diastolic blood pressures was noted with all three doses, with no observed difference seen between them.

In a placebo-controlled, open study of 53 patients, Tuomilheto[153] compared the antihypertensive efficacy of atenolol 100 mg twice daily,

200 mg once daily, and 100 mg once daily given successively over a 6-month period. Atenolol 100 mg twice daily produced a significant reduction in supine and standing blood pressure that decreased further with 200 mg once daily.

Upton et al.[154] conducted a multicenter, double-blind, randomized, crossover trial in 63 patients to assess the comparative efficacies of atenolol 50 mg twice daily for 4 weeks and 100 mg once daily for 4 weeks with an open 8-week follow-up phase using atenolol 100 mg once daily. Both regimens produced a highly significant reduction in mean systolic and diastolic blood pressures, with no difference between them. A further decrease in diastolic blood pressure was observed during the 8-week follow-up period.

Twenty-one patients received atenolol in doses of 50, 100, and 200 mg once daily over a 12-week period in a double-blind, placebo-controlled, randomized, crossover trial conducted by Jeffers, Petrie, and their associates.[155,156] All three dosing regimens caused significant reductions in supine, standing, and postexercise blood pressure.

To further assess the optimal dose and dosing frequency of atenolol, Marshall et al.[157] conducted a two-part trial. The first part was a double-blind, placebo-controlled, crossover, randomized trial in which 16 patient were given atenolol 50, 100, and 200 mg twice daily for 4 weeks each. Identical reductions in blood pressure were noted with each dosing regimen. Eleven patients then participated in a 4-week follow-up, during which they were given their most effective dose once daily. No significant difference was noted between the once- and twice-daily dosing regimens with regard to their effects on supine, standing, and postexercise blood pressures.

Gostick et al.[158] treated 98 patients with atenolol 50, 100, and 200 mg once daily for 4 weeks in a double-blind, randomized, placebo-controlled, crossover investigation with an 8-week follow-up phase using 100 mg once daily. All three dosing regimens led to a significant and comparable reduction in systolic and diastolic blood pressures, with 100 mg once daily producing the lowest pressures in the double-blind and follow-up phases.

Zacharias et al.[159] conducted a randomized, double-blind trial in which 57 patients previously controlled on atenolol 600 mg/day, and bendrofluazide 5 mg/day, were given atenolol 300 mg twice daily, 100 mg twice daily, or 100 mg once daily for 14 weeks. Bendrofluazide was continued throughout the trial. The investigators noted a significant and comparable blood pressure reduction for the three dosing regimens and the original dosage.

The efficacy of once-daily atenolol was further investigated by Ezra et al.[160] in a 6-month, placebo-controlled study of 41 patients. Each patient was given an initial dose of 100 mg once daily, with subsequent dose titration. A significant reduction in systolic and diastolic blood pressures was noted with once-daily dosing.

Danielson and Lindborg[161] confirmed these results in an open trial in which 191 patients (some of whom were concurrently receiving diuretics and/or hydralazine) received atenolol 100 mg once daily for 7 months. They also noted a significant decrease in systolic and diastolic blood pressures.

Comparative Studies Versus Diuretics and Combination Therapy. Petrie et al.[162] conducted a double-blind, randomized, crossover, placebo-controlled trial in order to assess the comparative antihypertensive efficacies of atenolol (200 and 400 mg/day) alone, bendrofluazide (5 mg/day) alone, and the combination of atenolol (200 mg/day) plus bendrofluazide (5 mg/day). Each therapeutic regimen was given for 4 weeks. Both dosages of atenolol used alone produced a comparable and greater reduction in blood pressure than bendrofluazide alone. The addition of bendrofluazide to the lower dose of atenolol caused a further decrease in blood pressure.

In a single-blind, placebo-controlled, randomized, crossover study of 20 patients. Douglas-Jones and Cruickshank[163] compared the antihypertensive efficacies of atenolol (100 mg twice daily for 4 weeks, 200 mg twice daily for 2 weeks) and bendrofluazide (5 mg twice daily for 4 weeks). There was no difference between the antihypertensive effect of the two atenolol doses. However, the larger atenolol dose produced a greater reduction in blood pressure than bendrofluazide, while the smaller atenolol dose only had greater effects on supine blood pressure.

Fifty-two patients participated in a double-blind, placebo-controlled, crossover study conducted by Fagard et al.[164] in which they received atenolol 200 mg three times daily for 3 weeks and bendrofluazide 5 mg three times daily for 3 weeks. A reduction in blood pressure was observed with both drugs, but the antihypertensive effect of atenolol was significantly greater.

Wilcox and Mitchell[165,166] conducted a double-blind, placebo-controlled, randomized, crossover trial in which 29 patients received various combinations of atenolol (50 mg or 100 mg twice daily), bendrofluazide (2.5 mg twice daily) and hydralazine (50 mg twice daily) over three 4-week periods. Following this double-blind phase, 11 patients were further treated with atenolol (100 mg once daily) and bendrofluazide (5 mg for 4 weeks) and then atenolol (50 mg once daily) and bendrofluazide (5 mg) for an additional 4 weeks. A significant reduction in blood pressure was noted for all treatment regimens when compared to placebo. No significant difference was noted between atenolol 50 mg twice daily or 100 mg twice daily used alone or in combination. Atenolol alone produced a significantly greater reduction in diastolic blood pressure than bendrofluazide alone, with no difference seen in systolic blood pressure. The combination of atenolol and bendrofluazide was significantly better than either agent used alone. Diastolic blood pressure was significantly decreased by the addition of hydralazine to the combination of atenolol and bendrofluazide. The combination of all three drugs given twice daily was found to have the greatest effect.

Rushford et al.[167] conducted a multicenter, double-blind, crossover trial in which the comparative antihypertensive efficacies of atenolol (100 mg once daily for 4 weeks) and bendrofluazide (5 mg once daily for 4 weeks) were assessed in 42 patients. Atenolol 100 mg once daily was then given in an 8-week open follow-up phase. Although both agents produced a highly significant reduction in systolic and diastolic blood pressure, atenolol's effect on diastolic blood pressure was significantly greater than that of bendrofluazide. The follow-up phase demonstrated continued blood pressure control with atenolol once daily.

The antihypertensive efficacies of atenolol (100 mg once daily for 4 weeks), chlorthalidone (25 mg once daily for 4 weeks) and atenolol (100 mg once daily) plus chlorthalidone (25 mg once daily for 4 weeks) were assessed in a placebo-controlled, double-blind, randomized, crossover study involving 21 patients.[168] Tenoretic, a preparation combining atenolol 100 mg and chlorthalidone 25 mg in a fixed combination (not available in the United States) was given once daily in an open 16-week follow-up treatment phase. Standing and supine diastolic blood pressures were reduced to a greater extent with atenolol than with chlorthalidone. The combination had a significantly greater effect than either agent used alone, without a difference in efficacy noted between tenoretic and the free combination.

The comparative effects of chlorthalidone (25 mg once daily), atenolol (100 mg once daily), and their combination was also investigated by Bateman et al.[169] in a 16-week, double-blind, randomized, crossover, placebo-controlled study with a 1 month open follow-up phase, during which tenoretic was given once daily. All three active treatments significantly reduced systolic and diastolic blood pressures. The combination was significantly better than the diuretic for all measurements but was only more effective than atenolol alone in decreasing supine systolic blood pressure. Tenoretic produced reductions in blood pressure that were similar to those of the free combination.

Teeuw et al.[170] conducted a two-part study to assess further the antihypertensive efficacy of the atenolol–chlorthalidone combination. In the first portion, 34 patients participated in a randomized, double-blind, placebo-controlled, crossover trial in which they received atenolol (100 to 300 mg twice daily for 3 weeks) and the combination of atenolol (100 to 300 mg twice daily) and chlorthalidone (25 mg twice daily for 3 weeks). These investigators determined that atenolol alone produced a significant reduction in blood pressure without significant differences between doses. The diuretic–β-blocker combination caused a significantly greater reduction in systolic and standing diastolic blood pressures than atenolol alone. In the second portion of this trial, six patients on chronic chlorthalidone (50 mg/day) therapy received atenolol (100 to 300 mg twice daily for three days at each dose) in a single-blind, placebo-controlled manner. A significant reduction in blood pressure was noted, with no difference seen between doses.

In a placebo-controlled study conducted by Velasco et al.,[171,172] 40 patients received atenolol 100 mg once daily for either 4 or 8 weeks, with chlorthalidone 50 mg/day added for 4 weeks, if the diastolic blood pressure was greater than 90 mm Hg on atenolol alone. These investigators noted a significant reduction in blood pressure with atenolol alone, with a further reduction in blood pressure once chlorthalidone was added.

Seedat[173] found the combination of chlorthalidone (25 mg once daily) and atenolol (100 mg once daily for 4 weeks) to be more effective in reducing mean supine and standing blood pressures than either agent used alone. Both drugs, when used alone, were found to be comparably effective in this double-blind, randomized, placebo-controlled, crossover study in 24 black South African patients.

Asbury et al.[174] conducted a multicenter, double-blind, randomized, crossover trial which consisted of two parts. In the first part, 261 patients received atenolol (100 mg once daily for 4 weeks), chlorthalidone (25 mg once daily for 4 weeks) and a combination of the two agents given in individual tablets. As had been noted previously, all three regimens produced a significant reduction in blood pressure, with the combination having a greater effect than either agent alone. In the second portion, the fixed combination tablet of atenolol (100 mg) and chlorthalidone (25 mg) used once daily was found to produce a reduction in systolic and diastolic blood pressures similar to that found with the free combination regimen.

Trials versus Other β-Blockers. Hansson et al.[175] conducted a double-blind, randomized study in which 30 patients received placebo for 12 weeks or atenolol (50, 100, and 200 mg, twice daily, each for 3 weeks). All patients then received propranolol 160 mg twice daily for 4 weeks.

Both active treatments produced significant reductions in supine and standing blood pressure, with no difference seen between them.

In a double-blind, randomized, crossover, placebo-controlled trial, Epstein and Lubbe[176] assessed the comparative antihypertensive efficacies of propranolol (80 mg twice daily for 4 weeks) and atenolol (100 mg twice daily for 4 weeks) in 15 patients who were being treated with the diuretic cyclopenthiazide (1 tablet once daily). Both β-blocking agents reduced sitting, standing, resting, and postexercise blood pressures, with no difference noted between the regimens.

Zacharias and Cowen[177,178] conducted a double-blind, randomized, crossover study comparing the antihypertensive efficacies of atenolol (100 to 600 mg twice daily for 8 weeks) versus propranolol (80 to 480 mg twice daily for 8 weeks) in 30 patients. These investigators determined that both β-blockers reduced systolic and diastolic blood pressure, however, in contrast to the findings of previous trials, atenolol was found to produce a slightly greater reduction in blood pressure.

The antihypertensive efficacies of atenolol (100 mg twice daily and 200 mg twice daily for 4 weeks) and metoprolol (100 mg twice daily and 200 mg twice daily for 4 weeks) were assessed by Jeffers et al.[179] in a double-blind, randomized, crossover, placebo-controlled trial in 20 patients. All active treatments were found to produce significant reductions in blood pressure compared to placebo without a significant difference between the regimens.

In a randomized, double-blind, placebo-controlled study of 55 patients, Lyngstam and Rydén[180] noted that metoprolol (100 to 200 mg once daily for 12 weeks) and atenolol (100 to 200 mg once daily for 12 weeks) had comparable antihypertensive effects.

Adams-Strump et al.,[181] in a placebo-controlled, double-blind, randomized study of 48 patients, also found that both metoprolol (100 to 200 mg once daily for 12 weeks) and atenolol (100 to 200 mg once daily for 12 weeks) produced parallel reductions in mean resting blood pressure.

Twenty-seven patients participated in a double-blind, randomized, placebo-controlled, crossover study[182] in which the antihypertensive efficacies of atenolol (50 and 100 mg twice daily for 4 weeks) and oxprenolol (80 and 160 mg twice daily for 4 weeks) were compared. All patients then received atenolol 100 mg once daily for an additional 16 weeks. No significant difference was noted in the antihypertensive effects with the different doses of each drug. Once-daily atentolol was found to be as effective as the twice-daily regimen. Systolic blood pressure was reduced by both drugs, but atenolol had a significantly greater effect on supine and standing diastolic blood pressures.

In an open, randomized, controlled, crossover study, Leary et al.[183]

determined that sotalol (160 to 800 mg once daily for 14 weeks) and atenolol (100 to 500 mg once daily for 14 weeks) had comparable antihypertensive effects on standing systolic and diastolic blood pressure, and supine diastolic blood pressure. Atenolol had a greater effect on supine systolic blood pressure.

In a 4-year open trial conducted by Zacharias et al.[184] 543 patients, a portion of whom were on previous propranolol or practolol therapy, received atenolol (50 to 200 mg twice daily) alone, or in combination with a diuretic and/or vasodilator and/or other antihypertensive drug. Significant reduction in systolic and diastolic blood pressure was noted with atenolol used alone or in combination. A greater decrease in blood pressure was observed in patients switched from either practolol or propranolol.

Wilcox[185] compared the antihypertensive efficacies of acebutolol (200 and 400 mg once daily), atenolol (100 and 200 mg once daily), bendrofluazide (5 and 10 mg once daily), labetalol (300 and 600 mg once daily), pindolol (5 and 15 mg once daily), propranolol (80 and 160 mg once daily), and timolol (10 and 20 mg once daily) in a single-blind, randomized, crossover, placebo-controlled trial in 15 patients. Each treatment period was 4 weeks. Bendrofluazide was found to be equal to or superior to all the β-blockers except atenolol in reducing resting blood pressure. Atenolol once daily was significantly better in decreasing resting and exercise blood pressure than any of the other agents administered once daily.

Waal-Manning[186] conducted a randomized, crossover study in 27 patients in which the antihypertensive efficacy of atenolol (dosage not specified) was compared to that of oxprenolol (20 to 480 mg/day in eight patients), propranolol (45 to 280 mg/day in eight patients) or pindolol (10 to 30 mg/day in 11 patients). Atenolol and one of the three abovementioned β-blockers were given over two consecutive 8-week periods. The decrease in supine and standing systolic blood pressures was comparable with these four agents.

Vaughan Williams et al.[187] found that the long-acting preparations of propranolol, pindolol, atenolol, and metoprolol, at initial doses of 160 mg once daily, 15 mg once daily, 100 mg once daily, and 200 mg once daily, respectively, produced significant and comparable reductions in diastolic and systolic blood pressure. They obtained their results in a 70-day double-blind, randomized study of 30 patients.

Twenty-three patients participated in a placebo-controlled, randomized, double-blind, crossover trial in which the comparative antihypertensive efficacies of atenolol (100 mg once daily for 4 weeks), sustained-release oxprenolol (160 mg once daily for 4 weeks), and long-acting propranolol (160 mg once daily for 4 weeks) were assessed.[188] The investigators found that long-acting propranolol and atenolol significantly reduced supine, standing, and postexercise systolic and diastolic blood pressure compared to placebo, while sustained-release oxprenolol did not. Atenolol and long-acting propranolol were also noted to cause a greater decrease in blood pressure than sustained-release oxprenolol. There were no significant differences in the antihypertensive effects of long-acting propranolol and atenolol.

The comparative antihypertensive efficacies of propranolol (mean dose 190 mg once daily for 4 weeks), pindolol (mean dose 17 mg once daily for 4 weeks) and atenolol (100 mg once daily for 4 weeks) were assessed in a randomized, double-blind, crossover, placebo-controlled investigation in 18 patients.[189] All active treatments significantly reduced systolic and diastolic blood pressure when compared to placebo. No significant difference was noted between the antihypertensive effects of propranolol and atenolol; pindolol produced a significantly smaller decrease in diastolic blood pressure.

Thulin et al.[190] assessed the comparative antihypertensive efficacies of atenolol (50, 100, and 200 mg, twice daily, each for 2 weeks) and labetalol (200, 400, and 600 mg twice daily each for 2 weeks) in a double-blind, crossover, multicenter, placebo-controlled, randomized trial in 33 patients. No significant differences in antihypertensive efficacies were noted between the doses of each drug. Atenolol and labetalol both reduced blood pressure when compared to placebo, with no significant difference between them in their effect on supine blood pressure. However, labetalol produced a greater reduction in standing blood pressure than atenolol.

Trials Versus Methyldopa and Combinations. In a double-blind, placebo-controlled, crossover trial in 14 patients on chlorthalidone therapy, Webster et al.[191] compared the antihypertensive efficacies of atenolol (50 mg three times daily and 100 mg three times day for 2 weeks), methyldopa (250 mg three times daily and 500 mg three times daily for 2 weeks) and atenolol (50 mg three times daily) plus methyldopa (250 mg three times daily) in combination for 4 weeks. No significant difference was noted between the doses of each drug. All active treatments were effective in reducing blood pressure. The antihypertensive effect of atenolol alone and the methyldopa–atenolol combination on supine and standing diastolic blood pressure was comparable, and greater than methyldopa alone.

Wilson et al.[192] conducted a 24-week double-blind, randomzied, crossover, placebo-controlled, trial in 24 patients on chlorthalidone therapy to assess the comparative antihypertensive effect of atenolol (150 and 300 mg/day), methyldopa (750 and 1500 mg/day), and the combination of atenolol (150 mg/day) and methyldopa (750 mg/day). No significant difference was noted between doses of each drug. Atenolol and methyldopa produced significant and comparable reductions in supine and standing blood pressure. The combination caused a significantly greater reduction in blood pressure than either agent alone.

Similarly, Basker et al.[193] found in a multicenter, double-blind, crossover, randomized study in 90 patients that atenolol (50 mg three times daily for 4 weeks) and methyldopa (250 mg three times daily for 4 weeks) produced a comparable reduction in blood pressure.

In a study by Tweed et al.,[194] 1428 patients who were receiving methyldopa (usually less than 1 g/day) were switched to atenolol (100 mg/day) in an 8-week multicenter, open study. A significant reduction in blood pressure was noted with atenolol.

Labetalol
Labetalol (Normodyne, Trandate) will be marketed soon in oral and parenteral form for the treatment of mild, severe, and accelerated hypertension. Multiple clinical trials have confirmed its safety and efficacy. This drug is reviewed in Chapters 7, 13, and 14.

Metoprolol
Metoprolol (Lopresor) is approved for both once and twice daily use in hypertension.

Open Studies. Haglund and Collste[195] studied the time course of reducing blood pressure and plasma renin activity in patients receiving metoprolol (100 mg twice daily for 3 months). A maximum decrease in blood pressure occurred within the first 2 days of metoprolol therapy. Plasma renin activity decreased from 2 ± 0.46 ng/ml/hr to 0.5 ± 0.09 ng/ml/hr and remained at that level throughout the 3-month period.

Bengtsson[196] followed 24 women between the ages of 50 and 64 with previously untreated hypertension for a 7-year period on metoprolol. The majority of patients were well controlled on once-daily regimens of 100 to 200 mg: however, a few patients were better controlled on 50 to 100 mg two times daily. There were also more side effects noted in the once-daily treatment group, which resolved when the same total dosage was taken twice daily.

Asplund and Ohman[197] compared conventional 200 mg metoprolol tablets to slow-release 200 mg tablets (not available in the United States) in 20 patients with essential hypertension. The peak plasma levels of slow-release metoprolol 2 hours postdose were 50 percent lower than those seen with conventional metoprolol. However, at 24 hours, the plasma drug concentrations with the long-acting metoprolol were 50 percent higher than that seen with conventional metoprolol. After 2 hours, despite the differences in plasma drug levels, both preparations reduced blood pressure during exercise compared to placebo, but conventional tablets produced a lower heart rate than the slow-release form.

Bengtsson et al.[198] followed the hemodynamic effects of withdrawing β-blockers in five hypertensive women. After 10 years of treatment with β-blockers, the agents were withdrawn for 1 year. Blood pressure remained low during the first year posttreatment, despite an increase in heart rate within the first few days. Hemodynamic studies demonstrated that cardiac output was increased, but total peripheral vascular resistance was unchanged. To account for the maintenance of good blood pressure control after stopping the medication, the investigators hypothesized that the small resistance vessels underwent structural changes, leading to normalization of hemodynamics.

Metoprolol Versus Diuretics and Combination Treatments. Velasquez et al.[199] studied 20 patients with thiazide-resistant hypertension and reported a wide range of plasma renin activity values with metoprolol treatment. Plasma renin activity decreased by 48 percent, but returned to baseline by the fourth week. Blood pressure control was achieved with metoprolol 200 mg/day in 12 patients at 1 week, while eight were controlled with both hydrochlorthiazide 100 mg/day added to metoprolol 300 to 400 mg/day. Since blood pressure control was maintained despite a return to baseline in plasma renin activity, the investigators postulated that the antihypertensive effects of metoprolol were separate from its ability to lower plasma renin activity.

Using a crossover design, Pederson[200] compared the antihypertensive effect of metoprolol to hydrochlorthiazide in 200 patients. Individually titrated doses of metoprolol or hydrochlorthiazide were administered for 18 weeks, followed by a placebo washout and a crossover period. He observed that both drugs produced a significant reduction in systolic and diastolic blood pressure, but that heart rate was reduced only by metoprolol.

Kubik et al.[201] compared the use of metoprolol with and without chlorthalidone in 24 patients with hypertension. In this double-blind, crossover study, 19 patients being treated with metoprolol 100 mg twice daily had their diastolic blood pressure reduced to less than 95 mm Hg. With the addition of chlorthalidone 50 mg, 33 patients had diastolic blood pressures of less than 95 mm Hg. They concluded that chlorthalidone is a safe and efficacious adjunct to metoprolol in the treatment of mild to moderate hypertension. Liedholm et al.[202] examined the antihypertensive effects of combining metoprolol and hydrochlorothiazide in the treatment of mild to moderate hypertension. Fifty-five patients were treated with metoprolol (100 mg twice daily) and randomized into Group A, which received an additional 12.5 mg twice daily of hydrochlorothiazide, and Group B, which received an additional 25 mg twice daily. Both diuretic β-blocker combinations were equally effective in reducing blood pressures. These investigators concluded that low-dose hydrochlorothiazide therapy was as effective as high-dose treatment, when combined with metoprolol.

Metoprolol Versus Other β-Blockers. Lameyer and Heese[203] compared the efficacy of metoprolol and propranolol in ten patients with essential hypertension and five with renal artery stenosis. Plasma renin activity was nearly twice as high in patients with renal artery stenosis as in the essential hypertension group. Unlike the study of Velasquez et al.[199] previously described, in patients with essential hypertension treated with metoprolol, a significant correlation was found between the reduction in blood pressure and the fall in plasma renin activity.

Svensson et al.[204] compared the hemodynamic effects of metoprolol and pindolol in 36 hypertensive patients. The patients were randomized to receive either 100 to 200 mg/day of metoprolol or 5 to 10 mg/day of pindolol. Both drugs reduced blood pressure. However, heart rate was reduced by metoprolol but not by pindolol. At rest, pindolol reduced vascular resistance by 14 percent, compared to the slight increase in resistance found in metoprolol-treated patients.

Additional comparative β-blocker studies with metoprolol are described in other sections of this chapter.

Nadolol

Nadolol (Corgard) is a long-acting β-blocker approved for once-daily use in patients with hypertension. There is also a diuretic–nadolol combination (Corzide) approved for clinical use.

Open Trials. Jackson et al.[205] assessed the efficacy of nadolol alone and in combination with a diuretic in a multicentric, open study of 10,711 patients. Patients received nadolol 40 to 240 mg once daily over a mean period of 10 weeks. A significant reduction in blood pressure was obtained in 66 percent of the patients studied.

Thirty-one patients with mild to moderate hypertension participated in an investigation where nadolol was administered in two divided doses, ranging up to 640 mg/day over a 3-month period.[206] Twenty-two patients had a reduction of 10 percent or more in supine diastolic pressure, with 12 patients becoming normotensive. During a 15 month follow-up period involving 23 patients, satisfactory control of blood pressure was obtained in 17 of these subjects.

Studies Versus Placebo. Frithz[207] investigated the antihypertensive efficacy of twice-daily nadolol in a 16-week single-blind, dose-ranging, placebo-controlled study involving 30 patients. Daily dosages of nadolol ranged from 20 mg to 280 mg twice daily. Using an average daily dose of 110 mg of nadolol, Frithz demonstrated a significant reduction in both systolic and diastolic blood pressures.

Studies with Diuretics. The antihypertensive efficacy of nadolol (40 to 240 mg once daily) combined with hydrochlorothiazide (50 or 100 mg once daily) was assessed by El Mehairy et al. in an open, 20-week study of 60 mild to moderately hypertensive patients.[208] On hydrochlorothiazide monotherapy, none of the patients achieved full control of their supine diastolic blood pressure (SDBP under 90 mm Hg), whereas on combined therapy, 91.7 percent of the patients demonstrated a full response.

In a follow-up article, El Mehairy et al.[209] reported that the significant decrease in average supine blood pressure that had been noted after 3 months of combined therapy was maintained over the following 21 months, without an increase in the nadolol or hydrochlorothiazide dosage.

Finnerty[210] utilized a randomized, crossover study design to assess the comparative antihypertensive efficacies of hydrochlorothiazide and nadolol in 55 patients. Both agents were found to be equally effective in reducing blood pressure.

In a recent study, Olerud[211] assessed the antihypertensive efficacy of nadolol (40 to 240 mg once daily) combined with hydrochlorothiazide (25, 50, or 100 mg once daily) in a 17-week placebo-controlled study of 30 patients. Hydrochlorothiazide treatment was noted to significantly reduce mean supine blood pressure from that on placebo. The addition of nadolol caused a further decrease in both mean supine systolic and diastolic blood pressures.

Studies Versus β-Blockers. In a study of 25 patients, Hill and Fand[212-214] found that nadolol (maximum dose 320 mg once daily) and propranolol (maximum dose 320 mg in four divided doses) produced similar reductions in blood pressure.

In a double-blind, randomized, placebo-controlled study, El Mehairy et al.[215] treated 75 patients with either nadolol (80 to 320 mg once daily for 12 weeks) or propranolol (80 to 320 mg four times daily for 12 weeks). Although both agents were effective in controlling blood pressure, nadolol was found to be better in reducing supine systolic blood pressure.

The comparative antihypertensive efficacies of nadolol (40 to 320 mg once daily) and propranolol (10 to 80 mg four times daily) were also assessed by Frithz[216] in a 15-week, double-blind, placebo-controlled, randomized study of 90 patients. A significant reduction in supine systolic and diastolic blood pressure was noted for both agents, with no difference noted between them.

Additional comparative β-blocker studies with nadolol are described in other sections of this chapter.

Studies Versus Methyldopa. Jenkins et al.[217] compared the antihypertensive efficacies of nadolol (160 to 240 mg once daily) and α-methyldopa (given three times daily in doses totaling 1000 to 2000 mg/day) in a 3-month open, randomized trial of 50 patients. The investigators noted a reduction in supine systolic and diastolic blood pressure for both agents, with nadolol producing a significantly greater decrease.

Oxprenolol

Oxprenolol (Trasicor, Iset) is not yet approved for clinical use in the United States.

Open Studies. Schlesinger and Barzilay[218] examined the effects of oxprenolol on blood pressure, pulmonary function, myocardial contractility and oxygen consumption in 66 hypertensive patients. Each patient received a course of oxprenolol with and without diuretics. Unlike propranolol, which decreases ventricular ejection fraction, oxprenolol did not hamper left ventricular function, perhaps due to its intrinsic sympathomimetic activity. Oxygen consumption and blood pressure were significantly reduced on both regimens. Oxprenolol had no effect on lung capacity volume, but increased airway resistance in some patients.

Resnekov and Harvard[219] compared conventional oxprenolol once and twice daily to slow-release tablets administered once daily in 15 hypertensive patients. Slow-release oxprenolol was more effective than conventional treatment, but the difference was not statistically significant. Conventional oxprenolol used once daily was significantly less effective than the twice daily regimen.

Oxprenolol in Combination and Other Antihypertensive Agents. Materson et al.[220] studied the efficacy of oxprenolol twice daily in 15 male patients who had been inadequately controlled on diuretics (diastolic blood pressures of more than 100 mm Hg). Using between 40 and 160 mg of oxprenolol twice daily in addition to hydrochlorothiazide, a significant drop in blood pressure was observed.

Farsang et al.[221] studied the hemodynamic effects of prazosin alone and in combination with oxprenolol in 48 hypertensive patients. Patients treated with prazosin alone experienced tachycardia, an increase in plasma renin activity, and a decrease in blood pressure. After 3 days of treatment, there was no further decrease in blood pressure and the level of plasma renin activity returned to baseline. When 40 mg oxprenolol thrice daily was added, there was a further decrease in blood pressure and a reduction in plasma renin activity.

Barret et al.[222] compared oxprenolol and methyldopa in a double-blind, crossover study in 24 patients. Fifty percent of the patients responded well to each drug regardless of whether low or high dosages were used. Therefore, it was recommended that if a patient did not adequately respond to a moderate dose of one medication, the use of an additional agent would be more beneficial than increasing the original treatment dosage.

Freeman and Knight[223] showed that the combination of oxprenolol and hydralazine was as effective as methyldopa in lowering blood pressure and was better tolerated.

Pindolol

Pindolol (Visken) is approved for twice and thrice daily use in the treatment of hypertension.

Open Studies. Gavras et al.[224] studied the effect of pindolol 45 mg/day in 11 hospitalized patients by assessing the effects of treatment on blood pressure, plasma renin activity, and plasma catecholamines. The blood pressure dropped significantly from an average of 160/111 to 144/101 mm Hg: however, the heart rate remained unchanged. The intrinsic sympathomimetic activity of pindolol was considered responsible for maintaining the heart rate. Plasma renin activity and epinephrine and norepinephrine levels did not change from baseline.

Toivonen et al.[225] examined the efficacy of using pindolol once daily in patients with hypertension. Of the 32 patients studied, 25 responded initially to pindolol three times daily. These 25 patients were then treated with a single dose of pindolol 20 to 40 mg/day—15 patients became normotensive (162/107 to 137/86 mm Hg) 5 had a fair response (158/104 to 143/93.6 mm Hg), 3 did not respond significantly, and 2 dropped out because of side effects.

Pindolol Versus Other Antihypertensive Drugs. McNeil et al.[226] compared metoprolol to pindolol in a double-blind, crossover study in 31 patients. Twenty-nine completed the study: the average daily dose of pindolol was 25 ± 2 mg and metoprolol 234 ± 22 mg. Metoprolol caused a decrease in heart rate of 18 beats per minute, which was significantly greater than that seen with pindolol (10 beats per minute). Both drugs were equally effective in lowering blood pressure but differed in the nature of their side effects. The most common side effects of pindolol were vivid dreams and insomnia, while eye discomfort, dry mouth, and mild Raynaud's complications caused by metoprolol.

Toumilheto et al.[227] later compared the long-term effects of metoprolol and pindolol in 44 patients. After 20 weeks of individually titrated dosages of pindolol, the mean blood pressure went from 159/103 to 141/94 mm Hg with 13/24 (54 percent) of the patients achieving a diastolic blood pressure lower than 95 mm Hg. The mean blood pressure with metoprolol went from 159/104 to 136/89, with 15/20 patients achieving a diastolic blood pressure lower than 95 mm Hg. The average heart rate reduction with treatment confirmed the results of McNeil et al.[226] that metoprolol-treated patients experienced greater decreases in their heart rates than those patients treated with pindolol.

Romo et al.[228] compared labetalol to pindolol in a double-blind, crossover study in 37 patients. After 2 weeks, both drugs caused a similar drop in blood pressure, although the pulse rate was slightly lower in the labetalol group.

Three hundred patients with mild to moderate hypertension were evaluated in double-blind clinical trials to determine the efficacy of pindolol in reducing blood pressure.[229] Pindolol-treated patients were compared to 65 patients on placebo, 52 on propranolol, 38 on hydrochlorothiazide, 62 on methyldopa, and 14 on chlorthalidone. Pindolol was significantly superior to placebo in lowering blood pressure and just as effective as propranolol, hydrochlorothiazide, α-methyldopa, or chlorthalidone treatment.

Combination Studies. Persson[230] examined 30 patients with essential hypertension on pindolol and hydralazine combination therapy. The patients were observed over an 11-week period, with placebo for the first 2 weeks, hydralazine 10 mg three times daily for 3 weeks, hydralazine 25 mg three times daily for 2 weeks, followed by hydralazine 25 mg three times daily plus pindolol in increasing doses ranging from 5 mg three times daily to 15 mg three times daily for 4 weeks. Compared to placebo, hydralazine caused a significant decrease in blood pressure and an increase in pulse rate. Hydralazine plus pindolol resulted in an additional fall in blood pressure, and a decrease in pulse rate when compared to hydralazine alone. Pindolol, with partial agonist activity, blunted the reflex tachycardia commonly seen with the vasodilator drug treatment.

Additional β-blocker comparative studies with pindolol are described in other sections of this chapter.

Propranolol
Propranolol (Inderal, Inderide, Inderal-LA) was the first β-blocker approved for systemic use in the treatment of hypertension.

There has been vast experience with the use of propranolol in hypertensive patients and the drug is currently available in a conventional tablet form for twice daily dosage, in a long-acting preparation for once-daily dosage, and in combination with a thiazide diuretic.

Trials Versus Placebo. Zacharias et al.[231] studied 109 patients receiving thiazide diuretics, and obtained good results in about 60 percent of his patients using an average propranolol dose of 290 to 320 mg/day (maximum 1000 mg/day). Only 20 percent of the patients required more than 600 mg/day. Other double-blind trials in propranolol responders have shown a significant difference in antihypertensive effectiveness between drug and placebo.[232]

In a double-blind study of Jamaican blacks with hypertension, Humphreys and Delvin,[233] using lower doses of propranolol (maximum 360 mg/day) without diuretics, demonstrated far less satisfactory results. This study raised the question of whether there is a decreased sensitivity of blacks to the effects of β-blockade.

The comparative antihypertensive efficacies of propranolol (90 to 240 mg) and placebo were assessed in ten hypertensive adolescents by Mongeau et al. in an 8-month, single-blind, randomized, crossover study.[234] These investigators noted a significant reduction in mean systolic and diastolic blood pressures with propranolol compared to placebo.

Dose-Finding and Dose Interval Studies. Galloway et al.[235] conducted a double-blind, randomized, placebo-controlled, crossover trial comparing the antihypertensive effects of propranolol 60, 120, and 240 mg/day (each dose used for 4 weeks) in 24 patients. A dosage of 60 mg/day was found to be no better than placebo in reducing blood pressure. However, the blood pressure–lowering effects of 120 and 240 mg/day were significantly different from placebo.

Once-daily propranolol doses of 80, 120, 160, 240, and 320 mg (used for 4 weeks each) were all noted to reduce supine and standing blood pressures in a double-blind, randomized, crossover, placebo-controlled trial in 23 patients.[236]

In a multicenter study of 63 patients, MacLeod et al.[237] found that there was no significant difference in the antihypertensive effects of comparable doses of propranolol administered twice daily and four times daily.

Propranolol 40 to 320 mg, given once daily and twice daily, was assessed by Patterson et al.[238] in a trial of seven patients. Both regimens produced comparable reductions in supine and standing systolic and diastolic blood pressures, and sitting diastolic blood pressure. The twice-daily regimen had a greater effect on sitting systolic pressure than the once-daily regimen.

In another crossover study, 26 patients receiving chlorthalidone 50 mg/day showed no significant difference between the antihypertensive effect of a once-daily or thrice-daily dosing regimen of propranolol.[239]

Serlin et al.[240] assessed the comparative antihypertensive efficacy of propranolol in twice-daily doses of 40, 80, 160, and 240 mg in a double-blind, crossover study in 24 patients. These investigators found no significant difference in the antihypertensive efficacies between the different dosage forms.

Conventional Propranolol Versus Sustained-Release Propranolol. Twenty-nine patients participated in a 10-week study comparing the antihypertensive effect of conventional propranolol given twice daily and a long-acting formulation (Inderal LA) given once daily.[241] No significant difference was noted in the blood pressure–lowering effects of these two dosage regimens.

In a double-blind, placebo-controlled, randomized, crossover trial in 19 patients, Woods[242] assessed the antihypertensive efficacies of long-acting propranolol (Inderal LA 160 mg once daily) and conventional propranolol (80 mg twice daily). Long-acting propranolol was noted to produce a greater reduction in diastolic and systolic blood pressures than the conventional preparation, although this difference was not statistically significant.

Studies Versus Diuretics and Combination Therapy. Berglund et al.[243] investigated the comparative efficacies of bendroflumethiazide and propranolol in a randomized study in 106 males previously untreated. A comparable reduction in blood pressure was noted with both active treatments.

Jaattele[244] conducted a double-blind, randomized, crossover, placebo-controlled trial in which 21 patients received propranolol (80 mg twice daily) and bendrofluazide (2.5 mg twice daily) individually and in free and fixed (Inderectic—not approved for clinical use) combinations for 4 weeks. Both the free and fixed combinations produced a greater reduction in systolic and diastolic blood pressures than the individual agents. There was no significant difference between the effects of the free and fixed diuretic–β-blocker combinations.

Karlberg et al.[245] conducted a 10-month randomized, crossover, placebo-controlled study in 27 patients to assess the comparative antihypertensive efficacies of spironolactone (200 mg/day), propranolol (320 mg/day), and the combination of both spironolactone (100 mg/day) and propranolol (160 mg/day). The individual agents significantly reduced supine and standing blood pressures, with the combination producing a further decrement.

The comparative antihypertensive effects of chlorthalidone, spironolactone, and propranolol were investigated in 11 patients by Drayer et al.[246] All three agents produced a significant and comparable reduction in blood pressure.

Vander Elst et al.[247] conducted a multicenter, double-blind, parallel, randomized, placebo-controlled study in 40 patients to compare the antihypertensive effects of propranolol (20 to 40 mg thrice daily) in combination with either furosemide (20 to 40 mg once daily) or hydrochlorothiazide (25 to 50 mg once daily). A significant reduction in supine, sitting, and standing blood pressures was noted, with both diuretic combinations without a significant difference seen between them.

Studies Versus Other β-Blockers. Many studies comparing propranolol to other β-blockers are illustrated in different sections of this chapter.

In a 2-year trial conducted by Nik-Akhtar et al.,[248] the antihypertensive efficacies of propranolol (20 to 200 mg four times daily) and alprenolol (25 to 75 mg four times daily) were compared in 107 patients. Both β-blockers produced a significant reduction in supine, sitting, and standing systolic and diastolic blood pressures.

Materson et al.[249] studied the antihypertensive effects of propranolol (20 to 80 mg three times daily) and oxprenolol (20 to 80 mg three times daily). They were compared in a 120-day randomized, double-blind, parallel, placebo-controlled study in 24 patients, all of whom continued to receive hydrochlorothiazide 50 mg once or twice daily. Both agents produced a comparable reduction in supine and standing systolic blood pressure.

Gavras et al.[250] carried out a double-blind, randomized, parallel, placebo-controlled trial comparing the antihypertensive effects of oxprenolol and propranolol (40 to 60 mg three times daily) in 20 patients receiving hydrochlorothiazide 50 mg/day. Both agents produced similar reductions in systolic and diastolic blood pressures.

Two hundred and sixty patients on hydrochlorothiazide (25 mg three times daily) participated in a multicenter, placebo-controlled, randomized, double-blind, parallel trial carried out by the Veterans Administration Cooperative Study Group,[251] in which propranolol (40 to 120 mg three times daily for 6 months) and oxprenolol (40 to 120 mg three times daily for 6 months) were compared with respect to their antihypertensive effects. The mean reduction of systolic and diastolic blood pressures was found to be significantly greater for propranolol.

Wilson et al.[252,253] observed in 11 patients that pindolol (15 to 45 mg/day) and propranolol (120 to 160 mg/day) produced similar control of blood pressure.

Salako et al.[254] conducted a double-blind, randomized, crossover, placebo-controlled study to assess the comparative antihypertensive effects of pindolol (20 mg/day) and propranolol (100 mg/day) in a group of nine hypertensive black Africans. Pindolol and propranolol produced comparable reductions in resting and exercise systolic blood pressure: however, neither agent produced a reduction in diastolic blood pressure.

Berglund[255] determined in a 32-week, double-blind, crossover, placebo-controlled comparison of sotalol (80 to 320 mg twice daily) and propranolol (40 to 160 mg twice daily) in 30 men that both agents caused a significant and comparable reduction in supine and standing systolic and diastolic blood pressures.

In a double-blind, crossover trial in 23 women, Bengtsson[256] noted that there was no significant difference between the antihypertensive effects of metoprolol and propranolol.

Bosman et al.[257] assessed the comparative antihypertensive efficacies of metoprolol (120 and 210 mg/day, each for 6 weeks), and propranolol (240 and 360 mg/day, each for 6 weeks) in a double-blind, placebo-controlled trial in 80 patients. All four active treatments reduced blood pressure. However, metoprolol, in both doses, was more effective in reducing diastolic blood pressure than both doses of propranolol.

Fifty patients participated in a 36-week, placebo-controlled, randomized, parallel study in which Sjoberg[258] compared the antihypertensive effects of metoprolol (50 to 200 mg twice daily) and propranolol (40 to 160 mg twice daily). It was found that although both agents significantly reduced supine and standing systolic and diastolic blood pressures, metoprolol has a significantly greater effect on supine diastolic blood pressure and standing systolic blood pressure.

In contrast to previous findings, Browning et al.,[259] in a multicenter, placebo-controlled, randomized, double-blind, crossover trial in 40 patients, found that metoprolol (100 mg twice daily for 4 weeks) and propranolol (80 mg twice daily for 4 weeks) reduced sitting and standing systolic and diastolic blood pressures without a difference in their effect noted between them.

Lohmoller and Frohlich[260] demonstrated in a double-blind trial of 22 patients that timolol (30 mg/day) and propranolol (120 mg/day) produced an equivalent reduction in blood pressure.

Similarly, Aronow et al.[261] also noted in a double-blind, randomized, placebo-controlled trial of 20 men that timolol 30 to 60 mg/day for 5 weeks) and propranolol (240 to 480 mg/day for 5 weeks) comparably reduced supine and standing systolic and diastolic blood pressures.

In a double-blind study in 24 patients, Nicholls et al.[262] found labetalol and propranolol to be similarly effective in reducing blood pressure.

Thirteen patients participated in a randomized, single-blind, crossover study comparing the antihypertensive effects of propranolol (mean dose 234 mg/day twice daily for 8 weeks) and labetalol (mean dose 585 mg/day twice daily for 8 weeks).[263] A reduction in systolic and diastolic blood pressures was obtained only with labetalol. However, the pretreatment blood pressure level for propranolol was significantly lower than for labetalol. The final blood pressure levels for both agents were the same.

Van der Veur et al.[264] assessed the antihypertensive efficacies of labetalol (mean dose 600 mg/day), and the combination of propranolol (median 120 mg/day) and hydralazine (median 60 mg/day) in a single-blind, randomized, crossover study in 34 patients who were receiving hydrochlorothiazide 50 mg/day. Both treatment regimens were noted to reduce blood pressure to the same extent and at the same rate.

Studies Versus Other Antihypertensive Agents. Vlachakis and Mendlowitz[265] assessed the efficacy of propranolol alone and in combination with phenoxybenzamine. Ten patients were started on propranolol (20 to 40 mg four times daily) and were then switched to the combination of propranolol (20 to 40 mg four times daily) and phenoxybenzamine (10 to 50 mg two to four times daily). Propranolol used alone significantly reduced supine and standing systolic and diastolic blood pressures; the combination was even more effective.

In a double-blind, randomized, crossover, placebo-controlled trial in 32 patients, Wilkinson and Raftery[266] compared the antihypertensive efficacies of clonidine and propranolol for 3 months. Both agents produced a significant reduction in blood pressure and were noted to be equipotent.

Weber et al.[267] conducted a two-part randomized, crossover trial in which 17 patients were divided into two groups. The patients in Group 1 received clonidine (0.3 mg/day) or propranolol (120 mg/day) during the first and third of three consecutive 6-week treatment periods. During the second treatment period, the two agents were combined. The protocol for Group 2 was the same as that for Group 1, except that prior to receiving clonidine or propranolol all patients received chlorthalidone 100 mg/day for 6 weeks, which was then continued throughout the trial period. In both groups, clonidine and propranolol reduced systolic and diastolic blood pressures, with clonidine having a slightly greater effect. The combination of clonidine and propranolol, with or without chlorthalidone, had a significantly greater effect than either agent alone.

In an open, randomized, placebo-controlled trial comparing the antihypertensive efficacies of captopril and propranolol, Friedlander[268] found that both agents produced a good response.

Seedat[269] found that captopril (maximal dose 450 mg/day) in combination with propranolol (maximal dose 360 mg/day) produced a significant reduction in blood pressure.

The comparative antihypertensive efficacies of captopril (25 to 150 mg three times daily for 12 weeks) and propranolol (20 to 120 mg three times daily for 12 weeks) were further assessed by Huang et al.[270] in a single-blind, placebo-controlled, randomized, parallel trial in 19 men. All 19 patients received the individual medications for 4 weeks. If the supine diastolic blood pressure was greater than 90 mm Hg at the end of 4 weeks, the other agent was added for 8 weeks. A significant reduction in supine diastolic and mean blood pressure was obtained in eight patients on captopril alone, and in four patients on propranolol alone. The remaining four patients in the captopril group had propranolol added without any further response. No further response was obtained when captopril was added to the three patients who had not initially responded to propranolol.

Eight patients participated in a placebo-controlled study comparing the antihypertensive efficacies of captopril and propranolol.[271] All patients received captopril (25, 50, and 100 mg three times daily, each for 1 week, and then three times daily for 4 weeks). Propranolol (20 mg three times daily) was added at the start of the fifth week, and was increased from 40 to 80 mg three times daily (each for a 1-week period). The mean supine blood pressure was significantly reduced with captopril. However, both the diastolic and mean supine blood pressures were reduced further when propranolol was added.

The antihypertensive effects of captopril (200 to 400 mg/day for 4 weeks), propranolol (120 to 160 mg/day for 4 weeks), and the combination of these two drugs for 4 weeks were assessed in a randomized, crossover trial in 13 patients conducted by Pickering et al.[272] A comparable reduction in supine, sitting, and standing systolic and diastolic blood pressures was obtained with both agents used alone. A further significant decrease was produced by the combination.

Studies Versus Calcium-Entry Blockers. Studies comparing the calcium-entry blockers to propranolol in the treatment of hypertension have recently been completed.

Aoki et al.[273] observed that the antihypertensive effects of nifedipine plus propranolol were greater than with nifedipine used alone.

In a double-blind, crossover study, Frishman et al.[274] observed that verapamil (480 mg/day) and propranolol (320 mg/day) were equally effective in reducing elevated blood pressure in patients with angina pectoris.

Studies Versus Multiple Drug Regimens. Prichard and Gillam,[275] using propranolol in a large number of patients previously treated with other antihypertensive regimens, found that propranolol achieved the best control of supine blood pressure, with the fewest side effects and the least incidence of postural hypotension. The average daily dose was 319 mg, with a maximum dose of 4000 mg/day.

Petrie et al.[276] conducted a double-blind, randomized, crossover, placebo-controlled comparison of the antihypertensive effects of methyldopa (750 mg/day for 4 weeks), propranolol (240 mg/day for 4 weeks), practolol (600 mg/day for 4 weeks), propranolol plus methyldopa (for 4 weeks), and methyldopa plus practolol (for 4 weeks) in 24 patients. The combination of methyldopa and propranolol was noted to be the most effective of the treatment regimens. Its effects were similar to the methyldopa–practolol combination, except that it produced a greater reduction in supine diastolic blood pressure. There was no difference in the antihypertensive efficacies of the individual agents.

West et al.[277] conducted a double-blind, crossover, randomized, placebo-controlled comparison of the antihypertensive effects of labetalol (300 mg twice daily for 6 weeks), propranolol (80 mg twice daily for 6 weeks), hydralazine (50 mg twice daily for 6 weeks), and propranolol plus hydralazine (for 6 weeks) in 12 patients who were receiving diuretics. Labetalol and propranolol produced comparable reductions in blood pressure. Labetalol was significantly better in reducing standing blood pressure than hydralazine. The combination of hydralazine and propranolol produced an equivalent reduction in standing blood pressure to that of labetalol alone. The combination had a greater effect than labetalol alone on supine blood pressure.

Sotalol
Sotalol (Betacardone, Sotacor) is not approved for hypertension in the United States.

Open Studies. In an open study by Gabriel,[278] 12 patients were controlled for three months on a once-daily sotalol regimen with a mean dose of 190 mg. Blood pressure control was maintained for at least 26 hours after the once-daily dose.

Pasquel[279] conducted an open study in which 15 patients received sotalol once daily (mean dose 341 mg/day). At the conclusion of the 12-week study period, a significant reduction in mean supine and standing systolic and diastolic blood pressures was noted for all 15 patients.

Double-Blind Trials. In a 24-week, double-blind, crossover, randomized trial conducted by Parvinen and Paukkala,[280,281] 30 patients whose blood pressure had been previously controlled with twice-daily sotalol (80 to 320 mg) were switched to the same dosage once daily for 8 weeks. No significant difference in blood pressure control was noted between the once-daily and twice-daily dosage regimens.

Studies Versus Other Antihypertensive Drugs. Jaattela[282] conducted a placebo-controlled, crossover trial in 25 patients comparing the antihypertensive effects of hydrochlorothiazide (25 to 100 mg/day for 1 month), sotalol (160 to 640 mg/day for 1 month), and the free and fixed combination (sotazide), each used for 1 month. Sotalol and hydrochlorothiazide used individually reduced supine and standing blood pressures when compared to placebo, without a difference noted in their effectiveness. The free and fixed combination produced an additional decrease in blood pressure, without any difference seen between the preparations.

In a follow-up study conducted by Jaattela,[283] 20 patients remained on their previously determined dosage of sotazide for 1 year. Mean supine and standing blood pressures at the end of the 12-month period were significantly reduced when compared to placebo but were unchanged from the end of the crossover period.

Eighteen patients participated in a placebo-controlled, crossover trial conducted by Basson and Myburgh.[284] The study was similar to that mentioned previously. Hydrochlorothiazide (25 mg to 100 mg once daily for 4 weeks) and sotalol (160 to 640 mg once daily for 4 weeks) were given individually as well as in free (for 4 weeks) and fixed combination (sotazide for 10 weeks). All blood pressure readings were taken 24 hours after the previous dose. Hydrochlorothiazide alone had no significant antihypertensive effect 24 hours postdose, whereas sotalol produced a significant reduction in blood pressure. Both combined preparations had a greater antihypertensive effect than either agent used alone.

The antihypertensive effect of the free combination of sotalol (160 mg once daily) and hydrochlorothiazide (25 mg once daily) for 3 months was assessed in a placebo-controlled study of 14 patients conducted by Reynaert.[285] A significant reduction in supine and standing systolic and diastolic blood pressures was noted with both regimens.

The antihypertensive efficacies of hydrochlorothiazide alone (25 to 50 mg once daily for 2 weeks) and the combination of hydrochlorothiazide (25 to 50 mg once daily) and sotalol (160 to 320 mg once daily) in a geriatric population (mean age 68 years) were assessed by Monsalvo[286] in a placebo-controlled study of 29 patients. Hydrochlorothiazide was found to significantly reduce mean supine diastolic blood pressure. The combination produced a further decrease in blood pressure.

Sundquist et al. found that on a weight basis, sotalol is significantly less potent than propranolol, with an effect on blood pressure that is closely dose-related in doses of 200 to 600 mg/day.[287]

The comparative antihypertensive efficacy of metoprolol (100 to 400 mg once daily for 16 weeks) and sotalol (160 to 640 mg once daily for 16 weeks) was assessed by Andersson et al. in a double-blind, randomized, crossover, placebo-controlled study in 26 patients.[288] Both drugs resulted in a significant reduction in standing and supine blood pressure, with no difference seen between them.

Comparative β-blocker studies with sotalol are also included in other sections of this chapter.

Saarima found that sotalol (80 mg twice daily) and clonidine (0.15 mg three times daily) used in combination had an antagonistic effect in six of ten elderly hypertensive patients studied.[289]

In contrast, Rowlands et al.[290] found that sotalol (40 mg three times daily—initial dose) in combination with bethanidine (5 mg three times daily—initial dose) was effective in reducing standing and supine systolic and diastolic blood pressures without a high incidence of side effects.

The comparative antihypertensive efficacies of sotalol (240 to 480 mg/day for 8 weeks) and methyldopa (750 to 3000 mg/day for 8 weeks) used individually and in combination (sotalol 160 to 400 mg plus methyldopa 250 to 2000 mg for 8 weeks), were assessed in 38 patients using a single-blind, crossover, randomized, placebo-controlled trial design.[291] The active treatments used alone and in combination produced significant and comparable reductions in supine and standing systolic and diastolic blood pressures.

Timolol

Timolol (Blocadren, Timolide) is approved for treatment of hypertension in a twice-daily dose and in a fixed diuretic combination.

Trials Versus Placebo. Rofman et al.[292] reported on a randomized, double-blind, multicenter trial of timolol in 355 patients with mild to moderate hypertension. After 12 weeks of treatment with either timolol 10 to 30 mg twice daily, or placebo, the mean supine blood pressure was 145/94 mm Hg (baseline 154/103) in the timolol group, and 155/102 mm Hg (baseline 156/103) in the placebo group. Fifty-seven percent (74/129) of the patients receiving timolol and 13 percent (15/114) of the patients receiving placebo had either a reduction in supine diastolic blood pressure to 90 mm Hg and below, or at least 10 mm Hg below baseline. The mean reduction in heart rate for the timolol group from baseline was 15 beats per minute.

Pawlowski[293] examined the efficacy of timolol used twice daily in a double-blind, randomized study in 30 hypertensive patients. The mean titrated dose of timolol was 24.6 mg, which reduced the supine systolic and diastolic blood pressures by an average of 40.2 and 24.3 mm Hg, respectively. The decrease in standing blood pressure was of the same magnitude, which indicates that there was no evidence of orthostatic hypotension. Timolol decreased the heart rate by 7.8 beats per minute.

Studies Versus Diuretics and Combination. Jennings et al.[294] compared the effectiveness of timolol administered once or twice daily with a diuretic in a double-blind trial in 15 patients with essential hypertension. The effectiveness of each regimen in reducing heart rate and blood pressure were similar.

LeBel et al.[295] added timolol to hydrochlorothiazide therapy to investigate the effect of combination therapy on blood pressure and plasma renin activity. In this double-blind study in 15 patients, combination therapy caused a significant decrease in supine and standing systolic and diastolic blood pressures and pulse rate. The mean plasma renin activity level was reduced from 6.7 to 1.6 ng/ml/hr. However, there were no significant correlations between changes in blood pressure and changes in plasma renin activity.

Oparil[296] compared the efficacy of timolol, hydrochlorothiazide, and the combination of both drugs in a double-blind, randomized trial in 97 patients with mild to moderate hypertension. The mean decreases in both supine and standing blood pressures were greater on the timolol-hydrochlorothiazide combination than either drug given alone.

Roginsky[297] evaluated the long-term efficacy of timolol combined with hydrochlorothiazide in 173 patients with mild to moderate hypertension. After 24 weeks, 86 percent of the patients had their diastolic blood pressure reduced by 10 mm Hg from baseline, or under 90 mm Hg. This good to excellent response continued with long-term follow-up in more than three-fourths of the patients. Eight patients (5 percent) were discontinued from treatment because of adverse side effects. Thirty-two of the patients had decreases in serum potassium of 0.5 mEq/L at various points, but clinical signs of hypokalemia were present in only one instance. An asymptomatic slowing of pulse rate by 10 to 15 beats per minute and a modest increase in mean blood urea nitrogen, blood sugar, cholesterol, and uric acid were observed.

In a double-blind, randomized, crossover trial in 38 patients with hypertension, Aronow et al.[298] compared the antihypertensive efficacies of the following regimens: hydrochlorothiazide 100 mg plus timolol 20 to 60 mg daily; hydrochlorothiazide alone; hydrochlorothiazide, timolol, plus hydralazine 40 to 200 mg daily; and hydrochlorothiazide plus hydralazine. Hydrochlorothiazide plus timolol was more effective than hydrochlorothiazide alone in lowering both supine and standing systolic and diastolic blood pressures. The hydrochlorothiazide, timolol, hydralazine combination also proved to be an effective regimen for lowering both supine and standing systolic and diastolic blood pressures. The patients also tolerated this regimen well, with a lower incidence of side effects, and greater hypotensive activity than with the hydrochlorothiazide–hydralazine combination.

ARRHYTHMIAS

β-Blockers are important drugs for the treatment of various cardiac arrhythmias (Table 5). A discussion of their possible modes of action in arrhythmia appears in Chapter 3. Before reviewing the results of the clinical trials with these agents, some general aspects regarding the individual arrhythmias in which β-blockade may have a role will be addressed. In general, β-blockers have been more effective for the treatment of supraventricular than ventricular arrhythmias. However, recent

TABLE 5. EFFECTS OF β-BLOCKERS IN VARIOUS ARRHYTHMIAS

Arrhythmia	Comment
Supraventricular	
Sinus tachycardia	Treat underlying disorder; excellent response to β-blocker, if need to control rate (e.g., ishcemia).
Atrial fibrillation	β-Blockers reduce rate, rarely restore sinus rhythm. May be useful in combination with digoxin.
Atrial flutter	β-Blockers reduce rate, sometimes restore sinus rhythm.
Atrial tachycardia	Effective in slowing ventricular rate, may restore sinus rhythm. Useful in prophylaxis.
Ventricular	
PVCs	Poor response to β-blockers, except digitalis-induced, exercise-(ischemia) induced, mitral valve prolapse, or hypertrophic cardiomyopathy.
Ventricular tachycardia	Usually not effective, except in digitalis toxicity or exercise-(ischemia) induced.
Ventricular fibrillation	Electrical defibrillation is treatment of choice. β-Blockers can be used to prevent recurrence in cases of excess digitalis or sympathomimetic amines. Appear to be effective in reducing the incidence of ventricular fibrillation and sudden death post-myocardial infarction.

studies in different postinfarction populations have clearly demonstrated the usefulness of β-blockers to treat ventricular tachyarrhythmias in the setting of myocardial ischemia.

Supraventricular Arrhythmias

These arrhythmias respond variably to β-blockade. β-Blockers may often be as useful diagnostically as they are therapeutically: by slowing a very rapid heart rate, the drug may allow for the establishment of an accurate ECG diagnosis of an otherwise puzzling arrhythmia.

Sinus Tachycardia. This arrhythmia usually has an obvious cause (e.g., hyperthyroidism, fever, congestive heart failure, etc.) and therapy should be addressed to correction of the underlying condition. However, if the rapid heart rate itself is compromising the patient, for example, causing recurrent angina in a patient with coronary artery disease, then direct intervention with β-blockers is effective and indicated therapy. Patients with heart failure, however, should not be treated with β-blockers unless they have been digitalized and placed on diuretic therapy, and then only with extreme caution.

Supraventricular Ectopic Beats. Again, specific treatment of these extrasystoles is seldom required, and is usually addressed to the underlying cause of the arrhythmia. These extrasystoles often herald the onset of atrial fibrillation, and there is no evidence to show that β-blockade can prevent its development. Supraventricular ectopic beats due to digitalis toxicity generally respond well to β-blockade. β-Blockers can be useful for those patients in whom supraventricular ectopic activity causes discomforting palpitations.

Paroxysmal Supraventricular Tachycardia. These may be divided into two groups: (1) those related to abnormal conduction (e.g., reciprocating AV nodal tachycardia; the reentrant tachycardias, as in the Wolff–Parkinson–White syndrome, in which there is abnormal conduction through an AV nodal bypass tract), and (2) those caused by ectopic atrial activity, as in digitalis toxicity. Since β-blockade delays AV conduction (increased AH interval in His bundle electrocardiograms) and prolongs the refractory period of the reentrant pathways, it is not surprising that many cases of paroxysmal supraventricular tachycardia respond to β-blockers. In acute episodes, vagal maneuvers after β-blockade may be effective in terminating an arrhythmia where they were unsuccessful without β-blockade. Even when β-blockers do not convert an arrhythmia to sinus rhythm, they will often slow the ventricular rate by increasing atrioventricular nodal refractoriness. Additionally, the use of β-blocking drugs still leaves the option of direct current countershock cardioversion (which would not be safe were digitalis in high doses used initially).

Atrial Flutter. β-Blockade can be used to slow the ventricular rate (by increasing AV block) and may restore sinus rhythm in a large percentage of patients. This is a situation in which β-blockade may be of diagnostic value: given intravenously, β-blockers slow the ventricular response and permit the differentiation of flutter waves, ectopic P-waves, or sinus mechanism.

Atrial Fibrillation. The major action of β-blockers in rapid atrial fibrillation is the reduction in the rapid ventricular response by increasing the refractory period of the AV node. All β-blocking drugs have been effective in slowing ventricular rates in patients with atrial fibrillation. However, they are less efficacious than quinidine or electrical cardioversion in the reversion of atrial fibrillation to sinus rhythm (although this can occur, especially when the atrial fibrillation is of recent onset). These drugs must be used cautiously when atrial fibrillation occurs in the setting of a severely diseased heart that is dependent on high levels of adrenergic tone to avoid myocardial failure. β-Blockers may be particularly useful in controlling the ventricular rate in situations where this is difficult to achieve with maximally tolerated doses of digitalis (e.g., thyrotoxicosis, hypertrophic cardiomyopathy, mitral stenosis, and the like).

Many patients who have paroxysmal atrial fibrillation or flutter may have "tachy-brady" or "sick sinus" syndrome, and administration of β-blockers may cause severe bradycardic episodes. These patients often require both antiarrhythmic therapy and a pacemaker.

Ventricular Arrhythmias

β-Blocking drugs can decrease the frequency of or abolish ventricular ectopic beats in various conditions. They are particularly useful if these arrhythmias are related to excessive catecholamines (e.g., exercise, halothane anesthesia, pheochromocytoma, exogenous catecholamines), myocardial ischemia, or digitalis.

Premature Ventricular Contractions. The response of these arrhythmias to β-blockade is variable. The best response can be expected to occur in ischemic heart disease, particularly when the arrhythmia is secondary to an ischemic event. Since β-blockers are effective in preventing ischemic episodes, they prevent the arrhythmias caused by the ischemia.

β-Blockers are also quite effective in controlling the frequency of premature ventricular contractions in hypertrophic cardiomyopathy and in mitral valve prolapse. In these situations, a β-blocker is generally the antiarrhythmic drug of first choice.

Ventricular Tachycardia. β-Blocking drugs should not be considered agents of choice in the treatment of acute ventricular tachycardia. Cardioversion or other antiarrhythmic drugs (lidocaine, quinidine, procainamide, or the like) should be the initial mode of therapy. β-Blockers have, however, been shown to be of benefit for prophylaxis against recurrent ventricular tachycardia, particularly if sympathetic stimulation appears to be a precipitating cause. There have been several reported studies showing the prevention of exercise-induced ventricular tachycardia by β-blockers; in many cases previously, there had been a poor response to digitalis or quinidine.[299–301]

Myocardial Infarction. There is now conclusive evidence to show that some β-adrenergic blockers will reduce the risk of mortality and reinfarction in survivors of an acute myocardial infarction.[302-304] Ventricular arrhythmias may also be favorably impacted. There is also preliminary data showing that β-blockers may reduce the amount of ischemic injury, the incidence of ventricular fibrillation and mortality during the hyperacute phase of myocardial infarction.[302,305-308] This subject is reviewed in greater detail in Chapter 10.

Clinical Studies

Acebutolol. Acebutolol (Sectral) is not approved for clinical use in arrhythmia.

In a double-blind study, Williams et al.[309] demonstrated the efficacy of treating supraventricular tachyarrhythmias with intravenous acebutolol in 15 patients. In the ten patients with atrial fibrillation, two with atrial flutter, two with multifocal atrial tachycardia, and one with premature atrial complexes, there was a significant reduction in heart rate 5 minutes after the drug was administered, with a peak reduction at 10 to 30 minutes. Two of ten patients with atrial fibrillation converted to normal sinus rhythm with β-blocker treatment.

Aronow et al.[310] demonstrated the efficacy of acebutolol in 20 patients with supraventricular tachyarrhythmias, five of whom had chronic obstructive pulmonary disease. All ten patients with atrial fibrillation and six with atrial flutter slowed their ventricular rates by more than 15 beats per minute. Atrial premature contractions were eliminated or reduced by greater than 75 percent in each of the two patients with this arrhythmia, and the one patient with multifocal atrial tachycardia converted to sinus rhythm. In this study, acebutolol was well tolerated by all five patients with chronic obstructive pulmonary disease.

De Soyza et al.[311] examined 60 patients by 24-hour ambulatory monitoring to determine the efficacy of acebutolol in treating ventricular arrhythmias. In a randomized, double-blind, placebo-controlled study using acebutolol 200 and 400 mg three times daily, these investigators showed a greater than 70 percent reduction in premature ventricular contractions per hour in greater than 50 percent of patients. The 400-mg dose appeared slightly more effective than the 200-mg dose in reducing ventricular ectopy.

In a double-blind, randomized study in 24 patients, Aronow et al.[312] compared intravenous acebutolol to propranolol for reducing premature ventricular contractions. In 10 of the 12 patients on propranolol or acebutolol, premature ventricular contractions were abolished or reduced by 75 percent or more. Singh et al.[313] confirmed the comparative efficacies of propranolol and acebutolol for decreasing premature ventricular contractions both at rest and with exercise.

In a randomized, double-blind, crossover trial in 20 patients, Shapiro et al.[314] compared the antiarrhythmic effects of acebutolol to slow-release quinidine sulfate, for reducing premature ventricular contractions. There was no significant difference between the two treatment groups, with 9 of 20 in the acebutolol group and 8 of 20 in the quinidine group demonstrating a reduction in premature ventricular contractions of greater than 75 percent.

Atenolol. Atenolol (Tenormin) is not approved for clinical use in arrhythmias.

Winchester et al.[315] treated 29 patients with supraventricular arrhythmias with two different intravenous β-blockers. Seventeen received intravenous atenolol 0.15 mg/kg for 20 minutes, and 12 received intravenous acebutolol 1.0 mg/kg for 15 minutes. Eleven of 12 patients with atrial flutter or fibrillation had their ventricular rate reduced to less than 100 beats per minute, including one conversion to sinus rhythm. Of the 16 patients with paroxysmal supraventricular tachycardia, four had their heart rate slowed to less than 100 beats per minute, five had no change in heart rate, and seven reverted to sinus rhythm. All six treatment failures occurred in patients with acute arrhythmias, whereas all patients with chronic arrhythmias responded. No differences in the antiarrhythmic efficacies of the two drugs were observed.

Rossi et al.[305] assessed the efficacy of intravenous atenolol in the treatment of ventricular arrhythmias in 182 patients suspected of an acute myocardial infarction. Ninety-five patients were randomized to receive intravenous atenolol followed by oral treatment, and 87 patients received placebo. The treated patients had significantly fewer ventricular extrasystoles. Repetitive ventricular arrhythmias were detected in 64 control patients (74 percent) and in 55 placebo-treated patients (58 percent). R on T wave arrhythmias occurred in 58 control patients (67 percent), compared with only 25 treated patients. These investigators confirmed that early intravenous atenolol prevents ventricular arrhythmias in patients with suspected acute myocardial infarction.

Roland et al.[316] used 24-hour electrocardiographic tape recordings to determine the incidence of arrhythmias in 388 patients with suspected myocardial infarction who were receiving either propranolol, atenolol, or placebo. Seventy-six percent of patients with a diagnosed myocardial infarction had ventricular arrhythmias compared to 24 percent of patients in whom a myocardial infarction was not substantiated. After monitoring patients for 6 weeks, the incidence of arrhythmias was similar with propranolol, atenolol, and placebo. There was no difference in the incidence or type of arrhythmias recorded between patients who died and those who were still alive at 6 weeks. These investigators hypothesized that since the β-blockers used in this study showed little evidence of antiarrhythmic activity, increasing the dosage would not be prudent because of the risk of hypotension.

With results different than those of Roland et al.,[316] Yusuf et al.[317] studied 477 patients suspected of having an acute myocardial infarction, and randomly assigned them treatment with intravenous and oral atenolol or placebo. Atenolol treatment significantly prevented the development of infarction compared to placebo in patients who presented with no electrocardiographic changes. One hundred eighty of these patients were analyzed for ventricular arrhythmias by 24-hour ECG monitoring. There was a significant reduction in the incidence of R on T ectopic beats in the atenolol-treated group (26 percent) compared to the 67 percent incidence in the placebo group. In the atenolol-treated patients, there was a significant reduction in repetitive ventricular arrhythmias, and a marginally significant reduction in supraventricular arrhythmias, most significantly in the incidence of atrial fibrillation. These investigators noted fewer cardiac arrests in the atenolol-treated group, but could not definitely implicate an antiarrhythmic effect for their observations.

Esmolol (ASL-8052). Esmolol is a new ultra-short-acting (half-life possibly 10 minutes) β$_1$-selective adrenergic blocker that is only available in intravenous form. It is still in the early stages of clinical testing and is not yet approved for clinical use in the United States.

Preliminary studies have shown the drug to be both effective and safe when used either as a pulse dose or drip infusion to treat various supraventricular and ventricular arrhythmias.[318,319]

Labetalol. Labetalol (Trandate, Normodyne) is a new α$_1$-blocking, nonselective β-adrenergic blocker that is not approved for clinical use in arrhythmia.

Preliminary studies have shown the drug to be both safe and effective for treating hypertensive patients with varied supraventricular and ventricular arrhythmias (see Chapter 7).[320,321]

Metoprolol. Metoprolol (Lopressor, Betacore) is not approved for clinical use in arrhythmia.

Moller and Ringquist[322] treated 21 patients with paroxysmal supraventricular tachyarrhythmias, atrial flutter, and atrial fibrillation. Using 2 to 20 mg of intravenous metoprolol, approximately 50 percent of the patients with paroxysmal supraventricular tachycardia and atrial flutter converted to normal sinus rhythm, compared to one of eight patients with atrial fibrillation. Of those patients who did not convert to normal sinus rhythm, there was still a significant lowering of the ventricular rate.

These findings were confirmed by Rehnquist,[323] who performed a multicenter study involving 142 patients; 28 had paroxysmal atrial tachycardia, 35 atrial flutter, and 79 atrial fibrillation. Given a regimen of 5 to 15 mg of metoprolol intravenously, 57 percent of the patients with paroxysmal atrial tachycardia, 23 percent with atrial flutter, and 13 percent with atrial fibrillation converted to normal sinus rhythm. A ventricular rate reduction of more than 25 percent, or less than 100 beats per minute was obtained in 68 percent of the patients, with an additional 18 percent showing a reduction of 10 percent in ventricular rate.

Metoprolol and its antiarrhythmic effects in 106 post-MI patients were studied by Olsson et al.[324] In a double-blind trial using placebo or oral metoprolol, 100 mg twice daily, the investigators followed patients for 6 months after their myocardial infarcts. There was a significant decrease in malignant premature ventricular contractions at one month with metoprolol, which was not observed at 6 months.

In a double-blind, placebo-controlled trial, Whitehead[325] followed 60 dental patients who underwent general anesthesia. After induction, he noted a lower mean heart rate in the metoprolol group (86 beats per minute), compared to placebo (98 beats per minute). Runs of ventricular premature contractions occurred in 12 patients on placebo and in only 4 on metoprolol.

Ryden et al.[306] analyzed the effects of intravenous and oral metoprolol on ventricular arrhythmias in 1395 patients suspected of having a myocardial infarction. In their double-blind, placebo-controlled, randomized study, patients received either placebo or 15 mg of metoprolol intravenously at the time of admission, and then 200 mg daily for 3 months. Metoprolol did not influence the occurrence of premature ventricular contractions or reduce the incidence of ventricular tachycardia episodes, but of the 23 patients with ventricular fibrillation in this study, only 6 were from the metoprolol group. It was suggested from these findings that metoprolol has a prophylactic effect against ventricular fibrillation in patients with acute myocardial infarction.

Nadolol. Nadolol (Corgard) is not approved for clinical use in arrhythmia.

Like other β-adrenoceptor blocking drugs, nadolol has antiarrhythmic properties that stem from its ability to antagonize the effects of catecholamines on cardiac automaticity and conductivity.[213,326,327] Although the electrophysiologic properties of nadolol are known, there are not enough clinical data on its effects in arrhythmia.

Vukovich et al.[328] treated 29 patients with ventricular and supraventricular arrhythmias with sequential oral doses of placebo and nadolol. A reduction or remission of arrhythmias was observed in approximately two-thirds of the patients. Arrhythmias that responded favorably to nadolol therapy included ventricular bigeminy and trigeminy, paroxysmal supraventricular tachycardia, and sinus tachycardia. The patients with atrial flutter or fibrillation did not convert to normal sinus rhythm with nadolol therapy, but did demonstrate a reduced ventricular response.

Nadolol might prove extremely useful in long-term management of cardiac arrhythmias because of its long plasma half-life that requires once daily administration; however, more clinical data are necessary to establish the efficacy of a single daily dose of nadolol or any other long-acting β-blocker in patients with arrhythmias.

Oxprenolol. Oxprenolol (Trasicor, Iset) is not approved for clinical use in arrhythmia.

Sandler et al.[329] studied the efficacy of intravenous and oral oxprenolol for the treatment of various cardiac arrhythmias in 43 patients with acute myocardial ischemia or infarctions. Thirteen of 27 episodes of paroxysmal supraventricular tachycardia were controlled. Only two of six episodes of supraventricular ectopia were abolished by oxprenolol. None of the seven episodes of atrial fibrillation reverted to sinus rhythm, and in only three of the seven patients did the ventricular rate fall below 100 beats per minute. Oxprenolol abolished premature ventricular contractions in 13 of 18 episodes, and two of three patients with idioventricular rhythm converted to normal sinus rhythm. Both patients with ventricular tachycardia failed to respond to oxprenolol treatment, and developed a hypotensive reaction.

Fuccella et al.[330] examined the efficacy of oral oxprenolol treatment in 98 patients with cardiac arrhythmias. Fifteen of 22 patients with sinus tachycardia converted to sinus rhythm and 6 of the remaining 7 had a decrease in heart rate. Of six patients with paroxysmal atrial fibrillation, the attacks completely disappeared in three, and decreased in frequency in another two. Only in 4 of the 28 patients with chronic atrial fibrillation did the fibrillation disappear, but in 19 a decrease in heart rate was observed. Since only six patients with atrial flutter were treated, no conclusion could be drawn regarding the efficacy of oxprenolol for this arrhythmia. Six of eight patients with supraventricular extrasystolies experienced a complete disappearance of this arrhythmia, with the two remaining patients experiencing a decrease in frequency. Of the 16 patients with ventricular extrasystoles, 5 had a complete disappearance of the arrhythmia, with 6 of the remaining patients experiencing a decreased incidence.

The effects of oxprenolol were examined in a large placebo-controlled trial in 1103 survivors of an acute myocardial infarction.[331] An antiarrhythmic effect with oxprenolol could explain the reduction in mortality observed when drug treatment was started within 4 months of infarction.

Pindolol. Pindolol (Visken) is not approved for the treatment of arrhythmia.

Multiple clinical trials have shown pindolol, with partial agonist activity, to be as efficacious as propranolol for the treatment of supraventricular arrhythmias.[92,332]

Frishman et al.[333] evaluated intravenous and oral pindolol in 18 patients with supraventricular tachyarrhythmias (paroxysmal atrial tachycardia, atrial fibrillation, and flutter) who had been responsive to propranolol treatment, but where long-term maintenance with propranolol was not possible because of drug-induced bronchospasm. All 18 patients failed to respond to an initial intravenous placebo, after which they received intravenous pindolol (0.4 to 1.4 mg). Six of seven patients with paroxysmal supraventricular tachycardia converted to normal sinus rhythm. In the six patients with atrial fibrillation, three converted to normal sinus rhythm, and three demonstrated only ventricular rate slowing. Of the two patients with atrial flutter, one converted to normal sinus rhythm, and one had no response. Both patients with junctional tachycardia converted to normal sinus rhythm, as did the one patient with multifocal atrial tachycardia. The 16 patients who responded to intravenous pindolol therapy received oral therapy (2.5 to 10 mg every 6 hours), and on this regimen a long-term antiarrhythmic benefit was maintained in 12 of 16 patients.

Aronow et al.[334] studied the efficacy of intravenous pindolol in 30 patients with various cardiac arrhythmias. All seven patients with atrial fibrillation reduced their ventricular rate, with two patients converting to normal sinus rhythm. A rapid ventricular rate was reduced in six of seven patients with atrial flutter. Three of these seven patients converted to atrial fibrillation, and two of these were converted to normal sinus rhythm. One patient with atrial tachycardia became hypotensive after the second dose of pindolol. Two patients with atrioventricular junctional tachycardia, three with sinus tachycardia, and three with atrial premature contractions were converted to normal sinus rhythm. Paroxysmal repetitive ventricular tachycardia due to digitalis toxicity was abolished in one patient. Pindolol abolished or greatly reduced frequent premature ventricular beats in 10 out of 14 patients. Thus, pindolol was useful for the treatment of cardiac arrhythmias in 24 of these 30 patients.

Podrid et al.[335] studied 43 patients to determine the efficacy of pindolol in treating ventricular arrhythmias. Of these patients, 23 had coronary heart disease, 5 had valvular disease, and 15 had no demonstrable heart disease. The efficacy of pindolol during acute and maintenance therapy was assessed by ambulatory ECG monitoring and treadmill exercise testing. Pindolol was most effective in preventing ventricular arrhythmias provoked by exercise, suppressing premature ventricular beats in 53 percent of patients. Eighty percent of patients without demonstrable heart disease had suppression of exercise-induced arrhythmias while they were receiving pindolol, whereas patients with coronary heart disease had a 50 percent suppression rate. These investigators concluded that pindolol was most effective when ventricular arrhythmias occur with exercise, especially in patients with no structural heart disease. However, pindolol has a limited role as a monotherapy for suppressing ventricular arrhythmias in patients with known coronary artery disease.

A recent electrophysiologic study demonstrated that pindolol's effect on the ventricular fibrillation threshold was not as pronounced as with other β-blockers. This study suggested that β-blockers with partial agonism may not be as effective in preventing sudden death.[336]

Propranolol. Propranolol (Inderal) is approved in intravenous and oral form for the treatment of supraventricular tachyarrhythmias. There have been multiple studies confirming the effectiveness of oral and intravenous propranolol for these arrhythmias.[337-340] Recent studies have also demonstrated the efficacy of the drug for treating ventricular arrhythmias.[307,308]

Frieden et al.[341] treated 30 patients with sustained or recurrent atrial arrhythmias who were treated unsuccessfully with agents such as digoxin, quinidine, diphenylhydantoin, and procainamide. In all ten patients with atrial fibrillation, the ventricular rate slowed to less than 100 beats per minute; three were converted to normal sinus rhythm. Seven of 12 patients with paroxysmal supraventricular arrhythmias were maintained in sinus rhythm with infrequent attacks, and the other five had no attacks for 22 months. Three of four patients with persistent sinus tachycardia were successfully treated with propranolol. Four patients in the study were unable to tolerate the drug because of gastrointestinal side effects and excessive bradycardia.

For the elective therapy of cardiac arrhythmias during an acute myocardial infarction, Lemberg et al.[342] reported favorably on the use of propranolol. The arrhythmias included atrial fibrillation, atrial flutter, paroxysmal tachycardia, and ventricular tachycardia. A majority of the patients responded to a total intravenous dose of less than 5 mg of propranolol.

Propranolol has also been shown to be an effective agent for preventing the supraventricular tachyarrhythmias that frequently occur after coronary artery bypass surgery.[343–346] Many of these arrhythmias are caused by the abrupt withdrawal of propranolol just prior to surgery (see Chapter 12).

In assessing the correct propranolol dose for arrhythmia treatment, Woosley et al. have suggested that higher oral doses of propranolol be used than those needed to treat hypertension.[347] In a study of 32 patients with chronic high-frequency ventricular arrhythmias, dosages were increased sequentially until arrhythmia suppression was achieved, side effects appeared, or a maximum dosage of 960 mg/day was reached. At dosages of less than 160 mg/day, only 33 percent responded with a 70 percent or greater decrease in ventricular ectopic beats. At daily dosages of 200 to 640 mg, an additional 40 percent responded. Since the response rate for this clinical trial was higher than that observed in other studies, the investigators stress the need for a more individualized approach to patient therapy.

These same investigators[347] also showed that the plasma concentration needed for ventricular arrhythmia treatment was higher than that needed for β-blockade. This raises the possibility that a mechanism such as membrane stabilization activity may be clinically important. It was also noted that suppression of renin release also occurs at the high dosage level and, therefore, might play a role in arrhythmia suppression.

Gibson and Sowton[348] reviewed 125 controlled cases of resting ventricular arrhythmia treated with propranolol 25 mg intravenously, or 30 to 120 mg orally per day. Ventricular arrhythmias were suppressed in 44 percent and decreased in an additional 13 percent of the patients.

Nixon et al.[349] studied the efficacy of propranolol in decreasing the frequency of exercise-induced ventricular ectopic activity in 15 patients. Using individually titrated doses, 10 patients had an effective reduction in exercise-induced ventricular ectopy. Propranolol therapy abolished ventricular tachycardia in four patients, and ventricular couplets in 8 of 12 patients.

Koppes et al.[307] evaluated the use of propranolol in treating premature ventricular beats in 32 patients within 2 months of an uncomplicated acute myocardial infarction. All patients at baseline had more than 30 premature ventricular beats per hour, with bigeminy, couplets, multifocal complexes, or ventricular tachycardia. With an average dose of 160 mg of propranolol daily, a significant decrease in the frequency and complexity of premature ventricular beats was noted compared to control. During treatment, 50 percent of patients had a 70 percent or greater suppression of premature ventricular beats, and in 41 percent of patients, a 90 percent or greater suppression of premature ventricular beats was observed. Koppes suggested that a decrease in ventricular arrhythmias induced by propranolol may have a favorable effect in reducing the risk of sudden cardiac death.

In the β-Blocker Heart Attack Trial, the largest controlled study of its kind to date, Lichstein et al.[350] evaluated the effects of propranolol and placebo on ventricular arrhythmias in survivors of an acute myocardial infarction. Ventricular arrhythmia was defined as a premature ventricular complex frequency of more than 10 per hour per day with ambulatory ECG monitoring. The ambulatory ECG was recorded at baseline before treatment, and again 6 weeks later. At baseline, 8.0 percent of patients randomized to propranolol and 9.1 percent of patients randomized to placebo had ventricular arrhythmias. The frequency of ventricular arrhythmias at six weeks in the propranolol-treated group was 14.9 percent compared to 27.3 percent in the placebo-treated group. In those patients with arrhythmias at baseline, only 56 percent (14/25) of the propranolol-treated patients compared to 69 percent (20/29) of the placebo-treated patients continued to have ventricular arrhythmias. It was also observed that at 6 weeks, 12 percent of the propranolol-treated patients compared to 23.5 percent of the placebo-treated patients developed arrhythmias that were not observed during the baseline study.

Hansteen et al.[351] studied 560 high-risk survivors of acute myocardial infarction at 12 Norwegian hospitals. The main purpose of this randomized, double-blind study was to determine the efficacy and safety of propranolol 160 mg/day on the incidence of sudden cardiac death over a 12-month treatment period. A 52 percent reduction in the rate of sudden cardiac death was noted with propranolol treatment compared to placebo (11 deaths in the propranolol group compared to 23 in the placebo group). The incidence of ventricular arrhythmias was also noted to be more frequent in the placebo-treated patients when compared to patients receiving propranolol.

Sotalol. Sotalol (Sotacor) differs electrophysiologically from other β-blockers, since, in high concentrations, it prolongs the duration of the action potential in ventricular muscle and Purkinje fibers. Sotalol thus possesses the properties of a Class III antiarrhythmic agent, in addition to the Class II antiarrhythmic actions shared by all other β-adrenoceptor blocking drugs. Sotalol prolongs the ECG QT interval, which can predispose to reentrant ventricular arrhythmias by enhancing temporal dispersion. The drug is not approved for clinical use in the United States.

Latour et al.[352] studied the efficacy of intravenous sotalol using doses of 20 to 60 mg in 20 patients with various cardiac arrhythmias. Sotalol was beneficial in two of two patients with sinus tachycardia and in four of seven patients with other supraventricular tachyarrhythmias. The drug was particularly efficacious in lidocaine-resistant ventricular arrhythmias, where it was effective in 9 of 11 patients.

Fogelman et al.[353] treated 34 patients with cardiac arrhythmias of varying etiology with 20 mg of intravenous sotalol. Five of the six patients with paroxysmal supraventricular tachycardia and none of the five patients with atrial flutter reverted to normal sinus rhythm. In the four patients with an acute onset of atrial ectopia, complete abolition of ectopic beats occurred in three, and in the fourth the incidence of ectopic beats was decreased from 50 to 4 ectopic beats per minute. In four of six patients with the acute onset of premature ventricular contractions, the ectopic beats were abolished, and, in the remaining two, they were reduced. Two of three patients with chronic ventricular arrhythmias demonstrated a reduced incidence of premature ventricular contractions, while the third patient had an increase in the ectopia from 9 to 20 beats per minute. Three of the five patients with the acute onset of atrial fibrillation converted to normal sinus rhythm, with the cardiac rate slowing in the remaining two. None of the nine patients with chronic atrial fibrillation converted to normal sinus rhythm, but the cardiac rate was significantly reduced in seven of the nine patients. No patient with ventricular tachycardia reverted to sinus rhythm with sotalol treatment. These investigators concluded that sotalol was effective for the treatment of supraventricular tachycardias, the acute onset of atrial and ventricular ectopias, and the acute onset of atrial fibrillation.

Prakash et al.[354] studied the antiarrhythmic efficacy of sotalol in 18 patients with supraventricular arrhythmias and in seven patients with ventricular arrhythmias. Four of six patients with paroxysmal supraventricular tachycardia converted to normal sinus rhythm. In an additional six patients with episodic supraventricular tachycardia, sotalol prevented further recurrences in two. Two of six patients with atrial flutter converted to normal sinus rhythm, but in the other four patients with atrial flutter and in another patient with atrial fibrillation, the ventricular response was slowed from an average of 150 to 60 beats per minute. In one patient with paroxysmal atrial fibrillation and in another with paroxysmal ventricular tachycardia, sotalol prevented recurrences in both. In one out of two patients, sotalol decreased the frequency of premature atrial contractions, and in five patients with premature ventricular contractions it abolished the arrhythmias in one and reduced the frequency of the ectopia in the other four. These investigators concluded that sotalol is a moderately effective antiarrhythmic drug.

Simon et al.[355] studied 38 patients with various cardiac arrhythmias for an average period of 5.9 months. Of the 38 patients, 16 received intravenous sotalol, electrocardioversion, or both, to restore sinus rhythm; 13 patients responded to intravenous sotalol alone. Eleven of these 13 (84.6 percent) converted to normal sinus rhythm. Nineteen of the 22 patients who received oral therapy were well controlled, with restoration of sinus rhythm; in nine of nine patients with paroxysmal supraventricular tachycardia, one of one with atrial flutter, three of four with atrial fibrillation, two of three with paroxysmal ventricular tachycardia, and four of five with premature ventricular contractions. Overall, 35 of 38 patients showed improvement of their arrhythmias on sotalol therapy. Of the three patients who did not improve, two had atrial fibrillation and one had premature ventricular contractions. After discontinuing oral sotalol therapy for 1 to 3 months, 14 of the original 38 patients were given a second course of sotalol treatment for an additional period of up to 9 months. Three of the six patients with paroxysmal supraventricular tachycardia abolished their arrhythmia, while the other three demonstrated a reduced frequency of the arrhythmia. Of the four patients with paroxysmal ventricular tachycardia, the severity of arrhythmic episodes decreased in one and disappeared in three. The three patients with atrial fibrillation and the one with atrial flutter were converted to normal sinus rhythm.

In a multicenter, double-blind, randomized study, Julian et al.[356] studied the effect of sotalol 320 mg once daily, compared with placebo in 1456 patients who survived an acute myocardial infarction. Treatment was started 5 to 14 days after infarction, and patients were followed for 12 months. The mortality rate was 7.3 percent in the sotalol group, compared to 8.9 percent in the placebo group. The mortality was 18 percent lower in the sotalol than in the placebo group, but the difference was not statistically significant. This study suggested that the Class III antiarrhythmic effects of sotalol are not clinically important, since β-blockers lacking this property appear to be as effective in post-MI therapy.

Timolol. Timolol (Blocadren) is not approved for clinical use in arrhythmia.

Timolol was shown to reduce the incidence of total mortality, nonfatal reinfarction, and sudden death after 1 year of treatment in survivors of an acute myocardial infarction. In this study, there were 17 patients with arrhythmia in the timolol treatment group who required withdrawal from the study versus 38 patients on placebo treatment.[303] These findings demonstrated a probable antiarrhythmic effect for the active drug.

In a sub-project of the above study, timolol appeared to reduce the incidence of complex ventricular arrhythmias in high-risk patients up to 6 months after infarction when compared to placebo treatment.[357]

OTHER CARDIOVASCULAR APPLICATIONS

Although β-blockers have been studied extensively in patients with angina pectoris, arrhythmia and hypertension, they have also been shown to be safe and effective for a host of other cardiovascular conditions (Table 1). Some of these conditions are described below.

Hypertrophic Cardiomyopathy

β-Adrenoceptor blocking drugs have been proven to be efficacious in the therapy of patients with hypertrophic cardiomyopathy or idiopathic hypertrophic subaortic stenosis (IHSS).[358–360] These drugs are useful in controlling the symptoms: dyspnea, angina, and syncope.[361] β-Blockers have also been shown to lower the intraventricular pressure gradient both at rest and with exercise.

The outflow pressure gradient is not the only abnormality in hypertrophic cardiomyopathy; more important is the loss of ventricular compliance, which impedes normal left ventricular functioning. It has been shown by invasive and noninvasive methods that propranolol can improve left ventricular function in this condition.[362] The drug also produces favorable changes in ventricular compliance while it relieves patient symptoms. Propranolol is approved for this condition and may be combined with the calcium-channel blocker verapamil in patients not responding to the β-blocker alone.

The salutary hemodynamic and symptomatic effects produced by propranolol derive from its inhibition of sympathetic stimulation to the heart.[363,364] However, there is no evidence that the drug alters the primary cardiomyopathic process; many patients remain in or return to their severely symptomatic state, and some die despite its administration.[359,360]

There has been limited experience, except for anecdotal reports with other β-blockers (other than practolol), in the therapy of hypertrophic cardiomyopathy. One might suspect that a β-blocker with partial agonist activity might be less efficacious than propranolol. This was suggested by the finding of less clinical improvement with practolol than propranolol in a comparative study of patients with hypertrophic cardiomyopathy.[362]

Mitral Valve Prolapse

This auscultatory complex, characterized by a nonejection systolic click, a late systolic murmur, or a midsystolic click followed by a late systolic murmur, has been studied extensively over the last 15 years.[365] Atypical chest pain, malignant arrhythmias, and nonspecific ST and T wave abnormalities have been observed with this condition. β-Adrenergic blockers, by decreasing sympathetic tone, have been shown to be useful for relieving the chest pains and palpitations that many of these patients experience and for reducing the incidence of life-threatening arrhythmias and other ECG abnormalities.[366]

Dissecting Aneurysms

β-Adrenergic blockade plays a major role in the treatment of patients with acute aortic dissection. During the hyperacute phase, the administration of β-blocking agents is mandatory to reduce the force and velocity of myocardial contraction (dp/dt) and, hence, progression of the dissecting hematoma.[6,367] Moreover, such administration must be initiated simultaneously with the institution of other antihypertensive therapy that may cause reflex tachycardia and increases in cardiac output, factors that could aggravate the dissection process. Initially, propranolol is administered intravenously to reduce the heart rate below 60 beats per minute. Once a patient is stabilized and long-term medical management is contemplated, the patient should be maintained on oral β-blocker therapy to prevent the recurrence.[368]

Recently, it has been demonstrated that long-term β-blocker therapy might also reduce the risk of dissection in patients prone to this complication (e.g., Marfan's syndrome). Systolic time intervals are used to assess the adequacy of β-blockade in children with Marfan's syndrome.

Tetralogy of Fallot

By reducing the effects of increased adrenergic tone on the right ventricular infundibulum in tetralogy of Fallot, β-blockers have been shown to be useful for the treatment of severe hypoxic spells and hypercyanotic attacks.[9] With chronic use, the drugs have also been shown to prevent prolonged hypoxic spells.[9] These drugs should only be looked at as palliative, and definitive surgical repair of this condition is usually required.

Q-T Interval Syndromes

The syndrome of ECG Q-T interval prolongation is usually a congenital condition associated with deafness, syncope, and sudden death.[8] Abnormalities in sympathetic nervous system functioning in the heart have been proposed as explanations for the electrophysiologic aberrations seen in these patients.[8] Propranolol appears to be the most effective drug for treatment of this syndrome. It reduces the frequency of syncopal episodes in the majority of patients, and may prevent sudden death.[8] The drug will reduce the ECG Q-T interval.

NONCARDIOVASCULAR APPLICATIONS

β-Blockers are now being used for a variety of noncardiovascular conditions (Table 2). Some of the conditions for which β-blocker treatment have been considered are described below.

Thyrotoxicosis

Many of the symptomatic and physical manifestations of thyrotoxicosis resemble those produced by the sympathetic nervous system or by the administration of catecholamines.[369–373] The physiologic basis for these sympathomimetic features of thyroid hormone excess is obscure, but there are a number of possible mechanisms: enhanced tissue sensitivity to catecholamines, due to increased numbers of β-receptors,[374] to more efficient coupling of catecholamine binding to activation of adenyl cyclase, or to inhibition of tissue phosphodiesterase activity[375]; increased delivery of circulating catecholamines, due to increased tissue perfusions; and the occurrence of similar but separate and additive effects of thyroid hormones and catecholamines.[373,376]

Despite the inability to define precisely the relationship between catecholamines and hyperthyroidism, certain antiadrenergic agents are capable of alleviating many of the sympathomimetic manifestations of the thyrotoxic state.[377,378] Since these drugs act within the peripheral tissues, their symptomatic effect is much more prompt than that of traditional approaches to treating hyperthyroidism, which achieve their effects by decreasing thyroid hormone synthesis or release.[373] Therefore, antiadrenergic agents like reserpine, guanethidine, and β-blockers have particular value in treating severely thyrotoxic patients.[377,378] Because of their relative freedom from side effects, ease of administration, and rapid onset of action, β-blockers are the agents of choice.[373] Although the largest experience has been garnered with propranolol, other β-blockers with and without β_1-selectivity have also proven useful.[379–383]

The exact mechanism of β-blocker benefit in hyperthyroidism is not fully defined. It is not definitely known whether the effects of β-blockade are mediated by adrenergic blockade or, as recently proposed, by blocking the peripheral conversion of T_4 to T_3.[384]

Particular benefit has been obtained with β-blocking drugs in the management of thyrotoxic excess (thyrotoxic storm).[385] In this situation, β-blockade produces a rapid reduction in fever, heart rate, and adverse central nervous system effects, such as restlessness and disorientation. Most of the experience with β-blockers to date in "thyroid storm" has been reported with propranolol, although other β-blockers may also be effective.[385] β-Blockers have also been used preoperatively in thyrotoxic patients undergoing partial thyroidectomy and other surgical procedures.[386,387]

As part of routine medical management for hyperthyroidism, β-blocking drugs are of less certain value. All are capable of reducing the heart rate, although drugs with partial agonist activity are probably less effective.[388] Other manifestations of thyrotoxicosis—tremor, hyperreflexia, agitation, hemodynamic changes, hyperkinesia and those eye signs attributable to sympathetically innervated smooth muscle—may be reduced by both $β_1$-selective and nonselective β-blockers.[373,387–391]

When employed chronically as the sole therapeutic agent, β-blockers alleviate but do not eliminate the symptomatic and physiologic manifestations of thyrotoxicosis.[373] The drugs have no effect on thyroid hormone secretion, the peripheral disposal of the hormone, or the thyrotropic or prolactin responses to thyrotropin-releasing hormone.[392] Patients fail to gain weight satisfactorily, and evidence for an increased metabolic rate persists.[393] Consequently, β-blockers cannot be considered a substitute for specific antithyroid therapies.

Prophylaxis of Migraine

The use of β-adrenergic blocking drugs to prevent migraine headache was first suggested by Rabkin et al. in 1966.[394] These investigators and others reported a beneficial effect of propranolol on migraine headaches in patients being treated for angina pectoris or arrhythmia. These early observations led to clinical trials that confirmed the safety and efficacy of propranolol for the prophylaxis of common migraine[395,396]; the FDA approved the drug for this indication in 1979. Propranolol is not approved for the treatment of migraine headache or for the prevention and treatment of cluster headaches.

The causes of vascular-headache syndromes, including common migraine, are not well defined.[397] Therefore, the exact mechanisms of propranolol activity in the prevention of migraine are not known. Other β-blockers may also be effective in migraine (nadolol), but they need more intensive study. The use of propranolol for migraine is based on the fact that the drug concentrates in the brain and presumably inhibits β-adrenoceptor-mediated vasodilatation. Dilatation of branches of the external carotid artery is assumed to be one source of pain during an episode of migraine. Propranolol may also prevent the uptake of serotonin by platelets and thereby increase the amount of extracellular serotonin, which is then available for vasotonic actions on cerebral blood flow.[398]

Propranolol decreases the frequency of common migraine and can completely suppress headaches in some patients. One-third of patients with common migraine have an excellent response to propranolol, with a more than 50 percent reduction in the number of attacks and a markedly reduced need for ergotamine and analgesic medication; another third have a smaller reduction in the number of attacks; and the remaining third either have no response or become worse.[399] In a recent comparative trial, propranolol was demonstrated to be as effective as methysergide in reducing the frequency and severity of migraine headaches.[400] However, fewer adverse reactions were seen during propranolol treatment.[400] Direct comparisons with other prophylactic regimens for migraine (cyproheptadine, tricyclic antidepressants, papaverine, and monoamine oxidase inhibitors) have not been made.[401]

Daily administration of any prophylactic medication is warranted only when headaches of moderate to severe intensity occur several times a month. For prevention of migraine, the initial amount is 80 mg daily in divided doses. The usual range of effective doses is 160 to 240 mg daily; the dose may be increased gradually to 480 mg daily to achieve a better response. Several reports have appeared on the combined use of propranolol and ergot preparations; this combination apparently had no untoward effects.[400] Severe migraine attacks have been reported to follow abrupt withdrawal from propranolol. It is recommended that the drug be gradually withdrawn over a 2-week period if the maximal dosage has not produced a satisfactory response within 4 to 6 weeks. Adverse reactions in patients receiving propranolol for migraine are similar to those in patients given this drug for hypertension or angina pectoris.[401]

Tremor

There is evidence that β_2-receptors are found in skeletal muscle, and that heightened adrenergic activity may play a role in some varieties of tremor.[402,403] Propranolol is reportedly useful in the treatment of action tremors, including essential, familial, and senile tremors, and familial essential myoclonus.[404-406] Most of the patients with benign action tremors noted clinical improvement with 60 to 240 mg of oral propranolol daily. A few patients showed virtually complete resolution of the tremor, while the majority of the patients reported mild improvement. The best responses were obtained in younger patients who had shorter histories of tremor.

There are, as yet, no good clinical studies evaluating the newer β-blocking drugs for treatment of tremor. Whether or not nonselective β-blockers will prove more efficacious than those with β_1-selectivity has yet to be determined.

Anxiety

Granville-Grossman[407] first suggested that β-blocking drugs might be of value in treating systematic anxiety. Since that time, several studies have appeared and they are reviewed in Chapter 17. Overall, the studies are rather inconclusive, even when the investigators utilize a satisfactory double-blind protocol. It was found that patients derived benefit from propranolol only if they presented initially with dominant somatic complaints (palpitations, shakiness, tremor), as opposed to psychic symptoms. β-Blockers effect the physiologic consequences of anxiety probably by blockade of a peripheral feedback loop of sympathetically mediated responses.[408]

Noncardioselective β-blockers (propranolol, nadolol) might be more useful in anxiety states than drugs with β_1-selectivity (which do not block peripheral receptors) or intrinsic sympathomimetic activity (which can activate peripheral receptors). This question has not yet been addressed in clinical trials.

Schizophrenia

The use of β-adrenoceptor blocking drugs for treatment of psychosis is highly controversial.[409,410] Several studies have reported the use of propranolol (up to 5800 mg/day) in patients with schizophrenia.[411,412]

In general, favorable results have been claimed in patients with acute psychotic states, while chronically affected patients do not seem to respond as well. In some cases the beneficial response to β-blockade became apparent within hours.[410]

Despite the apparent usefulness of β-blockers in some patients with acute psychosis, none of the clinical trials were based on a double-blind design. The possibility of spontaneous clinical remission and the concomitant use of other antipsychotic drugs were not taken into consideration.[413] The possible mechanism for a β-blocker response in patients with acute schizophrenia has not been elucidated. If it relates to a central nervous system effect, those drugs that rapidly cross the blood–brain barrier (metoprolol, propranolol) might prove more efficacious than β-adrenoceptor blocking agents that do not demonstrate this pharmacologic property.

Narcotic and Alcohol Withdrawal

Anecdotal reports suggest that propranolol reduces heroin-induced euphoria, ameliorates narcotic abstinence syndromes, and may be useful in treating narcotic addiction.[414,415] However, since no adequate clinical trials have been conducted with propranolol or the newer β-adrenoceptor blocking agents for treatment of narcotic addition, the effectiveness of these drugs in this condition is questionable.

Propranolol has been successfully used to manage patients undergoing acute alcohol withdrawal.[416] The drug's effect on alcohol withdrawal symptoms is thought to be due to blockade of central nervous system β-adrenoceptors, with a subsequent decrease in sympathetic outflow, or to blockade of increased β-receptor numbers. Patients with mild to moderate symptoms of alcohol withdrawal responded to 40 to 160 mg of oral propranolol daily over 6 days of therapy. Agitation and tremors lessened, none of the patients developed delirium tremens or withdrawal seizures, and all tolerated the drug well. At the time of this writing, there has been no published experience with the newer β-adrenoceptor blocking drugs for this indication.

Open-Angle Glaucoma

In treating systemic hypertension with β-adrenoceptor blocking drugs, it was fortuitously discovered that these agents reduced intraocular pressure in patients with concomitant glaucoma.[417] As early as 1968, topical application of propranolol was shown to reduce intraocular pressure[418]; however, its mild local anesthetic properties made investigators reluctant to use it for treatment of glaucoma. Topical application of timolol—a nonselective β-blocker without this local anesthetic property or partial agonist activity—also reduced intraocular pressure.[419] The mechanism of its ocular hypotensive effect has not been firmly established, but it may reduce the pressure by decreasing the production of aqueous humor.[419] Timolol maleate (Timoptic) was approved by the FDA in 1978 for the topical treatment of increased intraocular pressure in patients with chronic open-angle glaucoma. It is also approved for patients with aphakia and glaucoma, for some patients with secondary glaucoma, and for patients with elevated intraocular pressure who are at sufficient risk to require lowering of this pressure.

Timolol maleate has been studied primarily in comparative trials with topical epinephrine or pilocarpine in patients with open-angle glaucoma.[419,420] Its use in acute closed-angle glaucoma has not been reported in published studies. Timolol is at least as effective as pilocarpine and epinephrine in reducing intraocular pressure by 25 to 30 percent in up to 90 percent of patients.[419] Timolol does not affect pupil motility or accommodation, and for these reasons may be better tolerated than miotics. Although a slight reduction in the magnitude of the ocular hypotensive effect of timolol occurs during the first 1 to 2 weeks of treatment, serious tachyphylaxis has apparently not been a problem in long-term studies.[419,421]

There is little published information on the pharmacokinetic actions of timolol during ocular administration.[419] Such studies are needed to determine the extent of systemic absorption. That systemic absorption does occur through conjunctival and nasal muscosa has been suggested by lowered pressure in both treated and untreated eyes, and by the presence of small amounts of the drug in the plasma and urine.[419] In single-dose studies in rabbits, peak levels occur in blood and aqueous humor 30 minutes after administration of a 0.5 percent solution. In human beings, the start of the reduction in pressure can be detected within half an hour after a single dose. The maximal effect usually occurs in 1 to 2 hours, and appreciable lowering of pressure can be maintained for as long as 24 hours after a single dose. Systemically absorbed timolol is biotransformed in the liver, and its metabolites are excreted primarily in the urine.[419]

Timolol ophthalmic solution is available in concentrations of 0.25 and 0.5 percent. The recommended starting dose is one drop of 0.25 percent solution in each eye twice daily, increasing to one drop of 0.5 percent solution in each eye twice daily. The response of some patients to timolol may require a few weeks to stabilize. It is suggested that when intraocular pressure is controlled, a single dose per day can be tried, but there is no published evidence that such a regimen is effective. If a further reduction in intraocular pressure is considered necessary, concomitant therapy with miotics, epinephrine, or systemic carbonic anhydrase inhibitors may be instituted.[419]

Timolol ophthalmic solution is usually well tolerated. Mild eye irritation occurs occasionally, and a few patients have reported blurred vision after initial doses. Objective measurements of ophthalmic status during topical timolol treatment have shown few changes.[419] The oral dose of timolol maleate for treatment of systemic hypertension is 20 to 60 mg/day. In contrast, the amount of timolol in four drops of 0.5 percent ophthalmic solution (the maximal daily dose) is only about 1 mg.

Plasma levels of the drug after ocular administration are far below those of the cardiovascular therapeutic dose range. However, aggravation or precipitation of certain cardiovascular and pulmonary disorders have been reported and is presumably related to the systemic effects of β-adrenoceptor blockade.[419] These include bradycardia, hypotension, syncope, confusion, and bronchospasm (predominantly in patients with bronchospastic disease). Caution is recommended in prescribing timolol eyedrops when a systemic β-adrenergic blocking drug may be contraindicated, as in patients with preexisting asthmatic conditions, heart block or heart failure. Patients who are taking an oral β-adrenergic drug and are given topical timolol should be observed for a potential additive effect on intraocular pressure and on the known systemic effects of β-blockade.

Gastrointestinal Bleeding

Propranolol has been shown, by Lebrec et al., to reduce portal venous pressure and the risk of recurrent gastrointestinal bleeding in patients with Laennec's cirrhosis.[422–424] In a prospective controlled study, these investigators studied 74 patients with cirrhosis who had evidence confirmed by endoscopy for hemorrhage from esophageal and gastric varicies, or acute gastric erosions. These patients had minimal or no ascites and were randomized to propranolol treatment (20 to 180 mg twice daily) or control groups. The β-blocker was titrated to decrease the resting heart rate by 25 percent. The frequency of rebleeding after 1 year was 4 percent in the β-blocker groups, versus 50 percent in the control population.

Hillon et al.[425] demonstrated that a β_1-selective blocker was somewhat less effective than propranolol in reducing portal pressure, while it was as effective in reducing cardiac output. They suggested that the β_2-blocking properties of propranolol or other pharmacologic actions may contribute to the drug's ability to reduce portal pressure.

Since the other pharmacologic modalities used to treat gastrointestinal bleeding in patients with cirrhosis are administered in parenteral form, there would be a great advantage to an oral agent like propranolol in this situation. However, caution should still be exercised when considering propranolol for the treatment of active gastrointestinal bleeding or for long-term prophylactic use. β-Blockers should be compared to other procedures such as esophageal sclerosis. It should also be noted that none of Lebrec's patients had marked ascites. Patients with cirrhosis and ascites often have increases in plasma renin activity, which may be an important circulatory adjustment; this compensation could be adversely affected by propranolol treatment.[426,427]

REFERENCES

1. Frishman WH: Beta-adrenergic blockade in clinical practice. Hosp Prac 17:57, 1982
2. Frishman WH: The beta-adrenoceptor blocking drugs. Int J Cardiol 2:165, 1982
3. Frishman WH, Silverman R: Clinical pharmacology of the new beta-adrenergic blocking drugs. Part 3. Comparative clinical experience and new therapeutic applications. Am Heart J 98:119, 1979
4. Frishman WH, Kostis J, Strom J, et al: Clinical pharmacology of the new beta-adrenoceptor blocking drugs. Part 6. A comparison of pindolol and propranolol in treatment of patients with angina pectoris. The role of intrinsic sympathomimetic activity. Am Heart J 98:526, 1979
5. Cohn JN: Nitroprusside and dissecting aneurysms of aorta. N Engl J Med 295:567, 1976
6. Wheat MW Jr: Treatment of dissecting aneurysms of the aorta: current status. Prog Cardiovasc Dis 16:87, 1973
7. Turner JRB: Propranolol in the treatment of digitalis-induced and digitalis-resistant tachycardia. Am J Cardiol 18:450, 1966
8. Vincent GM, Abildskov JA, Burgess MJ: Q-T interval syndromes. Prog Cardiovasc Dis 16:523, 1974
9. Shah PM, Kidd L: Circulatory effects of propranolol in children with Fallot's tetralogy. Observations with isoproterenol infusion, exercise and crying. Am J Cardiol 19:653, 1967
10. Meister SG, Engel TR, Feitosa GS, et al: Propranolol in mitral stenosis during sinus rhythm. Am Heart J 94:685, 1977
11. Bhatia ML, Shrivastava S, Roy SG: Immediate haemodynamic effects of a beta-adrenergic blocking agent—propranolol—in mitral stenosis at fixed heart rates. Br Heart J 34:638, 1972
12. Svedberg K, Hjalmarson Å, Waagstein F, Beneficial effects of long-term beta-blockade in congestive cardiomyopathy. Br Heart J 44:117, 1980
13. Teuscher A, Bossi E, Imhof P, et al.: Effect of propranolol on fetal tachycardia in diabetic pregnancy. Am J Cardiol 42:304, 1978
14. Furberg C, Morsing C: Adrenergic beta-receptor blockade in neurocirculatory asthenia. Pharmacologia Clinica 1:168, 1969
15. Cumming GR, Mir GH: Effects of propranolol on the resting and exercise hemodynamics of pulmonary stenosis. Can J Physiol Pharmacol 47:137, 1969
16. Guntheroth WG, Kawabor I: Tetrad of Fallot, in Moss AJ, Adams FH, Emmanouilides GC (eds), Heart Disease in Infants, Children, and Adolescents, 2nd ed. Baltimore, Williams and Wilkins
17. Bada JL: Treatment of erythromegalia with propranolol. Lancet 2:412, 1977
18. Oka Y, Frishman W, Becker R, et al.: Clinical pharmacology of the new beta adrenergic blocking drugs. Part 10. Beta-adrenoceptor blockade and

coronary artery surgery. Am Heart J 99:255, 1980

19. Fox CA: Reduction in the rise of systolic blood pressure during human coitus by the beta-adrenergic blocking agent propranolol. J Reprod Fertil 22:587, 1970
20. Strang RR: Clinical trial with a beta-receptor antagonist in Parkinsonism. J Neurol Neurosurg Psychiatr 28:404, 1965
21. Brewer C: Beneficial effect of beta-adrenergic blockade on "exam nerves" (letter). Lancet 2:435, 1972
22. Sellers EM, Degani NC, Silm DH, MacLeod SM: Propranolol-decreased noradrenaline secretion and alcohol withdrawal. Lancet 1:94, 1976
23. Grosz HJ: Narcotic withdrawal symptoms in heroin users treated with propranolol. Lancet 2:564, 1972
24. Rapolt RT, Gay GR, Inaba DS: Propranolol: a specific antagonist to cocaine. Clin Toxicol 10:265, 1977
25. Linken A: Propranolol for LSD-induced anxiety states (letter). Lancet 2:1039, 1971
26. Kirk L, Baastrip PC, Schou M: Propranolol and lithium-induced tremor (letter). Lancet 1:839, 1972
27. Kales A, Soldatos CR, Cadieux R, et al: Propranolol in the treatment of narcolepsy. Ann Inter Med 93:741, 1979
28. Fournier A, Coevoet B, De Fremont JF, et al: Propranolol therapy for secondary hyperparathyroidism in uraemia. Lancet 2:50, 1978
29. Caro JF, Castro JH, Glennon JA: Effect of long-term propranolol administration on parathyroid hormone and calcium concentration in primary hyperparathyroidism. Ann Intern Med 91:740, 1979
30. Blum I, Aderka D, Doron M, Laron Z: Suppression of hypoglycemia by DL-propranolol in malignant insulinoma (letter). N Engl J Med 299:487, 1978
31. Baker L, Barcai A, Kaye R, et al.: Beta-adrenergic blockade and juvenile diabetes: acute studies and long-term therapeutic trial. J Pediatr 75:19, 1969
32. Caro JF, Besarab A, Burke JF, Glennon JA: A possible role for propranolol in treatment of renal osteodystrophy. Lancet 2:451, 1978
33. Prys-Roberts C, Kerr JH, Corbett JL, et al: Treatment of sympathetic overactivity in tetanus. Lancet 1:542, 1969
34. Cunliff WJ, Cotterill J: The effect of propranolol on acne-vulgaris and the rate of sebum excretion. Br J Dermatol 83:550, 1970
35. Douer D, Weinberger A, Pinkhas J, Atsmon A: Treatment of acute intermittent porphyria with large doses of propranolol. JAMA 240:766, 1978
36. Berk JL, Hagen JF, Beyer WH, et al: The treatment of endotoxin shock by beta adrenergic blockade. Ann Surg 169:74, 1969
37. Berk JL, Hagen JF, Beyer WH, et al: The treatment of hemorrhagic shock by beta-adrenergic receptor blockade. Surg Gynecol Obstet 125:311, 1967
38. Kobacz GJ: The role of adrenergic blockade in the treatment of uretheral colic. J Urol 107:949, 1972
39. Khanna OMP: Disorders of micturition. Neuropharmacologic basis and results of drug therapy. Urology 8:316, 1976

40. Oille WA: Beta adrenergic blockade and the phantom limb (letter). Ann Intern Med 73:1044, 1970

41. Coyne MJ, Bonorris GG, Chung A, et al: Propranolol inhibits bile acid and fatty acid stimulation of cyclic AMP in human colon. Gastroenterology 73:971, 1977

42. Lechin F, Van Der Dijs B, Bentolila A, Pena F: The spastic colon syndrome; therapeutic and pathophysiologic considerations. J Clin Pharmacol 17:431, 1977

43. Mitrani A, Oettinger M, Abinader EG, Sharf M: Use of propranolol in dysfunctional labor. Br J Obstet Gynecol 82:651, 1975

44. Szerkeres L, Papp J, Forster W: The action of adrenergic beta-receptor blocking agents on susceptibility to cardiac arrhythmias in hypothermia and hypoxia. Experientia 21:720, 1965

45. Moriau M, Noel H, Masure R: Effects of alpha and beta receptor stimulating and blocking agents on experimental disseminated intravascular coagulation. Throm Diath Haemorr 32:157, 1974

46. Szabuniewicz M, McCrady JD, Camp BJ: Treatment of experimentally induced oleander poisoning. Arch Int Pharmacodyn Ther 189:12, 1971

47. Frishman WH: Atenolol and timolol, two new systemic B-adrenoceptor antagonists. N Engl J Med 306:1456, 1982

48. Fiserova J, Hlavecek K, Vaura M, Holik F, Munz J: Acebutolol (sectral) in angina pectoris treatment. Acta Univ Carol 25:335, 1979

49. Rod JL, Admon D, Kimchi A, et al: Evaluation of the beta-blocking drug acebutolol in angina pectoris. Am Heart J 98:604, 1979

50. DiBianco R, Singh S, Singh J, et al: Effects of acebutolol on chronic stable angina pectoris—a placebo-controlled, double-blind randomized crossover study. Circulation 62:1179, 1980

51. Steele P, Gold F: Favorable effects of acebutolol on exercise performance and angina in men with coronary artery disease. Chest 82:40, 1982

52. DiBianco R, Singh S, Shah P, et al: Comparison of the antianginal efficacy of acebutolol and propranolol. A multicenter, randomized, double-blind, placebo-controlled study. Circulation 65:1119, 1982

53. DePonti C, DeBiase AM, Pirelli S, et al: Effects of nifedipine, acebutolol, and their association on exercise tolerance in patients with effort angina. Cardiology 68 (Suppl 2):195, 1981

54. Daltro LL, Lion MF: Treatment of angina pectoris with a new beta blocker atenolol (portuguese). Rev Bras Med 34 (Suppl 7):5, 1977

55. Langbehn AF, Burmeister G, Horst H, et al: Long-term effects of the beta-adrenergic blocking agents atenolol (tenormin) on coronary heart disease. Med Klin 73:101, 1978

56. Backman H, Normi H, Sano S: Atenolol in angina pectoris—preliminary results of an ergometric dose finding study. Acta Therapeutica 4:267, 1978

57. Roy P, Day L, Sowton E: Effect of new beta adrenergic blocking agent, atenolol (tenormin), on pain frequency, trinitrin consumption and exercise ability. Br Med J 3:195, 1975

58. Erikssen J, Osvik K, Dedichen J: Atenolol in the treatment of angina pectoris. Acta Med Scand 201:579, 1977

59. van der Vijgh WJF, Majid PA, deFeyter PJ, et al: Pharmacokinetics of atenolol and its clinical consequences in patients with angina pectoris. Int J Clin Pharmacol 18:375, 1980

60. Jackson G, Schwartz J, Kates RE, et al: Atenolol: once-daily cardioselective beta blockade for angina pectoris. Circulation 61:555, 1980

61. Schwartz J, Jackson G, Kates RE, Harrison DC: Long-term benefit of cardioselective beta blockade with once-daily atenolol therapy in angina pectoris. Am Heart J 101:380, 1981

62. Jackson G, Harry JD, Robinson C, et al: Comparison of atenolol with propranolol in the treatment of angina pectoris with special reference to once daily administration of atenolol. Br Heart J 40:998, 1978

63. Haghfelt T, Pindborg T, Thayssen P: Atenolol (tenormin) in the treatment of angina pectoris. Laeg 142:2475, 1980

64. Uusitalo A, Keyrilainen O, Johnsson G: A dose response study on metoprolol in angina pectoris. Ann Clin Res 13 (Suppl 30):54, 1981

65. Comerford MB, Besterman EMM: An eighteen months' study of the clinical response to metoprolol, a selective $beta_1$-receptor blocking agent, in patients with angina pectoris. Postgrad Med J 52:481, 1976

66. Borer JS, Comerford MB, Sowton E: Assessment of metoprolol, a cardioselective beta-blocking agent, during chronic therapy in patients with angina pectoris. J Int Med Res 4:15, 1976

67. Frick MH, Luurila O: Double-blind titrated-dose comparison of metoprolol and propranolol in the treatment of angina pectoris. Ann Clin Res 8:385, 1976

68. Thadani U, Davidson C, Chir B, et al: Comparison of the immediate effects of five β-adrenoreceptor blocking drugs with different ancillary properties in angina pectoris. N Engl J Med 300:750, 1979

69. Thadani U, Davidson C, Singleton W, Taylor SH: Comparison of five beta-adrenoceptor antagonists with different ancillary properties during sustained twice daily therapy in angina pectoris. Am J Cardiol 68:243, 1980

70. Arnman K, Rydén L: Comparison of metoprolol and verapamil in the treatment of angina pectoris. Am J Cardiol 49:821, 1982

71. Heel RC, Brogden RN, Pakes GE, et al: Nadolol: A review of its pharmacological properties and therapeutic efficacy in hypertension and angina pectoris. Drugs 20:1, 1980

72. Shapiro W, Park J, DiBianco R, et al: Comparison of nadolol, a new long acting beta-receptor blocking agent, and placebo in the treatment of stable angina pectoris. Chest 80:425, 1981

73. Ling AS, Groel JT: Improved physical performance as a therapeutic objective in patients with angina. Br J Clin Pharmacol 7 (Suppl 2):1615, 1979

74. Prager G: Angina pectoris: Effective therapy once daily. J Int Med Res 7:39, 1979

75. Furberg B, Dahlqvist A, Raak A, Wrege U: Comparison of the new beta-adrenoceptor antagonist, nadolol, and propranolol in the treatment of angina pectoris. Curr Med Res Opin 5:388, 1978

76. Jones GR, Mir MA: Comparison of antianginal efficacy of one conven-

tional and three long acting beta-adrenoceptor blocking agents in stable angina pectoris. Br Heart J 46:503, 1981

77. Watt M: Drug surveillance in general practice: A study of oxprenolol in the treatment of angina. N Z Med J 81:200, 1975

78. Burley DM: Monitored release studies with trasicor, in Schweizer W. (ed), Beta-Blockers—Present Status and Future Prospects Berne, Hans Huber, 1974, p. 140

79. Sandler G, Pistevos A: Clinical evaluation of oxprenolol in angina pectoris. Br Heart J 34:847, 1972

80. Bianchi C, Luchell PE, Starcich R: Beta-blockade and angina pectoris. A controlled multicentre clinical trial Pharmacologica Clinica 1:161, 1969

81. Wilson DF, Watson OF, Peel JS, Turner AS: Trasicor in angina pectoris: A double-blind trial. Br Med J 2:155, 1969

82. Taylor SH, Thadani U: Oxprenolol in angina pectoris. Br J Pharmacol 58:412P, 1976

83. Forrest WA: A double-blind clinical trial in angina pectoris. A comparison between oxprenolol, practolol, and placebo. Br J Clin Pract 29:343, 1975

84. Forrest WA: Experience with a sustained-release formulation of oxprenolol in the management of angina pectoris in hospital out-patient departments. Curr Med Res Opin 5:669, 1978

85. Majid PA, deFeiter PJ, Wardeh R, et al: Comparison of clinical effects of propranolol (inderal) with once-daily slow-release oxprenolol (slow trasicor) in angina pectoris. J Int Med Res 7:194, 1979

86. Olowoyeye JO, Thadani U, Parker JO: Slow release oxprenolol in angina pectoris: Study comparing oxprenolol, once daily, with propranolol, four times daily. Am J Cardiol 47:1123, 1981

87. Leary WP, Asmal AC: Treatment of coexistent angina pectoris and hypertension with pindolol. S Afr Med J 49:11, 1975

88. Storstein L: Effect of intravenous and oral pindolol on exercise tolerance and electrocardiographic changes in angina pectoris. J Cardiovasc Pharmacol 2:739, 1980

89. Dwyer EM Jr, Pepe AJ, Pinkernell BH: Effects of beta-adrenergic blockade with pindolol versus placebo in coronary patients with stable angina pectoris. Am Heart J 103:830, 1982

90. Harston WE, Friesinger GC: Randomized double-blind study of pindolol in patients with stable angina pectoris. Am Heart J 104:504, 1982

91. Harston WE, Friesinger GC: Variability of response to beta receptor blockade for angina pectoris in clinical trials: A study of pindolol. Am J Cardiol 50:722, 1982

92. Frishman WH: Pindolol: A new β-adrenoceptor antagonist with partial agonist activity. N Engl J Med 308:940, 1983

93. Cocco G, Strozzi C, Chu D, et al: Therapeutic effects of pindolol and nifedipine in patients with stable angina pectoris and asymptomatic resting ischemia. Eur J Cardiol 10:59, 1979

94. Cocco G, Strozzi C, Chu D, et al: Therapeutic effects of pindolol and ni-

fedipine in patients with stable angina pectoris and asymptomatic resting ischemia. Br J Clin Pract 34 (Suppl 8):59, 1980

95. Prichard BNC: β-adrenoceptor blocking drugs in angina pectoris, in Avery G (ed), β-Adrenoceptor Blocking Drugs. Baltimore, University Park Press, 1978, p 85

96. Prichard BNC: Propranolol in the treatment of angina: A review. Postgrad Med J 52 (Suppl 4):35, 1976

97. Prichard BNC, Gillam DMS: An assessment of propranolol in angina pectoris. A clinical dose response curve and the effect on the electrocardiogram at rest and on exercise. Br Heart J 33:473, 1971

98. Alderman EL, Davies RO, Crowley JJ, et al: Dose response effectiveness of propranolol for the treatment of angina pectoris. Circulation 51:964, 1975

99. Thadani U, Parker JO: Propranolol in angina pectoris: Duration of improved exercise tolerance and circulatory effects after acute oral administration. Am J Cardiol 44:119, 1979

100. Thadani U, Parker JO: Propranolol in the treatment of angina pectoris—comparison of duration of action in acute and sustained oral therapy. Circulation 59:571, 1979

101. Thadani U, Parker JO: Propranolol in angina pectoris—comparison of therapy given two and four times daily. Am J Cardiol 46:117, 1980

102. Halkin H, Vered I, Saginer A, Rabinowitz B: Once daily administration of sustained release propranolol capsules in the treatment of angina pectoris. Eur J Clin Pharmacol 16:387, 1979

103. Parker JO, Porter A, Parker JD: Propranolol in angina pectoris—comparison of long-acting and standard formulation propranolol. Circulation 65:1351, 1982

104. Leon MB, Rosing DR, Bonow RO, et al: Clinical efficacy of verapamil alone and combined with propranolol in treating patients with chronic stable angina pectoris. Am J Cardiol 48:131, 1981

105. Johnson SM, Mauritson DR, Corbett JR, et al: Double-blind, randomized, placebo-controlled comparison of propranolol and verapamil in the treatment of patients with stable angina pectoris. Am J Med 71:443, 1981

106. Subramanian B, Bowles MJ, Davies AB, Raftery EB: Combined therapy with verapamil and propranolol in chronic stable angina. Am J Cardiol 49:125, 1982

107. Frishman WH, Klein NA, Strom JA, et al: Superiority of verapamil to propranolol in stable angina pectoris: A double-blind randomized crossover trial. Circulation 65 (Suppl 1):51, 1982

108. Lynch P, Dargie H, Krikler S, Krikler D: Objective assessment of antianginal treatment: A double-blind comparison of propranolol, nifedipine, and their combination. Br Med J 48:131, 1981

109. Kenmure ACF, Scruton JH: A double-blind controlled trial of the antianginal efficacy of nifedipine compared with propranolol. Br J Clin Pract 8:49, 1980

110. Dargie HJ, Lynch PG, Krikler DM, et al: Nifedipine and propranolol: A beneficial drug interaction. Am J Med 71:676, 1981

111. Tweddel AC, Beattie JM, Murray RG, Hutton I: The combination of nifedipine and propranolol in the management of patients with angina pectoris. Br J Clin Pharmacol 12:229, 1981

112. Fox KM, Jonathan A, Selwyn AP: The use of propranolol and nifedipine in the medical management of angina pectoris. Clin Cardiol 4:125, 1981.

113. Toubes DB, Ferguson RK, Rice AJ, et al: β-Adrenergic blockade versus placebo in angina pectoris. Clin Res 18:345, 1970

114. Kentala E, Pyorala K, Frich MH: Sotalol in the treatment of angina pectoris: A double-blind crossover study. An Clin Res 6:253, 1974

115. Milei J, Fortunato MR: A new beta-adrenergic blocking agent, sotatol, in the treatment of angina pectoris. A double blind-crossed treatment study. Rev Bras Pesqui Med Biol 8:279, 1975

116. Slome R: Sotalol in angina pectoris. A double-blind study. S Afr Med J 50:469, 1976

117. Brailovsky D: Timolol Maleate (ML-950). A new beta-blocking agent for the prophylactic management of angina pectoris. A multicentre, multinational co-operative trial, in Magnani B (ed), Beta-Adrenergic Blocking Agents in the Management of Hypertension and Angina Pectoris. New York, Raven, 1974, p 117

118. Villa I, Dagenais GR, Dorian WD, Burford RG: Effects of timolol on exercise tolerance in patients with angina pectoris, in Magnani B (ed), Beta-Adrenergic Blocking Agents in the Management of Hypertension and Angina Pectoris. New York, Raven, 1974, p 153

119. Aronow WS, Turbow M, Van Camp S, et al: The effect of timolol vs placebo on angina pectoris. Circulation 61:66, 1980

120. DiSegni E, Fidelman E, David D, et al: The beneficial effect of the beta-blocker timolol in stable angina pectoris. Angiology 31:238, 1980

121. Aronow WS, Plasencia G, Wong R, Landa D: Exercise duration to angina at two and twelve hours after timolol. Clin Pharmacol Ther 29:155, 1981

122. Parmley WW: The combination of beta-adrenergic-blocking agents and nitrates in the treatment of stable angina pectoris. Cardiol Rev Rep 3:1425, 1982

123. Kirk ES, Sonnenblick EH: Newer concepts in the pathophysiology of ischemic heart disease. Am Heart J 103:756, 1982

124. Packer M, Leon MB, Bonow RO, et al: Hemodynamic and clinical effects of combined verapamil and propranolol therapy in angina pectoris. Am J Cardiol 50:903, 1982

125. Maseri A, L'Abbate A, Ballestra AM, et al: Coronary vasospasm in angina pectoris. Lancet 1:713, 1977

126. Maseri A: Pathogenic mechanisms of angina pectoris: Expanding views. Br Heart J 43:648, 1980

127. Mehta J, Conti CR: Verapamil therapy for unstable angina pectoris: Re-

view of double-blind placebo-controlled randomized trials. Am J Cardiol 50:919, 1982

128. Parodi O, Simonetti I, L'Abbate A, Maseri A: Verapamil versus propranolol for angina at rest. Am J Cardiol 50:923, 1982

129. Conti CR: Treatment of unstable angina: A model for step care therapy. Cardiol Rev Rep 3:1306, 1982

130. Oka Y, Frishman WH, Becker RM, et al: Clinical pharmacology of the new beta-adrenergic blocking drugs. Part 10. Beta-adrenergic receptor blockade and coronary artery surgery. Am Heart J 99:255, 1980

131. Frishman WH, Klein N, Strom J, et al: Comparative effects of abrupt withdrawal of propranolol and verapamil in angina pectoris. Am J Cardiol 50:1191, 1982

132. Alderman EL, Coltart J, Wettach GE, Harrison DC: Coronary artery syndrome after abrupt sudden propranolol withdrawal. Ann Intern Med 81:925, 1974

133. Miller RR, Olson HG, Amsterdam EA, Mason DT: Propranolol withdrawal rebound phenomenon. Exacerbation of coronary events after abrupt cessation of anti-anginal therapy. N Engl J Med 293:416, 1975

134. Shand DG, Wood AJJ: Propranolol withdrawal syndrome—Why? Circulation 58:202, 1978

135. Frishman WH, Christodoulou J, Weksler B, et al: Abrupt propranolol withdrawal in angina pectoris: Effects on platelet aggregation and exercise tolerance. Am Heart J 95:169, 1978

136. Nadeau J, Ogilvze R, Ruedy J, Brossard J: Acebutolol and hydrochlorthiazide in essential hypertension. Clin Pharmacol Ther 28:296, 1980

137. Franz IW: Differential antihypertensive effect of acebutolol and hydrochlorthiazide/amiloride hydrochloride combination on elevated exercise blood pressures in hypertensive patients. Am J Cardiol 46:301, 1980

138. Gorkin J, Elijovich F, Dziedzic S, Krakoff L: Addition of acebutolol to diuretics in hypertension. Clin Pharmacol Ther 30:739, 1981

139. Chatterji A: A randomized crossover comparison of acebutolol and methyldopa in the treatment of mild to moderate essential hypertension. Curr Med Res Opin 5:675, 1978

140. Hansson L, Henningsen NC, Karberg BE, et al: Hypertensive action of ICI 66.082, a new beta-adrenergic blocking agent. Int J Clin Pharmacol Ther Toxicol 10:206, 1974

141. Hansson L, Karlberg BE, Aberg H, et al: Clinical evaluation of atenolol in hypertension. Clin Sci Mol Med 51:513 1976

142. Hansson L, Karlberg BE, Aberg H, et al: Long-term hypotensive effect of atenolol (ICI 66.082), a new β-adrenergic blocking agent. Acta Med Scand 199:257, 1976

143. Hansson L, Henningsen NC, Karlberg BE, et al: Long-term trial of atenolol in hypertension 22:839, 1977

144. Gudbrandsson T, Hansson L: Combination therapy with saluretics and atenolol in essential hypertension. Effects on blood pressure, electrolytes, and uric acid. Acta Med Scand (Suppl) 625:86, 1979

145. Zacharias FJ: Long-term clinical experience with atenolol, in Cruickshank JM, McAinsh J, Caldwell ADS (eds), Atenolol and Renal Function: R Soc Med Int Congr Symp London 19:75, 1980

146. Hansson L, Alberg H, Karlberg BE, Westerlund A: Controlled study of atenolol in treatment of hypertension. Br Med J 2:367, 1975

147. Myers MG, Lewis GRJ, Steiner J, Dollery CT: Atenolol in essential hypertension. Clin Pharm Ther 19:502, 1976

148. Cilliers AJ: Atenolol as primary therapy in previously untreated hypertensives and as an adjuvant to other therapy. A South African multicenter study. S Afr Med J 55:321, 1979

149. DeTollenaere G, Verdonk G: Evaluation of atenolol administered once daily in the management of hypertension. Acta Therapeutica 2:317, 1976

150. Lehtonen A: Atenolol in hypertension. Acta Ther 2:125, 1976

151. Harris AM, Woolard KV, Tweed JA: A study of once daily tenormin (Atenolol) in hypertension: Some implications in patient compliance. J Int Med Res 4:347, 1976.

152. Douglas-Jones AP, Cruickshank JM: Once-daily dosing with atenolol in patients with mild or moderate hypertension. Br Med J 1:990, 1976

153. Tuomilehto J, Alasoini A, Koistinen A, Lamberg M: Atenolol in the management of hypertension. Acta Ther 3:131, 1977

154. Upton N, Tweed JA, Barker NP: A double-blind controlled comparison of once-daily and twice-daily atenolol in the treatment of hypertension. Acta Ther 3:15, 1977

155. Jeffers TA, Webster J, Petrie JC, Barker NP: Atenolol once-daily in hypertension. Br J Clin Pharm 4:523, 1977

156. Petrie JC, Galloway DB, Jeffers TA, Webster J: Clinical studies with atenolol in hypertension. Postgrad Med J 53:173, 1977

157. Marshall AJ, Barritt DW, Harry JD: Dose response and frequency of administration of atenolol in essential hypertension once-daily treatment with beta-blockade. Postgrad Med J 53:168, 1977

158. Gostick NK, Mayhew SR, Million R, et al: A dose-response study of atenolol in mild to moderate hypertension in general practice. Curr Med Res Opin 5:179, 1977

159. Zacharias FJ, Hayes PJ, Cruickshank JM: Atenolol in hypertension: A double-blind comparison of the response to three different doses. Postgrad Med J 53:114, 1977

160. Ezra D, Molho M, Rosenthal T: Atenolol in hypertension: A new cardioselective drug. Chest 77:662, 1980

161. Danielson M, Lindborg H: Long-term treatment of hypertension: Efficacy and tolerability of atenolol in clinical practice. Curr Ther Res 27:797, 1980

162. Petrie JC, Galloway DB, Webster J, et al: Atenolol and bendrofluazide in hypertension. Br Med J 4:133, 1975

163. Douglas-Jones AP, Cruickshank JM: Comparison of atenolol and bendrofluazide in mild to moderate hypertension. Acta Ther 2:221, 1976

164. Fagard R, Amery A, DePlaen JF, et al: Relative value of beta-blockers and

thiazides for initiating antihypertensive therapy. Beta-blockers or thiazides in hypertension. Acta Cardiol 31:411, 1976

165. Wilcox RG, Mitchell JRA: Contribution of atenolol, bendrofluazide, and hydralazine to management of severe hypertension. Br Med J 2:547, 1977.

166. Wilcox RG: Combination hypotensive therapy with atenolol, bendrofluazide and hydralazine. Postgrad Med J 53:128, 1977

167. Rushford WAI, Tweed JA, Barker NP: A comparison of atenolol and bendrofluazide in treating hypertension—A general practice study. Acta Ther 3:117, 1977

168. Sheriff MHR, Howard O, Warren DJ: Effects of atenolol, chlorthalidone and a new combined preparation, tenoretic, on blood pressure and total body potassium. Acta Ther 4:51, 1978

169. Bateman DN, Dean CR, Mucklow JC, Bulpitt CJ, Dollery CT: Atenolol and chlorthalidone in combination for hypertension. Br J Clin Pharm 7:357, 1979

170. Teeuw AH, Leenen FHH, Geyskes GG, Boer P: Atenolol and chlorthalidone on blood pressure, heart rate, and plasma renin activity in hypertension. Clin Pharm Ther 25:294, 1979

171. Velasco M, Guevara J, Morillo J, et al: Mechanism of the haemodynamic interaction between atenolol, a cardioselective β-adrenoreceptor-blocking agent, and chlorthalidone in hypertensive patients. Clin Sci 57:3635, 1979.

172. Velasco M, Guevara J, Morillo J, et al: Antihypertensive effect of atenolol alone or combined with chlorthalidone in patients with essential hypertension. Br J Clin Pharm 9:449, 1980

173. Seedat YK: Trial of atenolol and chlorthalidone for hypertension in black South Africans. Br Med J 281:1241, 1980

174. Asbury MJ, Wells FO, Barker NP: Once-daily combination therapy for hypertension. Practitioner 224:1306, 1980

175. Hansson L, Westerlund A, Aberg H, Karlberg BE: A comparison of the antihypertensive effect of atenolol (ICI 66,082) and propranolol. Eur J Clin Pharm 9:361, 1976

176. Epstein SE, Lubbe WF: Effects of propranolol and atenolol on blood pressure and plasma renin activity in patients with moderate hypertension. S Afr Med J 52:875, 1977

177. Zacharias FJ, Cowen KJ: Comparison of propranolol and atenolol in hypertension. Postgrad Med J 53:111, 1977

178. Zacharias FJ: Atenolol compared with other beta-blocking agents. Proc R Soc Med 70:24, 1977

179. Jeffers TA, Webster J, Reid B, Petrie JC: Atenolol and metoprolol in mild hypertension. Br Med J 2:1269, 1978

180. Lyngstam O, Rydén L: Metroprolol or atenolol for mild to moderate hypertension. Lancet 2:634, 1979

181. Adams-Strump BJ, Hayes J, Barber JH: A new approach to drug trials in general practice. Comparison of the antihypertensive efficacy of metoprolol and atenolol. Practitioner 224:541, 1980

182. Turner AS, Watson OF, Brocklehurst JE: Efficacy of atenolol and oxpren-

olol in the treatment of arterial hypertension. A comparison. Med J Aust 1:625, 1979

183. Leary WP, Asmal AC, Brayshaw P, Williams P: Antihypertensive effects of sotalol and atenolol given once daily. S Afr Med J 57:692, 1980

184. Zacharias FJ, Cowen KJ, Cuthbertson PJR, et al: Atenolol in hypertension: A study of long-term therapy. Postgrad Med J 53:102, 1977

185. Wilcox RG: Randomized study of six beta-blockers and a thiazide diuretic in essential hypertension. Br Med J 2:383, 1978

186. Waal-Manning HJ: Atenolol and three nonselective β-blockers in hypertension. Clin Pharm Ther 25:8, 1979

187. Vaughan Williams EM, Hassan MO, et al: Adaptation of hypertensives to treatment with cardioselective and non-selective beta-blockers. Absence of correlation between bradycardia and blood pressure control, and reduction in slope of QT/RR relation. Br Heart J 44:473, 1980

188. Petrie JC, Jeffers TA, Robb OJ, et al: Atenolol, sustained-release oxprenolol, and long-acting propranolol in hypertension. Br Med J 280:1573, 1980.

189. England JDF: Beta Adrenoreceptor-blocking drugs once-daily in essential hypertension: A comparison of propranolol, pindolol and atenolol. Aust NZ J Med 11:35, 1981

190. Thulin T, Henningsen NC, Karlberg BE, Nilsson OR: Clinical and metabolic effects of labetalol compared with atenolol in primary hypertension. Curr Ther Res 30:194, 1981

191. Webster J, Jeffers TA, Galloway DB, et al: Atenolol, methyldopa, and chlorthalidone in moderate hypertension. Br Med J 1:76, 1977

192. Wilson C, Scott ME, Abdel-Mohsen A: Atenolol and methyldopa in the treatment of hypertension. Postgrad Med J 53:123, 1977

193. Basker MA, Tweed JA, Barker NP: A double-blind comparison of atenolol (tenormin) and methyldopa in the treatment of moderate hypertension in general practice: A multicentre study. Curr Med Res Opin 4:618, 1977

194. Tweed JA, Mason B, Sleigh R: Multicentre general practitioner assessment of tenormin and methyldopa. J Int Med Res 7:324, 1979

195. Haglund K, Collste P: Time course of blood pressure, pulse rate, plasma renin, and metoprolol during treatment of hypertensive patients. Eur J Clin Pharm 17:321, 1980

196. Bengston C: Seven years on a selective β-blocker-metoprolol. Ann Clin Res 13:7, 1981

197. Asplund J, Ohman P: Metoprolol administered once-daily in the treatment of hypertension. Ann of Clinical Res 13:30, 1981

198. Bengtsson C, Larsson Y, Panfilov Y, et al: Hemodynamic effects of withdrawal of long-term treatment with β-adrenoreceptor blocking agents in subjects with essential hypertension. Clin Sci 61:4215, 1981

199. Velasquez M, Sukhanwan Maronder: Effects of metoprolol on blood pressure and plasma renin activity in thiazide resistant hypertensive patients. Clin Pharm Ther 26:555, 1976

200. Pederson DL: Comparison of metoprolol and hydrochlorthiazide as antihypertensive agents. Eur J Clin Pharm 10:381, 1976

201. Kubik M, Kendall M, Ebutt A, John V: Metoprolol with and without chlorthalidone in hypertension. Clin Pharm Ther 25:25, 1979

202. Liedholm H, Ursing O: Antihypertensive effect and tolerability of two fixed combinations of metoprolol and hydrochlorothiazide. Ann Clin Res 13:45, 1981.

203. Lameyer L, Hesse CJ: Metoprolol in high renin hypertension. Ann Clin Res 13:16, 1981

204. Svensson A, Gudbrandsson T, Sivertsson R, Hansson L: Metoprolol and pindolol in hypertension. Different effects on peripheral hemodynamics. Clin Sci 61:425s, 1981

205. Jackson DA: Nadolol, a once daily treatment for hypertension multicentre clinical evaluation. Br J Clin Pract 34:211, 1980.

206. Hitzenberger G: Initial experience with a new long-acting beta-blocker, nadolol, in hypertensive patients. J Int Med Res 7:33, 1979

207. Frithz G: Dose-ranging study of the new beta-adrenergic antagonist nadolol in the treatment of essential hypertension. Curr Med Res Opin 5:383, 1978

208. El-Mehairy MM, Shaker A, Ramadan M, et al: Long-term treatment of essential hypertension using nadolol and hydrochlorothiazide combined. Br J Clin Pharm 7:199s, 1979.

209. El-Mehairy MM, Shaker A, Ramadad M, et al: Long-term treatment of essential hypertension with nadolol and hydrochlorothiazide. A two-year follow-up. J Int Med Res 10:87, 1982

210. Finnerty FA Jr: Initial therapy of essential hypertension: Diuretic or beta-blocker? J Fam Pract 11:199, 1980

211. Olerud B: Hydrochlorothiazide and nadolol in the treatment of hypertension. Practitioner 226:785, 1981

212. Heel RC, Brogden RN, Pakes GE, et al: Nadolol: A review of its pharmacological properties and therapeutic efficacy in hypertension and angina pectoris. Drugs 20:1, 1980.

213. Frishman WH: Nadolol: A new β-adrenoceptor antagonist. N Engl J Med 305:678, 1981

214. Hill LS, Fand RS: A report on the clinical efficacy of nadolol—a new long-acting beta-blocker. Irish Med J 72:522, 1979

215. El Mehairy MM, Shaker A, Ramadan M, et al. Nadolol and propranolol in the treatment of hypertension: A double-blind comparison. J Int Med Res 8:193, 1980

216. Frithz G: Treatment of essential hypertension. A comparison between nadolol once-daily, and propranolol, four times daily. Practitioner 226:562, 1982

217. Jenkins AC, Rosenthal J, Stumpe KO: Mediation of blood pressure by nadolol and alpha methyldopa. Practitioner 225:405, 1981

218. Schlesinger Z, Barzilay J: Effect of oxprenolol on blood pressure pulmonary ventilatory function and myocardial contractility in hypertensive patients. Isr J Med Sci 16:420, 1980

219. Reskenov EB, Harvard CWH: A comparison of slow release oxprenolol with conventional oxprenolol in the treatment of hypertension. Eur J Clin Pharmacol 14:77, 1978
220. Materson B, Oster J, Michael V, Perez-Stable E: Antihypertensive effectiveness of oxprenolol administered twice daily. Clin Pharmacol Ther 19:325, 1975
221. Farsang C, Juhasz Z, Kapocsz J, et al: Effect of prazosin and oxprenolol on plasma renin activity and blood pressure in patients with essential hypertension. Cardiology 67:164, 1981
222. Barret DW, Marshall AJ, Heaton S: Comparison of oxprenolol and methyldopa in hypertension. Lancet 958:503, 1976.
223. Freeman JW, Knight LW: Oxprenolol and hydralazine in the treatment of hypertension. Med J Aust 1:12, 1975
224. Gavras I, Gavras H, Taft C, et al: Effect of pindolol on blood pressure, plasma renin activity and catecholamines in hypertensive patients. J Clin Pharm 21:79, 1981
225. Toivonen S, Mattila S, Tarpila S, Leirisalo M: The efficacy of single dose pindolol in hypertension. Ann Clin Res 9:93, 1977
226. McNeil J, Louis W, Doyle A, Vajda F: Comparison of metoprolol and pindolol in the treatment of mild to moderate hypertension. Med J Aust 1:431, 1979
227. Tuomilehto J, Pohjola M: A Comparison between metoprolol and pindolol in the treatment of essential hypertension. Ann Clin Res 10:24, 1979
228. Romo M, Halttunen P, Saarinen P, Sarna S: Labetalol and pindolol in the treatment of hypertension. Ann Clin Res 11:249, 1979
229. Gonasom L: Antihypertensive effects of pindolol. Am Heart J 104:374, 1982
230. Persson I: Combination therapy of essential hypertension with pindolol and hydralazine. Eur J Clin Pharmacol 9:91, 1975.
231. Zacharias FJ, Cowen KJ, Prestt J, et al: Propranolol in hypertension: A study of long-term therapy. Am Heart J 83:755, 1972
232. Zacharias FJ, Cowen KJ: Controlled trial of propranolol in hypertension. Br Med J 1:471, 1970.
233. Humphreys GS, Delvin DG: Ineffectiveness of propranolol in hypertensive Jamaicans. Br Med J 2:601, 1968.
234. Mongeau JG, Biron P, Pichardo ML: Propranolol efficacy in essential hypertension in adolescents. Can Med Assoc J 116:589, 1977
235. Galloway DB, Glover SC, Hendry WG, et al: Propranolol in hypertension: A dose–response study. Br Med J 2:140, 1976
236. Douglas-Jones AP, Baber NS, Lee A: Once daily propranolol in the treatment of mild to moderate hypertension: A dose range finding study. Eur J Clin Pharm 14:163, 1978
237. MacLeod SM, Hamet P, Kaplan H, et al: Antihypertensive efficacy of propranolol given twice daily. Can Med Assoc J 121:737, 1979
238. Patterson JH, Self TH, Wicke W, et al: Single daily dosing of propranolol in hypertension. Am Heart J 99:133, 1980

239. Van der Brink G, Boer P, van Asten P, et al: One and three doses of propranolol a day in hypertension. Clin Pharm Ther 27:9, 1980

240. Serlin MJ, Orme ML, Baber NS, et al: Propranolol in the control of blood pressure: A dose–response study. Clin Pharm Ther 27:586, 1980

241. Douglas-Jones AP: Comparison of a once daily long-acting formulation of propranolol given twice daily in patients with mild to moderate hypertension. J Int Med Res 7:221, 1979

242. Woods JO: Long-acting or conventional propranolol in hypertension. Practitioner 223:834, 1979

243. Berglund G, Andersson D, Larsson O, Wilhelmsen L: Antihypertensive effect and side-effects of bendroflumethiazide and propranolol. Acta Med Scand 199:499, 1976

244. Jaattela A: The fixed combination of propranolol and bendrofluazide in the treatment of hypertension. Ann Clin Res 11:80, 1979

245. Karlberg BE, Kagedal B, Tegler L, et al: Controlled treatment of primary hypertension with propranolol and spironolactone. A crossover study with special reference to initial plasma renin activity. Am J Cardiol 37:642, 1976

246. Drayer JI, Kloppenborg PW, Festen J, et al: Intrapatient comparison of treatment with clorthalidone, spironolactone and propranolol in normoreninemic essential hypertension. Am J Cardiol 36:716, 1975

247. Vander Elst E, Dombey SL, Lawrence J, Vlassak W: Controlled comparison of the effects of furosemide and hydrochlorothiazide added to propranolol in the treatment of hypertension. Am Heart J 102:734, 1981

248. NK Akhtar S, Rashed MA, Khakpour M: Effect of beta-adrenergic blocking agents (alprenolol and propranolol) in essential hypertension. Angiology 26:339, 1975

249. Materson BJ, Michael UF, Oster JR, Perez-Stable EC: Antihypertensive effects of oxprenolol and propranolol. Clin Pharm Ther 20:142, 1976

250. Gavras I, Gavras H, Sullivan PC, et al: A comparative study of the effects of oxprenolol versus propranolol in essential hypertension. J Clin Pharm 19:8, 1979

251. Veterans Administration Cooperative Study Group. Oxprenolol vs propranolol: A randomized, double-blind, multiclinic trial in hypertensive patients taking hydrochlorothiazide. Hypertension 3:250, 1981

252. Wilson M, Morgan G, Morgan T: The effect on blood pressure of beta-adrenoceptor blocking drugs administered once-daily and their duration of action when therapy is ceased. Br J Clin Pharm 3:857, 1976

253. Wilson M, Morgan G, Morgan T: The effect on blood pressure of β-adrenoreceptor-blocking drugs given once-daily. Clin Sci Mol Med 51:5275, 1976

254. Salako LA, Falase AO, Aderounmu AF: Comparative β-adrenoreceptor-blocking effects and pharmacokinetics of propranolol and pindolol in hypertensive Africans. Clin Sci 57:3935, 1979

255. Berglund G: Anti-hypertensive effect of sotalol and propranolol: A double-blind crossover study. Curr Ther Res 21:21, 1977

256. Bengtsson C: Comparison between metoprolol and propranolol as anti-

hypertensive agents. A double-blind cross-over study. Acta Med Scand 199:71, 1976

257. Bosman AR, Goldberg B, McKechnie JK, et al: South African multicentre study of metoprolol and propranolol in essential hypertension. S Afr Med J 51:57, 1977

258. Sjoberg CH: Metoprolol and propranolol in the treatment of essential hypertension—a long-term comparative study. Ann Clin Res 13:23, 1981

259. Browning RC, Ebbutt A, Russell JG, Mayhew SR: A multicenter study of cardioselective metoprolol (lopressor) and non-selective propranolol in the management of mild-moderate hypertension. Br J Clin Pract 35:399, 1981

260. Lohmöller G, Frohlich ED: A comparison of timolol and propranolol in essential hypertension. Am Heart J 89:437, 1975

261. Aronow WS, Ferlinz J, Del Vicario M, et al: Effect of timolol versus propranolol on hypertension and hemodynamics. Circulation 54:47, 1976.

262. Nicholls DP, Husaini MH, Bulpitt CJ, et al: Comparison of labetalol and propranolol in hypertension. Br J Clin Pharm 9:233, 1980

263. Hunyor SN, Baver GE, Ross M, Larkin H: Labetalol and propranolol in mild hypertensives: Comparison of blood pressure and plasma volume effects. Aust NZ J Med 10:162, 1980

264. Van der Veur E, ten Berge BS, Donker AJM, et al: Comparison of labetalol, propranolol, and hydralazine in hypertensive out-patients. Eur J Clin Pharm 21:457, 198?

265. Vlachakis ND, Mendlowitz M: An approach to the treatment of essential hypertension. Am Heart J 92:750, 1976

266. Wilkinson PR, Raftery EB: A comparative trial of clonidine, propranolol, and placebo in the treatment of moderate hypertension. Br J Clin Pharm 4:289, 1977

267. Weber MA, Drayer JIM, Laragh JH: The effect of clonidine and propranolol, separately and in combination, on blood pressure and plasma renin activity in essential hypertension. J Clin Pharm 18:233, 1978

268. Friedlander DH: Captopril and propranolol in mild and moderate essential hypertension: preliminary report. NZ Med J 90:146, 1979

269. Seedat YK: Comparison of captopril with propranolol in the treatment of mild and moderate essential hypertension. S Afr Med J 56:983, 1979

270. Huang CM, del Greco F, Quintanilla A, Molteni A: Comparison of antihypertensive effects of captopril and propranolol in essential hypertension. JAMA 245:478, 1981

271. MacGregor GA, Markandu ND, Banks RA, et al: Captopril in essential hypertension in contrasting effects of adding hydrochlorothiazide or propranolol. Br Med J 284:693, 1982

272. Pickering TG, Case DB, Sullivan PA, Laragh JH: Comparison of antihypertensive and hormonal effects of captopril and propranolol at rest and during exercise. Am J Cardiol 49:1566, 1982

273. Aoki K, Kondo S, Mochizaki, et al: Antihypertensive effect of cardiovascular Ca^{2+}-antagonist in hypertensive patients in the absence and presence of beta-adrenergic blockade. Am Heart J 96:218, 1978

274. Frishman WH, Klein NA, Klein P, et al: A comparison of oral propranolol and verapamil in patients with hypertension and angina pectoris: A placebo-controlled double-blind randomized crossover trial. Am J Cardiol 50:1164, 1982

275. Prichard BNC, Gillam PMS: Treatment of hypertension with propranolol. Br Med J 1:7, 1969

276. Petrie JC, Galloway DB, Jeffers TA, et al: Methyldopa and propranolol or practolol in moderate hypertension. Br Med J 2:137, 1976

277. West MJ, Wing LMH, Mulligan J, et al: Comparison of labetalol, hydralazine, and propranolol in the therapy of moderate hypertension. Med J Aust 1:224, 1980

278. Gabriel R: Control of hypertension with single daily doses of sotalol hydrochloride. Curr Med Res Opin 4:739, 1976

279. Pasquel R: Pharmacologic considerations in determining efficacy of once-daily sotalol administration to hypertensive patients. J Clin Pharm 19:523, 1979

280. Parvinen I, Paukkala E: Comparison of once and twice daily administration of sotalol in the treatment of hypertension. Eur J Clin Pharm 15:293, 1979

281. Parvinen I, Paukkala E: Thrice-daily blood pressure readings on sotalol in the treatment of hypertension: Once-versus twice daily regimen. J Clin Pharm 19:533, 1979

282. Jaattela A: The combination of sotalol and hydrochlorothiazide in the treatment of hypertension. J Clin Pharm 19:565, 1979

283. Jaattela A: Fixed combination of sotalol and hydrochlorothiazide in the treatment of uncomplicated hypertension. Eur J Clin Pharm 19:395, 1981

284. Basson W, Myburgh DP: Synergism of a beta-blocker and diuretic in the once a day treatment of essential hypertension. J Clin Pharm 19:571, 1979

285. Reynaert J: Once a day treatment with sotalol and hydrochlorothiazide in patients with essential hypertension. J Clin Pharm 19 (8–9 part 2) 579, 1979

286. Monsalvo HJ: Sotalol/hydrochlorothiazide in geriatric hypertensive patients. J Clin Pharm 19:584, 1979

287. Sundquist H, Anttila M, Arstila M: Antihypertensive effects of practolol and sotalol. Clin Pharm Ther 16:465, 1974

288. Andersson O, Bergland G, Descamps R, Thomis J: Sotalol and metoprolol comparison of their anti-hypertensive effect. Eur J Clin Pharm 21:87, 1981

289. Saarima H: Combination of clonidine and sotalol in hypertension. Br Med J 1:810, 1976

290. Rowlands G, McConachie NA, Currie WJC: Sotalol and bethanidine—An open general practice study in the combination therapy of hypertension. Br J Clin Pract 31:57, 1977

291. Scrazzolo JE, Queirol AG: Crossover comparison of sotalol plus methyldopa in hypertension. J Clin Pharm 19:540, 1979

292. Rofman B, Kulaga S, Gabriel M, et al: Multiclinic evaluation of timolol in the treatment of mild to moderate essential hypertension. Hypertension 2:643, 1980

293. Pawlowski GJ: Treatment of essential hypertension with a new β-blocking

drug, timolol: experience with a b.i.d. dosage regimen. Curr Ther Res 22:846, 1977

294. Jennings G, Bobik A, Korner P: Comparison of effectiveness of timolol administered once a day and twice a day in the control of blood pressure in essential hypertension. Med J Aust 2:263, 1979

295. LeBel M, Belleau LJ, Grose JH: Timolol as additive therapy in essential hypertension: effect on plasma renin activity. Curr Ther Res 24:591, 1978

296. Oparil S: Multiclinic double-blind evaluation of timolol combined with hydrochlorothiazide in essential hypertension. Curr Ther Res 27:527, 1980

297. Roginsky MS: Long-term evaluation of timolol maleate combined with hydrochorothiazide for the treatment of patients with essential hypertension: a cooperative multicenter study. Curr Ther Res 27:374, 1980

298. Aronow WS, Van Herick R, Greenfield R, et al: Effect of timolol plus hydrochlorothiazide plus hydralazine on essential hypertension. Circulation 57:1017, 1978

299. Taylor RR, Halliday EJ: β-adrenergic blockade in the treatment of exercise-induced paroxysmal ventricular tachycardia. Circulation 32:778, 1965

300. Sloman G, Stannard M: β-adrenergic blockade and cardiac arrhythmias. Br Med J 4:508, 1967

301. Gettes LS, Surawicz B: Long-term prevention of paroxysmal arrhythmias with propranolol therapy. Am J Med Sci 254:257, 1967

302. Hjalmarsson Å, Ehnfeldt D, Herlitz J, et al: Effect of mortality of metoprolol in acute myocardial infarction. Lancet 2:823, 1981

303. Norwegian Multicenter Study Group. Timolol induced reduction in mortality and reinfarction in patients surviving acute myocardial infarction. N Engl J Med 304:801, 1981

304. The β-blocker Heart Attack Trial Research Group. A randomized trial of propranolol in patients with acute myocardial infarction. JAMA 247:1707, 1982

305. Rossi PRF, Yusuf S, Ramsdale D, et al: Reduction of ventricular arrhythmias by early intravenous atenolol in suspected acute myocardial infarction by intravenous atenolol in suspected acute myocardial infarction. Br Med J 286:506, 1983

306. Rydén L, Ariniego R, Arnman K, et al: A double-blind trial of metoprolol in acute myocardial infarction. Effects on ventricular tachyarrhythmias. N Engl J Med 308:614, 1983

307. Koppes GM, Beckmann CH, Jones FG: Propranolol therapy for ventricular arrhythmias 2 months after acute myocardial infarction. Am J Cardiol 46:322, 1980

308. Morganroth J, Lichstein E, Hubble E, Harrist R: Effect of propranolol on ventricular arrhythmias in the beta-blocker heart attack trial. Circulation 66 (Suppl 2):328, 1982

309. Williams DO, Tatelbaum R, Most AS: Effective treatment of supraventricular arrhythmia with acebutolol. Am J Cardiol 44:521, 1979

310. Aronow WS, Wong R: Effect of acebutolol and propranolol on premature ventricular complexes. Clin Pharmacol Ther 28:28, 1980

311. DeSoyza N, Shapiro W, Chandraratna PA, et al: Acebutolol therapy for

ventricular arrhythmia: randomized placebo controlled double-blind multicenter study. Circulation 65:1129, 1982

312. Aronow WS, VanCamp S, Turbow M, et al: Acebutolol in supraventricular
arrhythmias. Clin Pharmacol Ther 25:149, 1979

313. Singh SN, DiBianco R, Davidov ME, et al: Comparison of acebutolol and
propranolol for the treatment of chronic ventricular arrhythmia. Circulation 65:1356, 1982

314. Shapiro W, Park J, Koch G: Variability of spontaneous and exercise induced ventricular arrhythmias in the absence and presence of treatment
with acebutolol or quinidine. Am J Cardiol 49:289, 1982

315. Winchester MA, Jackson G, Meltzer RS, et al: Intravenous atenolol and
acebutolol in the treatment of supraventricular arrhythmias. Circulation 58
(Suppl 2):49, 1978

316. Roland JM, Wilcox RG, Banks DC, et al: Effect of beta-blockers on arrhythmias during six weeks after suspected myocardial infarction. Br Med
J 11:518, 1979

317. Yusuf S, Sleight P, Rossi P: Reduction in infarct–size arrhythmias and
chest pain by early intravenous beta-blockade in suspected acute myocardial infarction. Circulation 67 (Suppl 1):32, 1983

318. Byrd RC, Sung RJ, Marks J, et al: Efficacy of ASL-8052 (a short-acting
beta-adrenergic blocking agent) for control of ventricular rate in atrial flutter or atrial fibrillation. Clin Res 31:172, 1983

·319. Byrd RC, Sung RJ, Marks J, Parmley WW: Safety and efficacy of ASL-
8052 (an ultrashort-acting beta-blocking agent) for control of ventricular
rate in supraventricular tachycardias. J Am Coll Cardiol (in press)

320. Romano S, Orfei S, Pozzoni L, et al: Preliminary clinical trial on hypotensive and antiarrhythmic effect of labetalol. Drugs Exptl Clin Res 7:65, 1981

321. Mazzola C, Ferrario N, Calzavara MP, et al: Acute antihypertensive and
antiarrhythmic effects of labetalol. Curr Ther Res 29:613, 1981

322. Moller B, Rehnquist N: Metoprolol in the treatment of supraventricular
tachyarrhythmias. Ann Clin Research 11:34, 1979

323. Rehnquist N: Clinical experience with I.V. metoprolol in supraventricular
tachyarrhythmias—a multicenter study. Ann Clin Research 13 (Suppl
30):68, 1981

324. Olsson G, Rehnquist N, Ludman L, Melcher A: Metoprolol after acute
myocardial infarction: Effects on ventricular arrhythmias and exercise
tests during 6 months. Acta Med Scand 210(1–2):59, 1981

325. Whitehead MH, Whitmarsh VB, Horton JN: Metoprolol in anaesthesia for
oral surgery. The effect of pre-treatment on the incidence of cardiac dysrhythmias. Anesthesia (8):779, 1980

326. Evans DB, Peschka MT, Lee RJ, Laffan RJ: Anti-arrhythmic action of nadolol, a β-adrenergic receptor blocking agent. Eur J Pharmacol 35:17, 1976

327. Chang M-S, Sung RJ, Tai T-X, et al: Nadolol and supraventricular tachycardia: an electrophysiologic study. J Am Coll Card 2:894, 1983

328. Vukovich RA, Sasahara A, Zombrano P, et al: Antiarrhythmic effects of a
new beta-adrenergic blocking agent, nadolol. Clin Pharmacol Ther 19:118,
1976

329. Sandler G, Pistevos AC: Use of oxprenolol in cardiac arrhythmias associated with acute myocardial infarction. Br Med J. 1:254, 1971

330. Fuccella LM, Imhoff P: Experience with a new beta-receptor blocking agent (transicor) in the management of cardiac arrhythmias. Pharmacol Clin 1:123, 1969

331. Taylor SH, Silke B, Ebbutt A, et al: A long-term prevention study with oxprenolol in coronary heart disease. N Engl J Med 307:1293, 1982

332. Levi GF, Proto C: Combined treatment of atrial fibrillation with quinidine and beta-blockers. Br Heart J 34:911, 1972

333. Frishman WH, Davis R, Strom J, et al: Clinical pharmacology of the new beta-adrenergic blocking drugs. Part 5. Pindolol (LB46) therapy for supraventricular arrhythmia: A viable alternative to propranolol in patients with bronchospasm. Am Heart J 98:393, 1979

334. Aronow WS, Uyeyama RR: Treatment of arrhythmias with pindolol. Clin Pharmacol Ther 13:15, 1972

335. Podrid PJ, Lown B: Pindolol for ventricular arrhythmia. Am Heart J 104:491, 1982

336. Anderson JL, Rodier HE, Green LS: Comparative effects of beta-adrenergic blocking drugs on experimental ventricular fibrillation threshold. Am J Cardiol 51:1196, 1983

337. Singh BN, Jewitt DE: β-adrenergic blocking drugs in cardiac arrhythmias. Drugs 7:426, 1974

338. Harrison DC, Griffin JR, Fiene TJ: Effects of beta-adrenergic blockade with propranolol in patients with atrial arrhythmias. N Engl J Med 273:410, 1965

339. Schamroth L: Immediate effects of intravenous propranolol on various cardiac arrhythmias. Am J Cardiol 18:438, 1966

340. Irons GV, Ginn WN, Orgain ES: Use of a beta-adrenergic receptor blocking agent (propranolol) in the treatment of cardiac arrhythmias. Am J Med 43:161, 1967

341. Frieden J, Rosenblum R, Enselberg CD, Rosenberg A: Propranolol treatment of chronic intractable supraventricular arrhythmias. Am J Cardiol 22:711, 1968

342. Lemberg L, Castellanos A, Aroebal AG: The use of propranolol in arrhythmias complicating acute myocardial infarction. Am Heart J 80:479, 1970

343. Salazar C, Frishman WH, Friedman S, et al: β-blockade for supraventricular tachycardia post-coronary artery surgery: A propranolol withdrawal syndrome. Angiology 30:816, 1979

344. Oka Y, Frishman WH, Becker R, et al: Clinical pharmacology of the new beta-adrenergic blockers. Part 10. Beta-adrenergic blockade and coronary artery surgery. Am Heart J 99:255, 1980

345. Mohr R, Smolinsky A, Goor D: Prevention of supraventricular tachyarrhythmia with low dose propranolol after coronary bypass. J Thorac Cardiovasc Surg 81:840, 1981

346. Silverman N, Wright R, Levitsky S: Efficacy of low dose propranolol in

preventing postoperative supraventricular tachyarrhythmias. Ann Surg 196:194, 1982

347. Woosley RL, Kornhauser D, Smith R, et al: Suppression of chronic ventricular arrhythmias with propranolol. Circulation 60:819, 1979

348. Gibson D, Sowton E: The use of beta-adrenergic receptor blocking drugs in dysrhythmias. Prog Cardiovasc Dis 12:16, 1969

349. Nixon JV, Pennington W, Ritter W, Shapiro W: Efficacy of propranolol in the control of exercise induced or augmented ventricular ectopic activity. Circulation 57:115, 1978

350. Lichstein E, Morganroth J, Harrist R, Hubble E: Effect of propranolol on ventricular arrhythmia. The beta-blocker heart attack trial. Circulation 67 (Suppl I):I-11, 1983

351. Hansteen V: Beta-blockade after myocardial infarction: The Norwegian propranolol study in high-risk patients. Circulation 67 (Suppl I):57, 1983

352. Latour Y, Dumont G, Brosseau A, LeLorie J: Effects of sotalol in twenty patients with cardiac arrhythmias. Int J Clin Pharmacol 15:275, 1977

353. Fogelman F, Lightman SL, Sillett RW, McNicol MW: The treatment of cardiac arrhythmias with sotalol. Eur J Clin Pharm 5:72, 1972

354. Prakash R, Allen HN, Condo F, et al: Clinical evaluation of the antiarrhythmic effects of sotalol. Am J Cardiol 26:654, 1970

355. Simon A, Berman E: Long-term sotalol therapy in patients with arrhythmias. J Clin Pharmacol 19:547, 1979

356. Julian DG, Presscott RJ, Jackson FS, Szekely P: Controlled trial of sotalol for one year after myocardial infarction. Lancet 1:1142, 1982

357. von der Lippe G, Lund-Johansen P: Effect of timolol on late ventricular arrhythmias after acute myocardial infarction. Acta Med Scand (Suppl.): 651; 253, 1981

358. Cohen LS, Braunwald E: Amelioration of angina pectoris in idiopathic hypertrophic subaortic stenosis with beta-adrenergic blockade. Circulation 35:847, 1967

359. Swan DA, Bell B, Oakley CM, Goodwin J: Analysis of symptomatic course and prognosis and treatment of hypertrophic obstructive cardiomyopathy. Br Heart J 33:671, 1971

360. Adelman AG, Wigle ED, Ragganathan N, et al: The clinical course in muscular subaortic stenosis—a retrospective and prospective study of 60 hemodynamically proved cases. Ann Intern Med 77:515, 1972

361. Cherian G, Brockington IM, Shah PM, et al: Beta-adrenergic blockade in patients with hypertrophic cardiomyopathy. Am Heart J 73:140, 1967

362. Hubner PJB, Ziady GM, Lane GK, et al: Double-blind trial of propranolol and practolol in hypertrophic cardiomyopathy. Br Heart J 35:1116, 1973

363. Harrison DC, Braunwald E, Glick G, et al: Effects of beta-adrenergic blockade on the circulation with particular reference to observations in patients with hypertrophic subaortic stenosis. Circulation 29:84, 1964

364. Epstein SE, Henry WL, Clark CE, et al: Asymmetric septal hypertrophy. Ann Intern Med 81:650, 1974

365. Jeresaty RM: Mitral-valve prolapse syndrome. Prog Cardiovasc Dis 15:623, 1973
366. Winkle RA, Lopes MG, Goodman DS, et al: Propranolol for patients with mitral valve prolapse. Am Heart J 93:422, 1970
367. Wheat MW, Palmer RF, Bartley TD, et al: Treatment of dissecting aneurysms of the aorta without surgery. Thorac Cardiovasc Surg 50:364, 1965
368. Slater EE, DeSanctis R: Dissection of the aorta. Med Clin N Amer 63:141, 1979.
369. Levey GS: Catecholamine hypersensitivity thyroid hormone and the heart—a reevaluation. Am J Med 50:413, 1971
370. Brewster WR, Isaacs JP, Osgood PF, King TL: The hemodynamic and metabolic interrelationships in the activity of epinephrine, norepinephrine, and the thyroid hormones. Circulation 13:1, 1956
371. Ramsay I: Adrenergic blockade in hyperthyroidism. Br J Clin Pharmacol 2:385, 1975
372. Landsberg L: Catecholamines and hyperthyroidism. Clin Endocrinol Metab 3:697, 1977
373. Ingbar SH: The role of antiadrenergic agents in the management of thyrotoxicosis. Card Rev Rep 2:683, 1981
374. Williams LT, Leibowitz RJ, Watanabe AM, et al: Thyroid hormone regulation of beta-adrenergic receptor numbers. J Biol Chem 252:2787, 1977
375. Malbon CC, Moreno FJ, Cabelli RJ, Fain JN: Fat cell adenylate cyclase and beta-adrenergic receptors in altered thyroid states. J Biol Chem 253:671, 1978
376. Levey GS, Epstein SE: Myocardial adenyl cyclase: Activation by thyroid hormones and evidence for two adenyl cyclase systems. J Clin Invest 48:1663, 1969
377. Canary JJ, Schaff M, Duffy BJ, Kyle LH: Effects of oral and intramuscular administration of reserpine in thyrotoxicosis. N Engl J Med 257:435, 1957
378. Wilson WR, Theilin FO, Fletcher FW: Pharmacodynamic effects of beta-adrenergic blockade in patients with hyperthyroidism. J Clin Invest 41:1697, 1967
379. Jones MK, John R, Jones GR: The effect of oxprenolol, acebutolol, and propranolol on thyroid hormones in hyperthyroid subjects. Clin Endocrin 13:343, 1980
380. How J, Khir ASM, Bewsher PD: The effect of atenolol on serum thyroid hormones in hyperthyroid patients. Clin Endocrin 13:299, 1980
381. Peden NR, Isles TE, Stevenson IH, Crooks J: Nadolol in thyrotoxicosis. Br J Clin Pharm 13(6):835, 1982
382. Nilsson OR, Karlberg BE, Kagedal B, et al: Non-selective and selective β_1-adrenoceptor blocking agents in the treatment of hyperthyroidism. Acta Med Scand 206:21, 1979
383. Wahlberg P, Carlsson SA: Long-term control of thyrotoxicosis with the beta-blocker sotalol—A model of untreated hyperthyroidism. Acta Endocrin 87:734, 1978

384. Wiersinga WM, Touber JL: The influence of β-adrenoceptor blocking drugs on plasma thyroxine and triiodothyronine. J Clin Endocrinol Metab 45:293, 1977
385. Mackin JF, Canary JJ, Pittman CS: Thyroid storm and its management. N Engl J Med 291:1396, 1974
386. Caswell HT, Marks AD, Channick BJ: Propranolol for the preoperative preparation of patients with thyrotoxicosis. Surg Gynecol Obstet 146(6):908, 1978
387. Lee TC, Coffey RJ, Currier BM, Ma XP, Canary JJ: Propranolol and thyroidectomy in the treatment of thyrotoxicosis. Ann Surg 195(6):766, 1982
388. Turner P, Hill RC: A comparison of three beta-adrenergic blocking drugs in thyrotoxic tachycardia. J Clin Pharmacol 8:268, 1968
389. Schelling JL, Scazziga B, Dufour RJ, et al: Effect of pindolol, a beta-receptor antagonist in hyperthyroidism. Clin Pharmacol Ther 14:158, 1973
390. Shanks RG, Hadden DR, Lowe DC, McDevitt DG: Controlled trial of propranolol in thyrotoxicosis. Lancet 1:993, 1969
391. Grossman W, Robin NI, Johnson LW, et al: The effect of beta-blockade on the peripheral manifestations of thyrotoxicosis. Ann Intern Med 74:875, 1971
392. Wartofsky L, Dimond RC, Noel GL, et al: Failure of propranolol to alter thyroid iodine release, thyroxine turnover, or the TSH and PRL responses to thyrotropin-releasing hormone in patients with thyrotoxicosis. J Endocrinol Metab 41:485, 1975
393. Georges LP, Santangelo RP, Machin JF, Canary JJ: Metabolic effects of propranolol in thyrotoxicosis. 1. Nitrogen, calcium, and hydroxyproline Metabolism 24:11, 1975
394. Rabkin R, Stables DP, Levin NW, Suzman MM: The prophylactic value of propranolol in angina pectoris. Am J Cardiol 18:370, 1966
395. Weber RB, Reinmuth OM: The treatment of migraine with propranolol. Neurology 22:366, 1972
396. Diamond S, Medina JL: Double blind study of propranolol for migraine prophylaxis. Headache 16:24, 1976
397. Caviness VS Jr, O'Brien P: Headache. N Engl J Med 302:446, 1980.
398. Borgesen SE: Propranolol for migraine. Compr Ther 3(4):53, 1977
399. Forssman B, Henriksson K-G, Johannsson V, et al: Propranolol for migraine prophylaxis. Headache 16:238, 1976
400. Behan PO, Reid M: Propranolol in the treatment of migraine. Practitioner 224:201, 1980
401. Frishman WH: B-adrenoceptor antagonists: new drugs and new indications. N Engl J Med 305:500, 1981
402. Marsden CD, Foley TH, Owen DAL, McAllister RG: Peripheral beta-adrenergic receptors concerned with tremor. Clin Sci 33:53, 1967
403. Young RR, Growdon JH, Shahani BT: Beta adrenergic mechanisms in action tremor. N Engl J Med 293:950, 1975
404. Murray TJ: Long-term therapy of essential tremor with propranolol. Can Med Assoc J 115:892, 1976

405. Winkler GF, Young RR: Efficacy of chronic propranolol therapy in action tremors of the familial, senile, or essential varieties. N Engl J Med 290:984, 1974

406. Ferro JM, Calhau ES: Treatment of familial essential myoclonus with propranolol. Lancet 2:143, 1977

407. Granville-Grossman KL, Turner P: The effect of propranolol on anxiety. Lancet 1:788, 1966

408. Editorial: Beta blockers in anxiety and stress. Br Med J 1:415, 1976

409. Whitlock FA, Price J: Use of beta adrenergic receptor blocking drugs in psychiatry. Drugs 8:109, 1974

410. Jefferson JW: Beta adrenergic blockade in psychiatry. Arch Gen Psychiatr 31:681, 1974

411. Atsmon A, Blim I, Steiner M, Latz A, Wijsenbeck H: Further studies with propranolol in psychotic patients. Relation to initial psychiatric state, urinary catecholamines and 3 methoxy 4 hydroxy phenyl glycol. Psycho Pharmacol 27:249, 1972

412. Yorkston NJ, Zaki SA, Malik MKU, et al: Propranolol in the control of schizophrenic symptoms. Br Med J 4:633, 1974

413. Editorial: New drugs for schizophrenia. Br Med J 4:614, 1975

414. Grosz HJ: Narcotic withdrawal symptoms in heroin users treated with propranolol. Lancet 2:564, 1972

415. Grosz HJ: Effect of propranolol on active users of heroin. Lancet 2:602, 1973

416. Sellers EM, Degani NC, Silm DH, MacLeod SM: Propranolol-decreased noradrenaline secretion and alcohol withdrawal. Lancet 1:94, 1976

417. Phillips CI, Howitt G, Rowlands DJ: Propranolol as ocular hypotensive agent. Br J Ophthalmol 51:222, 1967

418. Bucci MG, Missiroli A, Giraldi JP, Virno M: Local administration of propranolol in the treatment of glaucoma. Boll Oculist 47:51, 1968

419. Heel RC, Brogden RN, Speight TM, Avery GS: Timolol: A review of its therapeutic efficacy in the topical treatment of glaucoma. Drugs 17:38, 1979

420. Boger WP III, Steinert RF, Puliafito CA, Pavan-Langston D: Clinical trial comparing timolol ophthalmic solution to pilocarpine in open-angle glaucoma. Am J Ophthalmol 86:8, 1978

421. Steinert RF, Thomas JV, Boger WP III: Long-term drift and continued efficacy after multiyear, timolol therapy. Arch Opthal 99:100, 1981

422. Lebrec D, Nouel O, Corbic M, Benhamou J-P: Propranolol—a medical treatment for portal hypertension. Lancet 2:180, 1980

423. Lebrec D, Poynard J, Hillon P, Benhamou J-P: Propranolol for prevention of recurrent gastrointestinal bleeding in patients with cirrhosis. N Engl J Med 305:1371, 1981

424. Lebrec D, Hillon P, Munoz C, et al: The effect of propranolol on portal hypertension in patients with cirrhosis: a hemodynamic study. Hepatology 2:523, 1982

425. Hillon P, Lebrec D, Munoz C, et al: Comparison of a cardioselective and

a nonselective β-blocker on portal hypertension in patients with cirrhosis. Hepatology 2:528, 1982

426. Schroeder ET, Anderson GH, Goodman SH, et al: Effect of blockade of angiotensin II on blood pressure, renin, and aldosterone in cirrhosis. Kidney Int 9:511, 1976

427. Wilkinson SP, Bernardi M, Smith K, et al: Effect of β-adrenergic blocking drugs on the renin-aldosterone system, sodium excretion, and renal hemodynamics in cirrhosis with ascites. Gastroenterology 73:659, 1977

CHAPTER 5

Adverse Effects, Drug Interactions—
Choosing a β-Blocker

William H. Frishman

ADVERSE EFFECTS OF β-BLOCKERS

Comparing and tabulating adverse effects from different studies of β-adrenergic blockers is particularly difficult because of a number of factors. These include the use of different definitions of side effects, the kinds of patients studied, and study design features. Methods of ascertainment and reporting adverse side effects also differ from study to study.[1] Given these problems, the types and frequencies of adverse effects attributed to various β-blocker compounds appear to be similar.[2] The side effect profiles of β-blockers are also remarkably close to those seen with concurrent placebo treatments, attesting to the remarkable safety margin of the β-blockers as a group.[1,3]

The adverse effects of β-adrenoceptor blockers can be divided into two categories: (1) those that result from known pharmacologic consequences of β-adrenoceptor blockade; and (2) other reactions that do not appear to result from β-adrenoreceptor blockade.

Side effects of the first type are widespread because of the ubiquitous nature of the sympathetic nervous system in the control of physiologic and metabolic function. They include asthma, heart failure, hypoglycemia, bradycardia and heart block, intermittent claudication, and Raynaud's phenomenon. The incidence of these adverse effects varies with the type of β-blocker used.

Side effects of the second category are rare. They include an unusual oculomucocutaneous reaction and the possibility of carcinogenesis.

147

Major Clinical Experiences

There have been extensive clinical studies designed to identify the nature and frequency of side effects with β-blocking agents. The Boston Collaborative Drug Surveillance Program studied the effects of propranolol (nonselective, no partial agonism) in 800 hospitalized patients and practolol ($β_1$-selective, with partial agonism) in 199 patients.[4] Forrest reported on the adverse reaction seen with oxprenolol (nonselective, with partial agonism) in 4400 patients receiving the drug for angina pectoris.[5] Zacharias et al. reported on the side effects seen with long-term atenolol ($β_1$-selective, long-acting) treatment in patients with hypertension.[6] The side-effect profiles for pindolol (nonselective, with partial agonism)[7-9] and labetalol (nonselective, α-blocking, see Chapter 7)[10] have also been assessed in extensive clinical trials in hypertensive patients. The long-term β-blocker trials in thousands of myocardial infarct survivors have reported on the adverse reactions with different β-blocking compounds used in this clinical situation.[1,3,11-15]

In the Boston Collaborative Surveillance Program, propranolol was used for mixed clinical indications and adverse reactions were reported in 79 patients (9.9 percent).[4] These are summarized in Table 1. Ten adverse reactions were considered life-threatening, and all appeared to result from impaired cardiac function. Of the 69 other reactions, 43 also involved interference with cardiac performance but were not deemed life-threatening. The frequency of side effects was independent of the dose used. Adverse reactions were seen more commonly among older patients and those with azotemia.[4]

In the same study, of the 199 patients who received practolol ($β_1$-selective), adverse reactions were seen in 18 (9.0 percent). The nature and frequency of adverse reactions to practolol resembled those of propranolol (Table 2).[4]

In patients with hypertension, the frequency of adverse reactions with atenolol were reported to be approximately 15 percent in a four-year follow-up study (Table 3).[6] In an extensive literature survey in 15,753 patients receiving pindolol, a similar incidence of side effects was seen.[16] The frequency of side effects reported in labetalol-treated patients was similar to those described with atenolol and pindolol.[10]

Forrest reported a 13.7 percent incidence of side effects with oxprenolol in patients with angina pectoris (Table 4).[5] In 12 placebo-controlled long-term studies of patients surviving acute myocardial infarction, the incidence of side effects ranged from 7 to 20 percent.[3,11-15] The overall incidence of severe side effects was not much different from that seen with placebo treatment (Table 5).[3] The reasons for discontinuing treatment because of side effects in the largest of these trials (β-Blocker Post-Infarction Trial—BHAT) are shown in Table 6.

TABLE 1. ADVERSE REACTIONS TO PROPRANOLOL AMONG 800 HOSPITALIZED MEDICAL PATIENTS[*4]

Nature of Reaction	Number of Patients	Percent
Life-threatening		
Shock	5	0.6
Bradycardia and angina	1	0.1
Pulmonary edema	3	0.4
Complete heart block	1	0.1
Total	10	1.3
Non-life-threatening		
Bradycardia	17	2.1
Hypotension	16	2.0
Congestive heart failure or fluid retention	9	1.1
Gastrointestinal disturbances	9	1.1
CNS disturbances (headache, dizziness, fatigue, tinnitus, blurring of vision, paraesthesias, depression)	9	1.1
Bronchospasm	4	0.5
Sensitivity reactions (rash, fever)	3	0.4
2:1 heart block	1	0.1
Elevation in serum phenytoin level	1	0.1
Total	69	8.6
Total with adverse reactions	79	9.9

*With bradycardia in three cases and congestive heart failure in one; with syncope in five cases.

TABLE 2. ADVERSE REACTIONS TO PRACTOLOL AMONG 199 HOSPITALIZED MEDICAL PATIENTS[4]

Nature of Reaction	Number of Patients	Percent
Life-threatening		
Pulmonary edema	1	0.5
Complete heart block, bradycardia, and shock	1	0.5
Second-degree heart block and hypotension	1	0.5
Total	3	1.5
Non-life-threatening		
Congestive heart failure	3	1.5
Bradycardia	4	2.0
CNS disturbances (dizziness, confusion)	3	1.5
Sensitivity reactions (rash)	2	1.0
Hypotension	1	0.5
Gastrointestinal disturbances	1	0.5
Dyspnea	1	0.5
Total	15	7.5
Total with adverse reactions	18	9.0

TABLE 3. ADVERSE EFFECTS ATTRIBUTABLE TO ATENOLOL IN THE LONG-TERM (4 YEARS) TREATMENT OF SYSTEMIC HYPERTENSION ($N = 543$)[6]

	Leading to Treatment Withdrawal (Number of Patients)	Dose Limiting (Number of Patients)
Cold extremities	1	14
Indigestion	3	4
Fatigue	0	21
Vivid dreams	0	5
Hallucinations	0	0
Paresthesia	0	2
Dizziness	1	4
Ataxia	0	1
Depression	0	4
Impotence	0	1
Diarrhea	1	1
Constipation	0	1
Worsening claudication	1	6
Bronchospasm	2	16
Heart failure	2	0
Bradycardia	1	0
Rash	0	0
Total number	12	80
Percent incidence	2.2%	14.5%

TABLE 4. FREQUENCY AND TYPE OF SIDE EFFECTS REPORTED WITH OXPRENOLOL IN PATIENTS WITH ANGINA PECTORIS (10-MONTH FOLLOW-UP, 4400 PATIENTS)[5]

Side Effect	Total Number	%	Severe Number	%	Mild Number	%
Gastrointestinal	226	5.0	108	2.4	118	2.6
Dizziness–Giddiness	144	3.0	58	1.3	86	1.7
Cardiovascular						
Heart failure	30	0.7	22	0.5	8	0.2
Bradycardia	37	0.8	8	0.1	29	0.7
Worsened angina	27	0.7	27	0.7	—	—
Respiratory	49	1.0	25	0.5	24	0.5
Miscellaneous	114	2.5	61	1.3	53	1.2
Total percent incidence	627	13.7	309	6.8	318	6.9

TABLE 5. PERCENTAGE OF PATIENTS WHO STOPPED TAKING STUDY β-BLOCKERS IN VARIOUS LONG-TERM PLACEBO-CONTROLLED POSTINFARCTION TRIALS[1]

	Practolol[11]	Timolol[12]	Metoprolol[13]	Propranolol[3]	Sotalol[14]	Oxprenolol[15]
Heart failure	4.1/3.6*	2.9/2.1	0.6/1.0	4.0/3.5	2.6/3.8	1.8/1.2
Hypotension	0.6/0.1	2.8/1.2	4.2/1.9	1.2/0.3	2.1/0.7	0.3/0.2
Bradycardia	0.5/0.1	3.9/0.2	2.6/0.7	0.7/0.3	4.4/0	NA†
Depression	0.2/0.3	NA	0/0	0.4/0.4	0/0	1.8/0.4
Fatigue	0.3/0.1	0.4/0.1	0/0	1.5/1.0	0.9/0.7	0.5/0.7
Pulmonary problems	NA	1.1/0.4	0/0	0.9/0.7	0.5/0.2	NA

*Treatment group/placebo group.
†NA = not available.

TABLE 6. PERCENT OF PATIENTS WITHDRAWN FOR MEDICAL REASONS IN β-BLOCKER HEART ATTACK TRIAL[3]

Adverse Effect	Propranolol	Placebo	Significant Difference
Cardiopulmonary			
Congestive heart failure	4.0	3.5	No
Hypotension	1.2	0.3	Yes
Pulmonary problems	0.9	0.7	No
Sinus bradycardia	0.7	0.3	No
New or extended myocardial infarction	0.4	0.4	No
Serious ventricular arrhythmia	0.3	1.0	Yes
Heart block	0.1	0.1	No
Syncope	0.1	0.1	No
Neuropsychiatric			
Tiredness	1.5	1.0	No
Disorientation	0.6	0.6	No
Depression	0.4	0.4	No
Faintness	0.5	0.2	No
Nightmares	0.1	0.2	No
Insomnia	0.2	0.0	No
Reduced sexual activity	0.2	0.0	Yes
Other			
Gastrointestinal problems	1.0	0.3	Yes
Dermatologic problems	0.3	0.1	No
Cancer	0.2	0.1	No

Adverse Cardiac Effects Related to β-Adrenoceptor Blockade

Myocardial Failure. There are several circumstances by which blockade of β-receptors may cause congestive heart failure: (1) in an enlarged heart with impaired myocardial function where excessive sympathetic drive is essential to maintain the myocardium on a compensated Starling curve; and (2) if the left ventricular stroke volume is restricted and tachycardia is needed to maintain cardiac output.

Considering the factors noted above, any β-blocking drug may be associated with the development of heart failure. Furthermore, it is possible that an important component of heart failure may be accounted for by increases in peripheral vascular resistance produced by nonselective agents (e.g., propranolol, timolol, sotalol).[17] It has been claimed that β-blockers with intrinsic sympathomimetic activity are better in preserving left ventricular function and less likely to precipitate heart failure,[18] but there have been no human studies to support this contention. In dog-transplanted denervated heart preparations, β-blockers with intrinsic sympathomimetic activity have a positive rather than a negative inotropic effect.[19] The clinical significance of this effect in the intact organism is uncertain.

In patients with impaired myocardial function who require β-blocking agents, digitalis and diuretics can be used, preferably with drugs having intrinsic sympathomimetic activity or α-adrenergic blocking properties.

Sinus Node Dysfunction and Atrioventricular Conduction Delay. Slowing of the resting heart rate is a normal response to treatment with β-blocking drugs with and without intrinsic sympathomimetic activity. Healthy individuals can sustain a heart rate of 40 to 50 without disability, unless there is clinical evidence of heart failure.[20] Drugs with intrinsic sympathomimetic activity do not lower the resting heart rate to the same degree as propranolol[21]; however, all β-blocking drugs are contraindicated (unless an artificial pacemaker is present) in patients with the "sick sinus syndrome."[22]

If there is a partial or complete atrioventricular conduction defect, use of a β-blocking drug may lead to a serious bradyarrhythmia.[20] The risk of atrioventricular impairment is not the same with all β-blockers. Giudicelli et al.[23] showed that, in dogs, β-blockade and not membrane-stabilizing activity is responsible for atrioventricular conduction impairment. Compounds, like pindolol or oxprenolol, which have intrinsic sympathomimetic activity in dosages producing β-blockade, do not impair atrioventricular conduction to the same extent as propranolol. The clinical significance of this electrophysiologic difference among β-blockers in patients with atrioventricular conduction disease has not been determined.

β-Adrenoceptor Blocker Withdrawal. Following abrupt cessation of chronic β-blocker therapy, exacerbation of angina pectoris and, in some cases, acute myocardial infarction and death have been reported.[24–26]

Observations made in multiple double-blind randomized trials have confirmed the reality of a propranolol withdrawal reaction.[24–27] The exact mechanism for the propranolol withdrawal reaction is unclear. There is some evidence that the withdrawal phenomenon may be due to the generation of additional β-adrenoceptors or increased receptor sensitivity during the period of β-adrenoceptor blockade.[28,29] When the β-adrenoceptor blocker is then withdrawn, the increased β-receptor population, when stimulated, can result in excessive β-receptor stimulation, which will be clinically important when the delivery and use of oxygen is finely balanced, as occurs in ischemic heart disease. Other suggested mechanisms for the withdrawal reaction include heightened platelet aggregability,[26] an elevation in thyroid hormone activity,[30] and an increase in circulating catecholamines.[31]

As it seems possible that post–adrenoceptor blockade sensitivity may be due to the generation of additional β-adrenoceptors, a β-adrenoceptor blocking drug with some partial agonist activity might provide enough receptor stimulation to prevent the generation of additional β-adrenoceptors.[32] Studies with atenolol, metoprolol, pindolol, and propranolol in normal subjects and patients indicate that administration of pindolol is not associated with increased sensitivity to isoproterenol after pindolol is stopped, in contrast to the other β-adrenoceptor blocking drugs that do not possess partial agonist activity.[33,34] Despite this difference with pindolol, it is still prudent to discontinue all β-blockers with caution in patients with ischemic heart disease.[35]

Adverse Noncardiac Side Effects Related to β-Adrenoreceptor Blockade

Effect on Ventilatory Function. The bronchodilator effects of catecholamines on the bronchial β-adrenoreceptors ($β_2$) are inhibited by nonselective β-blockers (e.g., propranolol, nadolol).[36] Comparative studies have shown, however, that β-blocking compounds with partial agonist activity,[37] $β_1$-selectivity,[38,39] and α-adrenergic blocking actions[40] are less likely than propranolol to increase airways resistance in asthmatics. $β_1$-Selectivity, however, is not absolute and may be lost with high therapeutic doses, as shown with atenolol and metoprolol. It is possible in asthma to use a $β_2$-selective agonist (such as albuterol) in certain patients with concomitant low-dose $β_1$-selective blocker treatment.[41] In general, all β-blockers should be avoided in patients with bronchospastic disease.

Peripheral Vascular Effects (Raynaud's Phenomenon). Cold extremities and absent pulses have been reported to occur more frequently in patients receiving β-blockers for hypertension, compared to treatment with methyldopa.[42] Among the β-blockers, the incidence was highest with propranolol and lower with drugs having β_1-selectivity or intrinsic sympathomimetic activity. In some instances, vascular compromise has been severe enough to cause cyanosis and impending gangrene.[43] This is probably due to the reduction in cardiac output and blockade of β_2-adrenoceptor-mediated skeletal muscle vasodilation, resulting in unopposed α-adrenoceptor vasoconstriction.[44] β-Blocking drugs with β_1-selectivity or partial agonist activity will not affect peripheral vessels to the same degree as propranolol.

Raynaud's phenomenon is one of the more common side effects of propranolol treatment.[45,46] It is more troublesome with propranolol than practolol, probably due to the β_2-blocking properties of propranolol.

Patients with peripheral vascular disease who suffer from intermittent claudication often report worsening of the claudication when treated with β-blocking drugs.[47,48] Whether drugs with β_1-selectivity or partial agonist activity can protect against this adverse reaction has yet to be determined.

Hypoglycemia and Hyperglycemia. Several authors have described severe hypoglycemic reactions during therapy with β-adrenergic blocking drugs.[49,50] Some of the patients affected were insulin-dependent diabetics, but others were nondiabetic. Studies of resting normal volunteers have demonstrated that propranolol produces no alteration in blood glucose values,[51] although the hyperglycemic response to exercise is blunted.

In man, mobilization of muscle glycogen is a β-receptor-mediated function (β_2-mediated), while mobilization of liver glycogen depends on α-receptor stimulation.[52,53] As a result, β-receptor blocking drugs (especially nonselective β-blockers) may retard recovery from insulin-induced hypoglycemia. In humans, Abramson et al.[49] showed that propranolol delayed the return of blood glucose values to normal after insulin-induced hypoglycemia. If liver glycogen is reduced by fasting or illness, the concomitant use of nonselective β-blocking drugs may further prolong recovery from hypoglycemia, since alternative stores cannot be mobilized.[54,55] With propranolol, the normal hemodynamic response to hypoglycemia may be altered, with an elevation of diastolic blood pressure due to an α-constrictive response to reflex increases in plasma catecholamines.[55]

This enhancement of insulin-induced hypoglycemia and its hemodynamic consequences may be less with β_1-selective agents (where there is no blocking effect on β_2-receptors) and agents with intrinsic sympathomimetic activity (which may stimulate β_2-receptors).[56]

There is also a marked diminution in the clinical manifestations of sympathetic discharge associated with hypoglycemia (tachycardia).[57] These findings suggest that β-blockers interfere with compensatory responses to hypoglycemia and can mask certain "warning signs" of this condition. However, other hypoglycemic reactions, such as diaphoresis, are not affected by β-adrenergic blockade.

Central Nervous System Effects. Dreams, hallucinations, insomnia, and depression can occur during therapy with β-blockers (Chapter 15).[45,58] These symptoms are evidence of drug entry into the central nervous system (CNS) and are especially common with the highly lipid-soluble β-blockers (propranolol, metoprolol), which presumably better penetrate the CNS. It has been claimed that β-blockers with less lipid solubility (atenolol, nadolol) will cause fewer CNS side effects. This claim is intriguing, but its validity must be corroborated with more extensive clinical experiences.[39,59]

Clinical pharmacologic studies have generally supported the view that β-blockers do not have any marked sedative effects. No such action could be detected for propranolol, sotalol, oxprenolol, or atenolol.[58]

Skeletal Muscle Effects. In vitro studies demonstrate that ˌropranolol can produce neuromuscular blockade.[60] The direct actions of epinephrine on skeletal muscle are mediated probably through β_2-receptors and tremor is the most common side effect of β_2-stimulating drugs. Propranolol has been shown to attenuate the ankle jerk and a prolonged curare-like effect has been described in one patient.[61] Whether the β_1-selective blockers have similar effects remains to be determined.

Muscle cramps can also occur with pindolol[45] and have been described with practolol and propranolol.[62] The etiology of this side effect is unknown.

Miscellaneous Side Effects. Diarrhea, nausea, gastric pain, constipation and flatulence have been seen occasionally with all β-blockers (2 to 11 percent of patients) (see Chapter 14).[63]

Hematologic reactions are unusual: rare cases of purpura[64] and agranulocytosis[65] have been described with propranolol.

A devastating blood pressure rebound effect has been described in patients who discontinued clonidine while being treated with nonselective β-blocking agents. The mechanism for this may be related to an increase in circulating catecholamines and an increase in peripheral vascular resistance.[66,67] Whether β_1-selective or partial agonist β-blockers have similar effects following clonidine withdrawal remains to be determined. It has not been a problem with labetalol (see Chapter 7).[68]

Increases in patient weight may occur. Bengtsson[69] noted an average 1 kg weight increment in patients taking alprenolol. A similar weight gain in patients has also been noted with propranolol,[70] pindolol,[35,71] and oxprenolol. The mechanism of this weight gain has not been elucidated; however, treatment with diuretic agents will commonly relieve it.

Adverse Effects Unrelated to β-Adrenoceptor Blockade

Oculomucocutaneous Syndrome. A characteristic immune reaction—the oculomucocutaneous syndrome—affecting singly or in combination eyes, mucous and serous membranes, and the skin, often in association with a positive antinuclear factor, has been reported in patients treated with practolol and has led to the curtailment of its clinical use.[72,73] Close attention has been focused on this syndrome because of fears that other β-adrenoreceptor blocking drugs may be associated with this syndrome. In 19 patients with such a reaction with practolol, the lesions healed after switching to atenolol treatment.

The main features in this syndrome in 439 patients reviewed by Nichols[20] were as follows:

- Eye: A gritty feeling in the eye may progress to a panconjunctivitis, keratitis, and pannus formation. In Nichol's series, 18 patients manifested severe eye changes, 112 had corneal damage without loss of sight, and 146 had eye changes without corneal involvement. The average time to develop this syndrome was 23 months after initiating treatment.
- Skin: The skin changes usually begin with a pruritic rash involving the palms and the soles of the feet. Thickened plaques that resemble psoriasis may appear. Immunofluorescent studies have revealed granular deposits at the dermalectodermal junction in some cases.[74]
- Ear: Deafness with serious otitis media has been reported in some patients receiving practolol.

Sclerosing Peritonitis. Thirty-three patients with this syndrome were included in Nichol's report. Patients may present with colicky abdominal pain or with an abdominal mass. This condition may progress despite withdrawal of the drug and can first develop up to a year after the discontinuation of practolol. The peritoneum becomes covered with a film of white fibrous tissue with thicker plaques.[75] The natural history of this condition is unknown and the diagnosis has usually been made at laparotomy or autopsy. Most patients appear to improve with time after cessation of treatment. The mean time to diagnosis of sclerosing peritonitis after starting practolol was 37 months.

As with sclerosing peritonitis, many of the other practolol reactions are reversible by withdrawal of the drug, together with treatment with topical corticosteroids, artificial tear solutions, antibiotic eye drops, and oral corticosteroids.[76]

An important consideration is whether the practolol reaction is specific for practolol or is the direct and specific result of pharmacologically induced changes by β-blockade.[77] There have been few convincing published reports of the oculomucocutaneous reaction with oxprenolol[78,79] and propranolol.[80,81] In view of the extensive clinical use of both oxprenolol and propranolol, these reactions, even if drug induced, are exceedingly rare. There is need, however, for vigilance during therapy with the newer β-blockers.

Carcinogenicity. Pronethanol, the first β-adrenoceptor blocking drug to achieve widespread use, was withdrawn by its manufacturer because it caused thymic tumors and lymphosarcomata in mice, although it did not do so in rats or dogs.[82] The doses used to produce these tumors were ten times the maximum therapeutic concentration.

Recently, tolamolol and pamatolol, two cardioselective β-adrenoreceptor blocking drugs, were withdrawn from clinical trials because they caused mammary tumors in mice and rats at high doses.[83] Other β-blockers, alprenolol, practolol, and timolol, have given some indication of tumorigenicity in rodents.[39,83]

The relevance of these findings to causation of tumors in humans is difficult to evaluate.[39] The doses were high and the relationship between malignant tumors in animals and man is not defined.[39] A disturbing aspect has been the suggestion that this might be a pharmacologic property of β-adrenoceptor antagonism rather than carcinogenicity by another mechanism. Against the β-blocker theory of carcinogenesis is the fact that many β-blocking drugs (including many described in this book) have successfully undergone stringent carcinogenicity testing in animals and have been used safely in human beings.

DRUG INTERACTIONS

The wide diversity of diseases for which β-blockers are employed raises the likelihood of their concurrent administration with other drugs.[84] It is imperative, therefore, that familiarity be obtained regarding the interactions of β-blockers with other pharmacologic agents. The list of commonly used drugs with which β-blockers interact is extensive (Table 7).[85] The majority of the reported interactions have been associated with propranolol, the best studied of the β-blockers, and may not apply to other drugs in this class.

Antacid gels such as aluminum hydroxide impair absorption of β-blockers and decrease their therapeutic effects.[86] There may also be some variability in drug absorption related to food. It is probably prudent to advise patients to take these β-blocking doses in a consistent manner with regard to meals.[85]

Cimetidine has been shown to reduce liver blood flow and to inhibit hepatic enzymes used in drug metabolism.[87] These mechanisms probably account for the reports of its prolonging the serum half-life of propranolol and significantly decreasing the resting pulse rate when combined with the β-blocker. It is not known whether cimetidine has any interaction with β-blockers that are not metabolized in the liver (atenolol, nadolol, sotalol).

When lidocaine and propranolol are administered concurrently, lidocaine clearance is decreased and its steady-state plasma concentration increased.[88] This interaction may relate to a reduction in cardiac output and hepatic blood flow induced by propranolol. These findings suggest that the dose of lidocaine should be reduced to avoid intoxication when combined with propranolol. Similar interactions with lidocaine have not been described with pindolol, a β-blocker that may preserve cardiac output.[88]

The combination of the negatively inotropic calcium-entry blockers with β-blockers has the potential of decreasing myocardial contractile function sufficiently to precipitate congestive heart failure. However, calcium-entry blockers can be combined in many patients who have normal left ventricular function, and this is done with caution.[89,90] This combination also results in additive prolongation of atrioventricular and si-

TABLE 7. DRUG INTERACTIONS THAT MAY OCCUR WITH β-ADRENOCEPTOR BLOCKING DRUGS[85]

Drug	Possible Effects	Precautions
Aluminum hydroxide gel[86]	Decreases β-blocker absorption and therapeutic effect	Avoid β-blocker-aluminum hydroxide combination.
Aminophylline[95]	Mutual inhibition	Obseve patient's response.
Antidiabetic agents[93]	Enhanced hypoglycemia: hypertension	Monitor for altered diabetic response.
Calcium channel inhibitors (e.g., verapamil, diltiazem)[89,90]	Potentiation of bradycardia, myocardial depression and hypotension	Use with caution, although few patients show ill effects.
Cimetidine[87]	Prolongs half-life of propranolol	Combination should be used with caution.
Clonidine[66,91,92]	Hypertension during clonidine withdrawal	Monitor for hypertensive response; withdraw β-blocker before withdrawing clonidine.
Digitalis glycosides	Potentiation of bradycardia	Observe patient's response; interactions may benefit angina patients with abnormal ventricular function.
Epinephrine	Hypertension; bradycardia	Administer epinephrine cautiously; β₁-selective blocker may be safer.
Ergot alkaloids	Excessive vasoconstriction	Observe patient's response, few patients show ill effects.
Glucagon	Inhibition of hyperglycemic effect	Monitor for reduced response.
Halofenate	Reduced β-blocking activity; production of propranolol withdrawal rebound syndrome	Observe for impaired response to β-blockade.
Indomethacin	Inhibition of antihypertensive response to β-blockade	Observe patient's response.
Isoproterenol	Mutual inhibition	Avoid concurrent use or choose β₁-selective blocker.
Levodopa	Antagonism of levodopa's hypotensive and positive inotropic effects	Monitor for altered response; interaction may have favorable results.
Lidocaine[88]	Propranolol pretreatment increases lidocaine blood levels and potential toxicity	Combination should be used with caution; use lower doses of lidocaine.
Methyldopa	Hypertension during stress	Monitor for hypertensive episodes.

TABLE 7. CONTINUED

Drug	Possible Effects	Precautions
Monoamine oxidase inhibitors	Uncertain, theoretical	Manufacturer of propranolol considers concurrent use contraindicated.
Phenothiazines	Additive hypotensive effects	Monitor for altered response especially with high doses of phenothiazine.
Phenylpropranolamine	Severe hypertensive reaction	Avoid use, especially in hypertension controlled by both methyldopa and β-blockers.
Phenytoin	Additive cardiac depressant effects	Administer IV phenytoin with great caution.
Quinidine	Additive cardiac depressant effects	Observe patient's response; few patients show ill effects.
Reserpine[89]	Excessive sympathetic blockade	Observe patient's response.
Tricyclic antidepressants	Inhibits negative inotropic and chronotropic effects of β-blockers	Observe patient's response.
Tubocurarine[94]	Enhanced neuromuscular blockade	Observe response in surgical patients, especially after high doses of propranolol.

noatrial node conduction times, which can produce clinically important bradycardia and heart block, especially in patients prone to these problems.

HOW TO CHOOSE A β-BLOCKER

The various β-blocking compounds given in adequate dosage appear to have comparable, antihypertensive, antiarrhythmic, and antianginal effects. Therefore, the β-blocking drug of choice in an individual patient is determined by the pharmacodynamic and pharmacokinetic differences between the drugs, in conjunction with the patient's other medical conditions (Table 8).[96]

TABLE 8. CLINICAL SITUATIONS THAT WOULD INFLUENCE THE CHOICE OF A β-BLOCKING DRUG[96]

Condition	Choice of β-blocker
Asthma, chronic bronchitis with bronchospasm	Avoid all β-blockers if possible; however small doses of β_1-selective blockers (e.g. acebutolol, atenolol, metoprolol) can be used. β_1-Selectivity is lost with higher doses. Drugs with partial agonist activity (e.g. pindolol, oxprenolol) and labetalol with α-adrenergic blocking properties can also be used.
Congestive heart failure	Drugs with partial agonist activity and labetalol might have an advantage, although β-blockers are usually contraindicated.
Angina Pectoris	In patients with angina at low heart rates, drugs with partial agonist activity probably contraindicated. Patients with angina at high heart rates but who have resting bradycardia might benefit from a drug with partial agonist activity. In vasospastic angina, labetalol may be useful; other β-blockers should be used with caution.
Atrioventricular conduction defects	β-Blockers generally contraindicated but drugs with partial agonist activity and labetalol can be tried with caution.
Bradycardia	β-Blockers with partial agonist activity and labetalol have pulse-slowing effect and are preferable.
Raynaud's phenomenon, intermittent claudication, cold extremities	β_1-Selective blocking agents, labetalol, and those with partial agonist activity might have an advantage.
Depression	Avoid propranolol. Substitute a β-blocker with partial agonist activity.
Diabetes mellitus	β_1-Selective agents and partial agonist drugs are preferable.
Thyrotoxicosis	All agents will control symptoms but agents without partial agonist activity are preferred.
Pheochromocytoma	Avoid all β-blockers unless an α-blocker is given. Labetalol may be used as a treatment of choice.
Renal failure	Use reduced doses of compounds largely eliminated by renal mechanisms (nadolol, sotalol, atenolol) and of those drugs whose bioavailability is increased in uremia (propranolol, alprenolol). Also consider possible accumulation of active metabolites (alprenolol, propranolol).
Insulin and sulphonylurea use	Danger of hypoglycemia. Possibly less using drugs with β_1-selectivity.
Clonidine	Avoid sotalol (other non-selective β-blockers). Severe rebound effect with clonidine withdrawal.
Oculomucocutaneous syndrome	Stop drug. Substitute any other β-blocker.
Hyperlipidemia	Avoid nonselective β-blockers; use agents with partial agonism, β_1-selectivity or labetalol.

REFERENCES

1. Friedman LM: How do the various beta-blockers compare in type, frequency, and severity of their adverse effects? Circulation 67 (Suppl I):89, 1983.
2. Frishman W, Silverman R, Strom J, et al: Clinical pharmacology of the new beta-adrenoceptor blocking drugs. Part 4. Adverse effects. Choosing a β-adrenoceptor blocker. Am Heart J 98:256, 1979.
3. β-Blocker Heart Attack Trial Research Group. A randomized trial of propranolol in patients with acute myocardial infarction. 1. Mortality Results. JAMA 247:1707, 1982.
4. Greenblatt DJ, Koch-Weser J: Clinical toxicity of propranolol and practolol. A report from the Boston Collaborative Drug Surveillance Program, in Avery G (ed), Cardiovascular Drugs. Baltimore, University Park Press, 1978, vol II, pp 179–195.
5. Forrest WA: A monitored release study: a clinical trial of oxprenolol in general practice. Practitioner 208:412, 1972.
6. Zacharias FJ, Cowan KJ, Cuthbertson PJR, et al: Atenolol in hypertension. A study of long-term therapy. Postgrad Med J 53 (Suppl 3):102, 1977.
7. Collins IS, King IW: Pindolol (Visken LB 46), a new treatment for hypertension: Report of a multicentre open study. Cur Ther Res 14:185, 1972.
8. Morgan TO, Louis WJ, Dawborn JK, Doyle AE: The use of pindolol (Visken) in the treatment of hypertension. Med J Aust 2:309, 1972.
9. Gonason L, Langrall H: Adverse reactions to pindolol administration. Am Heart J 104 (Part 2):486, 1982.
10. Michelson EL, Frishman WH, Lewis JE, et al: Multicenter clinical evaluation of the long-term safety and efficacy of labetalol in the treatment of hypertension. Am J Med 75(4A):68, 1983.
11. Multicentre International Study: Improvement in prognosis of myocardial infarction by long-term beta-adrenoreceptor blockade using practolol. Br Med J 3:735, 1975.
12. The Norwegian Multicenter Study Group: Timolol-induced reduction in mortality and reinfarction in patients surviving acute myocardial infarction. N Engl J Med 304:801, 1981.
13. Hjalmarson Å, Herlitz J, Malek I, et al: Effect on mortality of metoprolol in acute myocardial infarction: A double-blind randomized trial. Lancet 2:823, 1981.
14. Julian DG, Prescott RJ, Jackson FS, Szekely P: Controlled trial of sotalol for one year after myocardial infarction. Lancet 1:1142, 1982.
15. Taylor SH, Silke B, Ebbutt A, et al: A long-term prevention study with oxprenolol in coronary heart disease. N Eng J Med 307:1292, 1982.
16. Krupp P, Fanchamps A: Pindolol: Experience gained in 10 years of safety monitoring. Am Heart J 104 (Part 2):486, 1982.
17. Vaughan Williams EM, Baywell EE, Singh BN: Cardiospecificity of beta-receptor blockade. A comparison of the relative potencies on cardiac and peripheral vascular beta-adrenoceptors of propranolol, of practolol and its

ortho-substituted isomer and of oxprenolol and its para-substituted isomer. Cardiovasc Res 7:226, 1973.

18. Taylor SH, Silke B, Lee PS: Intravenous beta-blockade in coronary heart disease: Is cardioselectivity or intrinsic sympathomimetic activity hemodynamically useful? N Engl J Med 306:631, 1982.

19. Nayler WG: The effect of beta-adrenergic receptor blocking drugs on myocardial function: an explanation of the subcellular level, in Simpson F (ed), Ciba Symposium Beta-Adrenergic Receptor Blocking Drugs. Sydney, Australasian Drug Information Services, 1970, pp 1–12.

20. Conolly ME, Kersting F, Dollery CT: The clinical pharmacology of beta-adrenoceptor blocking drugs. Prog Card Dis 19:203, 1976.

21. Frishman W, Kostis J, Strom J, et al: Clinical pharmacology of the new beta-adrenergic blocking drugs. Part 6. A comparison of pindolol and propranolol in treatment of patients with angina pectoris. The role of intrinsic sympathomimetic activity. Am Heart J 98:526, 1979.

22. Singh BN, Jewitt DE: β-Adrenoceptor blocking drugs in cardiac arrhythmias, in Avery G (ed), Cardiovascular Drugs. Baltimore, University Park Press, 1978, vol II, pp 119–159.

23. Giudicelli JF, Lhoste F: β-Adrenoceptor blockade and atrioventricular conduction in dogs. Role of intrinsic sympathomimetic activity. Br J Clin Pharmacol 13 (Suppl 2):167, 1982.

24. Alderman EL, Coltart DJ, Wettach GE, Harrison DC: Coronary artery syndromes after sudden propranolol withdrawal. Ann Intern Med 81:925, 1974.

25. Miller RR, Olson HG, Amsterdam EA, Mason DT: Propranolol withdrawal rebound phenomenon: Exacerbation of coronary events after abrupt cessation of anti-anginal therapy. N Engl J Med 293:416, 1975.

26. Frishman WH, Christodoulou J, Weksler B, et al: Abrupt propranolol withdrawal in angina pectoris: Effects on platelet aggregation and exercise tolerance. Am Heart J 95:169, 1978.

27. Frishman WH, Klein N, Strom J, et al: Comparative effects of abrupt propranolol and verapamil withdrawal in angina pectoris. Am J Cardiol 50:1191, 1982.

28. Lefkowitz R: Direct binding studies of adrenergic receptors: Biochemical, physiologic and clinical implications. Ann Intern Med 91:450, 1979.

29. Glaubiger G, Lefkowitz R: Elevated β-receptor number after chronic propranolol treatment. Biochem Biophys Res Commun 78:720, 1977.

30. Kristensen BO, Steiness E, Weeke J: Propranolol withdrawal and thyroid hormones in patients with essential hypertension. Clin Pharmacol Ther 23:624, 1978.

31. Rangno R, Nattel S: Prevention of propranolol withdrawal phenomena by gradual dose reduction. Clin Res 28:214A, 1980.

32. Molinoff PB, Aarons RD, Nies AS, et al: Effects of pindolol and propranolol on β-adrenergic receptors on human lymphocytes. Br J Clin Pharmacol 13 (Suppl 2):365S, 1982.

33. Prichard BNC, Walden RJ: The syndrome associated with the withdrawal of β-adrenoceptor blocking drugs. Br J Clin Pharmacol 13 (Suppl 2):337S, 1982.

34. Rangno RE, Langlois S: Comparison of withdrawal phenomena after propranolol, metoprolol and pindolol. Am Heart J 104 (Part 2):473, 1982.
35. Frishman WH: Pindolol: A new β-adrenoceptor antagonist with partial agonist activity. N Engl J Med 308:940, 1983.
36. Dunlop D, Shanks RG: Selective blockade of adrenoceptive beta receptors in the heart. Br J Pharmacol Chemother 32:201, 1968.
37. Ruffin RE, McIntyre ELM, Latimer KM, et al: Assessment of β-adrenoceptor antagonists in asthmatic patients. Br J Clin Pharmacol 13 (Suppl 2):325S, 1982.
38. Koch-Weser J: Metoprolol. N Engl J Med 301:698, 1979.
39. Frishman WH: Atenolol and timolol, two new systemic β-adrenoceptor antagonists. N Engl J Med 306:1456, 1982.
40. George RB, Manocha K, Burford J, et al: Effects of labetalol in hypertensive patients with chronic obstructive pulmonary disease. Chest 83:457, 1983.
41. Benson MK, Berrill WT, Cruickshank JM, Sterling GS: A comparison of four adrenoceptor antagonists in patients with asthma. Br J Clin Pharmacol 5:415, 1978.
42. Waal-Manning HJ: Hypertension: Which Beta-Blocker? Drugs 12:412, 1976.
43. Frohlich ED, Tarazi RC, Dustan HP: Peripheral arterial insufficiency: a complication of beta-adrenergic blocking therapy. JAMA 208:2471, 1969.
44. Lundvall J, Jarhult J: Beta-adrenergic dilator component of the sympathetic vascular response in skeletal muscle. Acta Physiol Scand 96:180, 1976.
45. Simpson FO: β-Adrenergic receptor blocking drugs in hypertension. Drugs 7:85, 1974.
46. Zacharias FJ, Cowen KJ, Prestt J, et al: Propranolol in hypertension: A study of long-term therapy: 1964–1970. Am Heart J 83:755, 1972.
47. George CF: Beta-receptor blocking agents. Prescriber's Journal 14:93, 1974.
48. Rodger J, Sheldon CD, Lerski RA, Livingston WR: Intermittent claudication complicating beta-blockade. Br Med J 1:1125, 1976.
49. Abramson EA, Arky RA, Woeber KA: Effects of propranolol on the hormonal and metabolic responses to insulin induced hypoglycemia. Lancet 2:1386, 1966.
50. Reveno WS, Rosenbaum H: Propranolol hypoglycemia. Lancet 1:920, 1968.
51. Allison SP, Chamberlain MI, Miller JE: Effects of propranolol on blood sugar, insulin, and free fatty acids. Diabetologia 5:339, 1969.
52. Porte D: Sympathetic regulation of insulin secretion. Its relation to diabetes mellitus. Arch Intern Med 183:252, 1969.
53. Antonis A, Clark ML, Hodge RL, et al: Receptor mechanisms in the hyperglycaemic response to adrenaline in man. Lancet 1:1135, 1967.
54. Dollery CT, Paterson JW, Conolly ME: Clinical pharmacology of beta-blocking drugs. Clin Pharmacol Ther 10:765, 1969.
55. Smith U: Effect of beta-adrenoceptor blocking agents on the reaction to hypoglycemia and the physical working capacity. Cardiovasc Rev Rep 2:563, 1981.
56. Deacon SP, Barnett D: Comparison of atenolol and propranolol during insulin-induced hypoglycaemia. Br Med J 2:7, 1976.

57. Lloyd-Mostyn RH, Oram S: Modification by propranolol of cardiovascular effects of induced hypoglycaemia. Lancet 2:1213, 1975.
58. Frishman WH, Razin A, Swencionis C, Sonnenblick EH: Beta-adrenoceptor blockade in anxiety states: A new approach to therapy? Cardiovasc Rev Rep 2:447, 1981.
59. Frishman WH: Nadolol: A new β-adrenoceptor antagonist. N Engl J Med 305:678, 1981.
60. Herishanu Y, Rosenberg P: Beta-blockers and myathenia gravis. Ann Intern Med 83:834, 1975.
61. Rozen MS, Whan FM: Prolonged curarization associated with propranolol. Med J Aust 1:467, 1972.
62. Greenblatt DJ, Koch-Weser J: Adverse reactions to β-adrenergic receptor blocking drugs: A report from the Boston Collaborative Drug Surveillance Program. Drugs 7:118, 1974.
63. Jacob H, Brandt LJ, Farhas P, Frishman W: Beta-adrenergic blockade and the gastrointestinal system. Am J Med 74:1042, 1983.
64. Stephen SA: Unwanted effects of propranolol. Am J Cardiol 18:463, 1966.
65. Nawabi IU, Ritz ND: Agranulocytosis due to propranolol. JAMA 223:1376, 1973.
66. Bailey R, Neale TJ: Rapid clonidine withdrawal with blood pressure overshoot exaggerated by beta-blockade. Br Med J 1:942, 1976.
67. Cairns SA, Marshall AJ: Clonidine withdrawal. Lancet 1:368, 1976.
68. Agabiti-Rosei E, Brown JJ, Lever AF, et al: Treatment of phaeochromocytoma and clonidine withdrawal hypertension with labetalol. Br J Clin Pharmacol 3 (Suppl 3):809, 1976.
69. Bengtsson C: Comparison between alprenolol and chlorthalidone as antihypertensive agents. Acta Med Scand 191:433, 1972.
70. Seedat YK, Stewart-Wynne E: Clinical experiences with pindolol (Visken) in the therapy of hypertension. South Afr Med J 46:1524, 1972.
71. Waal-Manning HJ, Simpson FO: Pindolol: A comparison with other antihypertensive drugs and a double-blind placebo trial. Aust NZ Med J 80:151, 1974.
72. Wright P: Untoward effect associated with practolol administration. Oculomucocutaneous syndrome. Br Med J 1:595, 1975.
73. Waal-Manning H: Problems with practolol. Drugs 10:336, 1975.
74. Felix RH, Ive FA, Dahl MCG: Cutaneous and ocular reactions to practolol. Br Med J 4:321, 1974.
75. Windsor WP, Durrein F, Dyer NH: Fibrinous peritonitis: a complication of practolol therapy. Br Med J 2:68, 1975.
76. Gaylarde PM, Sukany I: Side effects of practolol. Br Med J 2:435, 1975.
77. Zacharias FJ: Cross-sensitivity between practolol and other β-blockers. Br Med J 1:1213, 1976.
78. Holt PJA, Waddington E: Oculocutaneous reaction to oxprenolol. Br Med J 2:539, 1975.
79. Knapp MS, Gallaway HR, Clayden JR: Ocular reactions to beta-blockers. Br Med J 2:557, 1975.

80. Cubey RB, Taylor SH: Ocular reaction to propranolol and resolution on continued treatment with a different beta-blocking drug. Br Med J 4:327, 1975.
81. Harty RP: Sclerosing peritonitis and propranolol. Arch Intern Med 138:1424, 1978.
82. Paget GE: Carcinogenic actions of pronethalol. Br Med J 2:1266, 1963.
83. Status Report on Beta-Blockers. FDA Drug Bull 8:13, 1978.
84. Missri JC: How do beta-blockers interact with other commonly used drugs? Cardiovasc Med 8:668, 1983.
85. Hansten P: Drug Interactions, 4th ed. Philadelphia, Lea and Febiger, 1979, pp. 13–24.
86. Dobbs JH, Skoutakis VA, Acchiardo SR, Dobbs BR: Effects of aluminum hydroxide on the absorption of propranolol. Curr Ther Res 21:887, 1977.
87. Feely J, Wilkinson GR, Wood AJ: Reduction of liver blood flow and propranolol metabolism by cimetidine. N Engl J Med 304:692, 1981.
88. Svenden TL, et al: Effects of propranolol and pindolol on plasma lidocaine clearance in man. Br J Clin Pharmacol 13:223S, 1982.
89. Leon MB, Rosing DR, Bonow RO, et al: Clinical efficacy of verapamil alone and combined with propranolol in treating patients with chronic stable angina pectoris. Am J Cardiol 48:131, 1981.
90. Packer M, Leon MB, Bonow RO, et al: Hemodynamic and clinical effects of combined verapamil and propranolol therapy in angina pectoris. Am J Cardiol 50:903, 1982.
91. Crook JE, Nies AS: Drug interactions with anti-hypertensive drugs. Drugs 15:72, 1978.
92. Harris AL: Clonidine withdrawal and β-blockade. Lancet 1:596, 1976.
93. Lager I, Blohme G, Smith U: Effect of cardioselective and non-selective β-blockade on the hypoglycemic response in insulin dependent diabetes. Lancet 1:458, 1978.
94. Harrah MD, Way WL, Katzung BG: The interactions of d-tubocurarine with antiarrhythmic drugs. Anesthesiology 33:406, 1970.
95. Baumrucker J: Drug interaction—propranolol and cafergot. N Engl J Med 288:916, 1973.
96. Frishman WH: The beta-adrenoceptor blocking drugs. Int J Cardiol 2:165, 1982.

CHAPTER 6

Overdosage with β-Adrenoceptor Blocking Drugs: Pharmacologic Considerations and Clinical Management

William H. Frishman, Harold Jacob, Edward S. Eisenberg, and Carl R. Spivack

The extensive use of β-adrenoceptor blocking drugs in clinical practice has brought with it the problem of self-poisoning and deliberate intoxication with these agents. β-Adrenoceptor blocking drugs are now commonly employed in the treatment of arrhythmias of supraventricular and ventricular origin, angina pectoris, obstructive cardiomyopathy, essential hypertension, and thyrotoxicosis.[1] Additional uses of these drugs have included treatment of migraine syndrome, essential tremor, psychoses, hyperkinetic cardiac states, anxiety, and alcohol and narcotic withdrawal. Cases of suicidal ingestion and inadvertent overdosage, at first uncommon, have now been recorded in number. Furthermore, patients with massive ingestion have been studied and the optimal therapies debated.[2-5] It is likely that the pharmacologic properties of the ingested β-adrenoreceptor blocking agents—its β_1-selectivity, partial agonist effect, and membrane-stabilizing properties—determine the particular manifestations of overdosage. An understanding of the differences between these agents is central to the management of patients with life-threatening intoxication.

In this paper we (1) report four cases of propranolol overdosage encountered in our practice, (2) review the world literature on β-adreno-

Based on an article that appeared in The American Heart Journal, Volume 98, December 1979, pp 798–811, with permission.

receptor blocking agent overdosage, and (3) offer recommendations for management.

CASE REPORTS

The following four cases of massive intoxication with propranolol were seen at the Bronx Municipal Hospital Center in New York. The cases are summarized in Table 1.

TABLE 1. FOUR PATIENTS WITH PROPRANOLOL POISONING: CLINICAL DATA (BRONX MUNICIPAL HOSPITAL CENTER, NEW YORK)[53]

	#1	#2	#3	#4
Age	17	25	19	59
Sex	F	F	F	M
Plasma level (ng/ml)	449*	2300	2800	1800
Estimated ingestion (mg)	1200–1600		1600	2000
Heart rate (beats/min)	50	116→50	80→50	50
Blood Pressure (mm Hg)	Unobtainable	150/100→un-obtainable	130/80→90/60	120/70
Preantidote:				
Level of consciousness	comatose	alert/agitated	comatose	semi-delerious
Convulsions	Yes	Yes	Yes	No
Congestive heart failure	No	No	No	Yes
Bronchospasm	No	No	No	No
Blood sugar (mg/dl)	136	207	135	150
ECG findings	Regular rhythm, first-degree heart block IVCD†	NSR, IVCD	Regular rhythm, first-degree heart block IVCD	Regular rhythm, first-degree heart block IVCD
Treatment	Diazepam, Epinephrine	Atropine, Pheno-barbital, Iso-proterenol, Glucagon, Dopamine	Diazepam, Atropine, Glucagon, Isoprotere-nol	Pacemaker, Oxygen, Atropine, Glucagon, Isopro-terenol

*Obtained after 24 hours admission.
†Intraventricular conduction defect.

Case 1

A 17-year-old woman with no previous medical illness was brought to the emergency room 2 hours after ingestion of 30 to 40 propranolol pills, each containing 40 mg. The medication had been prescribed for a family member. The total quantity ingested was 1200 to 1600 mg. Within 90 minutes of ingestion, the patient became stuporous and experienced generalized seizures of several minutes duration. She was comatose with only avoidance responses to painful stimuli when she arrived at the hospital. Blood pressure was not obtainable, heart rate was 50 beats per minute, and respiratory rate 20 beats per minute with shallow excursions. Pupils were 4 mm and equal and reactive to light. There were rhonchi at both bases. The extremities were cool but not cyanotic; tendon reflexes were moderately active and symmetric. Several minutes after arriving at the hospital, the patient had a generalized tonic–clonic seizure that responded promptly to 5 mg of intravenous diazepam. She was then given two doses of 0.06-mg epinephrine intravenously with a resultant increase of heart rate to 70 beats per minute and blood pressure to 90/50 mm Hg. Electrolytes on admission to the hospital included a serum sodium of 138 mEq/L, potassium 4.5 mEq/L, calcium 8.1 mg/dl, bicarbonate 21 mEq/L, chloride 100 mEq/L, and glucose 136 mg/dl. Arterial pH was 7.30, Pco_2 was 26 mm Hg and Po_2 121 mm Hg. Routine toxicologic studies showed the presence of a barbiturate in the first of two specimens of gastric contents; however, urine screening was negative. The patient had no prior history of seizure or of cardiovascular disease. Her level of consciousness improved over the next several hours so that on the day following admission she was alert and oriented with an entirely normal neurologic examination. Serum propranolol levels were not drawn immediately upon arrival; however, 24 hours later the serum propranolol level measured spectrofluorometrically was 449 ng/ml, decreasing to 19 ng/ml at 48 hours following admission and to nondetectable levels at 96 hours. An ECG taken on admission showed normal sinus rhythm, first-degree AV block, and an intraventricular conduction defect. Twenty-four hours later, the electrocardiogram was normal. An electro-encephalogram performed on the eighth hospital day was also normal.

Case 2

A 25-year-old woman presented to the emergency room 30 minutes after ingestion of propranolol in a suicide attempt. "Two-handfuls" of 40-mg tablets were taken. She was alert and agitated with a pulse of 116 beats per minute and a blood pressure of 150/100 mm Hg. The patient received 30 ml of ipecac and several minutes later she vomited green pill fragments. Subsequently, she suffered a grand mal seizure. At that point, her blood pressure was unobtainable and her pulse 50 beats per minute. The patient was treated with 1 mg of atropine intravenously, 2 mg of intravenous isoproterenol, and 4 mg of intravenous glucagon. Subsequently she was placed on a continuous infusion of isoproterenol, glucagon, and dopamine, with a resultant increase in her pulse to 80 beats per minute and blood pressure to 80/50 mm Hg. Despite the injection of phenobarbital 250 mg intravenously, she then experienced two more generalized seizures, each of only seconds duration. Physical exam following this revealed a lethargic but arousable patient whose pupils were each 6 mm and reactive to light. The remainder of the physical examination was unremarkable. Electrolytes upon admission to the hospital revealed a serum sodium concentration of 139 mEq/L, potassium 3.5 mEq/L, bicarbonate 15 mEq/L, calcium 9.7 mg/dl, chloride 100 mEq/L, and glucose 207 mg/dl. An arterial blood gas specimen showed a pH of 7.41, Pco_2 of 20 mm Hg and a Po_2 of 75 mm Hg. Urine toxicology was negative. The serum propranolol level performed spectrofluorometrically was 2300 ng/ml on admission, falling to 800 ng/ml 5 hours later, and 300 ng/ml 1 day later. An electrocardiogram at the time of admission showed normal sinus rhythm with a QRS duration of 0.12 seconds. An electrocardiogram repeated 24 hours following admission was entirely normal. The remainder of the patient's hospital course was uneventful and her recovery was complete.

Case 3
A 19-year-old woman with a history of paroxysmal atrial tachycardia ingested 80 20-mg tablets of propranolol in a suicide attempt. She was brought to the emergency room 1 hour later in a semiconscious state. At that time the pulse rate was 80 beats per minute and the blood pressure 130/80 mm Hg. A nasogastric tube was inserted for gastric lavage, with recovery of pill fragments. Activated charcoal was also given. Fifteen minutes later the patient became delerious and then unresponsive and experienced a grand mal seizure. Her blood pressure at that time was 90/60 mm Hg and her heart rate 50 beats per minute. Treatment included 1 mg of intravenous atropine and 2 mg of intravenous isoproterenol with no response in either heart rate or blood pressure. Intravenous diazepam was given, after which the seizures stopped. An infusion of isoproterenol and glucagon was begun with a resultant increase in blood pressure to 110/60 mm Hg and of pulse to 70 beats per minute. Physical exam revealed a lethargic but arousable woman with reactive pupils. There was no abnormality on cardiac or pulmonary exam. Her admission sodium was 139 mEq/L, potassium 3.8 mEq/L, bicarbonate 17 mEq/L, calcium 9.4 mg/dl, chloride 99 mEq/L, and glucose 135 mg/dl.

Toxicologic scanning was negative for drugs. The initial plasma propranolol level was 2800 ng/ml. Five hours later it had fallen to 1100 ng/ml, and 24 hours after admission the level was 270 ng/ml. The admission electrocardiogram showed first-degree AV block, the PR interval being 0.24 seconds. Twelve hours later her electrocardiogram was normal, with a QRS duration of 0.06 seconds. Her chest x-ray upon admission showed no evidence of left ventricular dilation or pulmonary congestion. Subsequent neurologic examination was normal and the patient made an uneventful recovery.

Case 4

A 59-year-old man with long-standing hypertension but no other known cardiac disease ingested approximately 50 of his 40-mg propranolol tablets in a suicide attempt. He was brought to the emergency room in acute pulmonary edema, cyanotic, and semidelerious. Upon arrival in the emergency room he was found to have a blood pressure of 120/70 mm Hg and a weak pulse at 50 beats per minute. He was treated with oxygen, rotating tourniquets, and 80 mg of intravenous furosemide. The chest x-ray revealed fluffy alveolar infiltrates and cardiomegaly and the ECG demonstrated first-degree AV block, with a PR interval of 0.24 seconds and a heart rate of 50 beats per minute. The QRS duration was 0.11 seconds.

The patient was treated with 1 mg of intravenous atropine and 1 mg of intravenous isoproterenol with no increase in heart rate. A transvenous temporary pacemaker was inserted with the rate set at 70 beats per minute, and 10 mg of intravenous glucagon was injected intravenously. The patient responded within 10 to 15 minutes with improvement in his cardiovascular status and was then maintained on isoproterenol and glucagon intravenous infusions for a period of 8 hours. The pacemaker was removed after 1 day. Subsequent ECG revealed a heart rate of 76 beats per minute, with normal PR and QRS durations. A plasma propranolol level from the time of admission was 1800 ng/ml. An echocardiogram performed 72 hours after admission revealed left ventricular hypertrophy and a slightly diminished ejection fraction. The patient was discharged following psychiatric evaluation with no further cardiac disorder.

COMMENT

These four cases of massive propranolol poisoning exhibit a wide range of clinical effects. Hypotension, bradycardia, and prolonged AV conduction times are common and predictable consequences of sudden massive ingestion of a β-adrenoceptor blocking agent.[6] On the other hand, grand mal seizures, although reported, are unusual in this setting.[7] Metabolic causes of seizure activity such as hypoglycemia were excluded in our patients, and we are convinced that seizure activity is a direct effect of propranolol taken in massive quantity. Cerebral hypoperfusion may have contributed to the tendency to seizure, although two of our patients suffered generalized convulsions despite normal levels of blood pressure. The seizures responded to intravenous diazepam in two cases; in one of our patients, seizures could not be controlled by phenobarbital. Neurologic examination after recovery showed no disorder of any kind in our patients; none had had previous convulsions.

It is also significant that all of our patients had depression of sensorium, ranging from delerium to coma. Propranolol is extremely lipid soluble and crosses the blood–brain barrier with rapidity, concentrating in brain tissue. Propranolol is not β_1-selective and exerts a membrane-depressant action—a "quinidine-like" or local anesthetic effect.[8] In the usual dosage range, this membrane-depressant effect is of little importance, but with massive ingestion, it is possible that the effect becomes clinically manifest.[9] Depression of sensorium and grand mal seizure activity also occur with overdosage of lidocaine, another lipophilic local anesthetic agent.[10]

The second unusual effect of propranolol in massive dosages is widening of the QRS interval on the electrocardiogram—an intraventricular conduction defect. This effect is not seen when propranolol is used in the usual therapeutic dose.[1,11] It too may be due to the quinidine-like effect or membrane-depressant action of propranolol when taken in massive doses.

Of our four patients, none had definite evidence of bronchospasm and none developed hypoglycemia. Patient 4 went into pulmonary edema after a 2-g ingestion. Although higher doses of propranolol have been given over 24 hours to patients with normal hearts, the patient with occult cardiomyopathy may develop marked congestive heart failure after a single oral dose of 40 mg of propranolol.[12] It may be that our patient had occult or subclinical left ventricular dysfunction that became manifest after he ingested excessive quantities of propranolol.

REVIEW OF THE WORLD EXPERIENCE WITH β-ADRENOCEPTOR BLOCKER SELF-POISONING

For the physician caring for a patient with β-adrenoceptor blocking agent overdosage, the pharmacologic properties of these agents are of major importance. Special note should be taken of the β_1-selectivity of the drug, its membrane stabilizing properties, and elimination half-life.[2,8,13,14] The reported cases of β-adrenoceptor poisoning are reviewed below and summarized in Table 2.

Acebutolol

Acebutolol is a β_1-selective adrenergic blocking agent with partial agonist activity and membrane-depressant properties. Two cases have been reported: (1) A 32-year-old man ingested an unknown amount of acebutolol in a suicide attempt. He was dead upon arrival at the hospital. Levels of acebutolol were determined in body tissues at postmortem examination and were highest in urine and liver.[15] (2) A second case of massive fatal acebutolol ingestion (30 tablets) has been reported.[16]

Alprenolol

Alprenolol, a nonselective agent, has partial agonist activity and membrane-depressant properties. The following five cases of alprenolol self-poisoning have been reported:

1. A 32-year-old female who ingested 12.8 g of the drug (approximately 64 200-mg tablets) presented with hypotension, coma, and respiratory arrest. Despite the supportive measures implemented, the patient developed asystole and died. Her postmortem alprenolol blood level was 1300 ng/ml.[17]

2. A 58-year-old woman was admitted 3 to 4 hours after the ingestion of approximately 10 g of alprenolol and small quantities of ethanol, paracetamol, and dextropropoxyphene. She was comatose, with a heart rate of 48 beats per minute and no obtainable blood pressure. Treatment included dopamine infusion at 600 µg per minute, isotonic glucose, and deslanoside 1.2 mg intravenously. A temporary pacemaker was inserted as well. Her clinical state gradually improved so that 8 hours after admission her blood pressure was 120/80 mm Hg and heart rate 80 beats per minute. However, 10 hours following admission complete AV block suddenly appeared, with profound hypotension to 40 mm Hg systolic and massive congestive heart failure. Glucagon 8 mg was then given intravenously with rapid improvement in the clinical state over the next 30 minutes. A myocardial infarction occurred and was documented by LDH isoenzymes.[4]

3. Two additional cases of fatal alprenolol poisoning by suicidal ingestion had postmortem determination of body tissue levels.[18]

Atenolol

Atenolol is β_1-selective with neither partial agonist nor membrane-depressant effects. A single case of overdosage is on record: A 24-year-old female who was receiving atenolol for treatment of hypertension

TABLE 2.

TABLE 2. (PART I) SUMMARY OF WORLD EXPERIENCE WITH TREATMENT OF β-ADRENOCEPTOR BLOCKER INTOXICATION[53]

Drug	Pt. No.	Age	Sex	Estimated Ingested Dose (mg)	Other Drugs	Plasma Level (ng/ml)	Heart Rate (beats/min)
Alprenolol	1	32	F	12,800	0	1,300	
	2	58	F	10,000	Paracetamol Dextropro- poxyphene		48
Atenolol	1	24	F	1,200	0		80
Metoprolol	1	19	M	10,000	0	12,200	60–72
	2	17	F	10,000	Alcohol Diazepam	13,100	72
Nadolol	1	45	F	28,000	unknown	159 at 24 hrs	
Oxprenolol	1	38	F	6,080	Alcohol Pentazocine Paracetamol	8,200	60
	2	57	F	4,480	0	400	36
	3	62	M		Diazepam	3,100	0
	4	39	F	3,000	0		20
Pindolol	1	38	F	500	0	1,500	80
	2	24	F	250	Diazepam	660	110
Practolol	1	39	M	9,000	0	58,600	70
	2	39	F	5,000	0		100
Propranolol	1	47	F			2,462	50
	2	20	F	2,000		2,300	90
	3	14	M	8,000	0		0
	4	45	M	2,200	0		80
	5	35	F		0	28,000	
	6	34	F	6,000	Alcohol	14,000	
	7	38	F		Codeine	16,000	
	8	22	M	4,000	0		50

*Not obtainable—Blood pressure data are not available in report.
†Not measurable—Blood pressure measured but unable to record.

Blood Pressure (mmHg)	Level of Consciousness	Convulsions	Blood Sugar	Congestive Heart Failure	Broncho-Spasm	ECG
not obtainable*	Coma					Sinus bradycardia
150/110	Alert	0		No	No	Normal
not measurable†	Alert	0		Yes	No	Normal
80/60	Drowsy	0			No	Normal
not measurable†	Coma				Yes	Sinus bradycardia
90/50	Stupor	0		No	No	Normal sinus rhythm
not measurable†	Coma	0		Yes	No	Idioventricular rhythm
not measurable†	Coma	0		No	Yes	Asystole, sinus bradycardia
not measurable†	Coma	Yes		No	No	Bradycardia rate = 20
240/140	Alert	0		No	No	Normal
130/80	Coma	0	Normal	Yes	No	Sinus tachycardia, IVCD, QRS 0.11 sec.
90/60	Alert	0		No	No	Normal
110/60	Alert	0		Yes	No	LBBB
70/40	Coma	Yes		No	No	Sinus bradycardia
not measurable†	Coma	Yes				Widened QRS complex
not measurable†	Coma	Yes		No	No	Sinus bradycardia, RBBB, 2° AV block
120 systolic	Alert	0				Normal
110/70	Alert	0	Normal			Bradycardia

TABLE 2. (PART I) *continued*

Drug	Pt. No.	Age	Sex	Estimated Ingested Dose (mg)	Other Drugs	Plasma Level (ng/ml)	Heart Rate (beats/ min)
Propranolol (continued)	9	37	F	800	Imipramine		50
	10	24	F	1,000	Alcohol		40 → asystole
	11	41	M	5,100	Alcohol		50 → asystole
	12	65	M	800	0	1,536	50
	13	2	M	150	0		60
	14	3	F	150	0		120

ingested 1200 mg of the drug (a dose six times greater than the prescribed dose) in a suicide attempt. She was admitted to the hospital 2 to 3 hours later in good condition. Her pulse rate was 80 beats per minute, with a recumbent blood pressure of 150/110 mm Hg. There were no signs of cardiac decompensation and the ECG was normal. She was closely monitored over the next several days, during which time her pulse rate varied between 66 to 60 beats per minute in sinus rhythm. Her blood pressure was 190/120 mm Hg 5 days after ingestion. The clinical course was uncomplicated.[19]

Labetalol
Labetalol is a β-adrenoceptor blocking agent without β₁-selectivity or partial agonist activity. It possesses weak membrane-stabilizing properties and both α-adrenergic blocking and direct vasodilatory effects.[20] There have been no reported cases of self-poisoning with labetalol.

Metoprolol
Metoprolol is a β₁-selective adrenoceptor blocking agent with no partial agonist activity and weak membrane-suppressant activity. Two cases of nonfatal metoprolol intoxication have been recorded:

Blood Pressure (mmHg)	Level of Consciousness	Convulsions	Blood Sugar	Congestive Heart Failure	Broncho-Spasm	ECG
60 systolic				Yes		rate 42, transient atrioventricular block
not measurable†	Coma	0			Yes	Asystole
not measurable†	Coma	Yes				Bradycardia, then asystole
not measurable†	Coma	0				1st° AV block, RBBB
130 systolic	Coma		14 mg/dl	No		Sinus bradycardia, atrioventricular block
125/75	Drowsy	0	50 mg/dl	No		Normal

1. A 19-year-old man was admitted to the hospital after having ingested 200 50-mg tablets (10,000 mg total dosage). Upon arrival at the hospital he was conscious with peripheral cyanosis, weak heart sounds, and an unrecordable blood pressure. The electrocardiogram showed sinus rhythm at 60 to 70 beats per minute; AV conduction was normal. He was treated with metaraminol and glucagon following gastric lavage. Two hours after admission the plasma metoprolol level was 12,200 ng/ml. The patient recovered completely 12 hours after admission without signs of cardiac depression.[21]

2. A 17-year-old daughter of a hypertensive patient ingested over 10 g of metoprolol together with alcohol and diazepam. Upon admission to the hospital 1 hour later, she was conscious but drowsy. There was no cyanosis and respirations were normal. Her blood pressure was 80/60 mm Hg and her radial pulse 72 beats per minute and regular. Heart sounds and pupillary response were normal. A resting electrocardiogram on admission was within normal limits. She was admitted to the Intensive Care Unit and had normal sinus rhythm at all times. Treatment consisted of fluid administration in response to which blood pressure

TABLE 2. (PART II) SUMMARY OF WORLD EXPERIENCE WITH TREATMENT OF β-ADRENOCEPTOR BLOCKER INTOXICATION

Drug	Pt. No	Age	Sex	Treatment	Result	Reference
Alprenolol	1	32	F	Supportive	Death	Simonson and Worm[17]
	2	58	F	Dopamine, temporary pacemaker, glucagon	Recovery	Jacobsen et al[4]
Atenolol	1	24	F	Supportive	Recovery	Shanahan and Counihan[19]
Metoprolol	1	19	M	Gastric lavage, furosemide, metaraminol, glucagon	Recovery	Mollar[21]
	2	17	F	Supportive	Recovery	Sire[22]
Nadolol	1	45	F	Isoproterenol, dialysis	Recovery	Groel[23]
Oxprenolol	1	38	F	Atropine, glucagon, isoproterenol	Recovery	Illingworth[2]
	2	57	F	Unresponsive to atropine, isoproterenol, pacemaker	Death	Khan and Muscat-Baron[25]
	3	62	M	Unresponsive to atropine, epinephrine, responded to glucagon, bronchospasm treated with terbutaline	Recovery	Ward and Jones[26]
	4	39	F	Atropine, isoproterenol, epinephrine, pacemaker	Recovery	Mattingly[27]
Pindolol	1	38	F	None	Recovery	Thorpe[29]
	2	24	F	Fluids	Recovery	Offenstadt et al[30]
Practolol	1	39	M	Supportive	Recovery	Verdera Cosmelli et al[31]
	2	39	F	Supportive	Recovery	Karhunen and Hartel[32]

	Age	Sex	Treatment	Outcome	Reference
Propranolol					
1	47	F	Atropine, dopamine, isoproterenol, norepinephrine	Recovery	Halloren and Phillips[33]
2	20	F	Isoproterenol, dopamine, glucagon	Recovery	Salzberg & Gallagher[34]
3	14	M	Pacemaker, atropine, isoprenaline, calcium gluconate	Recovery	Tynan et al[35]
4	45	M	Supportive	Recovery	Wermut and Wojcicki[36]
5	35	F	None	Death	Gault et al[37]
6	34	F	None	Death	Kristonsson and Johanneson[38]
7	38	F	None	Death	Turner and Cravey[39]
8	22	M	Atropine, epinephrine	Recovery	Gydra et al[40]
9	37	F	Unresponsive to isoproterenol, responded to glucagon	Recovery	Kosinski and Malindzak[41]
10	24	F	Unresponsive to atropine, responded to epinephrine	Recovery	Frithz[42]
11	41	M	Epinephrine, isoproterenol, pacemaker	Recovery	Langerfelt and Matell[7]
12	65	M	Isoproterenol	Recovery	Ducret et al[43]
13	2	M	Glucose	Recovery	Hesse and Pedersen[44]
14	3	F	Glucose	Recovery	Hesse and Pedersen[44]

rose slowly during the first 3 hours to 90/80 mm Hg. Subsequently, the patient's normal level of blood pressure (115/70 mm Hg) returned. Pulse rate varied during monitoring from 80 to 85 beats per minute. Twelve hours after admission the patient was up and about in good condition. The concentration of metoprolol in plasma was 13,100 ng/ml measured 11 hours after ingestion. The patient made an uneventful recovery.[22]

Nadolol

Nadolol is neither β_1-selective nor does it have partial agonist activity or membrane-stabilizing activity. A single case of self-poisoning with nadolol has been reported. A 45-year-old female overdosed herself with 35 to 50 80-mg nadolol tablets. Two other unknown drugs were taken as well. The patient was admitted to the hospital with hypotension. Subsequently neither pulse nor blood pressure were obtainable. Treatment included isoproterenol infusion with good response. Dialysis was then performed, and albuterol administered because of bronchospasm. Blood sugar levels reported to be "erratic" and for this reason glucagon was given. Twenty-four hours after admission to hospital a blood specimen obtained for nadolol assay showed a concentration of 159 ng/ml. Two weeks thereafter the patient was still artificially ventilated and comatose and a blood specimen was negative for nadolol. Additional clinical data and follow-up on this patient are not available.[23]

Oxprenolol

Oxprenolol is nonselective with partial agonist activity and membrane-depressant effects. Eight cases of oxprenolol overdosage have been reported, with three fatalities:

1. A 38-year-old woman was admitted to the hospital 1 hour after taking 38 Slow-Trasicor tablets (6.08 g, oxprenolol HCl) prescribed earlier that day. In addition, she ingested alcohol (cider) and fortagesic (pentazocine and paracetamol) tablets. On admission she was unconscious but responded well to pain. She was pale, with central cyanosis and diaphoresis. Admission blood pressure was 90/50 mm Hg and pulse 60 beats per minute. Although 0.8 mg of intravenous naloxone restored consciousness, cyanosis and hypotension persisted. Gradually the patient lost consciousness. For a period of 2 hours, the patient had no palpable pulse and no detectable blood pressure, although the electrocardiogram showed normal sinus rhythm at 60 beats per minute and widespread elevation of the ST segment. Treatment

included atropine 1.2 mg intravenously, glucagon (2 mg intravenous and 1 mg boluses), and isoproterenol infusion at 30 μg per minute. None of these initial measures had any effect. A larger intravenous bolus of glucagon, 10 mg, produced recovery of consciousness, return of pulses and blood pressure, and immediate vomiting. Transient sinus tachycardia occurred. Thirty minutes later blood pressure was again undetectable and unconsciousness returned. A subsequent infusion of glucagon at a rate of 3 mg per hour for 4 hours, then 2 mg per hour for 3 hours, and finally 1 mg per hour restored consciousness. Pulses, blood pressure, and urinary output returned to normal levels. During glucagon infusion transient moderate hyperglycemia (205 mg/dl) was recorded, as was hypocalcemia (8.04 mg/dl). Plasma oxprenolol levels were first measured approximately 2 hours after the overdose (8200 ng/ml), falling to 500 ng/ml at 24 hours. The patient was discharged 2 days after admission with normal blood pressure. However, 4 days later she again ingested oxprenolol in large quantity, and became unconscious and asystolic. Cardiopulmonary resuscitation was not successful. Postmortem blood level was 84.30 ng/nl.[2]

2. A 29-year-old man committed suicide by ingesting in excess of 300 mg of oxprenolol after drinking 11 pints of beer.[24]

3. A 57-year-old woman ingested 112 40-mg tablets of oxprenolol (4480 mg total dosage). She was brought to the emergency room 20 minutes later in a coma. She was cold and clammy and had central cyanosis. Her pulse was not palpable and blood pressure unrecordable. Heart sounds were soft, with a ventricular rate of 36 beats per minute. Bibasilar rales were present. The electrocardiogram showed an idioventricular at a rate of 36. External cardiac massage and assisted respiration were carried out. There was no response in pulse rate to intravenous atropine and isoproterenol. A temporary transvenous pacemaker could not capture the ventricle. The patient died in asystole 1 hour after arrival at the hospital. An autopsy revealed no gross structural abnormality of the cardiovascular system. The postmortem plasma drug level was approximately 400 ng/ml.[25]

4. A 62-year-old man ingested a large amount of oxprenolol and diazepam. He was brought to the hospital pulseless with cold, cyanotic extremities after being supported by the ambulance crew. The admission electrocardiogram revealed asystole. After 35 minutes of resuscitation which included intravenous isoproterenol and epinephrine infusion, slow sinus rhythm at 32 beats per

minute was established. This increased to 68 beats per minute after 0.6 mg of intravenous atropine, and respirations also returned. The systolic blood pressure did not exceed 30 mm Hg. Further epinephrine administration by continuous infusion had no effect on heart rate or blood pressure in the next 1 and one half hours. Glucagon, 10 mg intravenously, produced an arterial blood pressure of 150 mm Hg within 60 seconds and an improvement in peripheral circulation. As cardiovascular status improved, severe bronchospasm developed, which was successfully treated with intravenous terbutaline. A continuous infusion of glucagon at 2 mg per hour was then given over the next 5 hours and improvement continued. The patient was eventually discharged after an uneventful recovery. The oxprenolol plasma level was 3100 ng/ml.[26]

5. A 39-year-old female ingested 3 g of oxprenolol. After arrival at the emergency unit she had a respiratory arrest and a mild generalized convulsion. The blood pressure was unrecordable and the pulse feeble. Spontaneous respirations returned and the cardiac monitor showed sinus rhythm at a rate of 60 beats per minute. Two further brief convulsions occurred. Following transfer to the Intensive Care Unit, she had a cardiopulmonary arrest, with the monitor showing a heart rate of 20 beats per minute. She was artificially ventilated and external cardiac message was maintained for a period of 2 hours. Treatment included atropine, epinephrine (intracardiac and intravenous), isoproterenol, and sodium bicarbonate. A pacemaker was inserted, with 100 percent capture. After 2 hours a blood pressure of 130/100 mm Hg was obtained and the rhythm reverted to sinus at 80 beats per minute. Within 48 hours she was fully conscious and by 72 hours after admission the patient was extubated. She made a full recovery.[27]

6. A 67-year-old man ingested 30 80-mg oxprenolol tablets (2400 mg) along with 25 thiazide–potassium (navidrex K) tablets. He presented with hyperkalemia. The oxprenolol may have delayed the excretion of potassium by reducing cardiac output and blood pressure. The patient made an uneventful recovery following supportive measures.[28]

Pindolol

Pindolol is a nonselective β-adrenoceptor blocking agent, possessing partial agonist activity and weak membrane-depressant activity. Two uncomplicated cases of pindolol self-poisoning have been recorded:

1. A 38-year-old woman ingested 500 mg of pindolol in a suicide attempt. She had received 30 to 40 mg of pindolol per day for treatment of hypertension. She presented 5 hours after massive ingestion with a blood pressure of 240/140 mm Hg and a pulse of 80 beats per minute. Her electrocardiogram was normal and she remained alert at all times. Her plasma pindolol level was 1500 ng/ml. No further complications of drug overdosage occurred.

2. A 24-year-old woman ingested 250 mg of pindolol together with 150 mg of diazepam. The following morning she presented to the hospital in a coma with a blood pressure of 80 mm Hg and a pulse of 110 beats per minute. With infusion of intravenous fluids, the systolic blood pressure rose to 130 mm Hg. The electrocardiogram showed a sinus rhythm of 110 beats per minute, with a QRS duration of 0.11 seconds. Her blood sugar was normal and pulmonary congestion was noted on chest x-ray. Twenty-four hours later the QRS duration on electrocardiogram was 0.06 seconds and the chest x-ray was normal. The plasma pindolol level was 660 ng/ml and the patient's recovery was uneventful.[30]

Practolol

Practolol is a selective β-adrenoceptor blocking agent with partial agonist activity and no membrane effect. Two nonfatal cases of practolol self-poisoning have been reported:

1. A 39-year-old man with mitral valve disease ingested 9 g of practolol. He had received 400 mg/day for control of arrhythmia. Three hours after the massive ingestion he was brought to the hospital with a heart rate of 70 beats per minute and blood pressure of 90/70 mm Hg. There was no change in the level of consciousness and no sign of cardiac decompensation. Over the next 2 hours his blood pressure rose to its usual level. The plasma level was 58.6 μg/ml. The patient's course was uncomplicated.[31]

2. A 39-year-old woman with mitral stenosis ingested 5000 mg of practolol and presented with clinical signs of mild congestive heart failure. Her blood pressure was 110/60 mm Hg and her heart rate was 100 beats per minute. Sequential electrocardiograms showed intermittent left bundle branch block. She made an uneventful recovery with resolution of the intraventricular conduction defect.[32]

Propranolol

Propranolol is nonselective, although it possesses membrane-depressant effects. Propranolol has no partial agonist activity. In addition to the four cases of propranolol intoxication seen at our institution, and presented in the paragraphs above, 14 other well-documented cases have been reported, with three fatalities. The substantial experience with propranolol intoxication reflects its widespread use in clinical practice.

1. A 47-year-old hypertensive female with a history of psychiatric depression ingested an unknown amount of propranolol in a suicide attempt. En route to the hospital two brief generalized seizures occurred. Upon arrival in the emergency room she was apneic and comatose. Heart rate was 50 beats per minute and blood pressure 70/40 mm Hg. The peripheral pulses were barely palpable. Course rhonchi were present in all lung fields and vomitus found in the trachea. Initial electrocardiogram revealed sinus bradycardia and a QRS of normal duration. Central venous pressure was 11. Initial treatment included atropine 3 mg intravenously administered over 30 minutes, dopamine infusion, and isoproterenol infusion, the latter at 32 μg/kg for 2 hours. In addition, 4 liters of D5NS were infused. The above treatment produced no improvements in mental status, heart rate, blood pressure, or urinary output. Norepinephrine was then infused intravenously at 12 μg per minute in place of isoproterenol. Response was prompt, with blood pressure rising from 70/40 to 100/80 mm Hg. Urine output increased. Peripheral pulses also increased in intensity. Twelve hours after admission, blood pressure, pulse, urine output, and mental status had returned to normal levels. Recovery of neurologic and cardiac function was complete. The admission propranolol level was 2462 ng/ml. It was 1194 ng/ml 17 hours later and 350 ng/ml 50 hours after admission. The urinary propranolol content was 64,015 ng/ml. The authors believe that the patient had the highest serum propranolol level ever reported with survival.[33]

2. A 20-year-old woman presented to the emergency department 30 minutes after ingesting 50 40-mg propranolol tablets in a suicide attempt. Medical history was significant for thyrotoxicosis in the past, which had been treated successfully 4 months earlier with I[131]. Thyroid function tests 3 weeks prior to admission were normal and propranolol had been stopped at that time. Admission physical examination revealed an alert patient with a blood pressure of 150/100 mm Hg and a heart rate of 110 beats per minute. Thirty minutes after arrival, she suddenly became unresponsive and blood pressure was not measurable. Cardiac monitor showed normal sinus rhythm at 90 beats per minute. A

generalized seizure occurred. Other complications included widening of the QRS complex (previous duration not stated), recurrent generalized seizures, and continued unobtainable blood pressure despite infusions of isoproterenol at 4 μg per minute and dopamine at 0.5 mg per minute. Isoproterenol was increased to 20 μg per minute and dopamine to 5 mg per minute. Subsequently a 3-mg glucagon bolus was given intravenously, with rapid conversion to normal sinus rhythm and an increase in blood pressure to 90/60 mm Hg. A glucagon drip at 5 mg per hour was established as dopamine and isoproterenol infusions were tapered. The patient made an uneventful recovery. Blood propranolol levels 90 minutes and 8 hours after ingestion were 2300 and 800 ng/ml.[34]

3. A 14-year-old boy ingested 8000 mg of propranolol 35 minutes before hospitalization. On admission he was alert, with a blood pressure of 130/70 mm Hg and a heart rate of 84 beats per minute. After vomiting pill fragments in response to ipecac, he collapsed, suffered a grand mal convulsion, and had neither palpable pulse nor blood pressure. Treatment included intubation, ventilation with 100 percent oxygen, and external cardiac compression. Lungs were clear, and pupils small, central and nonreacting. Peripheral cyanosis was present. Atropine (1.2 mg intravenously), isoproterenol (0.04 mg intravenously), and calcium gluconate (1 g) were administered, in response to which pressure rose to 50 mm Hg systolic. The electrocardiogram showed sinus bradycardia, right bundle branch block, and second-degree AV block. A temporary travenous pacemaker was then inserted. A second convulsion occurred, suppressed by intravenous diazepam. An isoproterenol infusion at 0.8 mg per minute restored blood pressure to 110/70 mm Hg. Seven hours after admission the isoproterenol was discontinued and the pacemaker removed. The patient recovered fully. In this case activated charcoal was instilled into the stomach and further gastric lavage was performed during the first hours of hospitalization.[35]

4. A 45-year-old man ingested 2000 mg of propranolol in a suicide attempt. He arrived at the hospital 2 hours later in good condition. Plasma levels were not measured. The heart rate was 80 beats per minue, with normal pulse contour and a systolic blood pressure of 120 mm Hg. Electrocardiogram showed normal sinus rhythm and the patient's course was uncomplicated.[36]

5. A 35-year-old woman with a past history of psychiatric illness was found dead at home. Toxicologic study showed a propran-

olol plasma level of 28,000 ng/ml, with 600 mg of ingested drug remaining in her stomach. An exact cardiovascular cause of death was not determined.[37]

6. A 34-year-old woman was found dead in bed, having allegedly ingested 6 g of propranolol with a large amount of alcohol. The plasma propranolol level was 14,000 ng/ml and there was a massive concentration in the brain. The exact anatomic cause for death was not ascertained.[38]

7. A 38-year-old woman with schizophrenia was found dead in bed, having ingested unknown quantities of propranolol and codeine. The plasma propranolol level was 16,000 ng/ml. An autopsy revealed no significant gross pathologic abnormality.[39]

8. A 22-year-old man ingested 4 g of propranolol in a suicide attempt. The blood pressure was 110/70 mm Hg and heart rate 42 to 50 beats per minute in sinus rhythm. There was no response to injection of epinephrine, but heart rate increased somewhat after atropine was given. There was no disorder of atrioventricular conduction. Hypoglycemia was not observed and the outcome was favorable.[40]

9. A 37-year-old woman attempted suicide with a mixed overdose of imipramine and 800 mg of propranolol. In the emergency room she was cold, cyanotic, with marked distention of her neck veins. The pulse rate was 50 beats per minute and regular, and the systolic blood pressure was 60 mm Hg. There was no response to isoproterenol infusion, but after a 10-mg intravenous bolus of glucagon blood pressure rose to 95 mm Hg and pulse to 70 beats per minute. Marked improvement was also observed in peripheral perfusion and the degree of neck vein distention. Her recovery was otherwise uncomplicated.[41]

10. A 24-year-old woman ingested 1000 mg of propranolol with beer and whiskey. Two hours later she was admitted to the hospital with a pulse of 35 to 40 beats per minute and no blood pressure. Rhonchi were heard over the lung fields. Treatment included atropine intravenously but asystole developed. Cardiopulmonary resuscitation was commenced with favorable response to intracardiac epinephrine. The patient's course thereafter was uncomplicated. Plasma propranolol levels were not measured.[42]

11. A 41-year-old man with a history of chronic alcoholism ingested 5.1 g of propranolol. He arrived in the emergency room 2 hours later and was found to be comatose and cyanotic, with a pulse rate of 50 beats per minute. Blood pressure could not be obtained and the patient experienced intermittent generalized con-

vulsions. The initial electrocardiogram showed bradycardia without identifiable P waves. The patient developed asystole requiring intensive supportive efforts, including 115 mg of isoproterenol administered over the next 2 and a half days, a temporary transvenous pacemaker, and intravenous epinephrine. The patient remained comatose for 18 hours but eventually made an uneventful recovery. The total duration of use of isoproterenol was 65 hours. Plasma propranolol levels were not measured.[7]

12. A 65-year-old man ingested 800 mg of propranolol. Two hours later he presented in coma with respiratory compromise. The blood pressure was unobtainable and the pulse rate was 50 beats per minute. The electrocardiogram showed first-degree AV block and a right bundle branch block. The response to intravenous isoproterenol was favorable, with return of normal blood pressure, ECG, and heart rate. The plasma renin activity was severely depressed during the acute intoxication but rose briskly as the drug effect wore off. Plasma propranolol level was 1536 ng/ml. The patient's ultimate course was unremarkable.[43]

13. Propranolol-induced hypoglycemia was seen in two healthy siblings, a boy aged 20 months and a girl aged 3 years. Together they ingested a total of 150 mg of propranolol. The boy presented in stupor, with a blood pressure of 130 mm Hg and a pulse of 60 beats per minute. His electrocardiogram showed sinus rhythm and periodic second-degree atrioventricular block. The plasma glucose was 14 mg/dl. He responded to intravenous glucose with dramatic improvement in his level of consciousness. The electrocardiogram reverted to normal after 3 days. The girl presented with drowsiness and diaphoresis. Her blood glucose level was 50 mg/dl. The electrocardiogram, pulse, and blood pressure were normal in her case. She rapidly recovered after milk and sugar were given orally. Ten days after admission, an oral glucose tolerance was performed in each child and was within normal limits.[44]

Sotalol

Sotalol is not β_1-selective. It has neither partial agonist nor membrane-depressant properties. However, it differs electrophysiologically from other β-blocking agents in clinical practice, as in high concentration it prolongs the duration of the action potential in ventricular muscle and Purkinje fibers.[45-47] Sotalol thus possesses the properties of a Class III antiarrhythmic agent in addition to the Class II antiarrhythmic action shared by all β-adrenoreceptor blocking agents. A total of seven cases of sotalol intoxication have been reported in the literature, six of them coming from Neuvonen's group in Finland.[48,49] The latter investigators have also mentioned two additional cases encountered by them. Two representative cases of sotalol intoxication are described as follows. A summary of all reported cases of sotalol poisoning is given in Table 3.

1. A 39-year-old man receiving 160 mg of sotalol per day for mild hypertension was admitted to the emergency room 2 hours after ingesting 2.4 g of sotalol (30 80-mg tablets) together with quantities of diazepam, chlordiazepoxide, and alcohol. He was drowsy but oriented, with a blood pressure of 130/80 mm Hg and a heart rate of 50 beats per minute. Gastric lavage yielded a tablet mass. Four hours after ingestion, blood pressure could be maintained at 80/50 mm Hg only with dopamine infusion at 0.5 mg per minute and heart rate by intracardiac pacing with a bipolar electrode. Nine hours after ingestion two episodes of ventricular fibrillation occurred, with transient loss of consciousness. The first episode ceased spontaneously and the second disappeared with pacing. Subsequently, lidocaine and pacing at 140 beats per minute were able to dispel numerous multifocal ventricular premature contractions. Pacing and dopamine infusion were required for up to 40 hours and lidocaine for up to 70 hours after ingestion. Thirteen hours after ingestion, the serum sotalol concentration was 16 mg/L (therapeutic concentrations approximately 1 to 2 ng/L). The electrocardiogram showed a maximum QT interval of 0.68 seconds (at a heart rate of 70 beats per minute, the normal QT is 0.37 seconds). The serum half-life of sotalol was 13 hours, the decline in concentration correlating closely with return of the normal QT interval.[50]

2. A 59-year-old man was admitted 3 hours after ingestion of 8 g of sotalol (100 tablets). The blood pressure was 85/55 mm Hg and the heart rate 60 beats per minute. Gastric lavage was performed and 50 g of activated charcoal given. The patient received an isoproterenol infusion; with this, blood pressure rose to 100/70 mm Hg. Six hours after ingestion, multifocal ventricular extrasystoles, up to 24 per minute, appeared. In addition, there were aberrantly conducted beats and short episodes of ventricular tachycardia. Twenty-two hours following ingestion the serum sotalol concentration was 7.5 mg/L, the half-life being 15 hours. The maximum QT interval was 0.70 seconds at a heart rate of 45

TABLE 3. SUMMARY OF SEVEN CASES OF SOTALOL POISONING[48,49]

Case #	Age	Sex	Dose of Sotalol (g)	Delay to Admission (h)	Serum Sotalol Highest Concentration (mg/L) Hours after Ingestion (hr)	Half-Life (hr)
1	39	M	2.4	2	16.8 (at 13 hr)	13
2	59	M	8.0	3	7.5 (at 22 hr)	15
3	16	F	4.0	1	not measured	
4	17	F	8.0	4.5	11.0 (at 17 hr)	11
5	48	F	4.5	4	not measured	
6	30	M	7.8	0.5	not measured	
7	47	M	3.2	1.5	40 µg/ml	

Case #	Longest Measured QT Interval % normal	(at hr)	Time to Normal QT Interval (h)	Occurrence of Negative T-wave	Occurrence of Severe Arrhythmias VES (at hr)	Bigeminy	VT (at h)	Lowest Systolic BP (mmHg)	Lowest Heart Rate (beats/min)
1	184	15 hr	100 hr	+	+(5–17 hr)*	+	+(9–17 h)*	80†	40
2	156	10 hr	90 hr	–	+(6–14 hr)	+	+(6–14 h)	85‡	45
3	206	6–7 hr	70 hr	+	+(4–24 hr)	+	+(4–20)*‡	110	60
4	172	11 hr	80 hr	+	+(4–28 hr)	+	–	95	50
5	159	7–8 hr	>16 hr (at 16h 131%)	+	–	–	–	60‡	5
6	153	4–13 hr	70 hr	–	+(8–36 hr)	+	+(9–10 h)*	90	44
7					+		+	60	
Mean ± SE	172 ± 8%	10 ± 1 hr	82 ± 6 hr	4/6	6/7	5/6	5/7	87 ± 7 mm Hg	49 ± 3.1 beats/min

*Lidocaine given (up to 70h in Case 1). †Dopamine or isoproterenol infusion. ‡Dopamine + intracardiac pacing up to 40 hr. "Atropine given; VES = ventricular extrasystoles; VT = ventricular tachycardia; + = yes; – = no.

beats per minute; this was recorded 10 hours after ingestion. The QT interval decreased with an apparent half-life of 14 hours, returning to normal 3 days after ingestion.[50]

Timolol
Timolol has neither β_1-selectivity nor membrane-stabilizing properties. It has no partial agonist effects. Cases of overdosage with this β-adrenoreceptor blocking agent have not been reported.[51]

DISCUSSION

Although self-poisoning with β-adrenoreceptor blocking drugs is uncommon, it is being reported with increasing frequency. This reflects the expanding indications and widespread use of these drugs. The principal manifestations of massive overdosage are bradycardia, hypotension, lowered cardiac output, left ventricular failure, and cardiogenic shock.[6] However, a large number of clinical signs can be seen, depending upon the drug ingested and the dose consumed. Bronchospasm, for example, may occur, although relatively few cases have been seen. Respiratory depression can occur, perhaps from severe circulatory impairment or central drug effect. In the most severe intoxications, the myocardium may be refractory to pharmacologic and electrical stimulation. Death then occurs in asystole. Sotalol, on the other hand, possesses unique cardiotoxicity, resulting in life-threatening ventricular arrhythmias.[50] Neurotoxocity can be seen as well. Such lipid-soluble β-adrenoreceptor blocking drugs as propranolol can cause alteration of mental and neurologic status, including grand mal seizures.[8] It is apparent, then, that β-adrenoceptor blocking drugs taken in massive doses have diverse manifestations.

Pharmacology
When properly administered, the β-adrenoreceptor blocking drugs are relatively safe, with a wide gap between therapeutic and toxic doses. There is individual variation in sensitivity. Some patients, however, tolerate therapeutic doses of up to 4 g of propranolol each day, while others have deliberately ingested both practolol and propranolol in large doses with no adverse effect.[12,32,36] On the other hand, individuals with preexisting cardiac failure may develop circulatory collapse after even a single small oral dose of β-adrenoreceptor blocking drug. Such patients are dependent upon sympathetic tone, which is then compromised.

The pharmacologic properties of the various β-adrenoceptor blocking agents affect both therapeutic effects and medical consequences of deliberate poisoning.[1,8,52,53] In the therapeutic dose range, these drugs primarily act as antiadrenergic agents. In high doses acebutolol, alprenolol, oxprenolol, and propranolol have membrane-stabilizing or "quinidine-like" properties in addition to the β-adrenoreceptor blocking effect.[8] It is this "quinidine-like" effect that was at first thought to explain the antiarrhythmic properties of β-blockers. At the usual dosage this effect is of minor significance.[8,9,54]

Certain β-adrenoceptor blocking agents have intrinsic sympathomimetic or partial agonist activities. Acebutolol, alprenolol, oxprenolol, pindolol, and practolol share this feature. These drugs both stimulate and block β-receptors. The action is dose-related, increasing in importance as the plasma drug concentration rises.[8,54]

The β_1-selective adrenoceptors (acebutolol, atenolol, metoprolol, and practolol) antagonize β-receptors in the heart at lower doses than are required for other tissues. This property is dose-related and is less important as plasma drug concentration increases.[8,54]

The lipid solubility, metabolic pathway, excretory route, and protein binding of the β-adrenoreceptor blocking drug also vary.[54]

Acute Toxicity

All β-adrenoreceptor blocking drugs are rapidly absorbed in the gastrointestinal tract.[8,54] The first critical signs of overdosage can appear 20 minutes after ingestion but are more commonly seen within 1 to 2 hours.[55] The half-life of most of these drugs is usually short, ranging from 2 to 13 hours.[8,54] Plasma half-life can, however, be significantly increased by diminished renal and kidney perfusion, as may be the case in the patient with drug-induced depression of cardiac output. This may explain the prolonged drug effect—at times in excess of 72 hours—reported in certain patients with massive overdosage and marked depression of cardiac function.[13]

In most reported instances of oxprenolol and propranolol self-poisoning, sinus heart rate was markedly slowed with hypotension and circulatory collapse. This may be contrasted with the two cases of pindolol intoxication in which hypertension and tachycardia were seen, reflecting the partial agonist effect of this drug. It is curious that intoxication with a β_1-selective adrenoreceptor blocking agent (atenolol, metoprolol, practolol) was not characterized by profound bradycardia. Frank pulmonary edema rarely occurred in patients with massive ingestion of β-adrenoreceptor blocking agent overdosage unless the patient had underlying heart disease or left ventricular dysfunction.[6,55]

Typically, patients with massive ingestion of these drugs have first-degree AV block and sinus bradycardia. With massive ingestion, the P wave may disappear,[55] asystole may occur, and intraventricular conduction delays may be seen. Three of our four patients with propranolol overdosage manifested prolongation of QRS interval, and this correlated temporally with the presence of high plasma propranolol levels. As the plasma drug level fell, so too did the QRS interval narrow to normal. As stated earlier, the appearance of an intraventricular conduction delay may be the consequence of a membrane-depressant or "quinidine-like" effect of propranolol which may become clinically significant at high plasma drug levels. Intraventricular conduction delay is seen with massive ingestion of other β-blocking agents possessing membrane depressant activities[10] but is rarely encountered in intoxication with beta-blockers lacking such membrane depresssant properties.[45–48,55]

Sotalol possesses unique electrophysiologic properties. In concentrations higher than those for β-blockade, it increases the time course of repolarization and lengthens the refractory period and duration of the action potential. The result is a prolonged QT interval corrected for rate. In contrast, propranolol and alprenolol accelerate repolarization and shorten action potential duration, causing the QT interval to shorten. It is likely that these differences in the electrophysiologic effect of sotalol explain the extraordinary manifestation of massive overdosage. In vitro sotalol concentrations of 10^{-4} to 10^{-5} M or 3 to 30 μg/L delay repolarization, lengthen the effective refractory period, and increase the duration of action potential in Purkinje fibers and atrial and ventricular muscles.

Sotalol prolongs the QT interval, thus predisposing to reentrant ventricular tachyarrhythmias. A substantially prolonged QT interval may also predispose to ventricular fibrillation by enhancing temporal dispersion, as is the case with quinidine.[56] It has been shown that serum sotalol levels correlate well with the extent of QT interval prolongation.[5] This has led to the suggestion that the width of the QT interval may serve as an index of the severity of overdosage.[50] Sotalol lacks intrinsic sympathomimetic activity. It has less of a myocardial depressant effect than propranolol and has even been thought to have a positive inotropic effect mediated by a nonadrenergic mechanism.[57] Of the six cases of sotalol overdosage reported by Neuvonen, three maintained satisfactory blood pressure and did not require pressor agents, although life-threatening arrhythmias occurred.[5] Prolongation of the QT interval may occur not only with sotalol poisoning, but also with high therapeutic doses of this drug.[5] Close monitoring of the length of the QT interval is appropriate for patients receiving moderate to high oral doses of sotalol. Eighty percent of the drug is excreted unchanged in the urine over 3 days and it may accumulate in renal insufficiency. Special caution is advised in this setting. Adequate diuresis is essential in the treatment of patients who have taken sotalol overdosage. As β-adrenoreceptor blocking drugs have been utilized with success in the treatment of prolonged QT interval syndromes, and prevention of torsades de point, it is important to remember that sotalol may further prolong the QT. It is prudent to use an alternate β-blocker in this situation. The long half-life of sotalol—13 hours—as well as its slow elimination partly explain the duration of symptoms with an overdose. Close monitoring for several days is in order, although toxicity is most serious in the first 20 hours.[5]

Bronchospasm is a well-known adverse effect in patients treated with β-adrenoreceptor blocking drugs and is more common with nonselective agents.[1,52] It is, however, seldom reported in patients with overdosage except in those with preexisting bronchospastic disease.[58] Respiratory arrest has been reported with β-blocker intoxication, and with propranolol in particular. It is generally regarded as a central drug effect.[6]

Hypoglycemia is uncommon in patients with β-blocker overdosage. This is surprising since propranolol interferes with the glycogen-mobilizing effects of catecholamines.[1] Individuals treated with both propranolol and insulin have developed hypoglycemia.[1] Some have suggested a special proclivity to hypoglycemia in children with β-blocker poisoning. This is based upon a single report of hypoglycemia in two nondiabetic children who ingested 150 mg of propranolol together.[44]

Propranolol is extremely lipid soluble and readily crosses the blood–brain barrier, concentrating in the brain.[8,54] Changes in mental and neurologic status were reported in patients treated with the usual therapeutic doses of propranolol. With overdosage, depressed sensorium, generalized convulsions, and coma have resulted. Seizure activity is a feature of self-poisoning with β-blockers such as propranolol, which has high lipid solubility and membrane-depressant properties. β-Blockers lacking these effects have not caused seizures even in massive overdosage. The alteration in mental status and seizure activity seen in propranolol overdosage have occurred with no cardiovascular compromise. It is true that massive ingestion of any of the β-blocking drugs may decrease cardiac output. Mental status changes on this basis may then follow. The central nervous system effects of massive propranolol overdosage are explained by membrane-depressant or "quinidine-like" actions that are apparent only at high plasma drug concentrations.[8,54] It is suggested that the mechanism of propranolol seizures may resemble that of lidocaine, another local anesthetic drug with membrane-depressant properties.[9]

Plasma Drug Levels

β-Adrenoreceptor intoxication may be difficult to recognize, particularly when the drug is taken in combination with other medicines. Al-the degree of β-adrenoreceptor blocker intoxication. Patients have different levels of sympathetic tone and different metabolic rates. A single blood level may be associated with different clinical signs in individual patients.[54,59] Drugs, such as alprenolol and propranolol, yield active metabolites that are not detected in the plasma assay.[8,54] It should be remembered that the β-adrenoreceptor blocking effect appears to last far longer than the plasma half-life might suggest.[54] It is, therefore, important that the physician recognize the clinical manifestations of β-adrenoreceptor blocker intoxication and not rely solely on plasma drug levels. An estimate of the plasma drug concentration can be made and will confirm the poisoning. This, however, is of limited value in the immediate patient management.[6]

THERAPY

Poisoning with β-adrenoreceptor blocking agents is a medical emergency that requires close collaboration between the cardiologist, the clinical pharmacologist, and others with experience in this area. It is always to be remembered that the patient with this drug intoxication may suddenly and precipitously deteriorate. The clinical manifestations of intoxication may occur within 20 minutes after drug ingestion, although they are usually seen 1 to 2 hours later.[5] The optimal management of the patient requires intensive supportive care with facilities for cardiac monitoring, ventilatory support, and transvenous electrical pacing. The approach to poisoning with all β-adrenoreceptor blocking agents is similar: (1) to rapidly remove any remaining ingested tablets; (2) to support cardiovascular and pulmonary status and counter the effect of β-blockade on these organs; and (3) to treat central nervous system disorders.

Removal of Drug
Gastric lavage may allow the ingested tablets to be identified, but is unlikely to be sufficient in preventing serious poisoning unless performed immediately. Since all β-adrenoreceptor blocking agents are rapidly absorbed. If the ingestion is recent, emesis should be induced unless coma, convulsion, or loss of gag reflex are present. If these conditions are present, endotracheal intubation is required, followed by gastric lavage with a large-bore tube. Activated charcoal in a dose of five to ten times the estimated ingested dose of 30 to 50 g then can be given orally or by lavage. Sodium or magnesium sulfate, 250 mg/kg, can be given orally as a cathartic.

Hemodialysis is unlikely to rid the body of propranolol, which is highly protein bound (greater than 95 percent). There are no well-documented reports of hemodialysis from massive ingestion nor is there experience with charcoal hemoperfusion. The rapidity of cardiovascular collapse in these patients may not allow sufficient time to establish hemoperfusion. However, the possibility exists that β-blockers, more water soluble and less protein bound than propranolol, may be treated by hemoperfusion. Nadolol and atenolol, for example, can be removed from the body by hemodialysis.[51,58,60] Tablets retrieved by gastric aspiration should be identified. Blood concentrations of the ingested β-blocking drug can be established and overdosage confirmed but this is of limited value in the immediate phase of support.

Bradycardia and Hypotension

Hypotension may be the direct consequence of bradycardia or may result from depression of myocardial contractility or a central nervous system effect.[9]

All patients with β-adrenoreceptor blocker overdosage should have continuous electrocardiographic monitoring. If clinically significant bradycardia or AV conduction defects occur, initial therapy should be with atropine 0.5 to 3 mg intravenously in adult or 50 μg/kg IV infusion in children.[61] This will reduce unopposed vagal tone. Ideally, most patients with serious overdosage with β-blocking drugs should have a temporary transvenous pacing catheter inserted.

Isoproterenol is a competitive antagonist of β-blocking drugs and should be given by continuous infusion with the dose monitored according to the response of blood pressure and pulse. At times, massive doses of isoproterenol have been required to treat β-blocker overdosage. In one case report, 115 mg was infused over 65 hours.[7] Isoproterenol may cause peripheral vasodilation and, thus, its administration as an antidote to β-blocker poisoning requires meticulous care. Our strategy is to advise temporary pacemaker placement for all serious, life-threatening overdosages with β-adrenoreceptor blocking agents. Hypotension, consequent to bradycardia, is treated with atropine and pacing. Hypotension that is not related to a slowed heart rate is first managed with isoproterenol infusion, titrated to the desired blood pressure. If isoproterenol itself causes vasodilation, we substitute a constant infusion of dobutamine, a β_1-selective adrenoreceptor agonist.[62] If hypotension is severe, an α-constricting catecholamine such as norepinephrine by continuous infusion, or dopamine at high dosage, may be necessary. On theoretical grounds, it seems that poisoning with β_1-selective blockers (such as atenolol and metoprolol) might best be treated with a selective β-adrenoreceptor agonist (such as dobutamine). Further experience is needed to evaluate such recommendations. It is likely that specific β-adrenoreceptor agonists will be developed in the future and will be employed in the treatment of specific β-blocker overdosage.

Glucagon

Glucagon, a polypeptide hormone, increases heart rate and improves atrioventricular conduction.[63] Its major inotropic action is not dependent on catecholamine stores or β-adrenoreceptor sites. Glucagon is thought to activate adenylcyclase and enhance myocardial contractility by mechanisms different from catecholamines. After β-adrenergic blockade with d,l-propranolol, the inotropic responses to glucagon is unchanged even at higher β-blocker dose levels. Nor does glucagon cause ventricular irritability or increase peripheral resistance.[63] These properties make glucagon an attractive pharmacologic means of combating β-adrenoreceptor blocking agent overdosage. Numerous reports attest to the favorable effect of glucagon in this situation, at times with immediate reversal of shock and bradycardia.[2,4,34,41] On the other hand, cases of massive β-blocker overdosage have responded successfully to isoproterenol and norepinephrine alone.[33,35] We believe that the evidence favoring the use of glucagon for massive β-blocker overdosage is impressive, but we are concerned that many skilled physicians do not yet have experience with this drug and its attendant problems. The physician caring for a patient with β-adrenoreceptor blocking agent overdosage should familiarize himself with dosage schedules (initial intravenous bolus of 50 μg/kg infused over 1 minute, followed by an intravenous infusion of one 5 μg/kg per hour) and side effects (hyperglycemia, mild hypocalcemia, and vomiting).[2] An initial bolus of 10 mg of intravenous glucagon therapy of β-adrenoreceptor blocking agent overdosage has been advocated[3] but initial bolus doses of 50 μg/kg have also been clinically successful.[41] The physician must be aware of the fact that glucagon, in certain preparations, is reconstituted with phenol. Thus, phenol toxicity can occur.[2,41] Reconstitution of glucagon should be with 5 percent dextrose, especially if large doses (as in constant infusion) are necessary. We also emphasize that glucagon is one further pharmacologic means of supporting the patient with β-adrenoreceptor blocker overdosage. It may be used together with isoproterenol or dobutamine but does not substitute for the most meticulous supportive care.

Such pharmacologic measures as the use of aminophylline in β-adrenoreceptor blocking overdosage are speculative and unsubstantiated at the present time.[64]

Support of the Patient with Sotalol Overdosage

Sotalol in massive dosage prolongs the QT interval, enhances temporal dispersion, and facilitates reentrant ventricular tachyarrhythmias.[48,50] Of the seven reported cases of sotalol intoxication, all had QT interval prolongation of 150 to 200 percent of normal, five developed ventricular tachycardia, three had ventricular fibrillation, and only one was free of high-grade ventricular ectopy.[48,49] Lidocaine was employed in three cases to suppress ventricular ectopic beats. One case required pacing for bradycardia and frequent VPCs. There is no reported experience with any measures but the above in the support of the sotalol-intoxicated patient. It is to be emphasized that procainamide and quinidine both prolong QT interval and are both best avoided in this setting. The role of such interventions as overdrive pacing (for ventricular tachycardia with a long QT interval) or bretylium (for high-grade ectopy not responsive to lidocaine) is not known. Perhaps because sotalol is a lesser myocardial depressant than is propranolol, and may even cause positive inotropic effects,[57] three of the seven reported sotalol intoxicated patients maintained adequate blood pressure despite the appearance of life-threatening ventricualr arrhythmia.[48] Patients who required blood pressure support received either dopamine or isoproterenol. No instances of glucagon use for sotalol intoxication are on record.

Pulmonary
Effective respiratory function should be assured and is essential in patients with overdosage of β-adrenoreceptor blocking agents. Endotracheal intubation should be performed if required. Adequate tidal volumes should be maintained and arterial blood gases sampled. Severe bronchoconstriction, although rare in self-poisoning, may require isoproterenol inhalation in larger than usual dosages. Such β-adrenoceptor stimulating drugs as terbutaline may be considered in this setting. Aminophylline may also be used for bronchoconstriction, given in an initial dosage of 5.6 mg/kg intravenously over 15 to 20 minutes, followed by a continuous infusion of 0.5 mg/kg per hour. Serum aminophylline levels should be maintained in the range of 10 to 20 μg/ml.

Hypoglycemia
Hypoglycemia, a rare complication of β-adrenoreceptor blocker self-poisoning, can be treated with either glucose or glucagon.

Seizures
Seizure activity can be seen in β-adrenoceptor blocking overdosage secondary to hypotension, hypoxia, or hypoglycemia. Each of these conditions should be corrected. Some β-blockers possess central nervous system depressant effects and may also produce seizures. Intravenous diazepam has proven effective in controlling seizure activity in several patients.

β-Blocker Withdrawal

Most patients who are successfully treated for self-poisoning will have no late sequelae. Certain patients, however, may be prone to β-adrenoceptor "withdrawal effects," including aggravation of chest pain or myocardial infarction in those with preexistent angina pectoris.[65,66] These patients should be closely observed for such complications.

Duration of Observation

This is highly dependent upon the ingested drug. Sotalol-intoxicated patients should be monitored in-hospital for several days, as the drug is slowly eliminated and duration of symptoms of intoxication is long.[48] Elimination half-time is also especially long for nadolol (urinary route of excretion); overdoses with this drug almost certainly will require in-hospital monitoring for several days. Other agents with prolonged half-times of elimination are practolol, atenolol, and acebutolol.

Concomitant Ingestions

The physician should consider the possibility of mixed or combined ingestions in all cases. Appropriate toxicologic sampling and blood alcohol levels should be performed. The time course and nature of intoxication with β-adrenoreceptor blocking agents may be modified by other ingested drugs or poisons (e.g., renal failure altering the excretion of sotalol, severe hypoglycemia with combined β-adrenoreceptor blocking agent overdosage, sulfonylurea overdosage, and so on).

Coincident Diseases

The presence of preexistent heart or lung disease, such as congestive heart failure, atrial fibrillation, bronchospastic disease, and so forth, may radically alter the clinical manifestations of the β-adrenoreceptor blocking agent overdosage.

REFERENCES

1. Frishman W, Silverman R: Clinical pharmacology of the new beta-adrenergic blocking drugs. Part 3. Comparative clinical experience and new therapeutic applications. Am Heart J 98:119, 1979.
2. Illingworth RN: Glucagon for beta-blocker poisoning. Practitioner 223:683, 1979.
3. Robson RH: Glucagon for β-blocker poisoning (letter). Lancet 1:1357, 1980.
4. Jacobsen D, Helgeland A, Koss A: Treatment of beta-blocker poisoning (letter). Lancet 1:1031, 1980.

5. Editorial: Beta-blocker poisoning. Lancet 803, 1980.
6. Editorial: Self-poisoning with beta-blockers. Br Med J 1:1010, 1978.
7. Lagerfelt J, Matell G: Attempted suicide with 5.1 G of propranolol. A case report. Acta Med Scand 199:517, 1976.
8. Frishman W: Clinical pharmacology of the new beta-adrenergic blocking drugs. Part 1. Pharmacodynamic and pharmacokinetic properties. Am Heart J 97:663, 1979.
9. Nies AS, Shand D: Clinical pharmacology of propranolol. Circulation 52:6, 1975.
10. Nies AS: Pathophysiologic and pharmacological considerations in drug administration (cardiovascular disorders), in Melmon K, Morelli H (eds), Clinical Pharmacology. New York, Macmillan, 1978, p 242.
11. Buiumsohn A, Eisenberg ES, Jacob H, et al: Seizures and intraventricular conduction defect in propranolol poisoning. Ann Intern Med 91:860, 1979.
12. Boakes AJ, Boerre BH: Suicidal attempts with beta-adrenoceptor blocking agents. Br Med J 4:675, 1973.
13. Waal-Manning J: Hypertension: Which beta-blocker? Drugs 12:412, 1976.
14. Johnsson G, Regardh CG: Clinical pharmacokinetics of β-adrenoceptor blocking drugs. Clin Pharmacokinet 1:233, 1976.
15. Klug E, Schneider V: Tödliche vergiftung mit acebutolol. Z Rechtsmed 83:325, 1979.
16. Harzer K: Tödliche vergiftung mit acebutolol (Prent). Toxichem 7:58, 1979.
17. Simonsen J, Worm K: Acute fatal alprenolol poisoning. Ugeskrift for Laeger 139:2817, 1977.
18. Dickson SJ, Miurhead JM, Nelson PE: The gas chromotographic determination of alprenolol in human postmortem liver and blood samples. J Anal Toxicol 2:242, 1978.
19. Shanahan FL, Counihan TB: Atenolol self-poisoning (letter). Br Med J 2:773, 1978.
20. Frishman WH, Halprin S: New horizons in beta-adrenoceptor blocking therapy: labetalol. Am Heart J 98:660, 1979.
21. Moller BHM: Massive intoxication with metoprolol (letter). Br Med J 1:222, 1976.
22. Sire S: Metoprolol intoxication (letter). Lancet 2:1137, 1976.
23. Groel JT: Personal communication. Pol Arch Med Wewn 1981.
24. Editorial: Death from an overdose of oxprenolol. Pharm 208:143, 1972.
25. Khan A, Muscat-Baron JM: Fatal oxprenolol poisoning. Br Med J 1:52, 1977.
26. Ward DE, Jones B: Glucagon and beta-blocker toxicity. Br Med J 2:151, 1976.
27. Mattingly PC: Oxprenolol overdose with survival (letter). Br Med J 1:776, 1977.
28. Hume L, Forfar JC: Hyperkalemia and overdosage of antihypertensive agents (letter). Lancet 2:1182, 1977.
29. Thorpe P: Pindolol in hypertension. Med J Aust 58:1242, 1971.
30. Offenstadt G, Hericord P, Amstutz P: Voluntary poisoning with pindolol (letter). Nouv Presse Med 5:1539, 1976.

31. Verdera Cosmelli JT, Garcia del Pozo JM, Lopez Morales J: Attempted suicide with practolol. Rev Esp Cardiol 29:195, 1976.
32. Karhunen P, Hartel G: Suicidal attempt with practolol. Br Med J 2:178, 1973.
33. Halloran TJ, Philips CE: Propranolol intoxication: a severe case responding to norepinephrine therapy. Arch Intern Med 141:810, 1981.
34. Salzberg MR, Gallagher EJ: Propranolol overdosage. Ann Emerg Med 9:26, 1980.
35. Tynan RF, Fisher MM, Ibels LS: Self-poisoning with propranolol. Med J Aust 1:82, 1981.
36. Wermut W, Wojcicki M: Suicidal attempt with propranolol. Br Med J 3:591, 1973.
37. Gault R, Monforte JR, Khasnabis S: A death involving propranolol (Inderal). Clin Toxicol 11:295, 1977.
38. Kristinsson J, Johannesson T: A case of fatal propranolol intoxication. Acta Pharmacol Toxicol 41:190, 1977.
39. Turner JE, Cravey RH: A fatal case involving propranolol and codeine. Clin Toxicol 8:271, 1975.
40. Gdyra D, Billip-Tomecka A, Szajewsky JM: Case of poisoning with a 4 gram dose of propranolol. Pol Arch Med Wewn 50:1341, 1973.
41. Kosinski EJ, Malindzak GS Jr: Glucagon and isoproterenol, in reversing propranolol toxicity. Arch Intern Med 132:840, 1973.
42. Frithz G: Toxic effects of propranolol on the heart. Br Med J 1:769, 1976.
43. Ducret F, Zech P, Perrot D, et al: Deliberate self-overdose with propranolol. Change in serum levels. Nouv Presse Med 7:27, 1978.
44. Hesse B, Pedersen JT: Hypoglycemia after propranolol in children. Acta Med Scand 193:551, 1973.
45. Singh BN, Vaughan Williams EM: A third class of antiarrhythmia action. Effects on atrial and ventricular intracellular potentials and other pharmacological actions on cardiac muscle of MJ 1999 and AH 3474. Br J Pharmacol 39:675, 1970.
46. Strauss HC, Bigger JT Jr, Hoffman BF: Electrophysiological and beta-receptor blocking effects of MJ 1999 on dog and rabbit cardiac tissue. Circ Res 21:661, 1970.
47. Wit AL, Hoffman BF, Rosen MR: Electrophysiology and pharmacology of cardiac arrhythmias. IX. Cardiac electrophysiological effects of beta-adrenergic receptor stimulation and blockade. Part C. Am Heart J 90:795, 1975.
48. Neuvonen PJ, Elonen E, Vuorenman T, Laako M: Prolonged QT interval and severe tachyarrhythmias, common features of sotalol intoxication. Eur J Clin Pharmacol 20:85, 1981.
49. Montagna M, Groppi A: Fatal sotalol poisoning. Arch Toxicol 43:221, 1980.
50. Elonen E, Neuvonen P, Tarssanen L, Kala R: Sotalol intoxication with prolonged QT interval and severe tachyarrhythmias. Br Med J 1:1184, 1979.
51. Frishman WH: Atenolol and timolol—two new systemic β-adrenoceptor antagonists. N Engl J Med 306:1456, 1982.
52. Frishman W, Silverman R, Strom J, et al: Clinical pharmacology of the new

beta-adrenergic blocking drugs. Part 4. Adverse effects. Choosing a β-adrenoceptor blocker. Am Heart J 98:256, 1979.

53. Frishman W, Jacob H, Eisenberg E, Ribner H: Clinical pharmacology of the new beta-adrenergic blocking drugs. Part 8. Self-poisoning with beta-adrenoceptor blocking agents. Recognition and management. Am Heart J 98:798, 1979.

54. Frishman WH: β-Adrenoceptor antagonists. New drugs and new indications. N Engl J Med 305:500, 1981.

55. Gabinski C: Toxicite aigue des beta-bloquants. Bord Med 11:2623, 1978.

56. Deglin SM, Deglin JM, Chung EK: Drug-induced cardiovascular diseases. Drugs 14:29, 1977.

57. Parmley WW: Inotropic and Antiarrhythmic Effects of Sotalol. In Smart AG (ed), Advances in Beta-adrenergic Blocking Therapy. Vol 3: Sotalol. Proceedings of the International Symposium, Rome, Italy, May 1974. Excerpta Medica, Amsterdam, 1974, p 11.

58. Williams IP, Millard FJC: Severe asthma after inadvertant ingestion of oxprenolol. Thorax 35:160, 1980.

59. Frishman W, Smithen C, Befler B, et al: Noninvasive assessment of clinical response to oral propranolol. Am J Cardiol 35:635, 1975.

60. Frishman WH: Nadolol: A new β-adrenoceptor antagonist. N Engl J Med 305:678, 1981.

61. Richards DA, Prichard BN: Self-poisoning with beta-blockers. Br Med J 1:1623, 1978.

62. Sonnenblick EH, Frishman WH, LeJemtel TH: Dobutamine: a new synthetic cardioactive sympathetic amine. N Engl J Med 300:17, 1979.

63. Parmley WW, Glick G, Sonnenblick EH: Cardiovascular effects of glucagon in man. N Engl J Med 279:12, 1968.

64. Jones B: Treatment of beta-blocker poisoning (letter). Lancet 10:1031, 1980.

65. Frishman WH, Christodoulou J, Weksler B, et al: Abrupt propranolol withdrawal in angina pectoris: effects on platelet aggregation and exercise tolerance. Am Heart J 95:169, 1978.

66. Frishman WH, Klein N, Strom J, et al: Comparative effects of abrupt withdrawal of propranolol and verapamil in angina pectoris. Am J Cardiol 50:1191, 1982.

CHAPTER 7

Labetalol: A New β-Adrenergic Blocker-Vasodilator

William H. Frishman, E. Paul MacCarthy, Bruce Kimmel, Eliot Lazar, Eric L. Michelson, and Saul S. Bloomfield

Labetalol hydrochloride is the forerunner of a new group of β-adrenergic blockers that act as competitive pharmacologic antagonists at both α- and β-adrenoceptors.[1] Agonists, acting at one or both types of adrenoceptor, have been available for years. However, the situation with regard to adrenergic antagonists is different. Before labetalol, only antagonists acting at either α- or β-adrenoceptors, but not at both, were available. In addition, labetalol is also a prototype for β-blockers with ancillary vasodilatory properties, whether direct or mediated via $β_2$-agonist activity.

The pharmacology of labetalol was first described in 1972 and an extensive worldwide experience has since been gathered regarding its clinical applications.[2] Labetalol has been developed as an oral and intravenous agent. It has been used for the treatment of patients with essential hypertension, hypertensive emergencies, hypertension associated with pheochromocytoma and pregnancy, and angina pectoris.[3-5] It has also been used as a hypotensive agent during general anesthesia.[3]

Initial attempts to treat hypertension with the combination of α- and β-blocking agents proved impractical due to unacceptable side effects, most commonly postural hypotension and tachyphylaxis due to α-blockers. The use of phenoxybenzamine, a noncompetitive, nonselective α-antagonist, with propranolol, was associated with marked orthostatic

Based on an article that appeared in Pharmacotherapy, Volume 3, July–August, 1983, pp 193–219, with permission.

hypotension.[6] When phentolamine, a competitive, nonselective α-antagonist, was combined with β-blockers, the results varied.[7] The combination of a β-blocker with either the postsynaptic $α_1$-blocker prazosin or the arteriolar vasodilator hydralazine, has been more consistently efficacious, but is usually reserved for more refractory or moderately severe hypertensive patients. Labetalol, a single drug with selective postsynaptic $α_1$-blocking and nonselective β-blocking activities, is associated with a low incidence of postural hypotension and tachyphylaxis and appears to be a clinically useful agent.[1,3,8] In this chapter, the pharmacology of labetalol will be reviewed, and recommendations regarding its clinical use will be presented.

CHEMISTRY

Labetalol hydrochloride is 2-hydroxy-5 {1-hydroxy-2-(1-methyl-3-phenylpropyl) aminoethyl} benzamide hydrochloride. Its chemical structure is shown in Figure 1. It has two optical centers and is an equal mixture of four diastereoisomers.[9] The RR stereoisomer is a nonselective, competitive β-adrenoceptor antagonist which is virtually devoid of α-blocking activity, but has direct vasodilator activity. The SR stereoisomer is an α-blocker with minimal β-blocking activity. The SS and RS stereoisomers have weak α- and β-adrenoceptor activity, respectively. The presence of the large *N*-alkyl substitution is essential for labetalol's combined α-β-blocking properties.[10] In this chapter, the mixture of stereoisomers is being discussed when labetalol is mentioned.

EXPERIMENTAL MODELS AND CLINICAL PHARMACOLOGY

The basic pharmacology of labetalol in experimental models has been reviewed in a number of excellent reports.[2,11–13] Its known pharmacologic effects are listed in Table 1. Labetalol possesses competitive pharmacologic blocking activity at both α- and β-adrenergic receptors[2,11,13] but appears to be a more potent inhibitor at β-receptors than α-adrenoceptors.[10,13] The degree of potency at α- and β-adrenergic receptors is

LABETALOL

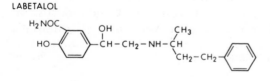

Figure 1. Chemical structure of labetalol.

TABLE 1. PHARMACOLOGIC PROPERTIES OF LABETALOL[13]

Adrenoceptor Blockade

β-Blockade (β_1 and β_2)
α-Blockade (α_1)

Agonist Activity

β_2-Agonist activity producing vasodilatation and tracheal and uterine relaxation.
Minimal α- or β_1-agonist activity—not clinically apparent

Other Adrenergic Interactions

Inhibition of neuronal uptake mechanism

influenced by the experimental conditions and the mode of administration, with differences in animal species or tissue preparations affecting the affinity of labetalol for adrenoceptors. Over the range of in vitro and in vivo tests used, labetalol has been shown to be 6 to 10 times less potent than phentolamine at α-adrenoceptors, 1.5 to 4 times less potent than propranolol at β-adrenoceptors, and was itself 4 to 16 times less potent at α- than at β-adrenoceptors.[11] The drug has also been shown to have partial β_2-agonist properties,[13-16] as well as the ability to cause direct vasodilation.[13,17,18]

The pharmacologic properties of labetalol and the pure β-adrenoceptor blocking drugs in human subjects are compared in Chapter 2.

Blockade of Receptors

Actions at β-Adrenoceptors in Experimental Models. In isolated tissue preparations, labetalol was found to be a competitive, nonselective β-adrenoceptor antagonist (Fig. 2, left), having a similar order of blocking potency at atrial β_1- and tracheal β_2-adrenoceptors.[19] In anesthetized dogs, labetalol was about 4 times less potent than propranolol in blocking cardiac β_1-receptors and 11 to 17 times less potent than propranolol in blocking β_2-receptors in the lung and vascular bed. This difference in potency at β_1- and β_2-receptors as compared to propranolol is probably related to labetalol's partial agonist activity at β_2-adrenoceptors.[13-16]

Labetalol has been shown to inhibit spontaneous contractions and acetylcholine-induced contractions of isolated rat uteri,[14,15] and to cause relaxation of guinea pig isolated trachealis muscle preparations.[16] This partial agonist property may also contribute to the direct peripheral vasodilation seen with labetalol, an effect that is discussed in greater detail later.[13,17,18] Unlike its effects at β_2-adrenoceptors, labetalol has been shown to have little, if any, agonist activity at β_1-adrenoceptors.[11,20]

Labetalol blocks α- and β-adrenoceptor mediated sympathetic nerve stimulation to approximately the same extent as it does with exogenously administered catecholamines.[2,11]

Actions at α-Adrenoceptors in Experimental Models. The stimulation of α-adrenoceptors by exogenous catecholamines or sympathetic nerve activation is competitively inhibited by labetalol (Fig. 2, right).[2,11,13,19,21] Like prazosin, labetalol appears to be a selective α_1-blocker.[22] α_1-Adrenoceptors mediate the effect or organ response to noradrenergic stimulation, for example, vasoconstriction, whereas α_2-adrenoceptors mediate the negative feedback inhibition of neurotransmitter release.[23]

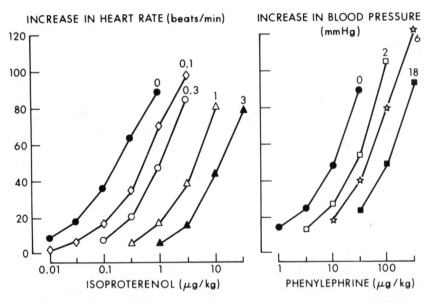

Figure 2. β- and α-adrenoceptor blocking activity of labetalol in pentobarbital-anesthetized vagotimized dogs. Left panel: increases in heart rate in response to intravenous doses of isoproterenol before (0) and after increasing doses (0.1 to 3 mg/kg intravenous) of labetalol in 6 dogs. Baseline heart rates averaged 163 ± 7 beats per minute before and 156 ± 7, 151 ± 9, 148 ± 8, and 144 ± 8 after the 4 doses of labetalol. Right panel: increases in diastolic blood pressure produced by phenylephrine before (0) and after increasing doses of labetalol (2 to 18 mg/kg) in 6 dogs. Baseline blood pressures averaged 128 ± 7 mm Hg before and 76 ± 5, 67 ± 3, and 58 ± 4 after the 3 doses of labetalol. Dose–response curves were obtained to isoproterenol and phenylephrine (injected at 5 to 15-minute intervals) starting at 5 to 15 minutes after each dose of labetalol. [Reprinted from Baum TS, Sybertz EJ: Am J Med (Suppl):75(4A): 17, 1983, with permission.[13]]

There are many experimental studies supporting the α_1-selectivity of labetalol. In the guinea pig ileum, α-adrenoceptor agonists act by reducing the release of acetylcholine and thus, inhibiting the twitch response. In this tissue preparation, Drew demonstrated that labetalol did not antagonize the inhibitory effect of clonidine. Labetalol increased norepinephrine transmitter outflow with splenic nerve stimulation in the isolated cat spleen.[24] Supramaximal doses of the prosynaptic α_2-adrenoceptor antagonist piperoxan produced a further increase in transmitter overflow. Labetalol, given after catecholamine reuptake blockade in sympathetic nerve endings by either cocaine or desmethylimipramine, produced no further increase in transmitter overflow. Blakely and Summers thus concluded that labetalol has no α_2-adrenoceptor blocking action in this tissue preparation.[21] Drew et al. showed that labetalol was ineffective in blocking the α_2-receptor mediated sedation by clonidine seen in rats.[25]

Labetalol has also been shown to block the reuptake of catecholamines by sympathetic nerve endings, which is partly responsible for removal of circulating norepinephrine at the synaptic junction. This is a property labetalol shares with such drugs as cocaine and desmethylimipramine.[21]

Unlike its actions at β_2-receptors, labetalol does not appear to possess significant agonist effects at α-adrenoceptors.[2,11,13,21] In humans, however, labetalol has been reported to cause scalp tingling, an effect that is reported to be a sensitive index of α-receptor stimulation.[12,26,27]

The α- and β-adrenoceptor blockade produced by labetalol is highly specific.[28] In rabbit aortic strips, labetalol has been shown to displace the norepinephrine concentration-effect curve to the right by 200-fold but has been shown not to inhibit contractile responses to histamine, angiotensin II, bradykinen, 5-hydroxytryptamine, acetylcholine, and barium chloride, both in vitro and in vivo.[11,26] Similarly, in the guinea pig left atrium, labetalol displaced the isoproterenol concentration–effect curve by 1300-fold, but had no effect on the positive inotropic response to calcium chloride.[11]

Blockade of Adrenoceptors in Human Studies. In human studies, as in the animal experiments, labetalol has been shown to be an extremely effective competitive antagonist at both α- and β-adrenoceptors. In the earliest studies in human volunteers, Boakes et al. demonstrated that the cumulative log dose–response curves of isoproterenol-induced tachycardia and the phenylephrine-induced rise in blood pressure were both shifted to the right in a parallel manner after intravenous labetalol administration, indicating competitive antagonism at α- and β-adrenoceptor sites.[29]

Collier et al. examined the effect of labetalol infused both locally into superficial hand veins and systemically through peripheral veins and the brachial artery. The blockade of norepinephrine-induced vasoconstriction by labetalol was dose-dependent and increased progressively up to an infusion rate of 32 μg/min. When isoproterenol and labetalol were infused together into preconstricted superficial hand veins, β-adrenergic blockade was dose-dependent and appeared to be competitive. Labetalol infused into the brachial artery at 40 μg/min showed no effect on the heart rate response to isoproterenol infusion; however, at 400 μg/min, it produced consistent competitive blockade. The pharmacologic effect of systemic drug administration was longer in duration than that seen following local infusion. Labetalol was found to be 40 times more potent at blocking β- than α-adrenoceptors when administered locally in veins, and 200 times more potent at β- than α-receptors when administered systemically. Labetalol was 10 to 20 times less potent than propranolol in peripheral vessels and four times less potent than propranolol in inhibiting isoproterenol-induced tachycardia.[26]

Richards et al.[30] also demonstrated that labetalol is a competitive antagonist at both α- and β-adrenoceptors in human beings. After either oral or intravenous administration, labetalol causes a parallel shift to the right of the cumulative log dose–response curves of isoproterenol-induced increases in heart rate and reductions in diastolic blood pressure. The shifts of the heart rate–response curves were similar in magnitude to those of reductions in diastolic blood pressure, thus implying that labetalol has nonselective β-adrenoceptor blocking properties. Labetalol and propranolol were qualitatively similar in their β-blocking effects; however, propranolol was found to be 4 to 6 times more potent on a milligram for milligram basis. The dose–response curve of the increase in cardiac output produced by graded doses of isoproterenol was also shifted to the right by labetalol. This effect is not enhanced by the administration of phentolamine in doses sufficient to produce further α-adrenoceptor blockade. It is therefore due to the β-blocking effects of labetalol. After either oral or intravenous administration, labetalol causes a parallel shift to the right of the cumulative log dose–response curves of phenylephrine and norepinephrine-induced increases in blood pressure, showing that it is a competitive α-adrenoceptor antagonist. After oral administration, labetalol was 3 times less potent at α- than at β-adrenoceptors. After intravenous administration, labetalol was 6.9 times less potent at α- than at β-adrenoceptors. There is no clear-cut evidence that the ratio between α- and β-adrenergic blocking properties of labetalol changes with the dosage of the drug.[30-35]

Mehta and Cohn studied the effects of labetalol in phenylephrine-induced diastolic hypertension and isoproterenol-induced tachycardia in hypertensive patients. They found that at an oral dose of 800 to 1600 mg/day, labetalol appeared to be 4 to 6 times more potent as a β-adrenoceptor antagonist than as an α-adrenoceptor antagonist.[36] These results agree with those obtained by Richards et al.[30]

As in the animal experiments in which labetalol was shown to block adrenergic responses mediated by sympathetic nerve stimulation, labetalol in humans causes blockade of endogenous sympathetic activity caused by standardized physiologic stresses. Immersion of a hand in ice cold water for 60 seconds elevates blood pressure through α-adrenergic stimulation; labetalol blocks this cold pressor respose in normal humans.[37] This is in contrast to observed cold pressor responses with phentolamine and suggests that prejunctional α-blockade does not occur with labetalol. The drug also produced a sustained dose-related reduction of blood pressure and heart rate in response to treadmill and bicycle exercise after either oral or intravenous administration.[32,38] It inhibited the tachycardia induced by the Valsalva maneuver,[33] and the reflex tachycardia related to amyl nitrate-induced hypotension was attenuated.[36] The overshoot of arterial blood pressure following the Valsalva maneuver was also blocked by labetalol.[36] Finally, the tachycardia induced by 80 degree tilting was inhibited.[30] Propranolol was found to be more potent than labetalol in inhibiting all β-adrenoceptor mediated responses.[30]

Hemodynamic and Antihypertensive Effects

Direct Vasodilator Action. Labetalol has been shown to exert direct vascular effects that are not attributable to peripheral α- or β-adrenoceptor blockade. Johnson et al. observed in anesthetized dogs that labetalol caused a fall in blood pressure despite pretreatment with large intravenous doses of propranolol plus phentolamine. Labetalol also caused relaxation of barium contracted rabbit portal vein strips in the presence of phentolamine and propranolol.[17]

Dage and Hsieh showed in anesthetized dogs that intraarterial labetalol caused a dose-related direct vasodilation of resistance blood vessels similar to that seen with hydralazine.[18] Again, these effects were observed despite the presence of propranolol and phentolamine.

Later experiments by Baum and Sybertz have confirmed the accuracy of these observations, and, in addition, have shown that the dilator effect of labetalol may be mediated by activation of vascular β_2-adrenoceptors. Using anesthetized dogs, acute intraarterial labetalol infusions were shown to cause a dose-related increase in femoral blood flow in the

dog hind limb. These effects on the femoral blood flow were also seen
after phentolamine and prazosin injections; however, the effects of these
latter two agents were eliminated following acute sympathetic denervation. In contrast, labetalol's effect on peripheral blood flow was even
greater in denervated limbs (Fig. 3).[13,39] This effect was abolished by the
administration of intravenous propranolol, suggesting again a β_2-
mediated mechanism may be contributing to the direct vasodilator effect
(Fig. 4).[13,39]

Hemodynamic Effects in Normotensive Animals. The hemodynamic effects
of labetalol are attributed to its adrenergic receptor blocking activity and
direct vasodilator effects.[5,7,11,13,39] The observed responses to labetalol,

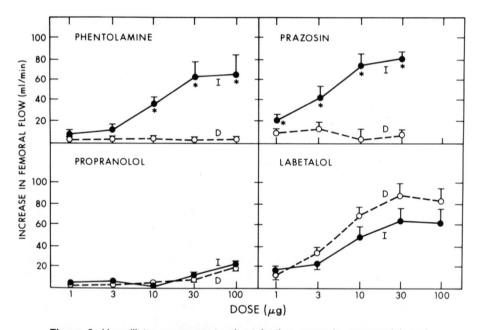

Figure 3. Vasodilator responses to phentolamine, prazosin, propranolol, and
labetalol in the dog hind limb. Test drugs were administered intraarterially via a
cannulated branch of the femoral artery at intervals of 10 to 30 minutes in intact
and acutely sympathetically denervated limbs (5 to 7 pentobarbital-anesthetized
dogs per group). I: innervated limb. D: denervated limb. Baseline blood flows
ranged from 39 ± 8 to 63 ± 12 ml/min in innervated limbs and from 88 ± 10 to
126 ± 24 in denervated limbs. An asterisk indicates that increases in femoral
blood flow are significantly different in innervated and denervated preparations.
[Reprinted from Baum TS, Sybertz EJ: Am J Med (Suppl):75(4A): 19, 1983, with
permission.[13]]

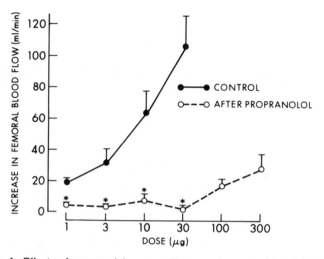

Figure 4. Effects of propranolol on vasodilator responses to labetalol in dener-vated limbs of anesthetized dogs. Labetalol was administered intraarterially be-fore and after intravenous propranolol (0.3 mg/kg followed by infusion of 0.1 mg/kg/hr). Baseline flow averaged 136 ± 31 ml/min before propranolol and 99 ± 17 afterwards (4 dogs). An asterisk indicates that response after propranolol is sig-nificantly different from that beforehand ($p<0.05$). [Reprinted from Baum TS, Sy-bertz EJ: Am J Med (Suppl):75(4A): 20, 1983, with permission.[13]]

especially the heart rate response, vary according to the experimental situation and autonomic nervous system influences. In barbital-anesthe-tized dogs with high sympathetic tone and low vagal tone, labetalol, like propranolol, reduced the heart rate, cardiac contractility, cardiac out-put, and work-effects, all of which are attributable to β-adrenergic blockade.[11] In contrast to propranolol, however, labetalol reduced total peripheral vascular resistance and produced larger decrements in blood pressure at equipotent β_1-blocking doses.[11] These differences between propranolol and labetalol were attributed to the peripheral vasodilator effects of labetalol. In conscious normotensive dogs, where sympathetic tone is low and vagal tone high, labetalol caused prolonged falls in blood pressure and increased heart rate. The increase in heart rate was attrib-uted to reflex withdrawal of vagal inhibition, in response to the fall in blood pressure.[11] In intact normotensive anesthetized dogs with normal levels of sympathetic tone, intravenous labetalol caused a fall in blood pressure and a decrease in peripheral vascular resistance.[39,40]

Antihypertensive Effects in Hypertensive Animals. In conscious dogs with renal hypertension, oral labetalol caused dose-dependent falls in systolic blood pressure. Heart rate was either unchanged or increased slightly, usually in animals with low initial heart rates. The increase in heart rate was attributed to a reflex response to peripheral vasodilation.[28] Propranolol, however, did not lower systolic blood pressure in this animal model despite a marked decrease in heart rate. Thus, the antihypertensive effect of labetalol did not appear to be related to a β-adrenoceptor blocking action.

In the DOCA (deoxycorticosterone-salted) hypertensive rat, labetalol caused a dose-dependent fall in systolic blood pressure but had little effect on heart rate. The antihypertensive effect of labetalol was evident only at doses producing significant α-adrenoceptor blockade.[41] Thus, in hypertensive animals, labetalol's effect probably results from vasodilation mediated by its α-adrenoceptor blocking action and/or partial β₂-agonist activity.

Hemodynamic Effects in Humans (Table 2). Traditional β-adrenergic blocking drugs such as propranolol cause a decrease in heart rate and cardiac output, a widening of arteriovenous oxygen difference, and an increase in total systemic vascular resistance, which prevents lowering of blood pressure after acute intravenous or oral administration. Left ventricular filling pressures and stroke volume remain unchanged or become slightly elevated. With chronic administration, the total peripheral vascular resistance tends to regress towards pretreatment levels and blood pressure falls.[42]

Table 3 summarizes a number of studies examining the hemody-

TABLE 2. COMPARATIVE EFFECTS ON HEMODYNAMIC VARIABLES AND IN PLASMA RENIN ACTIVITY USUALLY OCCURRING DURING TREATMENT WITH β-ADRENOCEPTOR ANTAGONISTS, α-ADRENOCEPTOR ANTAGONISTS, AND α-β-ADRENOCEPTOR BLOCKERS[42]

	β-Adrenoceptor Blockade (Propranolol)	α-Adrenoceptor Blockade (Prazosin)	α-β-Adrenoceptor Blockade (Labetalol)
Heart rate	↓	↔ ↑	↔ ↓
Cardiac output	↓	↔ ↑	↔
Stroke volume	↔ ↑	↔ ↑	↔ ↑
Systemic vascular resistance	↔ ↑	↓	↓
Arteriovenous oxygen difference	↑	↔ ↓	↔ ↑
Left ventricular filling pressure	↑	↓	↔
Plasma renin activity (PRA)	↓	↔ ↑	↓

↔ Unchanged
↑ Increased
↓ Decreased

TABLE 3. HEMODYNAMIC EFFECTS OF INTRAVENOUS LABETALOL IN HYPERTENSIVE PATIENTS

Author	# Pts.	Labetalol Dose		BP*	HR	CO	SV	SVR
Prichard et al. (1975)[47]	12	0.5 mg/kg	Supine	↓	≈	≈	≈	↓
Joekes et al. (1976)[44]	14	0.5–1 mg/kg	Supine	↓	≈	≈	≈	↓
Koch (1979)[45]	13	50 mg	Supine	↓	≈	≈	≈	≈
			Upright	↓	↓	↓	≈	↓
			Exercise	↓	↓	↓	↑	↓
Bahlmann et al. (1979)[48]	9	0.6–1.6 mg/kg	Supine	↓	≈	≈	≈	↓
Svendsen et al. (1980)[46]	10	50 mg	Supine	↓	≈	≈	≈	↓
			Upright	↓	↓	≈	≈	↓
			Exercise	↓	↓	≈	≈	≈
Trap-Jensen et al. (1980)[49]	8	0.75 mg/kg	Supine	↓	≈	≈	NR	↓
			Psychic Stress	↓	↓	↑	NR	≈
Agabiti-Rosei et al. (1982)[43]	18	100 mg	Supine	↓	↓	≈	≈	↓
Omvik, Lund-Johansen (1982)[50]	11	0.2–0.8 mg/kg	Supine	↓	↓	↓	≈	↓

Modified from MacCarthy EP, Bloomfield SS: Labetalol: A review of its pharmacology, pharmacokinetic clinical uses, and adverse effects. Pharmacotherapy 3(4):193, 1983

*BP = blood pressure; HR = heart rate; CO = cardiac output; SV = stroke volume; SVR = systemic vascular resistance. ↓ = significant reduction; ↑ = significant increase; ≈ = no significant change; NR = not reported namic effects of acute intravenous administration of labetalol.[43–50] Unlike the responses seen with β-blockers, blood pressure and peripheral vascular resistance fall after acute intravenous administration of labetalol. Cardiac output and stroke volume are usually not affected. Heart rate is either unchanged or decreases slightly. Falls in cardiac output are due entirely to decreases in heart rate when it occurs. Heart rate usually falls in the standing position, and increases are blunted during exercise. This hemodynamic profile is similar to that seen with the combination of intravenous propranolol and hydralazine or prazosin.[47,51]

Antihypertensive Effects in Humans. The effects of oral labetalol in hypertensive patients have been studied for periods of from 1 week to 6 years.[36,45,46,51–54] These investigations are summarized in Table 4. After chronic dosing (range 300 to 2400 mg daily), heart rate in the supine and

TABLE 4. HEMODYNAMIC EFFECTS OF ORAL LABETALOL IN HYPERTENSIVE PATIENTS

Author	Duration (wk)	# Pts.	Max. Dose (g/day)		BP*	HR	CO	SV	SVR	PVR
Edwards et al. (1976)[52]	4	11	0.8	Supine	↓	↓	≃	↑	≃	NR
				Exercise	↓	↓	↓	≃	≃	NR
Mehta et al. (1977)[36]	1	6	1.6	Supine	↓	↓	≃	NR	↓	NR
				Upright	↓	↓	≃	NR	↓	NR
				Exercise	↓	↓	NR	NR	NR	NR
Fagard et al. (1979)[53]	2.5	18	0.3–2.4	Supine	↓	↓	↓	≃	≃	≃
				Upright	↓	↓	↓	≃	↓	≃
				Exercise	↓	↓	↓	↑	↓	≃
Lund-Johansen et al. (1979)[51]	52	14	0.2–0.8	Supine	↓	↓	≃	↑	↓	NR
				Upright	↓	↓	↓	≃	≃	NR
				Exercise	↓	↓	↓	↑	↓	NR
Koch (1979)[45]	85	9	0.6–2.4	Supine	↓	↓	≃	↑	↓	↓
				Upright	↓	↓	≃	↑	↓	≃
				Exercise	↓	↓	≃	↑	↓	↑
Svendsen et al. (1980)[46]	13	8	0.6–0.9	Supine	↓	↓	≃	↑	↓	≃
				Upright	↓	↓	≃	≃	↓	NR
				Exercise	↓	↓	↓	≃	≃	↑
Lund-Johansen (1983)[54]	6 yr.	15	0.2–0.8	Supine	↓	↓	≃	≃	↓	NR
				Upright	↓	↓	≃	≃	↓	NR
				Exercise	↓	↓	≃	≃	↓	NR

Modified from Prichard EP, SS Bloomfield, Labetalol: A review of its pharmacology, pharmacokinetic clinical uses and adverse effects, Pharmacotherapy 3(4):193, 1983
*BP = blood pressure; HR = heart rate; CO = cardiac output; SV = stroke volume; SVR = systemic vascular resistance; PVR = pulmonary vascular resistance; ↑ = significant increase; ↓ = significant reduction; ≃ = no significant change; NR = not reported; max = maximal.

standing positions was lowered and blood pressure remained reduced. In the two longest hemodynamic follow-up studies, Koch after 20 months and Lund-Johansen after 6 years showed that stroke volume in the supine and standing positions had risen to compensate for the decreased heart rate, thus returning cardiac index towards normal. Peripheral vascular resistance had fallen further with chronic dosing[45]; cardiac index was not significantly affected. During exercise, increases in heart rate were reduced and exercise-induced blood pressure increases blunted (see Fig. 5).[54] This decrement in the double-product may provide a favorable hemodynamic profile for hypertensive patients with coronary artery disease.[4]

The effects of labetalol on the pulmonary circulation have been studied both at rest and during exercise. After intravenous administra-

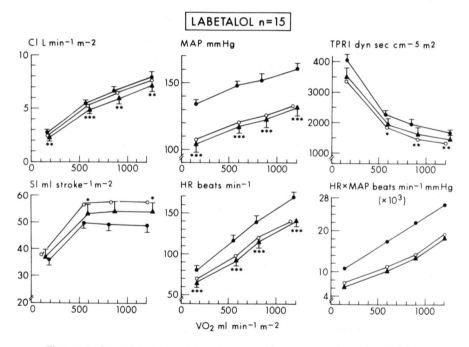

Figure 5. Central hemodynamics at rest and during exercise before therapy (solid circle), after 1 year (solid triangle), and after 6 years (open circle) on labetalol therapy (200 to 800 mg/day). Mean values and SEM (at first and second study). VO_2 = oxygen consumption; CI = cardiac index; MAP = mean arterial pressure; TPRI = total peripheral vascular resistance index; SI = stroke index; HR = heart rate. An asterisk indicates level of statistical significance between first and second study. $* = p < 0.05$, $** = p < 0.01$, $*** = p < 0.001$. [Reprinted from Lund-Johansen P: Am J Med (Suppl):75(4A): 28, 1983, with permission.[54]]

tion of labetalol, pulmonary artery pressures at rest decreased in both the supine and standing positions, but no effect on pulmonary artery pressures during exercise was observed.[45] After oral administration, pulmonary vascular resistance in the sitting position was unaffected and pulmonary artery pressure and wedge pressure were reduced.[55] Central blood volume has been observed to be reduced after intravenous labetalol.[56]

When labetalol was administered to patients with coronary artery disease and stable angina pectoris, heart rate, mean arterial pressure, pressure–rate product, and pulmonary vascular resistance all fell. No significant change in cardiac output or pulmonary wedge pressures were noted. Coronary sinus blood flow increased significantly (Table 5).[57] In a randomized study on patients with angiographically proven coronary artery disease, propranolol induced significantly greater depression of left ventricular function both at rest and during exercise than did labetalol.[58] This difference was attributed to labetalol's vasodilatory activity and the concomitant afterload reduction caused by the drug.

The effect of chronic oral labetalol therapy on cerebral blood flow has also been studied. Labetalol and a number of β-adrenoceptor blocking drugs did not reduce cerebral blood flow despite significant reductions in blood pressure with these treatments.[59]

Effects on Renin–Angiotensin–Aldosterone System. Chronic oral administration of labetalol in doses ranging from 150 to 2400 mg daily has been reported to produce decrements in both supine and upright plasma renin activity in a number of clinical studies (see Chapter 11).[60-64] In most of these studies, the net renin-suppressive effect was evident even at low doses of labetalol and was proportional to basal renin values. The increase in plasma renin activity that occurs with exercise was also suppressed by oral labetalol therapy.[61] Significant reductions in plasma angiotensin II concentration, especially in patients with high basal values, have been reported following acute intravenous administration of labe-

TABLE 5. HEMODYNAMIC EFFECTS OF INTRAVENOUS LABETALOL IN PATIENTS WITH CORONARY ARTERY DISEASE[57]

BP	HR	MPAP	W	CO	SVR	PVR	CSF	CVR
↓	↓	↓	≃	≃	↓	↓	↑	↓

* = supine position; BP = blood pressure; HR = heart rate; MPAP = mean pulmonary arterial pressure; W = mean pulmonary wedge pressure; CO = cardiac output; SVR = systemic vascular resistance; PVR = pulmonary vascular resistance; CSF = coronary sinus flow; CVR = coronary vascular resistance; ↑ = significant increase; ↓ = significant reduction; ≃ = no significant change.

talol.[65-67] Likewise, Lijnen and associates[61] found a significant decrement in plasma aldosterone concentration with oral labetalol, as did Trust and colleagues[65] after intravenous administration of the drug. Urinary aldosterone excretion has also been reported to be suppressed by oral labetalol therapy.[63]

In contrast to these findings, a number of investigators have been unable to show an influence of oral labetolol administration on the renin–angiotensin–aldosterone system. Several studies, for instance, failed to demonstrate a significant effect of oral labetalol on supine plasma renin activity.[36,68-70] Louis and colleagues administered the labetalol intravenously and still found no significant effect on supine plasma renin activity.[68] Other studies have failed to produce a significant change in plasma aldosterone concentration.[62,67]

Effects on Plasma and Urinary Catecholamines. A recently identified metabolite of labetalol interferes with the fluorometric assay for catecholamines and the photometric assay for metanephrine, giving falsely high values for these substances in some patients during labetalol therapy.[71] Caution, therefore, must be exercised in interpreting apparently elevated levels of plasma catecholamines during labetalol therapy. Since fluorometric methods may lead to false-positive findings, it has been recommended that either urinary vanillylmandelic acid (VMA) or urinary 4-hydroxy-3-methoxymandelic acid (HMMA) be measured when screening for pheochromocytoma in patients who are being treated with labetalol.[72,73]

When highly specific methods for catecholamine estimation such as high-pressure liquid chromatographic or radioenzymatic techniques are employed, chronic oral treatment with labetalol does not appear to increase plasma or urinary norepinephrine or epinephrine levels.[61,72-75]

Antiarrhythmic Action

Experimental Systems. Farmer et al. demonstrated that intravenous labetalol eliminated both catecholamine and ouabain-induced arrhythmias in barbitone-anesthesized dogs.[2] Labetalol exhibits weak membrane-stabilizing activity, a property it shares with some other β-blocker drugs; propranolol has much more membrane-stabilizing activity.[76]

Vaughan Williams et al. reported on the electrophysiologic effects of labetalol on rabbit atrial, ventricular, and Purkinje cells under normal and hypoxic conditions.[77] Labetalol was shown to possess substantial Class I antiarrhythmic activity on atrial and ventricular tissues. A significant slowing of all phases of repolarization in normal ventricular tissue was also observed (Class III antiarrhythmic activity). In addition, the drug demonstrated no negative inotropic activity, and there was no slowing of the atrioventricular conduction time. These findings contrast somewhat from those made by Ambie, who demonstrated in anesthetized dogs that labetalol caused the functional refractory period of the atria, atrioventricular node, and ventricles to increase.[78]

More recent studies in the chloralose-anesthetized cat and isolated rat heart have demonstrated that labetalol reduced the number of premature contractions and the incidence of ventricular fibrillation induced by coronary artery occlusion and reperfusion.[79,80] In the treated rat hearts, the levels of high-energy phosphate were significantly higher and lactate, adenosine, and hypoxanthine levels were significantly lower in the ischemic myocardium when compared to control hearts.[80] These studies suggest that labetalol may prove to be an effective agent in the prevention and treatment of ventricular dysrhythmias associated with acute myocardial ischemia.

Electrophysiologic and Antiarrhythmic Effects in Humans. The effects of intravenous labetalol on human cardiac electrophysiology were studied using His bundle electrocardiography in 12 patients who had normal left ventricular function and no clinical or electrocardiographic evidence for significant conduction system disease.[81] Generally, labetalol appears to have less effect on either the SA node or the AV node than propranolol, atenolol, or acebutolol.[82–84] Labetalol has inconsistent effects on AV nodal refractoriness, but slightly prolongs the AV nodal conduction time and atrial effective refractory period, with only small changes in heart rate. No effects on the His Purkinje system have been noted. The effects on sinus cycle length and sinoatrial conduction time are small and variable.[81] Clinically, labetalol appears less likely than conventional β-blockers to produce pathologic bradycardia or heart block. It remains to be seen whether the electrophysiologic effects of labetalol are modified in patients with myocardial ischemia and/or with conduction system disease.

A recent clinical study confirmed an antiarrhythmic effect of labetalol in ten patients with essential hypertension and frequent premature ventricular contractions (PVCs). Labetalol (800 mg daily) significantly lowered blood pressure and produced a significant reduction in PVCs after 2 weeks of oral therapy, with nearly complete extinction of PVCs at the end of the fourth week of treatment.[85] There is also a report demonstrating that intravenous labetalol was successful in restoring sinus rhythm in approximately 80 percent of patients with severe hypertension and a variety of dysrhythmias.[86]

Other Clinical Effects

The effects of intravenous labetolol on a number of other metabolic functions have been studied in hypertensive patients.[87] A number of these effects are discussed in this section.

Plasma Glucose. Plasma glucose was shown to rise significantly following labetalol administration, while no changes were observed in serum free fatty acids, insulin, C-peptide, and growth hormone levels. Trap-Jensen and coworkers also reported a significant increase in plasma glucose concentration following intravenous labetalol, which they attributed to a possible increase in glycogenolysis from the β_2-adrenoceptor agonist action of labetalol.[88] Oral administration of labetalol 300 to 1200 mg/daily to hypertensive males for 4 weeks was reported to produce a small increase in mean fasting blood glucose level, but no alteration in insulin activity or response to an oral glucose tolerance test.[89]

No clinically significant effects on blood glucose levels have been reported in either normal or noninsulin-requiring diabetics with chronic oral labetalol administration, either in clinical practice or in long-term trials.

The effects of labetalol on plasma lipids have been evaluated by multiple investigators, with no adverse effects on lipids being seen.[90–93] Frishman and colleagues performed a double-blind randomized placebo-controlled study comparing the efficacies of labetalol and metoprolol in 70 hypertensive patients.[93] After 4 months of therapy with labetalol (300 to 1200 mg/daily), there were no significant alterations in plasma cholesterol, triglyceride, HDL-cholesterol, LDL-cholesterol, or the HDL/total cholesterol ratio (see Chapter 13). Thus, long-term administration of labetalol appears to have no unfavorable effects on plasma lipid levels.

Respiratory Function. Due to its nonselective β-adrenoceptor blocking activity, labetalol might be expected to have an adverse effect on respiratory function in patients with chronic obstructive pulmonary disease. α-Adrenoceptor antagonists, however, may have a bronchodilating action of their own, and have been shown to enhance the bronchodilator actions of isoproterenol and salbutamol.[94,95] It is therefore conceivable that the α-adrenoceptor blocking property of labetalol or its mild β_2-agonist activity could mitigate some of the possible adverse effects on bronchial tone caused by its β-adrenoceptor blocking action.

In healthy human volunteers treated with propranolol, forced expiratory volume in 1 second (FEV_1) was reduced and the fall in FEV_1 induced by inhalation of histamine was enhanced. Postexercise peak expiratory flow rates were also observed to decline after propranolol administration. These effects on respiratory function were not observed after labetalol administration.[96,97]

In asthmatic patients given equipotent β-blocking doses, resting FEV_1 was reduced significantly after administration of intravenous propranolol (5 mg), but there were no significant changes noted after intravenous labetalol (20 mg) or placebo. In this same study, there was no difference in the response to inhaled salbutamol with either propranolol or labetalol.[98,99] Recent studies have demonstrated no deleterious effect on midexpiratory flow rates, FEV_1, or forced vital capacity (FVC) when oral doses of labetalol, up to 1200 mg daily, were used in patients with chronic obstructive pulmonary disease.[100–102] Adam et al. demonstrated that propranolol was the only medication that significantly affected respiratory function in hypertensive patients with chronic obstructive pulmonary disease when compared to labetalol, atenolol, and metoprolol.[103]

Labetalol has, however, been reported to cause bronchospasm.[104] When labetalol, 200 mg orally twice daily for 6 weeks, was compared to verapamil in patients with chronic obstructive airways disease, labetalol before and after albuterol administration caused a statistically significant decrease in FEV_1 and FVC. Only one of nine patients, however, showed subjective worsening.[105] When the effects of atenolol (100 mg) were compared to labetalol (300 mg) in patients with hypertension and asthma, no significant differences in FEV_1 were noted between the two drugs. Both medications, however, did cause a fall in FEV_1 from baseline, and labetalol significantly reduced the expected beneficial effect of inhaled salbutamol on FEV_1.[106]

Thus, despite the majority of studies that demonstrate no clinically significant deterioration in respiratory status after labetalol administration, bronchospasm can be induced by this drug, although less frequently than with propranolol. It is still prudent to avoid this medication in patients with clinically overt bronchospasm. Labetalol should be used with the same caution as the $β_1$-selective adrenoceptor blocking drugs.

Body Fluid Volumes and Renal Function. Findings to date are mixed. Weidmann et al. observed that labetalol, given alone in increasing doses during a 6-week period, produced increments in body weight, plasma volume, and blood volume of 1.7, 21, and 17 percent, respectively.[62] These results were confirmed in another study where an increase in plasma volume (mean 294 ml) was found after 8 weeks of labetalol monotherapy (average daily dose 585 mg) in 13 patients with essential hypertension.[107] In the same study, propranolol monotherapy failed to increase plasma volume. Other studies have not confirmed these observations. In a large long-term study of 337 hypertensive patients, Michelson and colleagues could not demonstrate any major changes in body weight or fluid accumulation with chronic labetalol therapy.[108] In another study, a 4- to 15-week course of labetalol monotherapy (300 to 1200 mg/day) was shown to produce insignificant increases in plasma volume and extracellular fluid volume in 12 patients with essential hypertension.[109] Thus, it is possible that fluid retention may occur with labetalol monotherapy, and that the addition of diuretic agents could be considered in the event of an inadequate blood pressure response with the drug.

A number of investigations have shown that the short- or long-term administration of labetalol to patients with essential hypertension is not associated with a reduction in glomerular filtration rate or renal plasma flow.[44,110-115] Three groups found no substantial alterations in glomerular filtration rate, renal plasma flow, filtration fraction or free-water clearance, after short- and long-term labetalol therapy with patients receiving up to 2400 mg labetalol daily.[110,112,113] One group reported glomerular filtration rate actually increased during labetalol therapy.[116] This is in contrast to reports of diminished renal plasma flow and glomerular filtration rate during treatment observed with many pure β-blockers.[112,117] It thus appears that the concomitant α-blockade of labetalol plays an important role in preventing deleterious alterations in renal hemodynamics. Labetalol has been used successfully in patients with chronic renal failure and hypertension, and the drug has not been implicated in producing a deterioration in renal function in such patients.[111,114,118,119]

PHARMACODYNAMIC PROPERTIES

Following oral administration of labetalol to normal subjects or patients with hypertension, a hypotensive response is seen within 2 hours and is maximal within 3 hours.[38,120,121] Richards demonstrated that the fall in blood pressure was dose-related and that the effect after a single 400-mg oral dose was still apparent 8 hours later. Continuous intraarterial blood pressure monitoring in patients receiving chronic labetalol orally three times daily showed that labetalol achieved smooth blood pressure control over a 24-hour period, and that there was no increase in blood pressure during the dosing interval.[122,123] Recent reports have shown that labetalol is equally effective when administered twice daily in controlling blood pressure over a 24-hour period.[124-126] Breckenridge et al. found that labetalol could be administered once daily: however, side effects associated with the large single dose (greater than 1 g) required would possibly limit its effectiveness, so that twice daily administration was an acceptable compromise.[127] Wilcox, however, found that a single dose of labetalol was not effective at lowering blood pressure over a 24-hour period.[128]

Richards et al. showed in normotensive healthy men a significant drop in supine systolic and diastolic blood pressure within 3 minutes, using an intravenous labetalol dose of 1.5 mg/kg.[30] In hypertensive patients, multiple studies have shown a significant fall in supine systolic and diastolic blood pressures within 5 minutes after bolus dose intravenous administration of 1 to 2 mg/kg labetalol.[43,65,66,129-131] This was followed by a prolonged (up to 6 hours) reduction in blood pressure. Using an intravenous infusion of 0.5 to 1 mg/kg of labetalol over 10 to 20 minutes, Joekes and Thompson reported a maximum hypotensive effect between 20 to 40 minutes after cessation of the infusion. The hypotensive effect lasted on the average of 3 hours.[44]

Richards et al. also showed that there was a clear relationship between the dose of labetalol administered and the plasma concentration achieved.[30] Other investigators have also confirmed this result.[126,132] Richards et al. showed that there was a linear correlation between the plasma labetalol concentration 2 hours after oral drug administration and the degree of inhibition of exercise tachycardia, and inhibition of exercise systolic blood pressure.[38] Sanders et al. found no correlation between steady-state labetalol concentrations and anithypertensive response; however, in 13 of 16 patients, there appeared to be a significant correlation between steady-state labetalol concentrations and β-blockade.[132] In a recent study, a close correlation was found between log plasma levels of free and conjugated labetalol and its effect on mean blood pressure decline. Wide interpatient variation limits the predictive value of labetalol plasma levels with respect to expected blood pressure lowering effects.[126] In another study in which 12 moderately hypertensive patients received doses of labetalol ranging from 100 to 600 mg every 12 hours, log–linear relationships were shown between dose and mean arterial blood pressure, and also area under the plasma concentration time curve and mean arterial blood pressure.[133] In the study by McNeil et al., patients with lower steady-state levels on a fixed dose of labetalol usually required higher maintenance doses to control blood pressure.[134]

PHARMACOKINETIC PROPERTIES

The pharmacokinetic properties of labetalol are summarized in Chapter 2.

The absorption, distribution, and metabolism of labetalol has been extensively studied in rats, rabbits, dogs, and humans. Using radioactively labeled [^{14}C] labetalol, it has been shown that after a large oral dose, radioactivity is quickly taken up by the tissues and rapidly cleared from the body via the kidneys and bile. After oral tritiated labetalol, 60 percent of the radioactivity is recovered in the urine, and 40 percent in the feces. Plasma levels of radioactivity show that labetalol is rapidly and almost completely absorbed after oral administration.[135]

In hypertensive patients, following administration of labetalol by mouth, peak plasma concentrations of the drug occurred 20 to 60 minutes after a 100mg dose, and 40 to 90 minutes after a 200-mg dose.[136] Labetalol undergoes extensive first-pass metabolism with a large proportion of the drug being converted to inactive metabolites by the gut wall and liver; a 1 mg/kg intravenous dose of labetalol is less extensively metabolized than a similar oral dose.[135] In humans, the major metabolite of labetalol is an alcoholic glucuronide of the secondary alcohol group, whose formation is catalyzed by UDP glucuronyl transferase. Smaller proportions of the N-glucuronide and o-phenyl glucuronide of labetalol are also produced. Only 3 percent of the drug is excreted unchanged in the urine.[22,135] There are no active metabolites of the drug.

Food ingestion appears to increase the bioavailability of orally administered drug by as much as 38 percent.[137,138] The bioavailability of labetalol is also increased by concomitant cimetidine administration.[139] The high plasma clearance of the drug probably reflects its extensive hepatic degradation since plasma clearance approaches hepatic blood flow.[140] In individuals with significant hepatic dysfunction, dosages should therefore by adjusted.[141] The large volume of distribution of labetalol (9.4 L/kg) reflects the extensive tissue uptake of the drug.[135] In humans, only 50 percent of labetalol in plasma is protein bound.[135] No adjustment of dosage is necessary in patients in renal failure.[118,140,142] Data on the dialyzability of labetalol are not available as yet. In elderly subjects, there is a significant increase in both the bioavailability and elimination half-life of labetalol.[143]

Labetalol is much less lipid soluble than propranolol. The partition coefficient of labetalol between chloroform and pH 7.4 buffer is 1.2 as compared to 9 for propranolol and 10 for oxprenolol.[135] Studies using tritiated labetalol in the rat and dog have shown that negligible amounts enter the brain.[135] Like the passage across the blood–brain barrier, passage of a drug across the placental barrier is dependent on lipid solubility. After oral administration of radioactively labeled [^{14}C] labetalol to pregnant rats and rabbits, little radioactivity was found to cross the placental barrier.[135] Levels of labetalol in cord blood from the human fetus at delivery have revealed that the levels were well below the therapeutic plasma levels found in the mother, except at extremely high daily dosages.[143] Fetal bradycardia has not been observed with maternal labetalol treatment. Labetalol is found in breast milk at much lower concentrations than the mean maternal plasma drug levels.

Original estimates of the plasma terminal elimination half-life for labetalol was 4 ± 0.5 hours.[136] High-precision liquid chromatographic techniques are now available for measuring labetalol concentrations in plasma.[144,145] Using these methods, it has been found that the pharmacokinetic data best fit a two-compartment pharmacokinetic model with first-order absorption. The true terminal elimination half-life of the drug is closer to 6 hours (5.5 to 8 hours) with these new assay techniques.[126] The absolute bioavailability of labetalol has been found to be 25 percent due to its first-pass metabolism in the liver.

CLINICAL USES

Essential Hypertension

Labetalol, in both fixed and individually titrated doses, has been used abroad since 1975 for the management of mild, moderate, and severe hypertension.[127,146–148] A number of investigators using labetalol have reported the drug to be at least as effective in lowering blood pressure as a wide range of other antihypertensive drugs. Labetalol administered alone, or with a diuretic, is often effective in lowering blood pressure when other regimens, including β-blockers, have failed.[149,150]

In addition, a majority of studies comparing labetalol to placebo have shown a significant antihypertensive effect of labetalol when compared with placebo (Fig. 6).[27,69,151,152] Most comparative studies comparing labetalol to diuretics in management of hypertension have shown labetalol to be equivalent or superior to thiazide diuretics.[64,153] The addition of labetalol to a diuretic regimen produces a further dose related fall in blood pressure (Fig. 7).[154,157] Michelson et al. recently demonstrated the long-term antihypertensive effectiveness of labetalol, used alone or in combination with a diuretic in patients with mild, moderate, and severe hypertension (see Chapter 14).[108]

A number of studies have compared labetalol to other β-adrenoceptor blockers in the treatment of hypertension.[107,158–166] In 18 previously untreated patients with severe hypertension, labetalol and propranolol produced similar decreases in supine blood pressure, but labetalol produced a greater decrease in standing blood pressure and less bradycardia.[165] In a randomized crossover study in 24 hypertensive patients who were receiving thiazide diuretic therapy, the antihypertensive effects of labetalol (maximum dose 2400 mg/day) and propranolol (maximum dose

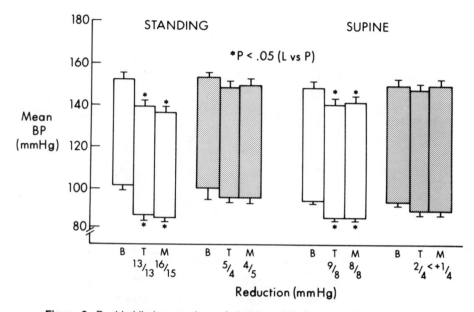

Figure 6. Double-blind comparison of placebo to labetalol in patients with mild hypertension. The figure shows standing and supine systolic/diastolic blood pressure and the mean ± SEM reductions from baseline (B) to the end of labetalol titration (T) 200 to 1200 mg, and to the monotherapy end point (M) for the labetalol (open) n = 38 and placebo (shaded) n = 36 treatment groups. L = labetalol; P = placebo. [Reprinted from Davidov ME, et al: Am J Med (Suppl):75(4A): 50, 1983, with permission.[151]]

960 mg/day) were comparable, but labetalol was associated with a greater incidence of side effects. A study using smaller doses found that the antihypertensive effect of labetalol (average daily dose 585 mg) was greater than that of propranolol (average daily dose 234 mg).[107]

Labetalol and pindolol have demonstrated similar efficacy in blood pressure control and a similar incidence of side effects in comparative studies.[160,164] A variable dose, comparative trial of atenolol, pindolol, labetalol, and metoprolol demonstrated that all four drugs provide similar blood pressure control.[159] Reported side effects were similar, but numerically less with labetalol than atenolol or pindolol. Frishman and colleagues, compared labetalol (mean dose 995 mg) to metoprolol (mean dose 342 mg) in patients with mild-moderate systemic hypertension (see Chapter 14).[163] Both drugs were equally effective in reducing supine and standing blood pressure. However, metoprolol caused a greater reduction in resting heart rate. The foregoing comparative studies indicate

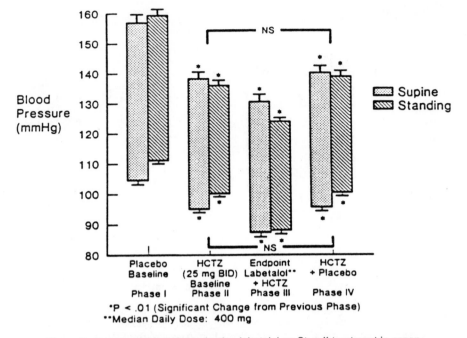

Figure 7. Double-blind study evaluating labetalol as Step II treatment in essential hypertension. Mean ± SEM supine and standing blood pressure at the end of each phase of a four-phase study comparing placebo treatment (4 weeks), hydrochlorothiazide (HCTZ 4 weeks) plus labetalol (4 weeks), and HCTZ plus placebo (2 weeks). [Reprinted from Bloomfield S, et al: Am J Med (Suppl):75(4A): 84, 1983, with permission.[157]]

that labetalol is at least as effective an antihypertensive agent as pure β-adrenoceptor blocking drugs.

Other studies have compared labetalol monotherapy to the combination of β-adrenoceptor blockers plus direct-acting vasodilators. A double-blind comparative study found that labetalol 600 mg twice daily was approximately equivalent to the combination of pindolol 15 mg twice daily plus hydralazine 150 mg daily in mild to moderately severe hypertensive patients.[167] In a fixed-dose randomized study, labetalol 600 mg daily was as effective as propranolol 160 mg daily plus hydralazine 100 mg daily in lowering standing blood pressure; however, the drug combination reduced supine blood pressure more effectively.[168] In a randomized crossover trial, labetalol plus hydrochlorothiazide was found to be as effective as the combination of propranolol, hydralazine, and hydrocholorothiazide.[169] In two other studies, labetalol was equivalent to the combination of β-adrenoceptor blockers plus dihydralazine in reducing standing blood pressure. However, the combination drug treatment was shown to be more effective in reducing supine blood pressure.[170,171]

Labetalol has compared favorably with various combinations of pure α- and β-adrenoceptor blocking drugs in controlled studies. In one such study, labetalol produced significantly greater reductions in both supine and standing blood pressure than the combination of oxprenolol and phentolamine.[172] In another study of 31 hypertensive patients, labetalol alone appeared to be as effective as a previously used combination of different β-adrenoceptor blocking drugs and the α-adrenoceptor blocker prazosin in lowering blood pressure.[173]

As an antihypertensive agent, labetalol has also been shown to be at least as effective as methyldopa, a methyldopa–diuretic combination, clonidine, various adrenergic neuronal blockers, and the calcium-channel blocker verapamil. Prichard and Boakes compared labetalol to methyldopa and to the sympathetic inhibitory drugs bethanidine, debrisoquine, and guanethidine. They found labetalol to be similar.[158] Dargie and colleagues obtained satisfactory clinical results when they substituted labetalol for methyldopa, clonidine and adrenergic neuronal blockers in patients with severe resistant hypertension.[149] Wallin et al. observed that labetalol 200 to 2400 mg/day with or without furosemide was as effective as a methyldopa (500 to 2000 mg/day)–furosemide combination in a large, parallel-design, dose-titration study.[174] In a randomized dose titration study, it was reported that labetalol 1200 to 1800 mg/daily was more effective than the adrenergic neuronal blocker bethanidine 30 to 45 mg/daily at lowering blood pressure in the supine, sitting, and standing positions and after exercise.[175] A variable-dose crossover trial comparing placebo, labetalol, and methyldopa in 20 patients using a maximum dose of 1000 mg three times daily of each active drug demonstrated similar antihypertensive results and incidence of adverse effects.[176] In a randomized crossover study comparing labetalol to clonidine in 17 patients being treated with a thiazide diuretic, doses of each agent were titrated until normotension or intolerable side effects occurred.[177] At mean daily doses of 476-mg labetalol and 0.355-mg clonidine, 12 patients complained of tiredness and dry mouth during clonidine therapy; two patients had unsteadiness, one a rash, and one limb weakness during labetalol administration. In a double-blind comparative study of labetalol and the calcium-entry blocker verapamil, labetalol 200 mg twice daily was similar to verapamil 160 mg twice daily in reducing blood pressure.[105]

Initial studies in black hypertensive patients appeared to demonstrate no response to labetalol when doses up to 3200 mg daily were employed.[178] These results, however, may reflect an element of noncompliance. Recent studies show that labetalol is equally effective as a monotherapy in the black, white, and Indian population.[179-181] In a recent study comparing oral labetalol to the β-blocker propranolol in hypertensive patients, the addition of a diuretic was frequently necessary in black patients treated with propranolol to attain adequate blood pressure control, as compared to labetalol where monotherapy was often effective.[181]

These studies indicate that labetalol, when administered alone or in combination with diuretics and vasodilators, is as effective an antihypertensive agent as are most other currently available antihypertensive drugs.[155,156,177] Tolerance to the antihypertensive actions of labetalol does not seem to develop during prolonged administration up to 6 years.[54,182,183]

Hypertensive Emergencies

Because of its α-adrenoceptor blocking activity, labetalol abruptly lowers elevated blood pressure when given via the oral or intravenous routes and has been used effectively in the management of various hypertensive emergencies. In severe hypertension, blood pressure has been observed to decline within 2 hours of oral treatment with labetalol 300 or 400 mg, and occasionally with doses as low as 100 to 200 mg. An oral regime has also been shown to be efficacious in hypertensive emergencies such as accelerated hypertension or hypertensive encephalopathy.[184,185]

Intravenous administration is feasible in circumstances where a very prompt reduction in blood pressure is indicated or when the patient cannot take the drug by mouth. In contrast to alternative parenteral antihypertensive agents, labetalol permits controlled, steady lowering of blood pressure without significant alteration in heart rate or cardiac output. Thus, the drug may be administered safely in patients with concomitant coronary artery disease. In addition, intravenous labetalol does not produce a significant reduction in cerebral blood flow and may therefore be preferable to other agents in patients who also have cerebrovascular disease.[186]

In one multicenter study conducted in the United States, 59 patients with supine blood pressures averaging 211/134 mm Hg, 36 of whom had symptomatic accelerated hypertension, were treated with intravenous pulse doses of labetalol, starting with a 20-mg dose and gradually increasing it to a total of up to 300 mg.[187] The effects of intravenously administered labetalol in severe hypertension in this study are shown in

Table 6 and Figure 8. Of the 59 patients treated, 53 reached the study's therapeutic goal, which consisted of a reduction of supine diastolic blood pressure to less than 95 mm Hg or a decrease of at least 30 mm Hg. No serious adverse effects were encountered, even in patients with concomitant diagnoses of left ventricular failure, myocardial infarction, stable congestive heart failure, angina pectoris, stroke, and encephalopathy.[187] Labetalol offers the advantage of being used parenterally in emergent situations, and then orally when continued long-term blood pressure control is necessary.

Many other reports support the use of labetalol in the treatment of severe hypertension and hypertensive emergencies.[43,65-67,129-131,188-191] On the other hand, in a small number of investigations, use of intravenous labetalol has not produced satisfactory blood pressure responses in a significant number of patients.[192-195] In these studies, the drug was usually administered as a single bolus and the majority of the nonresponders were already receiving other antihypertensive drugs, including

TABLE 6. EFFECTS OF INTRAVENOUS LABETALOL IN PATIENTS WITH SEVERE HYPERTENSION[187]

Variable	Mean
Age (years)	49.4 (range 21–28)
Male	31
Female	28
Symptomatic	23
Asymptomatic	36
Baseline BP	211/134 mmHg
BP after 20 mg of labetalol IV	188/120 mmHg
BP after last injection	143/93 mmHg
Mean BP decrement	68/41 mmHg
Mean Total Dose	197 mg (range 20 to 300 mg)

Significant Adverse Experiences

Signs/Symptoms	# Pts.
Nausea	8
Vomiting	4
Paresthesia	6
Sweating	4
Flushing	2
Dizziness	2
Headache	2
Somnolence	2
Symptomatic Hypotension	2
Arrhythmias	2

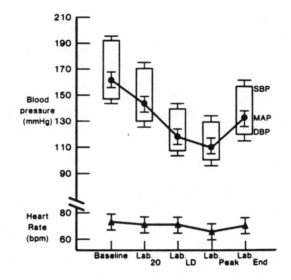

Figure 8. Intravenous labetalol in severe hypertension. Supine systolic (SBP), diastolic (DBP), mean arterial blood pressure (MAP), and heart rate (HR) at baseline after the first 20-mg mini-bolus of labetalol (lab_{20}), after the last dose of labetalol (lab_{LD}), the lowest blood pressure (BPs) recorded after the last injection (lab_{PEAK}), and the BPs and HR just prior to initiation of oral labetalol (lab_{END}) for the total study population ($n = 59$). [Reprinted from Wilson et al: Am J Med (Suppl):75(4A): 95, 1983, with permission.[187]]

β-adrenoceptor blockers, prazosin, or other sympatholytic agents. Still, Pearson and Havard, as well as Wilson et al., were able to attain good results in patients who were receiving concomitant β-adrenoceptor blocking therapy.[191,196] Thus, the hypotensive response to intravenously administered labetalol may be reduced in patients who are already receiving treatment with other β- and α-adrenoceptor blocking drugs.

Following intravenous bolus administrations of labetalol, most responding patients show a hypotensive response after 5 minutes, and a maximum response 10 minutes after administration.[65] The antihypertensive effect has been shown to persist for 6 hours or more after a single intravenous bolus of the drug.[196] Either a fast (over one minute) or slow (over 15 minutes) intravenous injection can be effective.[131] The extent of the reduction in arterial pressure is independent of the rate of injection, but the rate of reduction does vary with the rate of injection. The degree of blood pressure reduction after intravenous labetalol appears to relate to pretreatment basal norepinephrine concentration and also to the patient's age.[43,189] One series of 70 hypertensive patients has received intravenous labetalol without adverse neurologic or cardiovascular sequelae.[182] However, there is one report of a hemiparesis developing 36 hours after bolus administration of labetalol.[197] A pressor response has also been reported following intravenous bolus administration of labetalol to a patient who was already receiving other antihypertensive agents.[198]

A number of studies have compared intravenously administered labetalol to other parenteral antihypertensive therapies. For instance, a report published in 1976 showed that labetalol 100 to 125 mg intravenously was more effective than propranolol 10 mg intravenously in five patients in lowering blood pressure, but less effective in reducing pulse rate.[65] In another study, the short-term effects of labetalol 1 to 2 mg/kg intravenously were comparable to those of diazoxide 3 to 5 mg/kg intravenously in a randomized crossover study in severely hypertensive patients.[188] There was a similar result in a study comparing intravenous labetalol 150 mg to diazoxide 300 mg intravenously.[186] In contrast, Yeung and associates found that labetalol, 100 mg intravenously, was less effective than diazoxide, 300 mg intravenously, or clonidine, 300 μg intravenously.[195] Although this study and another[192] suggest that labetalol may not be as effective a parenteral antihypertensive agent as diazoxide, it would also appear less likely to induce profound hypotension and adverse neurological, metabolic, or cardiovascular sequelae.

Use of Labetalol to Treat Pheochromocytoma and Chronic Clonidine Withdrawal

The use of labetalol has been reported in the preoperative management of patients with pheochromocytoma[199] and in clonidine withdrawal hypertension,[200,201] two clinical situations in which catecholamine excess is manifest, and in which peripheral blockade of both α- and β-adrenergic receptors may be desirable. Indeed, there have been several reports describing the successful use of labetalol in the management of pheochromocytoma.[199,202–205] In one study, labetalol treatment achieved good blood pressure control in 21 of 30 patients with pheochromocytoma.[205] In that study, Takeda and colleagues also noted that labetalol was more effective in patients with predominantly epinephrine-secreting tumors and in those patients with sustained rather than paroxysmal hypertension. Although the combined α- and β-adrenoceptor blockade with labetalol appears useful in patients with pheochromocytoma, there are at least two reports that oral labetalol may provoke a hypertensive crisis in such patients.[206,207] Subsequent treatment with phentolamine and phenoxybenzamine achieved satisfactory control of blood pressure in these two cases. The pressor response to labetalol in these case studies may be the result of the preponderance of β-adrenoceptor blockade after oral dosing that leaves α-adrenoceptor stimulation relatively unopposed. An alternative explanation may be the failure of labetalol, a selective postsynaptic α_1-adrenoceptor antagonist, to prevent catecholamine-induced vasoconstriction via stimulation of peripheral α_2-adrenoceptors. Such postsynaptic α_2-adrenoceptors have been demonstrated in vascular smooth muscle.[208]

As mentioned earlier, labetalol has been used successfully in the management of hypertensive crisis following clonidine withdrawal, and has also been used prophylactically to prevent such crises during withdrawal from clonidine therapy.[188,200,202] However, there has been one report of severe rebound hypertension developing during gradual clonidine withdrawal and concurrent oral labetalol administration.[201] Thus, oral labetalol may have similar disadvantages in clonidine withdrawal as observed in some patients with pheochromocytoma. Like other β-adrenoceptor blockers, oral labetalol should be avoided unless α-adrenergic blockers have already been given in the form of intravenous phentolamine.

Hypertension in Pregnancy

Studies reporting on the use of labetalol in pregnant women with severe hypertension are encouraging (see Chapter 15).[143,209–219] Not only does labetalol satisfactorily control blood pressure in the pregnant woman, but it may also exert a beneficial effect on fetal pulmonary maturity.[209] This effect of labetalol on lung maturation may be mediated through a partial β_2-adrenoceptor agonist action. Nicholas and coworkers found a similar effect with salbutamol in rabbits.[217] Although labetalol has been shown to cross the placental barrier, it does not appear to produce adverse effects on the fetus antenatally, during labor, or postpartum.[209,212] To date, there have been no reports of clinically significant fetal hypoglycemia, fetal bradycardia, or fetal respiratory depression with maternal labetalol therapy. One study using a radioactive indium technique indicates that labetalol effectively reduces maternal blood pressure without diminishing uteroplacental blood flow.[220]

Hypertension in pregnancy can be controlled effectively by oral administration of labetalol in doses ranging from 330 to 1800 mg daily.[209,211,213] In two randomized studies, labetalol compared favorably with methyldopa for the treatment of hypertension in pregnancy. In one such study, labetalol 400 to 800 mg daily provided better blood pressure control than methyldopa 750 to 1500 mg daily. Furthermore, perinatal mortality was 4.4 percent and there were no congenital malformations in any of the infants delivered to labetalol-treated patients.[213] Redman reported that blood pressure control was similar in two groups of patients treated with either labetalol 300 to 1200 mg daily or methyldopa 1 to 4 g daily.[214]

In a situation where rapid reduction of blood pressure is required, such as in severe preeclampsia or eclampsia, intravenous labetalol gives satisfactory results.[213,218–220] In a study comparing intravenous labetalol to intravenous dihydralazine, the labetalol infusion appeared to offer significant advantages in the management of severe hypertension in pregnancy.[215]

Despite these favorable reports on the use of labetalol in the treatment of hypertension in pregnancy, its use under these circumstances must be regarded as investigational until more extensive studies confirm its safety and clearly demonstrate its superiority over the more established antihypertensive drugs being used in pregnancy.

Ischemic Heart Disease

The α-adrenoceptor blocking component of labetalol may minimize the propensity for coronary artery spasm to develop with β-adrenoceptor blockade alone, while the β-blocking component may offset any tendency for arrhythmias to develop secondary to α-adrenoceptor stimulation. In addition, labetalol has demonstrated favorable hemodynamic effects in normotensive patients with documented coronary artery disease, and appears to be less likely to cause myocardial depression than conventional β-adrenoceptor blockers.[57,58,221] The hemodynamic rationale for using labetalol in ischemic heart disease is illustrated in Table 5.[57]

Earlier investigations of labetalol in patients with ischemic heart disease were encouraging. Acute injection of propranolol, pindolol, or labetalol produced similar increases in exercise tolerance in normotensive patients with angina pectoris.[222] More recently, Condorelli and associates examined the effect of labetalol 100 mg twice daily on exercise tolerance in 19 normotensive subjects with angiographic evidence of coronary artery disease.[223] Compared to placebo, labetalol produced significant reductions in systolic and diastolic blood pressure, heart rate, and rate–pressure product. In addition, ST segment depression was reduced by labetalol, and exercise tolerance was increased. Oral labetalol has also been used effectively in hypertensive patients with coexisting angina pectoris.[224–226] Lubbe and White substituted labetalol for existing β-adrenoceptor blockers in the treatment regimens of six hypertensive patients with angina pectoris and found that labetalol produced a significant reduction in blood pressure while reducing the frequency of angina pectoris.[224] Our experience with labetalol in the treatment of hypertensive patients with angina has also been favorable and is described in Chapter 11.[4] When labetalol therapy is withdrawn abruptly, there does appear to be a sharp increase in blood pressure or anginal symptoms. This contrasts with the situation following abrupt cessation of many conventional β-adrenoceptor blocking drugs.[227] At this juncture, studies comparing labetalol to conventional β-adrenoceptor blockers, nitrates, and calcium-entry blockers are still needed to clearly define the role of labetalol in the management of angina pectoris.

Other reports describe the successful use of labetalol in the management of hypertension associated with acute myocardial infarction. Incremental infusion of labetalol lowered blood pressure safely and effectively in 15 hypertensive patients with acute myocardial infarction.[228] Timmis and colleagues confirmed this finding and also showed that labetalol did not produce adverse hemodynamic effects.[229] These investigators concluded that labetalol infusion in patients with acute myocardial infarction is unlikely to precipitate heart failure and is likely to be of value in reducing myocardial oxygen requirements.

Overall, the initial studies reporting on the use of labetalol in patients with myocardial infarction are encouraging, but more extensive and definitive clinical trials are required before the drug can be recommended for routine use in such circumstances.

Use in General Anesthesia

The established and potential roles for labetalol in anesthetic practice have been reviewed recently.[230] The drug is useful for correcting uncontrolled hypertension before anesthesia, during surgery, and in the immediate postoperative period, when it can be administered either orally or intravenously.[231]

Induced hypotension is a useful technique to minimize blood loss during certain surgical procedures. However, the typically utilized agents, e.g., ganglionic blockers and nitroprusside, are frequently accompanied by tachyphylaxis and undesirable tachycardia. Labetalol has been used effectively with halothane and other anesthetic agents for controlled hypotensive anesthesia during a variety of surgical procedures, including otological operations and coarctation repair, with no such undesirable effects.[232–234] Stable blood pressure and heart rate are maintained throughout anesthesia with the combination of labetalol and halothane, and the degree of hypotension can be adjusted by altering the concentration of the anesthetic. However, a high concentration of halothane (3 percent or more) used with labetalol may produce large reductions in cardiac output.[235] Blood pressure and heart rate can be restored to normal levels postoperatively by the administration of atropine sulfate. Although Cope[232] reports that patients with ischemic heart disease may receive labetalol during anesthesia without any untoward effect, there is a conflicting report of severe myocardial depression and death in such a patient during labetalol therapy and 0.5 percent halothane anesthesia.[236]

Labetalol may also be used effectively to counter acute hypertensive responses during laryngoscopy and various surgical procedures, including pheochromocytoma removal.[203] A recent study reported that labetalol may be effective for the treatment of cancer pain when administered through a peridural catheter.[237]

SIDE EFFECTS AND CONTRAINDICATIONS

Multiple reports identify the nature and frequency of side effects with labetalol.[1,108,147,163,183,205] Side effects are generally mild and self-limited. They fall into three categories: (1) non-specific; (2) related to α-adrenoceptor blockade; and (3) related to β-adrenoceptor blockade.

Non Specific Side Effects
Gastrointestinal side effects have been reported in up to 15 percent of patients; complaints include nausea, dyspepsia, flatulence, vomiting, diarrhea, and abdominal pain. Less frequent complaints include fatigue and headache. A variety of skin rashes, including a maculopapular erythematous rash, urticaria, atypical lichen planus, and bullous lichen planus, have been described during labetalol treatment; these occurrences have been rare.[152,183,238-240] Myositis has been described, and there is one report of Peyronie's disease, which developed in a 58-year-old male after eight months of labetalol therapy.[241]

Side Affects Related to α-Adrenoceptor Blockade
The most bothersome side effect reported with labetalol treatment is dizziness, which occurs in about 5 percent of patients. It tends to occur more frequently in the early stages of treatment, in patients receiving concomitant diuretic therapy, with higher drug doses, and with large dose increments.[146] Other less frequent side effects, which are probably related to α-blockade, include scalp tingling, nasal stuffiness, and genitourinary disorders.[183] Scalp tingling, or formication, has been reported after both oral and intravenous labetalol use.[26,27] Circumoral paresthesia has also been reported. Side effects such as decreased libido and impotence are relatively uncommon with the drug, whereas delayed and/or retrograde ejaculation, also attributed to α-blockade, occurs with some frequency in male patients.

Side Effects Related to β-Adrenoceptor Blockade

Adverse side effects related to the β-adrenoceptor blocking actions of labetalol include vivid dreams,[183] asthma,[183,205] Raynaud's phenomenon,[183] intermittent claudication,[183] muscle cramps,[89,183] and heart failure. The side effects from β-blockade are generally less troublesome during labetalol treatment than during therapy with pure β-blocking drugs.[159,179] The frequency and type of side effects with labetalol therapy, in our experience from double-blind trials and open-label studies, are described in Chapters 13 and 14.[108,163]

Alterations During Chronic Labetalol Therapy

Antinuclear antibody tests may become positive at a low titer during chronic labetalol therapy, but they are not accompanied by any symptoms or signs of immunologic disease. A lupus-type illness, however, has been reported in a single patient during labetalol therapy.[242] Antimitochondrial antibodies may also develop during chronic labetalol therapy, but they do not appear to be of clinical significance.[243,244] There have been no reports of ophthalmologic side effects related to labetalol therapy.

In our long-term labetalol study, 8 percent of treated patients developed reversible, asymptomatic transaminase elevations to greater than twice normal at some time during the study.[108] In half of these patients, the alterations resolved while on continued labetalol therapy, but in five (2 percent) patients, the elevations led to drug discontinuation.[108]

Kane reviewed the results of labetalol treatment in 8573 hypertensive patients for periods of up to 5 years.[148] The withdrawal rate attributable to side effects was between 6 and 13 percent in his report. In our long-term study of labetalol in 337 patients, a 9 percent withdrawal rate was reported.[108] Takeda et al.[205] reported that approximately 5 percent of patients withdraw from labetalol therapy due to side effects, whereas Waal-Manning and Simpson reported an unusually high side effect withdrawal rate of 25 percent.[183] Overall, labetalol appears to be well-tolerated, with a low incidence of side effects; in some instances, side effects reported by patients have been less than on previous treatment regimens.

Labetalol should be used with caution, or avoided, in instances where the β-adrenoceptor blocking action of the drug could prove harmful, although with therapeutic doses, labetalol appears less likely than propranolol to exacerbate various serious conditions. Such conditions include heart failure, which should first be controlled with conventional agents, such as digitalis and diuretics, before administration of labetalol. The drug is probably best avoided in patients with asthma until further information is available on its effects on respiratory function in asthmatics. In order to diminish the potential for a pressor response to the drug in patients with pheochromocytoma, it seems preferable to establish α-adrenoceptor blockade with intravenous labetalol or some other α-blocking agent before commencing with oral labetalol therapy.

Dosage

The recommended starting dose for oral labetalol, used alone or in combination with a diuretic, is 100 mg twice daily. The dose may be increased to 200 mg twice daily after 2 days, and further dose increments may be made every 1 to 3 days until an optimum response is obtained. Slower upward titration may be preferable, because it is less likely to result in bothersome side effects including orthostatic symptoms. The usual maintenance dose of labetalol is 200 to 400 mg twice daily. However, some patients with severe hypertension may require 1200 to 2400 mg of labetalol daily in two or three divided doses, possibly with a thiazide diuretic in addition, in order to achieve a satisfactory therapeutic response.

Labetalol may be administered intravenously either by slow continuous intravenous or by repeated bolus injection. If given by slow infusion, a solution should be made by diluting 200-mg labetalol (40 ml) to 200 ml with a standard intravenous solution such as 5 percent dextrose. The recommended rate of infusion is 2-mg labetalol (2 ml of infusion solution) per minute, until a satisfactory response is obtained; the infusion should then be stopped. The usual effective dose range is 50 to 200 mg, and the infusion may be repeated every 6 to 8 hours to maintain satisfactory blood pressure control. If given by bolus injection, a dose of 20-mg labetalol should be given intravenously over a period of 2 minutes. Additional bolus injections of 40 to 80 mg may be given at 10-minute intervals, until an optimum response is obtained. The maximum recommended total dose of labetalol by either of the methods of administration is 300 mg. Patients should remain supine when given labetalol intravenously, and should not assume the upright position for 3 hours after drug administration in order to avoid excessive postural hypotension.[146]

After the blood pressure has been adequately reduced by parenteral labetalol, maintenance oral dosing may begin when it has been established that the supine blood pressure has begun to rise.

CONCLUSION

Labetalol is the prototype agent of a new class of antihypertensive agents—β-blockers with ancillary α-blocking and/or direct vasodilating activity. The drug appears to be safe and effective as an oral antihypertensive agent in the management of mild, moderate, and severe hypertension. It is also effective and safe when used parenterally to achieve rapid control of blood pressure in hypertensive emergencies. Side effects are usually only mild, and the most troublesome of these (dizziness) appears to attenuate with time. In comparison to conventional β-blockers, labetalol has favorable hemodynamic effects that render it less likely to compromise myocardial function. The antihypertensive efficacy of labetalol is superior to diuretic therapy in many subsets of patients, and is at least comparable, if not superior, to that of pure β-blockers, methyldopa, clonidine, and various adrenergic neuronal blockers. Preliminary studies also indicate that labetalol may be of value for hypotensive anesthesia, hypertension of pregnancy, ventricular arrhythmias, and in the management of ischemic heart disease.

REFERENCES

1. Frishman W, Halprin S: Clinical pharmacology of the new beta-adrenergic blocking drugs. Part 7. New horizons in beta-adrenoceptor blockade therapy: Labetalol. Am Heart J 98:660, 1979
2. Farmer JB, Kennedy I, Levy GP, Marshall RJ: Pharmacology of AH5158: a drug which blocks both α- and β-adrenoceptor blocking drugs. Br J Clin Pharmacol 45:660, 1972
3. Wallin JD, O'Neill WM: Labetalol. Arch Intern Med 143:485, 1983
4. Frishman WH, Strom JA, Kirschner M, et al: Labetalol therapy in patients with systemic hypertension and angina pectoris: effects of combined alpha and beta-adrenoceptor blockade. Am J Cardiol 48:917, 1981
5. MacCarthy EP, Bloomfield SS: Labetalol: A review of its pharmacology, pharmacokinetic clinical uses and side effects. Pharmacotherapy 3:193, 1983
6. Berlin LJ, Juel-Jensen BE: α- and β-adrenoceptor blockade in hypertension. Lancet 1:979, 1972
7. Majid PA, Meeran MK, Benaim ME, et al: α- and β-adrenoceptor blockade in the treatment of hypertension. Br Heart J 36:588, 1974
8. Michelson EL, Frishman WH: Labetalol: An alpha-beta adrenergic blocker. Ann Intern Med 99:553, 1983
9. Brittain RT, Drew GM, Levy GP: The α- and β-adrenoceptor blocking potencies of labetalol and its individual stereoisomers in anesthetized dogs and in isolated tissues. Br J Pharmacol 77:105, 1982
10. Aggerbick M, Guellaen G, Hanoune J: N-alkyl substitution increases the affinity of adrenergic drugs for the α-adrenoceptor in rat liver. Br J Pharmacol 65:15, 1979
11. Brittain RT, Levy GP: A review of the animal pharmacology of labetalol, a combined α- and β-adrenoceptor blocking drug. Br J Clin Pharmacol 3 (Suppl 3):681, 1976

12. Blakeley AG, Summers RJ: The pharmacology of labetalol, an α- and β-adrenoceptor blocking agent. Gen Pharmacol 9:399, 1978
13. Baum T, Sybertz EJ: Pharmacology of labetalol in experimental animals. Am J Med (Suppl): 75(4A):15, 1983
14. Carey B, Whalley ET: Labetalol possesses β-adrenoceptor agonist action on the isolated rat uterus. J Pharm Pharmacol 31:791, 1979
15. Carey B, Whalley ET: β-adrenoceptor agonist activity of labetalol on the isolated rat uterus. Br J Pharmacol 67:13, 1979
16. Carpenter JR: Intrinsic activity of labetalol on guinea pig isolated trachea. J Pharm Pharmacol 33:806, 1981
17. Johnson GL, Prioli NA, Ehrreich SJ: Antihypertensive effects of labetalol (SCH 15719W, AH5158A) (Abstr). Fed Proc 36:1049, 1977
18. Dage RC, Hsieh CP: Direct vasodilatation by labetalol in anesthetized dogs. Br J Pharmacol 70:287, 1980
19. Sybertz EJ, Sabin CS, Pula KK, et al: Alpha- and beta-adrenoceptor blocking properties of labetalol and its R-R isomer, SCH 19927. J Pharmacol Exp Ther 218:435, 1981
20. Katano Y, Takeda K, Nakagawa Y, et al: α- and β-adrenoceptor blocking actions of labetalol and effects on the myocardial function, coronary circulation and myocardial energy metabolism thereof. Folia Pharmacol Jpn 74:819, 1978
21. Blakeley AG, Summers RJ: The effects of labetalol (AH5158) on adrenergic transmission in the cat spleen. Br J Pharmacol 59:643, 1977
22. Levy GP, Richards DA: Labetalol, in Scriabine A (ed), Pharmacology of Antihypertensive Agents. New York, Raven Press, 1980, pp 325–347
23. Hoffman BB, Lefkowitz R: Alpha-adrenergic receptor subtypes. N Engl J Med 302:1390, 1982
24. Drew GM: Pharmacological characterization of the presynaptic α-adrenoceptors regulating cholinergic activity in the guinea pig ileum. Br J Pharmacol 64:293, 1978
25. Drew GM, Gower AJ, Marriott AS: Pharmacological characterization of α-adrenoceptors which mediate clonidine-induced sedation (Abstr). Br J Pharmacol 61:468P, 1977
26. Collier JG, Dawnay NAH, Nachev CH, et al: Clinical investigation of an antagonist at α- and β-adrenoceptors AH 5158A. Br J Pharmacol 44:286, 1972
27. Frick MH, Porsti P: Combined alpha and beta-adrenoceptor blockade with labetalol in hypertension. Br Med J 1:1046, 1976
28. Brittain RT, Harris DM, Jack D, et al: Labetalol, in Goldberg ME (ed), Pharmacological and Biochemical Properties of Drug Substances. Am Pharm Assoc Acad Pharm Sci 1979, pp 229–254
29. Boakes AJ, Knight EJ, Prichard BNC: Preliminary studies of the pharmacologic effects of 5-1-hydroxy-2-(1-methyl-3 phenylpropyl) amino ethyl salicyolamide (AH 5158) in man. Clin Sci 40:188, 1971
30. Richards DA: Pharmacologic effects of labetalol in man. Br J Clin Pharmacol 3 (Suppl 3):721, 1976

31. Richards DA, Prichard BNC, Dobbs RJ: Adrenoceptor blockade of the circulatory responses to intravenous isoproterenol. Clin Pharmacol Ther 24:264, 1978

32. Richards DA, Woodings EP, Stephen MDB, et al: The effects of oral AH 5158, a combined α- and β-adrenoceptor antagonist in healthy volunteers. Br J Clin Pharmacol 1:505, 1974

33. Richards DA, Prichard BNC, Boakes AJ, et al: Pharmacological basis for antihypertensive effects of intravenous labetalol. Br Heart J 39:99, 1977

34. Richards DA, Prichard BNC, Hernandez R: Circulatory effects of noradrenaline and adrenaline before and after labetalol. Br J Clin Pharmacol 7:371, 1979

35. Richards DA, Tuckman J, Prichard BNC: Assessment of alpha and beta-adrenoceptor blocking action of labetalol. Br J Clin Pharmacol 3:849, 1976

36. Mehta J, Cohn JN: Hemodynamic effects of labetalol, an alpha and beta adrenergic blocking agent, in hypertensive subjects. Circulation 55:370, 1977

37. Maconochie JG, Richards DA, Woodings EP: Modification of pressor responses induced by "cold" (Abstr). Br J Clin Pharmacol 4:389P, 1977

38. Richards DA, Maconochie JG, Bland RE, et al: Relationship between plasma concentrations and pharmacological effects of labetalol. Eur J Clin Pharmacol 11:85, 1977

39. Baum T, Watkins, Sybertz, et al: Antihypertensive and hemodynamic actions of SCH 19927, the R-R isomer of labetalol. J Pharmacol Exper Ther 218:444, 1981

40. Maxwell GM: The effects of a new alpha and beta-adrenoceptor antagonist (AH 51581) upon the general and coronary hemodynamics of intact dogs. Br J Clin Pharmacol 49:370, 1973

41. Drew GM, Hilditch A, Levy GP: The relationships between the cardiovascular effects, α and β-adrenoceptor blocking actions and plasma concentration of labetalol in DOCA hypertensive rats. Clin Exp Hypertens 1:597, 1979

42. Koch G: Hemodynamic changes after acute and long-term combined alpha–beta adrenoceptor blockade with labetalol as compared with beta-receptor blockade. J Cardiovasc Pharmacol 3 (Suppl 1):s30, 1981

43. Agabiti-Rosei E, Alicandri CL, Beschi M, et al: The acute and chronic hypotensive effect of labetalol and the relationship with pretreatment plasma noradrenaline levels. Br J Clin Pharmacol 13 (Suppl 1):87s, 1982

44. Joekes AM, Thompson FD: Acute haemodynamic effects of labetalol and its subsequent use as an oral hypotensive agent. Br J Clin Pharmacol 3 (Suppl 3):789, 1976

45. Koch G: Cardiovascular dynamics after acute and long-term α- and β-adrenoceptor blockade at rest, supine and standing, and during exercise. Br J Clin Pharmacol 8 (Suppl 2):101s, 1979

46. Svendsen TL, Rasmussen S, Hartling OJ: Sequential haemodynamic effects of labetalol at rest and during exercise in essential hypertension. Postgrad Med J 56 (Suppl 2):21, 1980

47. Prichard BNC, Thompson FO, Boakes AJ, et al: Some haemodynamic effects of compound AH 5158 compared with propranolol, propranolol plus hydralazine, and diazoxide: the use of AH 5158 in the treatment of hypertension. Clin Sci Mol Med 48:97s, 1975

48. Bahlmann J, Brod J, Hubrich W, et al: Effect of an α- and β-adrenoceptor blocking agent (labetalol) on haemodynamics in hypertension. Br J Clin Pharmacol 8 (Suppl 2):113s, 1979

49. Trap-Jensen J, Clausen JP, Hartling OJ, et al: Immediate effects of labetalol on central, splanchnic-hepatic, and forearm haemodynamics during pleasant emotional stress in hypertensive patients. Postgrad Med J 56 (Suppl 2):37, 1980

50. Omvik P, Lund-Johansen P: Acute hemodynamic effects of labetalol in severe hypertension. J Cardiovasc Pharmacol 4:915, 1982

51. Lund-Johansen P: Comparative haemodynamic effects of labetalol, timolol, prazosin and the combination of tolamolol and prazosin. Br J Clin Pharmacol 8 (Suppl 2):107s, 1979

52. Edwards RC, Raftery EB: Haemodynamic effects of long-term oral labetalol. Br J Clin Pharmacol 3 (Suppl 3):733, 1976

53. Fagard R, Amery A, Reybrouck T, Linjen P, Billiet L: Response of the systemic and pulmonary circulation to alpha- and beta-receptor blockade (labetalol) at rest and during exercise in hypertensive patients. Circulation 60:1214, 1979

54. Lund-Johansen P: Acute and chronic (six years) hemodynamic effects of labetalol in essential hypertension. Am J Med (Suppl):75(4A): 24, 1983

55. Fagard R, Lijnen P, Amery A: Response of the systemic pulmonary circulation to labetalol at rest and during exercise. Br J Clin Pharmacol 13 (Suppl 1):13s, 1982

56. Dunn FG, Olgman W, Messerli FH, et al: Hemodyanamic effects of intravenous labetalol in essential hypertension. Clin Pharmacol Ther 33:139, 1983

57. Gagnon RM, Morissette M, Presant S, et al: Hemodynamic and coronary effects of intravenous labetalol in coronary artery disease. Am J Cardiol 49:1267, 1982

58. Taylor SH, Silke B, Nelson GIC, et al: Haemodynamic advantages of combined alpha-blockade and beta-blockade over beta-blockade alone in patients with coronary heart disease. Br Med J 285:325, 1982

59. Griffith DNW, James IM, Newbury PA, Woolard ML: The effect of β-adrenergic receptor blocking drugs on cerebral blood flow. Br J Clin Pharmacol 7:491, 1979

60. Koch G: Combined α- and β-adrenoceptor blockade with oral labetalol in hypertensive patients with reference to haemodynamic effects at rest and during exercise. Br J Clin Pharmacol 3 (Suppl 3):729, 1976

61. Lijnen PJ, Amery AK, Fagard RH, et al: Effects of labetalol on plasma renin, aldosterone, and catecholamines in hypertensive patients. J Cardiovasc Pharmacol 1:625, 1979

62. Weidmann P, DeChatel R, Zeigler WH, et al: Alpha and beta-adrenergic

blockade with orally administered labetalol in hypertension. Am J Cardiol 41:570, 1978

63. Salvetti A, Pedrinelli R, Sassano P, Arzilli F: Effect of increasing doses of labetalol on blood pressure, plasma renin activity and aldosterone in hypertensive patients. Clin Sci 57:401s, 1979

64. Dawson A, Johnson BF, Smith IK: Comparison of the effects of labetalol, bendrofluazide and their combination in hypertension. Br J Clin Pharmcol 8:149, 1979

65. Trust PM, Agabiti-Rosei E, Brown JJ, et al: Effect on blood pressure, angiotensin II, and aldosterone concentrations during treatment of severe hypertension with intravenous labetalol: Comparison with propranolol. Br J Clin Pharmacol 3 (Suppl 3):799, 1976

66. Agabiti-Rosei E, Trust PM, Brown JJ, et al: Effects of intravenous labetalol on blood pressure, angiotensin II and aldosterone in hypertension: comparison with propranolol. Clin Sci Mol Med 51:497s, 1976

67. Cummings AM, Brown JJ, Fraser R, et al: Blood pressure reduction by incremental infusion of labetalol in patients with severe hypertension. Br J Clin Pharmacol 8:359, 1979

68. Louis WJ, Christophidis N, Brignell M, et al: Labetalol: Bioavailability, drug plasma levels, plasma renin, and catecholamines in acute and chronic treatment of resistant hypertension. Aust NZ J Med 8:602, 1978

69. Larochelle P, Hamet P, Hoffman B, et al: Labetalol in essential hypertension. J Cardiovasc Pharmacol 2:751, 1980

70. Kornerup HJ, Pedersen EB, Christensen NJ, et al: Effect of oral labetalol on plasma catecholamines, renin, and aldosterone in patients with severe arterial hypertension. Eur J Clin Pharmacol 16:305, 1979

71. Mihano L, Kolloch R, DeQuattro V: Increased catecholamine excretion after labetalol therapy: A spurious effect of drug metabolites. Clin Chim Act 95:211, 1979

72. Hamilton CA, Jones DH, Dargie HJ, Reid JL: Does labetalol increase excretion of urinary catecholamines. Br Med J 2:800, 1978

73. Richards DA, Harris DM, Martin LE: Labetalol and urinary catecholamines (letter). Br Med J 1:685, 1979

74. Keusch G, Weidmann P, Ziegler WH, et al: Effects of chronic alpha and beta-adrenoceptor blockade with labetalol on plasma catecholamines and renal function in hypertension. Klin Wochenschr 58:25, 1980

75. Kolloch R, Mihano L, De Quattro V: Labetalol and urinary catecholamines (letter). Br Med J 1:268, 1979.

76. Frishman WH: β-adrenoceptor antagonists: new drugs and new indications. N Engl J Med 305:500, 1981

77. Vaughan Williams EM, Millar JS, Campbell TJ: Electrophysiological effects of labetalol on rabbit atrial, ventricular and Purkinje cells, in normoxia and hypoxia. Cardiovasc Res 16:233, 1982

78. Ambie JP: A study of the labetalol-induced changes in conductivity and refractoriness of the dog heart in situ. Cardiovasc Res 12:646, 1978

79. Pogwizd SM, Sharma AD, Corr PB: Influence of labetalol, a combined

α and β-adrenergic blocking agent on the dysrhythmias induced by coronary occlusion and reperfusion. Cardiovasc Res 16:398, 1982

80. Lubbe WF, Nguyen T, Edwards MF: Antiarrhythmic action of labetalol and its effect on adenosine metabolism in the isolated rat heart. J Am Coll Cardiol 1:1296, 1983

81. Harley A, Coverdale HA: The electrophysiological effect of intravenous labetalol in man. Eur J Clin Pharmacol 20:241, 1981

82. Seides SF, Josephson ME, Batsford WP, et al: The electrophysiology of propranolol in man. Am Heart J 88:733, 1974

83. Robinson C, Birkhead J, Crook B, et al: Clinical electrophysiological effects of atenolol, a new cardioselective beta-blocking agent. Br Heart J 40:14, 1978

84. Mason JW, Winkle RA, Meffin PJ, Harrison DC: Electrophysiological effects of acebutolol. Br Heart J 40:35, 1978

85. Romano S, Orfei S, Pozzoni L, et al: Preliminary clinical trial on hypotensive and antiarrhythmic effect of labetalol. Drugs Exptl Clin Res 7:65, 1981

86. Mazzola C, Ferrario N, Calzavara MP, et al: Acute antihypertensive and antiarrhythmic effects of labetalol. Curr Ther Res 29:613, 1981

87. Barbieri C, Ferrari C, Caldara R, Crossignani RM, Endocrine and metabolic effects of labetalol in man. J Cardiovasc Pharmacol 3:986, 1981

88. Riley AJ: Some further evidence for partial agonist activity of labetalol (letter). Br J Clin Pharmacol 9:517, 1980

89. Andersson O, Berglund G, Hansson L: Antihypertensive action, time of onset and effects on carbohydrate metabolism of labetalol. Br J Clin Pharmacol 3 (Suppl 3):757, 1976.

90. Sommers DEK, De Villiers LS, Van Wyk M, Schoeman HS: The effects of labetalol and oxprenolol on blood lipids. S Afr Med J 60:379, 1981

91. Pagnan A, Pessina AC, Hlede M, et al: Effects of labetalol on lipid and carbohydrate metabolism. Pharmacol Res Commun 11:227, 1979

92. McGonigle RJS, Williams L, Murphy MJ: Labetalol and lipids (letter). Lancet 1:163, 1981

93. Frishman W, Michelson E, Johnson B, et al: Effects of beta-adrenergic blockade on plasma lipids: A double-blind randomized placebo-controlled multicenter comparison of labetalol and metoprolol in patients with hypertension (Abstr). Am J Cardiol 49:984, 1982

94. Patel KR, Kerr JW: Alpha-receptor blocking drugs in bronchial asthma. Lancet 1:348, 1975

95. Geumei A, Miller JR, Miller WF: Effects of phentolamine inhalation on patients with bronchial asthma. Br J Clin Pharmacol 2:539, 1975

96. Richards DA, Woodings EP, Maconochie JG: Comparison of the effects of labetalol and propranolol in healthy men at rest and during exercise. Br J Clin Pharmacol 4:15, 1977

97. Maconochie JG, Woodings EP, Richards DA: Effects of labetalol and propranolol on histamine-induced bronchoconstriction in normal subjects. Br J Clin Pharmacol 4:157, 1977

98. Skinner C, Gaddie J, Palmer KNV: Comparison of intravenous AH 5158 (labetalol) and propranolol in asthma. Br Med J 2:59, 1975

99. Skinner C, Gaddie J, Palmer KNV: Comparison of effects of intravenous AH 5158, a combined alpha and beta-adrenoceptor antagonist and propranolol in asthmatics. Scot Med J 20:41, 1957

100. George RB, Manocha K, Burford J, et al: Effects of labetalol in hypertensive patients with chronic obstructive pulmonary disease. Chest 83:457, 1983

101. Mazzola C, Guffanti E, Vacarella A, et al: Respiratory effects of labetalol in anginous or hypertensive patients. Curr Ther Res 31:219, 1982

102. Light RW, Chetty KG, Stansbury DW: Comparisons of the effects of labetalol and hydrochlorothiazide on the ventilatory function of hypertension patients with mild chronic obstructive pulmonary disease. Am J Med (Suppl):75(4A): 109, 1983

103. Adam WR, Meagher EJ, Barter CE: Labetalol, beta-blockers and acute deterioration of chronic airway obstruction. Clin Exp Hyper A4 (8):1419, 1982

104. Larsson K: Influence of labetalol, propranolol and practolol in patients with asthma. Eur J Respir Dis 63:221, 1982

105. Anavekar SN, Barter C, Adam WR, Doyle AE: A double-blind comparison of verapamil and labetalol in hypertensive patients with coexisting chronic obstructive airways disease. J Cardiovasc Pharmacol 4:s374, 1982

106. Jackson SHD, Bievers DG: Comparison of the effects of single doses of atenolol and labetalol on airways obstruction in patients with hypertension and asthma. Br J Clin Pharmacol 15:553, 1983

107. Hunyor SN, Bauer GE, Ross M, Larkin H: Labetalol and propranolol in mild hypertensives: comparison of blood pressure and plasma volume effects. Aust NZ J Med 10:162, 1980

108. Michelson EL, Frishman WH, Lewis JE, et al: Multicenter clinical evaluation of the long-term efficacy and safety of labetalol in the treatment of hypertension. Am J Med (Suppl): 75(4A); 68, 1983

109. Rasmussen S, Nielson PE: Blood pressure, plasma volume, extracellular volume and glomerular filtration rate during treatment with labetalol in essential hypertension. Postgrad Med J 56 (Suppl 2):33, 1980.

110. Rasmussen S, Nielsen PE: Blood pressure, body fluid volumes and glomerular filtration rate during treatment with labetalol in essential hypertension. Br J Clin Pharmacol 12:349, 1981

111. Thompson FD, Joekes AM, Hussein MM: Monotherapy with labetalol for hypertensive patients with normal and impaired renal function. Br J Clin Pharmacol 8 (Suppl 2):129s, 1979

112. Pedersen EB, Larsen JS: Effect of propranolol and labetalol on renal haemodynamics at rest and during exercise in essential hypertension. Postgrad Med J 56 (Suppl 2):27, 1980

113. Cruz F, O'Neill WM, Clifton G, Wallin JD: Effects of labetalol and methyldopa on renal function. Clin Pharmacol Ther 30:57, 1981

114. Valvo E, Previato G, Tessitore N, et al: Effects of the long-term adminis-

tration of labetalol on blood pressure, hemodynamics and renal function in essential and renal hypertension. Curr Ther Res 29:634, 1981

115. Malini PL, Strocchi E, Negroni S, et al: Renal haemodynamics after chronic treatment with labetalol and propranolol. Br J Clin Pharmacol 13 (Suppl 1):123s, 1982

116. Watson A, Maher K, Keogh JAB: Labetalol and renal function. Irish J Med Sci 150:174, 1981

117. Epstein M, Oster JR: Beta-blockers and the kidney. Mineral Electrolyte Metab 8:237, 1982

118. Bailey RR: Labetalol in the treatment of patients with hypertension and renal function impairment. Br J Clin Pharmacol 8 (Suppl 2):135s, 1979

119. Wallin JD: Antihypertensives and their impact on renal function. Am J Med (Suppl):75(4A): 87, 1983

120. Serlin MJ, Orme MC, Maciver M, et al: Rate of onset of hypotensive effect of oral labetalol. Br J Clin Pharmacol 7:165, 1979

121. Rossi A, Ziacchi V, Lomanto B: The hypotensive effect of a single daily dose of labetalol: a preliminary study. Int J Clin Pharmacol Ther Toxicol 20:438, 1982

122. Bala-Subramanian V, Mann S, Raftery EB: The effect of labetalol on continuous ambulatory blood pressure. Br J Clin Pharmacol 8 (Suppl 2):119s, 1979

123. Sanders GL, Murray A, Rawlins MD: Interdose control of β-blockade and arterial blood pressure during chronic oral labetalol treatment. Br J Clin Pharmacol 8 (Suppl 2):125s, 1979

124. Mancia G, Pomidossi G, Parati G, et al: Blood pressure responses to labetalol in twice and three times daily administration during a 24 hour period. Br J Clin Pharmacol 13 (Suppl 1):27s, 1982

125. Ferrari A, Buccino N, DiRienzo M, et al: Labetalol and 24 hour monitoring of arterial blood pressure in hypertensive patients. J Cardiovasc Pharmacol 3 (Suppl 1):42s, 1981

126. Maronde RF, Robinson D, Vlachakis N, et al: A study of single and multiple dose pharmacokinetic/pharmacokinetic modeling of the antihypertensive effects of labetalol. Am J Med (Suppl):75(4A): 40, 1983

127. Breckenridge A, Orme M, Serlin MJ, Maciver M: Labetalol in essential hypertension. Br J Clin Pharmacol 13 (Suppl 1):37s, 1982

128. Wilcox R: Randomized study of six beta-blockers and a thiazide diuretic in essential hypertension. Br Med J 2:383, 1978

129. Ronne-Rasmussen JO, Andersen GS, Bowal Jensen N, et al: Acute effect of intravenous labetalol in the treatment of systemic arterial hypertension. Br J Clin Pharmacol 3 (Suppl 3):805, 1976

130. Cumming AMM, Brown JJ, Lever AF, et al: Treatment of severe hypertension by repeated bolus injections of labetalol. Br J Clin Pharmacol 8 (Suppl 2):199s, 1979

131. Pearson RM, Havard CWH: Intravenous labetalol in hypertensive patients given by fast and slow injection. Br J Clin Pharmacol 5:401, 1978

132. Sanders GL, Routledge PA, Ward A, et al: Mean steady state plasma con-

centrations of labetalol in patients undergoing antihypertensive therapy. Br J Clin Pharmacol 8 (Suppl 2):153s, 1979

133. Gural RP, Leitz F, Patrick J, et al: Rising multiple dose study of labetalol in hypertensive patients: Pharmacodynamic profile (Abstr). World Cong Clin Pharm and Therap (in press)

134. McNeil JJ, Anderson AE, Louis WJ, et al: Labetalol steady-state pharmacokinetics in hypertensive patients. Br J Clin Pharmacol 13 (Suppl 1):75s, 1982

135. Martin LE, Hopkins R, Bland R: Metabolism of labetalol by animals and man. Br J Clin Pharmacol 3 (Suppl 3):695, 1976

136. McNeil JJ, Anderson AE, Louis WJ: Pharmacokinetics and pharmacodynamic studies of labetalol in hypertensive subjects. Br J Clin Pharmacol 8 (Suppl 2):157s, 1979

137. Mantyla R, Allonen H, Kanto J, et al: Effect of food on the bioavailability of labetalol (letter). Br J Clin Pharmacol 9:435, 1980

138. Daneshmend TK, Roberts CJC: The influence of food on the oral and intravenous pharmacokinetics of a high clearance drug: a study with labetalol. Br J Clin Pharmacol 14:73, 1982

139. Daneshmend TK, Roberts CJC: Cimetidine and bioavailability of labetalol (letter). Lancet 1:565, 1981

140. Wood AJ, Ferry DG, Bailey RR: Elimination kinetics of labetalol in severe renal failure. Br J Clin Pharmacol 13 (Suppl):81s, 1982

141. Homeida M, Jackson L, Roberts CJC: Decreased first-pass metabolism of labetalol in chronic liver disease. Br Med J 2:1048, 1978

142. Williams LC, Murphy MJ, Parsons V: Labetalol in severe and resistant hypertension. Br J Clin Pharmacol 8 (Suppl 2):143s, 1979

143. Kelly JG, McGarry K, O'Malley K, O'Brien ET: Bioavailability of labetalol increases with age. Br J Clin Pharmacol 14:304, 1982

144. Woodman TF, Johnson B: High pressure liquid chromatography of labetalol in serum or plasma. Ther Drug Monitor 3:371, 1981

145. Dusci LJ, Hackett JP: Determination of labetalol in human plasma by high-performance liquid chromatography. J Chromatogr 175:208, 1979

146. Brogden RN, Heel RC, Speight TM, Avery GS: Labetalol: A review of its pharmacology and therapeutic uses in hypertension. Drugs 15:251, 1978

147. Prichard BNC, Richards DA: Comparison of labetalol with other antihypertensive drugs. Br J Clin Pharmacol 13 (Suppl 1):41s, 1982

148. Kane JA: Labetalol in general practice. Br J Clin Pharmacol 13 (Suppl 1): 59s, 1982

149. Dargie HJ, Dollery CT, Daniel J: Labetalol in resistant hypertension. Br J Clin Pharmacol 3 (Suppl 3):751, 1976

150. Milne BJ, Logan AG: Labetalol: Potent antihypertensive agent that blocks both α- and β-adrenergic receptors. Can Med Assoc J 123:1013, 1980

151. Davidov ME, Moir GD, Poland MP, et al: Monotherapy with labetalol in the treatment of hypertension. A double-blind study. Am J Med (Suppl):75(4A): 47, 1983

152. Kane J, Gregg I, Richards DA: A double-blind trial of labetalol. Br J Clin Pharmacol 3 (Suppl 3):737, 1976

153. Horvath JS, Caterson RJ, Collett P, et al: Labetalol and bendrofluazide: comparison of their antihypertensive effects. Med J Aust 1:626, 1979

154. Lifshitz AA, McMahon FG, Jain AK, et al: Combined trichlormethiazide and labetalol therapy in moderate to severe hypertension (abstr.). Clin Pharmacol Ther 23:118, 1978

155. Bloomfield S, Sinkfield A, Bichlmeir G, et al: Labetalol with hydrochloro-thiazide for moderate essential hypertension. (Abstr.) Clin Pharmacol Ther 31:204, 1982

156. Lechi A, Pomari S, Berto R, et al: Clinical evaluation of labetalol alone and combined with chlorthalidone in essential hypertension: a double-blind multicentre controlled study. Eur J Clin Pharmacol 22:289, 1982

157. Bloomfield SS, Lucas CP, Gantt CL, et al: Step II treatment with labetalol for essential hypertension. Am J Med (Suppl):75(4A): 81, 1983

158. Prichard BNC, Boakes AJ: Labetalol in long-term treatment of hypertension. Br J Clin Pharmacol 3 (Suppl 3):743, 1976

159. McNeil JJ, Louis WJ: A double-blind crossover comparison of pindolol, metoprolol, atenolol, and labetalol in mild to moderate hypertension. Br J Clin Pharmacol 8 (Suppl 2):163s, 1979

160. Romo M, Halttunen P, Saarinen P, Sarna S: Labetalol and pindolol in the treatment of hypertension: a comparative study. Ann Clin Res 11:249, 1979

161. Pugsley DJ, Nassim M, Armstrong BK, Beilin L: A controlled trial of la-betalol (Trandate), propranolol, and placebo in the management of mild to moderate hypertension. Br J Clin Pharmacol 7:63, 1979

162. Kofod P, Kjaer K, Vejlo S, Hvidt S: Labetalol and alprenolol. A compar-ative investigation of antihypertensive effect. Postgrad Med J 56 (Suppl 2):69, 1980

163. Frishman WH, Michelson EL, Johnson BF, Poland M: A multiclinic com-parison of labetalol to metoprolol in the treatment of mild-moderate sys-temic hypertension. Am J Med (Suppl):75(4A): 54, 1983

164. Bjerle P, Fransson L, Koch G, et al: Pindolol and labetalol in hyperten-sion: Comparison of their antihypertensive effects with particular respect to conditions in the upright posture and during exercise. Curr Ther Rest 27:516, 1980

165. Pugsley DJ, Armstrong BK, Nassim MA, et al: Controlled comparison of labetalol and propranolol in the management of severe hypertension. Br J Clin Pharmacol 3 (Suppl 3):777, 1976

166. Nicholls DP, Husaini MH, Bulpitt CJ, et al: Comparison of labetalol and propranolol in hypertension. Br J Clin Pharmacol 9:233, 1980

167. Barnett AJ, Kalowski S, Guest C: Labetalol compared with pindolol plus hydralazine in the treatment of hypertension. A double-blind crossover study. Med J Aust 65:105, 1978

168. West MJ, Wing LMH, Mulligan J, et al: Comparison of labetalol, hydral-

azine, and propranolol in the therapy of moderate hypertension. Med J Aust 1:224, 1980

169. Van der Veur E, ten Berge BS, Donker AJ, Wesseling H: Comparison of labetalol, propranolol, and hydralazine in hypertensive out-patients. Eur J Clin Pharmacol 21:457, 1982

170. Lehtonen A, Allonen H, Kleimola T: Antihypertensive effect and plasma levels of labetalol. A comparison with propranolol and dihydralazine. Int J Clin Pharmacol Biopharm 17:71, 1979

171. Thibonnier M, Lardoux MD, Corvol P: Comparative trial of labetalol and acebutolol, alone or associated with dihydralazine in treatment of essential hypertension. Br J Clin Pharmacol 9:561, 1980

172. Johnson BF, LaBrooy J, Monroe-Faure AD: Comparative antihypertensive effects of labetalol and the combination of oxprenolol and phentolamine. Br J Clin Pharmacol (Suppl 13):783, 1976

173. MacDonald I, Hua ASP, Thomas GW, et al: Use of labetalol in moderate to severe hypertension. Med J Aust 1:325, 1980

174. Wallin JD, Wilson D, Winer N, et al: Treatment of severe hypertension with labetalol compared to methyldopa and furosemide: Results of a long-term, double-blind, multicenter trial. Am J Med (Suppl):75(4A): 87, 1983

175. Chalmers AG, Hunter J, Lees CD, et al: A comparison and an investigation of a potential synergistic effect of labetalol and bethanidine in patients with mild hypertension. Br J Clin Pharmacol 8 (Suppl 2):183s, 1979

176. Sanders GL, Davies DM, Gales GM, et al: A comparative study of methyldopa and labetalol in the treatment of hypertension. Br J Clin Pharmacol 8:149s, 1979

177. Whiting G, Craswell P, Boyle P, Bett N: Minoxidil and labetalol. Very effective antihypertensive combination. Med J Aust 1:225, 1980

178. Jennings K, Parsons V: A study of labetalol in patients of European, West Indian and West African origin. Br J Clin Pharmacol 3 (Suppl 3):773, 1976

179. Seedat YK: Labetalol in the treatment of Black and Indian hypertensive patients. Med Proc 25:53, 1979

180. Olivier LR, Retief JH, Buchel EH, et al: Evaluation of labetalol hydrochloride (Trandate) in hospital out-patients. Clin Trials J 17:75, 1980

181. Flamenbaum W, McMahon FG, et al: Monotherapy with labetalol compared with propranolol: Differential effects by race. Manuscript submitted for publication.

182. Prichard, BNC, Boakes AJ, Hernandez R: Long-term treatment of hypertension with labetalol. Br J Clin Pharmacol 8 (Suppl 2):171s, 1979

183. Waal-Manning HJ, Simpson FO: Review of long-term treatment with labetalol. Br J Clin Pharmacol 13 (Suppl 1):65s, 1982

184. Ghose RR, Sampson A: Rapid onset of action of oral labetalol in severe hypertension. Curr Med Res Opin 5:147, 1977

185. Davies AB, Bala Subramanian V, Gould B, Raftery EB: Rapid reduction of blood pressure with acute oral labetalol. Br J Clin Pharmacol 13:705, 1982

186. Pearson RM, Griffith DNW, Woollard M, et al: Comparison of effects on

cerebral blood flow of rapid reduction in systemic arterial pressure by diazoxide and labetalol in hypertensive patients: preliminary findings. Br J Clin Pharmacol 8 (Suppl 2):195s, 1979

187. Wilson DJ, Wallin JD, Vlachakis ND, et al: Intravenous labetalol in the treatment of severe hypertension and hypertensive emergencies. Am J Med (Suppl):75(4A): 95, 1983

188. Cumming AMM, Brown JJ, Lever AF, Robertson JI: Intravenous labetalol in treatment of severe hypertension. Br J Clin Pharmacol 13 (Suppl 1):93s, 1982

189. Rumboldt Z, Bagatin J, Vidovic A: Diazoxide vs labetalol: A crossover comparison of short-term effects in hypertension. (Abstr.) Clin Pharmacol Ther 29:278, 1981

190. Papademetriou V, Notargiacomo AV, Khatri IM, et al: Treatment of severe hypertension with intravenous labetalol. Clin Pharmacol Ther 32:431, 1982

191. Dal Palu C, Pessina AC, Semplicini A, et al: Intravenous labetalol in severe hypertension. Br J Clin Pharmacol 13 (Suppl 1):97s, 1982

192. MacCarthy EP, Frost GW, Stokes GS: Labetalol in hypertensive emergencies. Med J Aust 1:399, 1978

193. McGrath BP, Matthews PG, Walter NM, et al: Emergency treatment of severe hypertension with intravenous labetalol. Med J Aust 2:410, 1978

194. Anderson CC, Gabriel R: Poor hypotensive response and tachyphylaxis following intravenous labetalol. Curr Med Res Opin 5:424, 1978

195. Yeung CK, Thomas GW, Whitworth JA, Kincaid-Smith P: Comparison of labetalol, clonidine, and diazoxide intravenously administered in severe hypertension. Med J Aust 2:499, 1979

196. Pearson RM, Havard CWH: Intravenous labetalol in hypertensive patients treated with β-adrenoceptor blocking drugs. Br J Clin Pharmacol 3 (Suppl 3):795, 1976

197. Solomons R: Hemiparesis after single minibolus of labetalol for hypertensive encephalopathy (letter). Br Med J 2:672, 1979

198. Crofton M, Gabriel R: Pressor response after intravenous labetalol. Br Med J 2:737, 1977

199. Bailey RR: Labetalol in the treatment of a patient with phaeochromocytoma: a case report. Br J Clin Pharmacol 8 (Suppl 2):141s, 1979

200. Rosenthal T, Rabinowitz B, Boichis H, et al: Use of labetalol in hypertensive patients during discontinuation of clonidine therapy. Eur J Clin Pharmacol 20:237, 1981

201. Hurley DM, Vandongen R, Beilin LJ: Failure of labetalol to prevent hypertension due to clonidine withdrawal. Br Med J 1:1122, 1979

202. Agabiti Rosei E, Brown JJ, et al: Treatment of phaeochromocytoma and of clonidine withdrawal hypertension with labetalol. Br J Clin Pharmacol 3 (Suppl 3):809, 1976

203. Kaufman L: Use of labetalol during hypotensive anesthesia and in the management of phaeochromocytoma. Br J Clin Pharmacol 8 (Suppl 2):229s, 1979

204. Reach G, Thibonnier M, Chevillard C, et al: Effect of labetalol on blood pressure and plasma catecholamine concentrations in patients with phaeochromocytoma. Br Med J 1:1300, 1980

205. Takeda T, Kaneko Y, Omae T, et al: The use of labetalol in Japan: results of multicentre clinical trials. Br J Clin Pharmacol 13 (Suppl 1):49s, 1982

206. Briggs RSJ, Birtwell AJ, Pohl JEF: Hypertensive response to labetalol in phaeochromocytoma (letter). Lancet 1:1045, 1978.

207. Feek CM, Earnshaw PM: Hypertensive response to labetalol in phaeochromocytoma (letter). Br Med J 2:387, 1980.

208. Starke K, Docherty JR: Types and functions of peripheral α-adrenoceptors. J Cardiovasc Pharmacol 4 (Suppl 1):s3, 1982.

209. Michael CA: Use of labetalol in the treatment of severe hypertension during pregnancy. Br J Clin Pharmacol 8 (Suppl 2):211s, 1979.

210. Riley AJ: Clinical pharmacology of labetalol in pregnancy. J Cardiovasc Pharmacol 3 (Suppl 1):s53, 1981.

211. Coevoet B, Leuliet P, Comoy E: Labetalol for hypertension in pregnancy. Second Congress of the International Society for the Study of Hypertension in Pregnancy, Cairo 1980.

212. Lamming GD, Symonds EM: Use of labetalol and methyldopa in pregnancy-induced hypertension. Br J Clin Pharmacol 8 (Suppl 2):217s, 1979.

213. Lamming GD, Broughton Pipkin F, Symonds EM: Comparison of the alpha and beta-blocking drug, labetalol, and methyldopa in the treatment of moderate and severe pregnancy-induced hypertension. Clin Exp Hypertens 2:865, 1980.

214. Redman CWG: A randomized comparison of methyldopa (Aldomet) and labetalol (Trandate) for the treatment of severe hypertension in pregnancy. (Abstr.) Clin Exp Hypertens B1:345, 1982.

215. Garden A, Davey DA, Dommisse J: Intravenous labetalol and dihydralazine in severe hypertension in pregnancy. Clin Exp Hypertens B1:371, 1982.

216. Walker J, Crooks A, Houston A, et al: Fetal and neonatal cardiovascular effects of maternal labetalol therapy used in the treatment of pregnancy induced hypertension. (Abstr.) Clin Exp Hypertens B1:223, 1982

217. Rotmensch HH, Elkayam U, Frishman W: Antiarrhythmic drug therapy during pregnancy. Ann Intern Med 98:487, 1983

218. Jorge CS: Labetalol in the hypertensive states of pregnancy. I. Emergency treatment of severe hypertension in a pregnant patient. The European Society of Cardiology. Drug Symposium on Labetalol. 1979, p 131

219. Lilford RJ: Letter. Br Med J 281:1635, 1980

220. Lunell NO, Hjemdahl P, Fredholm BB, et al: Circulatory and metabolic effects of a combined α- and β-adrenoceptor blocker (labetalol) in hypertension of pregnancy. Br J Clin Pharmacol 12:345, 1981

221. Silke B, Nelson GI, Ahuja RC, Taylor SH: Comparative haemodynamic dose response effects of propranolol and labetalol in coronary heart disease. Br Heart J 48:364, 1982

222. Boakes AJ, Prichard BNC: The effect of AH 5158, pindolol, propranolol,

d-propranolol on acute exercise tolerance in angina pectoris. (Abstr.) Br J Pharmacol 47:673P, 1973.

223. Condorelli M, Brevetti G, Chiarello M, et al: Effects of combined α- and β-blockade by labetalol in patients with coronary artery disease. Br J Clin Pharmacol 13 (Suppl 1):101s, 1982.

224. Lubbe WF, White DA: Labetalol in hypertensive patients with angina pectoris: Beneficial effect of combined α- and β-adrenoceptor blockade. Clin Sci Mol Med 55:283s, 1978.

225. Besterman EMM, Spencer M: Open evaluation of labetalol in the treatment of angina pectoris occurring in hypertensive patients. Br J Clin Pharmacol 8 (Suppl 2):205s, 1979.

226. Nyberg G, Bjuro, Hagman M, Smith U: Relation between ST-depression and chest pain in patients with coronary heart disease receiving no treatment and after β-blockade and combined α–β-blockade. Acta Med Scand (Suppl 644):30, 1981.

227. Prichard BNC, Walden RJ: The syndrome associated with the withdrawal of β-adrenergic receptor blocking drugs. Br J Clin Pharmacol 13 (Suppl 2):337s, 1982.

228. Marx PG, Reid DS: Labetalol infusion in acute myocardial infarction with systemic hypertension. Br J Clin Pharmacol 8 (Suppl 2):233s, 1979.

229. Timmis AD, Fowler MB, Jaggarao NSV, et al: Role of labetalol in acute myocardial infarction. Br J Clin Pharmacol 13 (Suppl 1):111s, 1982.

230. Scott DB: The use of labetalol in anesthesia. Br J Clin Pharmacol 13 (Suppl 1):133s, 1982.

231. Morel DR, Forster A, Suter PM: Labetalol in the treatment of hypertension following coronary artery surgery. Br J Anaesth 54:1191, 1982.

232. Cope DHP, Crawford MC: Labetalol in controlled hypotension. Administration of labetalol when adequate hypotension is difficult to achieve. Br J Anaesth 51:359, 1979.

233. Jones SEF: Coarctation in children. Controlled hypotension using labetalol and halothane. Anaesthesia 34:1052, 1979.

234. Kanto J, Pakkanen A, Allonen H, et al: The use of labetalol as a moderate hypotensive agent in otological operations—plasma concentrations after intravenous administration. Intl J Clin Pharmacol Ther Toxicol 18:191, 1980.

235. Cope DHP: Use of labetalol during halothane anesthesia. Br J Clin Pharmacol 8 (Suppl 2):223s, 1979.

236. Hunter JM: Synergism between halothane and labetalol. Anesthesia 34:257, 1979.

237. Margaria E, Gagliardi M, Palieri L, et al: Analgesic effect of peridural labetalol in the treatment of cancer pain. Int J Clin Pharmacol Ther Toxicol 21:47, 1983.

238. Gange RW, Wilson Jones E: Bullous lichen planus caused by labetalol. Br Med J 1:816, 1978.

239. Finlay AY, Waddington E: Cutaneous reactions to labetalol. (Letter.) Br Med J 1:987, 1978.

240. Branford WA, Hunter JAA, Muir AL: Cutaneous reaction to labetalol. Practitioner 221:765, 1978
241. Kristensen BO: Labetalol-induced Peyronie's disease? Acta Med Scand 206:511, 1979
242. Griffiths ID, Richardson J: Lupus-type illness associated with labetalol. Br Med J 2:496, 1979
243. Stevenson CJ: Antimitochondrial antibodies associated with labetalol. Lancet 2:924, 1980
244. Wilson JD, Booth RJ, Bullock JY, Campbell DG: Antimitochondrial antibodies associated with labetalol. Lancet 2:312, 1980

PART TWO

β-Blockers in Ischemic Heart Disease

CHAPTER 8

β-Adrenergic Blocking Drugs in Ischemic Heart Disease

William H. Frishman

Ischemic heart disease is the most serious health problem of contemporary Western society. In the United States, more than 675,000 patients die each year from complications of ischemic heart disease. Approximately 1.3 million have a myocardial infarction, and many more suffer from angina pectoris and congestive heart failure secondary to ischemic myocardial damage.[1] β-Adrenergic blockers were introduced over 20 years ago for the treatment of angina pectoris[2] and recently have been demonstrated to reduce the risk of mortality and nonfatal reinfarction in survivors of acute myocardial infarction.[3] The antiischemic effects of β-adrenergic blockers are most likely contributory to their observed benefits in these disorders. In this presentation, the current concepts regarding the pathophysiology of myocardial ischemia are reviewed and the mechanisms by which β-adrenergic blockers are thought to modify and relieve ischemia are discussed.

PATHOPHYSIOLOGY OF MYOCARDIAL ISCHEMIA

Under normal circumstances, an increase in oxygen demand is followed, through a process of local autoregulation,[4] by increased coronary blood flow and, with it, increased oxygen supply. In patients with restricted

From Circulation, Volume 67 (Supplement I), June 1983, pp 11–18, by permission of The American Heart Assoc, Inc.

coronary flow, increases in the determinants of myocardial oxygen demand cannot be met with increased supply. The basis of myocardial ischemia is the loss of this balance between oxygen requirements and oxygen supply to the heart (Fig. 1).[1,4]

Determinants of Myocardial Oxygen Needs

Myocardial oxygen needs are determined by many factors of varied importance.[5,6] Of lesser quantitative importance are the basal metabolism of the myocardium, external contractile element work, and the activation energy required for depolarization and electromechanical coupling.[5,6] Myocardial oxygen consumption is also influenced by the metabolic substrate available to the heart for use in energy production and by transmembrane calcium fluxes.[7]

Probably the most important hemodynamic factor determining myocardial oxygen consumption is tension development, which is determined by the product of systolic pressure and ventricular volume (La Place phenomenon).[4] Almost as important is the heart rate, which also enters the supply part of the supply–demand equation by setting the time for coronary flow to occur (Fig. 2). Contractility is much less important, and its role can be unpredictable when changes in heart size significantly alter wall tension. These hemodynamic factors are greatly influenced by the activity of the sympathetic nervous system. For example, with exercise, sympathetic tone is enhanced and leads to an increase in heart rate, contractility and blood pressure. All of these factors lead to an increase in the oxygen needs of the heart.[8] These hemodynamic changes enable augmented cardiac performance during exer-

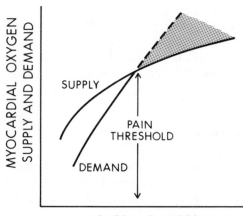

Figure 1. Basis of myocardial ischemia—loss of the balance between oxygen requirements and oxygen supply to the heart.

BALANCE BETWEEN OXYGEN REQUIREMENTS
AND SUPPLY

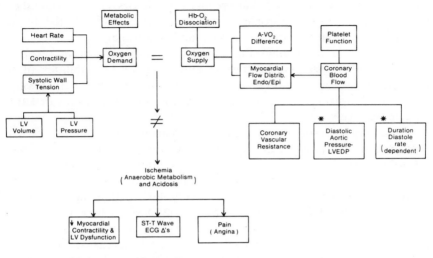

* Limiting only in presence of coronary obstruction

Figure 2. Balance between oxygen requirements and supply.

cise in normal persons but may be detrimental in the presence of coronary artery disease because the increased oxygen demand may outstrip the available supply, leading to myocardial ischemia.[8]

Determinants of Myocardial Oxygen Supply—Coronary Blood Flow
Myocardial oxygen supply depends directly on coronary blood flow, because the heart maximally extracts oxygen from the blood flowing through it.[1,4,7] The most important metabolic determinant of coronary blood flow is myocardial oxygen demand.[9] As demand is increased, adenosine is released and dilates the coronary arteries appropriate to the increased needs of the heart. The coronary circulation can autoregulate its flow over a wide range in response to changes in myocardial oxygen demand. Although adenosine has been identified as the primary mediator of this autoregulatory functioning, other hormonal factors have also been suggested.[9,10]

Vascular tone is being studied as a potential determinant of coronary blood flow, specifically, as the back pressure to coronary flow.[9] The major drop in arterial pressure occurs at the arteriolar level, which probably represents the major site for regulating vascular tone and coronary resistance. However, in some situations, spasm occurs in large epicardial vessels and can markedly diminish coronary blood flow.[9,10]

Superimposed on these autoregulatory factors is the sympathetic nervous system.[9] The coronary arteries are richly innervated by adrenergic nerve endings and contain α_1- and β_1-adrenergic receptors. The neurotransmitter norepinephrine stimulates the α-constrictor receptors and can slightly modify the normal autoregulatory capabilities of the vessels. The precise importance of this superimposed adrenergic tone is uncertain, but it may be of significance in the presence of elevated catecholamine levels.[9,10]

The major coronary arteries are primarily epicardial vessels that send penetrating arteries through the myocardium and end in a subendocardial complex. When there is a substantial obstruction of a large coronary artery by an atheroma or spasm, reduced flow will occur.[4] Since endocardial wall stress is relatively higher than epicardial wall stress, the subendocardium is at greatest jeopardy when blood flow is reduced.[1,4,9] The percent reduction in maximum coronary flow becomes more important as myocardial oxygen demand increases. Conversely, reduction of oxygen demand lessens the impact of coronary artery stenosis.[4]

With a major coronary vessel obstruction, dilation of the peripheral vascular bed occurs and local autoregulatory controls are lost.[4] At that point, the severity and extent of the coronary artery pathology and other mechanical factors become the primary determinants of coronary blood flow to the affected region (Fig. 2). One of these mechanical factors is the pressure gradient, which forces blood into the heart during diastole, when most coronary blood flow occurs. This pressure gradient is related to the difference between diastolic aortic pressure and the filling pressure in the left ventricle. In the normal heart, a coronary perfusion pressure of approximately 60 mm Hg and above is required to maintain appropriate flow to meet myocardial oxygen needs.[9,11] In patients who have coronary artery disease with relatively low diastolic aortic pressures, increasing aortic pressure can increase perfusion pressure and coronary artery supply. However, marked increases in aortic pressure may increase myocardial oxygen demand more than supply and may be deleterious.

Another major physical factor that determines coronary blood flow is the time in diastole when flow can occur. The diastolic time for coronary blood flow is inversely related to the heart rate, and when tachycardia occurs the diastolic time is seriously reduced.[4] In addition, variable amounts of smooth-muscle spasm in the large arterial walls may occur over partially obstructed atheromatous lesions, further reducing coronary blood flow.[10] Flow from collateral vessels may augment compromised coronary flow distal to the obstruction.[4] An important goal of any antiischemic drug therapy is to preserve or increase the flow from collateral vessels to the ischemic region.

Other Factors Possibly Contributing to Myocardial Ischemia

Platelet Function. Heightened platelet activity has been described in patients with coronary and cerebral vascular diseases[12-14] and in conditions associated with ischemic heart disease, such as diabetes mellitus,[15] hyperlipidemia,[16] cigarette smoking, and hypertension.[17] Therefore, platelets may have an important role in acute and chronic cardiovascular events.[18] Myocardial ischemia may result during the sequence of platelet activation, reactions of adhesion, aggregate formation, release of granular constituents, microembolization and local thromboxane A_2-induced vasospasm. If the microemboli disaggregate and the vasospasm is transient, only angina pectoris may be manifest. However, myocardial infarction may follow extensive permanent occlusion or localized narrowing by vasospasm of small vessels and extension of platelet thrombus formation at the site of intimal thickening.[18] Sudden death may occur if the platelet vascular occlusions lead to significant ventricular arrhythmias. Direct experimental and indirect clinical studies support the concept that platelets are important in ischemic cardiovascular events, but the exact relationship of heightened platelet activity to coronary spasm and to other ischemic events is unclear.[18-21] The hypothesized importance of platelets in the pathogenesis of ischemic heart disease has stimulated interest in drugs that modify platelet behavior.[22]

Oxyhemoglobin Equilibrium Curve. Alterations in the oxyhemoglobin equilibrium curve may also influence oxygen supply to the myocardium. Decreased hemoglobin affinity for oxygen, reflected in a rightward shift in the oxyhemoglobin equilibrium curve, results in increased oxygen delivery to tissues.[23] Increased erythrocyte 2,3-diphosphoglycerate is one means by which the oxyhemoglobin equilibrium curve is shifted to the right. Decreased hemoglobin affinity for oxygen would permit increased oxygen delivery to the myocardium compromised by inadequate coronary perfusion and benefit the ischemic state. On the other hand, physiologic variables that shift the oxyhemoglobin equilibrium curve to the left would increase the affinity of hemoglobin for oxygen and reduce tissue oxygen delivery, aggravating myocardial ischemia.

The Ischemic State

When myocardial ischemia occurs because of supply–demand imbalances, the heart shifts from normal aerobic metabolism to anaerobic metabolism, resulting in incomplete oxidation of substrate, with local production of lactic acid and development of acidosis.[4,7] Once blood flow is limited, the supply is reduced to a greater extent in the subendocardium.[4] Ischemia, therefore, develops first in the subendocardium and with increasing demand or decreasing supply of oxygen, extends out to the epicardium. The segment of myocardium involved is determined by the distribution of flow from the primary vessel, whereas the intensity of the ischemia is determined by the relative disproportion of demand and supply of oxygen. When the ischemic state occurs in the myocardium, it may result in pain, which may be variable in nature, very rapid failure of myocardial contraction, which is segmental, impaired ventricular relaxation with diastolic stiffness, and localized changes in the ECG, characterized by shifts in the ST segment (Fig. 2).[1,4] The major goal of antiischemic therapy is to prevent or reverse this pathologic process and to protect the patient from irreversible or fatal myocardial injury.

β-ADRENERGIC BLOCKERS IN ISCHEMIC HEART DISEASE

The findings that the relative potency of a series of sympathomimetic amines varied with the effector organs or systems led Ahlquist,[24] in 1948, to conclude that there were two types of adrenergic receptors, which he classified as α and β. Ten years later, Black searched for an antianginal compound that could improve myocardial ischemia by reducing the effects of sympathetic nervous stimulation on the heart. The discovery and clinical application of β-adrenoceptor antagonists by Black and others gave strong support to Ahlquist's initial hypothesis and initiated one of the most important advances in the pharmacotherapy of ischemic heart disease.[2,25]

Although β-blockers were initially intended as treatment for symptomatic angina pectoris of effort,[8] it soon became clear that they had much to offer as therapies for other myocardial ischemic disorders, including the "intermediate" syndrome and myocardial infarction, and for long-term antiischemic prophylaxis.[3,8] As a class, the β-adrenergic blockers have been so successful that scores of them have been synthesized. The application of these agents has been accelerated by the development of drugs that possess a degree of selectivity for the two subgroups of the β-adrenoceptor population: β_1 receptors in the heart and β_2 receptors in the peripheral circulation and bronchi.[2,8] More controversial has been the introduction of β-blocking agents with α-adrenergic blocking properties, varying degrees of intrinsic sympathomimetic activity (partial angonist effect), and nonspecific membrane-stabilizing action.[2,8,25–29]

β-Adrenergic blockers are competitive inhibitors of catecholamine binding at β-adrenoceptor sites. They reduce the effect of any concentration of a catecholamine agonist on a sensitive tissue.[2,25] The dose–response curve of the agonist is shifted to the right; a given tissue response then requires a higher concentration of the agonist in the presence of a β-blocking drug. Despite extensive experience with the β-blockers inside and outside of the United States, no clinical studies suggest that any one of these drugs has major advantages or disadvantages over any other in the treatment of arrhythmia, hypertension, and angina pectoris.[8,25] However, one β-blocking drug may be better than another with regard to inducing fewer side effects in certain patients and in specific clinical situations.[25,30]

The Effects of β-Blockers on Determinants of Myocardial Oxygen Consumption

β-Blockers may be expected to protect the heart from the deleterious effects of physiologic or psychologic stresses.[8] By reducing catecholamine-induced increments in heart rate, velocity, and extent of myocardial contraction, and blood pressure, β-blockers reduce the oxygen requirements of the heart at any level of activity (Fig. 3). These pharmacologic effects are especially important for reducing or preventing ischemia in patients with compromised coronary blood flow.

The β_1-receptors in the heart mediate increases in both heart rate and contractility and are blocked by both β_1-selective and nonselective β-blockers.[8] Thus, β-blockers frequently cause reductions in the resting heart rate, although their most beneficial effect in relieving angina may be by blunting the heart rate response to exercise. This fact is exemplified by the newer β-blockers that have intrinsic sympathomimetic activity (partial agonist activity).[8,29] These drugs have little or no effect on resting heart rate and, therefore, are probably less useful for angina at rest.[31] However, they do limit the heart rate response to exercise and are effective in exercise-induced angina pectoris.

The direct effects of β-blockers on myocardial contractility are probably minimal. Since the β-blockers interfere with the actions of catecholamines, they have their greatest effect on exercise-induced increments in contractility.[8] This effect on contractility will reduce myo-

EFFECTS OF β- BLOCKERS

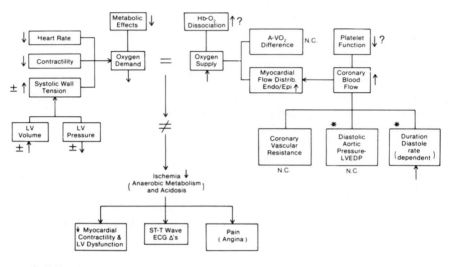

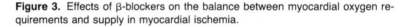

❋ *Limiting only in presence of coronary obstruction*

Figure 3. Effects of β-blockers on the balance between myocardial oxygen requirements and supply in myocardial ischemia.

cardial oxygen demand and may be beneficial in patients with angina pectoris. By reducing heart rate and contractility, β-blockers lead to a reduction in cardiac output both at rest and during exercise. These effects may limit the increase in exercise tolerance seen in patients receiving these drugs.

β-Blockers are effective in reducing left ventricular wall tension because of their ability to reduce systolic blood pressure while having minimal effects on heart size in normal subjects. However, in patients with overt heart failure, they can increase the heart size by blocking the sympathetic tone to the heart, which is necessary for cardiac compensation.[8,25] By increasing left ventricular fiber length and end-diastolic pressure in heart failure, myocardial oxygen requirements may be increased.[8] At the same time, increments in left ventricular end-diastolic pressure may compromise an already limited subendocardial blood flow.[8,32]

In some patients with intrinsic conduction disease of the heart, cardiac impulse formation may be impaired by β-blockade and atrioventricular conduction diminished to a degree that causes cardiac arrest.[30,32]

In general, β-blockers should be avoided in patients with myocardial failure and intrinsic sinus node and atrioventricular conduction disease, who may be dependent on sympathetic tone to maintain their left ventricular integrity and heart rhythm.[25] Whether the new β-blockers with intrinsic sympathomimetic activity or α-blocking activity are useful in these situations has yet to be determined.[28,29]

Effects on Coronary Blood Flow

The effects of β-blocking drugs on coronary blood flow are not well defined. The reduction in myocardial oxygen demands with β-blockade leads to an increase in coronary vascular resistance through metabolic autoregulation. This increase in coronary resistance may not be detrimental. Rather, it reflects the autoregulatory response of the coronary circulation to a reduction in myocardial oxygen demands.[9] In patients prone to coronary spasm (angina at rest or variant angina), increased myocardial ischemia and symptoms may occur when β-blockers are given, resulting from[10,33] unopposed α and other vasoconstrictive influences can lead to increased spasm.[9,10,33–35] However, since the coronary circulation in most humans is influenced more by local autoregulatory stimuli than by adrenergic tone,[9] the potentially harmful effects of β-adrenergic blockade in most patients with ischemic heart disease are probably minimal.

There is also evidence to suggest that coronary blood flow may be augmented, or at least maintained, by β-blockade. By reducing the heart rate at rest and with exercise, the diastolic time for coronary perfusion to occur will increase (Fig. 3).[4,36] In experimental studies, some β-blockers have improved collateral blood flow and caused a favorable redistribution of blood flow favoring the ischemic subendocardium.[37–40] Other investigators have not been able to reproduce these findings.[41] The marked differences in total and regional coronary blood flow seen experimentally with different β-blockers may be accounted for, in part, by the other pharmacologic properties of these drugs: $β_1$-selectivity, intrinsic sympathomimetic activity, and α-adrenergic blocking properties.[40] The actual effects of β-adrenergic blockade on the coronary collaterals and regional blood flow in humans has not been determined.

Overall, except for the patients with rest angina who are prone to coronary vasospasm, β-blockers have beneficial effects on coronary blood flow relative to the reduction in myocardial oxygen consumption in patients with obstructive coronary artery disease. Thus, these drugs appear to favorably affect both the supply and demand sides of the supply-demand equation.

Effects on Myocardial Substrate Utilization

β-Blockers can also reduce oxygen demands and ischemia by altering the metabolic substrate utilized by the heart.[42] During myocardial infarction, adrenergic activity stimulates lipolysis, resulting in increased circulating free fatty acids. This, in turn, may augment free fatty acid uptake by the heart, which increases myocardial oxygen consumption and the risk of malignant arrhythmias.[1,7,42,43] During experimental myocardial infarction, β-adrenergic blockers decrease lipolysis and myocardial free fatty acid uptake, thereby shifting the utilization of myocardial substrate from fatty acids to glucose.[42,43] Moreover, β-blockers may decrease glycogenolysis.[42] In patients with acute myocardial infarction, Mueller et al.[43] found that propranolol shifted myocardial metabolism from free fatty acids to carbohydrates and decreased myocardial oxygen consumption, while causing lactate production to revert to extraction. The degree to which alterations in myocardial metabolism contribute to the beneficial effects of β-adrenergic blocking drugs in human ischemic heart disease is not known.

Effects on Platelets

The effects of β-blockers on platelets are described in Chapter 10.

Propranolol, when added to normal platelets in vitro, inhibits platelet aggregation induced by ADP, epinephrine, collagen, thrombin, and the inophore A23187.[44,45] The drug affects mainly the secondary phase of aggregation and serotonin release but has little effect on primary aggregation. Platelet adhesion to collagen and the availability of platelet factor 3 are also inhibited by the drug. In vitro measurements of platelet activity in peripheral venous and coronary sinus blood have shown that therapeutic doses of propranolol can normalize the heightened platelet aggregability in patients with angina pectoris and can also inhibit thromboxane A_2 release.[12,13,46] Platelets return to their hyperaggregable state after treatment withdrawal.[12,47] In vivo experiments in rats showed that propranolol prevented isoproterenol and stress-induced platelet aggregation in the microcirculation.[22]

In in vitro experimental studies, platelets accumulate 14C-propranolol 10- to 30-fold over plasma drug concentrations.[44,45] Preferential accumulation of the drug by platelets in vivo may relate to its high degree of lipid solubility, accounting for altered platelet responsiveness at the therapeutic plasma–propranolol concentrations measured in vivo.[44,45]

Several lines of evidence suggest that propranolol alters platelet behavior through mechanisms other than β-adrenergic blockade. First, only α-adrenergic receptors are found on platelet membranes.[48] Second, platelet aggregation in vitro is inhibited to the same extent by both optical isomers of propranolol although the levorotatory stereoisomer has 100 times the β-blocking potency of the dextrorotatory isomer.[25] Third, some β-blockers have no effects on platelet aggregation.[44,45] The nonspecific membrane effect of propranolol, rather than its β-adrenergic blocking property, apparently contributes to the drug's antiplatelet activity. In vitro platelet studies in normal subjects have shown that propranolol binds to platelets and renders the platelet membrane less sensitive to the actions of aggregating substances. The clinical importance of the antiplatelet activity of propranolol has not been determined.

Effects on the Oxyhemoglobin Equilibrium Curve

Propranolol, when added to a red cell suspension, has a direct effect on the cell membrane, leading to an altered Gibbs–Donnan equilibrium and a decrease in intraerythrocyte pH.[49,50] By the classic Bohr effect, this could result in a shift of the oxyhemoglobin equilibrium to the right, apparently without a quantitative change in total 2,3-diphosphoglycerate. Oski et al.[51] found that approximately 30 percent of 2,3-diphosphoglycerate may be normally bound to red cell membranes, and therefore may be incapable of binding to deoxyhemoglobin. They reported that propranolol administration in vitro released membrane-bound 2,3-diphosphoglycerate. This, they postulated, then combined with deoxyhemoglobin and decreased the affinity of hemoglobin for oxygen.

Not all reported data confirm a shift to the right of the oxyhemoglobin dissociation curve with propranolol. Lichtman et al.[52] concluded, on the basis of studies in six normal subjects and two patients with coronary artery disease, that propranolol had no significant effects on P_{50}. Frishman et al.,[53,54] in a placebo-controlled, double-blind study of 19 patients with angina pectoris and coronary artery disease, found no effects of propranolol on P_{50} or 2,3-diphosphoglycerate when measured at rest or during exercise. Thus, it is still unresolved whether the antiischemic effect of β-adrenergic blockers is accounted for, in part, by alterations in the oxyhemoglobin equilibrium curve.

Effects on the Microvasculature

Using colloidal carbon black as a marker, Kloner et al.[55] demonstrated that propranolol reduced ischemic microvascular damage during experimental myocardial infarction in dogs. This marker, which identifies damage to vessels, was injected intravenously 5 minutes after release of a 1-hour coronary occlusion in control and in propranolol-treated dogs. The intravascular carbon was allowed to circulate for 2 hours, during which time it is normally cleared by the reticuloendothial system unless it is retained by damaged vessels. Significantly fewer vessels labeled by carbon black were found in propranolol-treated groups, suggesting decreased microvascular injury. However, since significant microvascular damage occurs only after myocardial cell injury, it appears unlikely that propranolol's primary action is through protection of the microvasculature.

Other Actions of β-Adrenergic Blockade

All β-blockers exert a powerful suppressive effect on plasma renin secretion both at rest and during stress activation. Owing to the attendant aldosterone-lowering effect, β-blockers slightly improve plasma potassium and may protect patients with myocardial ischemia from the dangers of hypokalemia.[56]

Welman and co-workers[57] showed that low plasma concentrations for propranolol (0.1 mg/ml/cell) can stabilize cardiac lysosomal membranes in the presence of acute anoxia. In a subsequent study, they found that patients on long-term propranolol therapy have a delayed release of plasma lysosomal and cytosolic enzymes after an acute myocardial infarction.[58] These changes may lead to a reduction in electrical instability and myocardial injury.

Finally, serious questions have been raised as to whether long-term β-blocker use in ischemic heart disease might accelerate atherosclerosis by reducing plasma high-density lipoprotein levels and increasing triglycerides.[54-61] Although this issue needs further clarification, especially if β-blockers are to be considered for long-term use in patients with ischemic heart disease, recent data suggest that some of these drugs have no detrimental effects on plasma lipids.[62]

CLINICAL APPLICATIONS

The beneficial effects of β-adrenergic blockers on the myocardial supply–demand relationship have had a great impact on the therapy of many ischemic heart disease syndromes. Ninety percent of patients with angina pectoris resulting from obstructive coronary artery disease demonstrate improved exercise tolerance and a reduced chest pain with β-blocker therapy.[8] With increased exercise capabilities, the secondary benefit of training can be obtained in some patients. This result may allow even greater increments in exercise performance for a given degree of ischemic heart disease. β-Blockers have also been used in patients with "intermediate" syndromes in combination with nitrates and calcium-entry blockers, in part to prevent the undesirable consequences of increased sympathetic tone seen with the latter agents.[32]

The antiischemic effects of β-blockers can best explain their effi-

cacy in reducing the risks of cardiovascular mortality and nonfatal reinfarction in patients who survive an acute myocardial infarction.[3] The use
of β-adrenoceptor blockade in the early stage of acute myocardial infarction may also be beneficial in salvaging jeopardized tissue and improving immediate mortality and long-term ventricular function.[63] The
value of β-adrenergic blocker therapy within 6 to 12 hours of myocardial infarction in humans is being addressed in four cooperative acute-
phase trials being carried out in Europe and the United States.[3] Whether
β-blockers protect patients with occult or symptomatic ischemic heart
disease from their first myocardial infarction has yet to be determined.

REFERENCES

1. Hillis LD, Braunwald E: Myocardial ischemia. N Engl J Med 296:971, 1034, 1093, 1977.
2. Frishman WH: Clinical pharmacology of the new β-adrenergic blocking drugs. 1. Pharmacodynamic and pharmacokinetic properties. Am Heart J 97:663, 1979.
3. Braunwald E, Muller JE, Kloner R, Maroko PR: Role of beta-blockade in the therapy of patients with myocardial infarction. Am J Med 74:113, 1983.
4. Kirk ES, Sonnenblick EH: Newer concepts in the pathophysiology of is-chemic heart disease. Am Heart J 103:756, 1982.
5. Sonnenblick EH, Ross J Jr, Braunwald E: Oxygen consumption of the heart. Newer aspects of its multifactorial determination. Am J Cardiol 22:328, 1968.
6. Sonnenblick EH, Skelton CL: Myocardial energetics. Basic principles and clinical implications. N Engl J Med 285:668, 1971.
7. Opie LH: Myocardial infarct size. Part 1. Basic considerations. Am Heart J 100:355, 1980.
8. Frishman WH, Silverman R: Clinical pharmacology of the new β-adrener-gic blocking drugs. Part 2. Physiologic and metabolic effects. Am Heart J 97:797, 1979.
9. Rubio R, Berne R: Regulation of coronary blood flow. Prog Cardiovasc Dis 18:105, 1975.
10. Maseri A, Chierchia S: Coronary artery spasm: demonstration, definition, diagnosis and consequences. Prog Cardiovasc Dis 25:169, 1982.
11. Stowe DF, Mathey DG, Moores WY, et al: Segment stroke and metabolism depends on coronary blood flow in the pig. Am J Physiol 234:H597, 1978.
12. Frishman WH, Weksler B, Christodoulou J, et al: Reversal of abnormal platelet aggregability and change in exercise tolerance in patients with an-gina pectoris following oral propranolol. Circulation 50:887,1974.
13. Mehta J, Mehta P, Pepine C: Differences in platelet aggregation in coronary artery sinus and aortic blood in patients with coronary artery disease: effect of propranolol. Clin Cardiol 1:96,1978.

14. Walsh PN, Pareti FI, Corbett JJ: Platelet coagulant activities and serum lipids in transient cerebral ischemia. N Engl J Med 295:854, 1976.

15. Kwaan HC, Colwell JA, Cruz S, et al: Increased platelet aggregation in diabetes mellitus. J Lab Clin Med 80:236, 1972.

16. Carvalho AC, Colman RW, Lees R: Platelet function in hyperlipidemia. N Engl J Med 290:434, 1974.

17. Poplawski A, Skorolska M, Niewiarowski S: Increased platelet adhesiveness in hypertensive cardiovascular disease. J Atheroscler Res 8:721, 1968.

18. Harker LA, Ritchie JL: The role of platelets in acute vascular events. Circulation 62 (Suppl V):V-13, 1980.

19. Jorgensen L, Roswell HC, Hovig T, et al: Adenosine diphosphate induced platelet aggregation and myocardial infarction in swine. Lab Invest 17:616, 1967.

20. Haft JI, Gershengorn K, Kranz PD, Oestreicher R: Protection against epinephrine-induced myocardial necrosis by drugs that inhibit platelet aggregation. Am J Cardiol 30:838, 1972.

21. Folts J, Gallagher K, Rowe GG: Blood flow reductions in stenosed canine coronary arteries: vasospasm or platelet aggregation? Circulation 65:248, 1982.

22. Haft J: Role of blood platelets in coronary artery disease. Am J Cardiol 43:1197, 1979.

23. Schrumph J, Sheps DS, Wolfson S, et al: Altered hemoglobin-oxygen affinity with long-term propranolol therapy in patients with coronary artery disease. Am J Cardiol 40:76, 1977.

24. Ahlquist RP: A study of the adrenotropic receptors. Am J Physiol 153:586, 1948.

25. Frishman WH: β-adrenoceptor antagonists—new drugs and new indications. N Engl J Med 305:500, 1981.

26. Frishman WH: Nadolol—a new β-adrenoceptor antagonist. N Engl J Med 305:678, 1981.

27. Frishman WH: Atenolol and timolol—two new orally active β-adrenoceptor antagonists. N Engl J Med 306:1456, 1982.

28. Frishman WH, Halprin S: Clinical pharmacology of the new β-adrenergic blocking drugs. 7. New horizons in β-adrenoceptor blocking therapy: labetalol. Am Heart J 98:660, 1979.

29. Frishman WH: Pindolol: a new β-adrenoceptor antagonist with partial agonist activity. N Engl J Med 308:940, 1983.

30. Frishman WH, Silverman R, Strom J, et al: Clinical pharmacology of the new β-adrenergic blocking drugs. 4. Adverse Effects. Choosing a β-adrenoceptor blocker: Am Heart J 98:256, 1979.

31. Kostis J, Frishman W, Hossler MH, et al: Treatment of angina pectoris with pindolol: the significance of intrinsic sympathomimetic activity of beta-blockers. Am Heart J 104:491, 1982.

32. Frishman WH: Clinical pharmacology of the new β-adrenoceptor blocking drugs. Part 12. Beta-adrenoceptor blockade in myocardial infarction: the continuing controversy. Am Heart J 99:528, 1980.

33. Parodi A, Simonetti I, L'Abbate A, Maseri A: Verapamil vs propranolol for angina at rest. Am J Cardiol 50:923, 1982.
34. Downey JM: An evaluation of the coronary constriction following propranolol. Eur J Pharmacol 46:119, 1977.
35. Gunther S, Muller J, Mudge GH, Grossman W: Therapy of coronary vasoconstriction in patients with coronary artery disease. Am J Cardiol 47:157, 1981.
36. Boudoulas H, Lewis RP, Rittgers SE, et al: Increased diastolic time: a possible important factor in the beneficial effect of propranolol in patients with coronary artery disease. J Cardiovasc Pharmacol 1:503, 1979.
37. Becker LC, Fortuin NJ, Pitt B: Effect of ischemia and antianginal drugs on the distribution of radioactive microspheres in the canine left ventricle. Circ Res 28:263, 1971.
38. Vatner SF, Baig H, Manders WT, Ochs H: Effects of propranolol on regional myocardial function, electrograms, and blood flow in conscious dogs with myocardial ischemia. J Clin Invest 60:353, 1977.
39. Vatner SF, Baig H, Manders WT, Murray PA: Effects of cardiac glycosides in combination with propranolol on the ischemic heart of conscious dogs. Circulation 57:568, 1978.
40. Berdeaux A, Guidicelli JF: Intrinsic sympathomimetic activity and coronary blood flow. Br J Clin Pharmacol 13:175s, 1982.
41. Kloner RA, Reimer K, Jennings R: Distribution of coronary collateral flow in acute myocardial ischemic injury: effect of propranolol. Cardiovasc Res 10:81, 1976.
42. Kjekshus JK, Mjos OD: Effect of inhibition of lipolysis on infarct size after experimental coronary occlusion. J Clin Invest 52:1770, 1973.
43. Mueller HS, Aryes SM, Religa A, Evans RG: Propranolol in the treatment of acute myocardial infarction: effect on myocardial oxygenation and hemodynamics. Circulation 49:1078, 1974.
44. Weksler B, Gillick M, Pink J: Effect of propranolol on platelet function. Blood 49:185, 1977.
45. Frishman WH, Weksler BB: Effects of β-adrenoceptor blocking drugs on platelet function in normal subjects and patients with angina pectoris. In Advances in β-blocker Therapy: Proceedings of an International Symposium, edited by Roskamm H, Graefe KH. Amsterdam, Excerpta Medica, 1980, p. 165.
46. Tai E, Berezow J, Weksler B, et al: Comparative effects of oral verapamil and propranolol on platelet activation in angina pectoris: a placebo-controlled double-blind crossover study. (abstr) Circulation 66 (Suppl II): II-322, 1982.
47. Frishman WH, Christodoulou J, Weklser B, et al: Abrupt propranolol withdrawal in angina pectoris: effects on platelet aggregation and exercise tolerance. Am Heart J 95:169, 1978.
48. Lefkowitz R: Identification of α-drenergic receptors in human platelets by ^{3}H dihydroergocryptine binding. J Clin Invest 61:395, 1978.
49. Pendleton R, Newman DJ, Sherman SS, et al: Effect of propranolol upon

the hemoglobin-oxygen dissociation curve. J Pharmacol Exp Ther 180:647, 1972.

50. Manninen B: Movement of sodium and potassium on their tracers in propranolol-treated red cells and diaphragm muscle. Acta Physiol Scand (Suppl 325):1, 1970.

51. Oski F, Miller L, Delivoria-Papadopoulous M, et al: Oxygen affinity in red cells. Changes induced in vivo by propranolol. Science 175:1372, 1972.

52. Lichtman MA, Cohen J, Murphy MS, et al: Effect of propranolol on oxygen binding to hemoglobin in vitro and in vivo. Circulation 49:881, 1974.

53. Frishman WH, Wilner G, Smithen C, et al: Effects of exercise and propranolol on hemoglobin oxygen affinity in patients with angina pectoris. Clin Res 24:614, 1976.

54. Frishman WH, Smithen C, Christodoulou J, et al: Medical management of angina pectoris: multifactorial actions of propranolol. In Coronary Artery Medicine and Surgery: Concepts and Controversies, edited by Norman JC, Cooley D. New York, Appleton Century Crofts, 1975, p 285.

55. Kloner RA, Fishbein MC, Cotran RS, et al: The effect of propranolol on microvascular injury in acute myocardial ischemia. Circulation 55:872, 1977.

56. Buhler FR, Laragh JH, Vaughan ED, et al: Anti-hypertensive action of propranolol. Am J Cardiol 32:511, 1973.

57. Welman E, Fox KM, Selwyn AP, Carroll BJ: The effect of established β-adrenoceptor blocking therapy on the release of cytosolic and lysosomal enzymes after acute myocardial infarction in man. Clin Sci Mol Med 55:549, 1978.

58. Welman E: Stabilization of lysosomes in anoxic myocardium by propranolol. Br J Pharmacol 65:479, 1979.

59. Leren P, Helgeland A, Holme I, et al: Effects of propranolol and prazosin on blood lipids. The Oslo study. Lancet 2:4, 1980.

60. Johnson B: The emerging problem of plasma lipid changes during antihypertensive therapy. J Cardiovasc Pharmacol 4 (Suppl 2):S-213, 1982.

61. Shulman RS, Herbert PN, Capone R, et al: Effects of propranolol on blood lipids and lipoproteins in myocardial infarction. Circulation 67 (Suppl I): I-19, 1983.

62. Frishman W, Michelson E, Johnson B, et al: Effects of beta-adrenergic blockade on plasma lipids: a double-blind, randomized, placebo-controlled, multi-center comparison of labetalol and metoprolol in patients with hypertension. (Abstr) Am J Cardiol 49:984, 1982.

63. Gold HK, Leinbach RC, Maroko PR: Propranolol-induced reduction of signs of ischemic injury during acute myocardial infarction. Am J Cardiol 38:689, 1976.

CHAPTER 9

Effects of β-Adrenoceptor Blocking Agents on Platelet Function

William H. Frishman and Babette B. Weksler

There is increasing evidence to suggest that blood platelets may contribute to the development of occlusive vascular disease both by mechanical obstruction of the microcirculation and by release of vasoactive mediators that affect the blood vessel wall.[1] These vasoactive materials in turn can alter permeability and lead to proliferative changes[2] or to deposition of materials in the vascular wall.[3] The platelets of patients with vascular diseases show increased turnover rates[4-6] and augmented responses to a variety of aggregating substances.[7-10] These observations suggest a pathophysiologic process characterized by increased platelet consumption. Clinical interest has therefore developed in using pharmacologic interventions to control increased platelet reactivity and in the mechanisms by which drugs might normalize platelet function. Our group has demonstrated that platelets from patients with angina pectoris and coronary artery disease have increased aggregability, responses that become normal during propranolol therapy.[9-11] The studies presented here were undertaken to examine the in vitro effects of propranolol upon platelets of normal subjects, and to elucidate the mechanism by which the drug alters platelet responsiveness.[12] The effects of chronic propranolol treatment and its withdrawal on the platelets of patients with angina pectoris were also assessed.[11]

From Advances in β-Blocker Therapy, Proceedings of an International Symposium, 1980, Excerpta Medica, Amsterdam, Oxford, Princeton, pp 164–190, with permission.

MATERIALS AND METHODS

In Vitro Studies in Platelets from Normal Subjects

Blood was drawn from healthy, fasting, normal subjects who had not ingested acetylsalicyclic acid-containing compounds for at least one week. The blood was mixed with 10 volume percent of 3.2 percent sodium citrate in polypropylene tubes and centrifuged at 240 g for 15 minutes at room temperature to yield platelet-rich plasma (PRP). PRP was used at platelet counts of 300,000 to 400,000/μl. Platelet counts were performed with a Coulter County Model ZBI (Coulter Electronics). Washed platelet suspensions were prepared from PRP by the method of Mustard et al.[13] and were used at a concentration of 300,000/μl.

Aggregation Studies. Platelet aggregation was carried out by a modification of the method of Born[14] using a dual-channel Payton aggregation module and Riken-Denshi recorder (Payton Associates). Light transmission was set at zero percent with PRP and 100 percent with platelet-poor plasma. All tests were performed in duplicate. Aggregating agents [adenosine diphosphate (ADP), epinephrine, collagen, and thrombin] were diluted in Tris-buffered saline, pH 7.35. The ionophore A23187 was dissolved in 25 percent dimethyl sulfoxide (DMSO) and 75 percent absolute ethanol and diluted in Tris-saline. The DMSO-ethanol solution at similar dilutions (final concentrations less than 0.1 percent) did not affect platelet function.

The effect of propranolol on the aggregation of platelets was measured by adding propranolol in vitro to a suspension of platelets prior to addition of the threshold concentration of aggregating agent.

The threshold for ADP-induced aggregation was defined as the minimum concentration of ADP producing a biphasic aggregation response that resulted in a final optical density within 10 percent of that of platelet-poor plasma (complete aggregation). The threshold for epinephrine was the minimum concentration that produced a complete biphasic aggregation, even if delayed. The threshold for collagen or thrombin was the minimum concentration producing complete aggregation. All platelet preparations used produced biphasic responses with ADP and epinephrine.

Platelet shape change was assessed visually and by changes in oscillation pattern on the aggregation module recorder.

Serotonin Labeling and Release. ^{14}C-serotonin (as 5-hydroxy-2-^{14}C-tryptamine creatinine sulfate, specific activity 57 mCi/mmol) was incubated with PRP or washed platelet suspensions at a final concentration of 0.45 μmol at 37°C for 15 minutes with gentle shaking. Samples of labeled platelets were stirred with aggregating agents in the aggregation module; aggregation responses were recorded and the cuvettes were rapidly placed in a melting ice bath. The platelets were sedimented by centrifugation at 4°C at 4340 g for 10 minutes. Then 50 μl of supernatant was added to 0.5 ml of 2 N NaOH and 10 ml PCS (liquid scintillation cocktail). Radioactivity was measured in a liquid scintillation counter. Release was expressed as the percentage of total radioactivity in the platelet suspension (radioactivity of supernatant of experimental samples minus radioactivity of control supernatants divided by total radioactivity).

In some experiments platelets were also labeled with ^{3}H-adenine (specific activity 19 Ci/mmol, final concentration 1.06 nmol). The total ^{3}H count in the supernatant of experimental samples was measured and corrected for residual counts in control supernatants.

Uptake of Propranolol. PRP or washed platelets were incubated with ^{14}C-propranolol (5.42 mCi/mmol) at concentrations of 0.1 to 10×10^{-6} mol for up to 15 minutes at 0, 25, or 37°C. In PRP studies, 0.8 mg/ml ^{3}H-insulin (175 μCi/mg), which is not taken up by platelets, was included as a plasma marker. The platelets were sedimented by centrifugation through silicone oil for 2 minutes at 8000 g. Supernatant radioactivity was measured as described. The platelet pellets were dissolved overnight in 0.5 ml NCS (tissue solubilizer) and the entire pellet counted in PCS scintillant. In calculating the ^{14}C-propranolol associated with the platelets, a correction was made for trapped plasma in the platelet pellet using the ^{3}H-inulin counts in the pellet.

Platelet subcellular fractionation following incubation of washed platelets with 5×10^{-5} mol of ^{14}C-propranolol was carried out by the method of Marcus et al.[15]

Uptake of ^{45} CaCl$_2$. Washed platelets were incubated for 5 to 15 minutes at 37°C with a final concentration of 3.9 μmol ^{45}CaCl$_2$ (29.1 mCi/mg Ca) in 2 mmol unlabeled CaCl$_2$ in the presence or absence of 0.5×10^{-6} mol A23187 and/or $2.5 - 5 \times 10^{-5}$ mol propranolol. The tubes were then placed in ice and the platelets separated by centrifugation. Platelet pellets were dissolved in NCS and counted as described above.

Platelet Adhesion to Collagen. The capacity of platelets to adhere to collagen was measured by the method of Cazenave et al.[16] using new glass tubes coated with collagen. Washed platelets were labeled with ^{14}C-serotonin and were suspended in Tyrode's buffer containing apyrase (0.5 mg/ml) to inhibit aggregation. The platelet suspensions were rotated in the tubes at 25°C for 10 minutes at 17 rpm, poured into fresh tubes, and centrifuged; the supernatants were tested for serotonin release. The collagen-coated tubes were then rinsed four times in saline, drained, and treated with 0.5 ml NCS per tube in order to solubilize the residual radioactivity, representing platelets adherent to collagen. Aliquots of NCS were then counted in Toluene-Liquifluor.

Platelet Factor 3 Availability. The method of Spaet and Cintron[17] was used, employing the Stypven clotting time. Platelets were activated by Celite, ADP or collagen in the presence or absence of propranolol.

Studies in Patients with Angina Pectoris

Patients. This study population consisted of 20 patients, 14 men and six women, aged 35 to 69 years of age (mean 54). Criteria for inclusion were: at least three attacks of angina pectoris per week with no evidence of an accelerated course ('unstable angina') in the 6 months prior to study; absence of valvular heart disease, hypertension, congestive heart failure, chronic obstructive pulmonary disease, diabetes, lipoprotein abnormalities, anemia, smoking history, or myocardial infarction within six months of the study; and angiographic narrowing of at least 70 percent of one or more of the coronary arteries and definite ECG evidence of myocardial ischemia associated with chest pain during submaximal exercise stress testing.

Ten age- and sex-matched healthy subjects with a negative exercise stress test were also studied. These subjects had no evidence of ischemic vascular disease, lipid abnormalities, or diabetes, and each had a negative history for cigarette smoking and drug ingestion of any sort.

Experimental Design. All healthy subjects had platelet aggregation studies and exercise tests as described below.

The patients with angina pectoris were seen every 2 weeks by the same physician. Informed consent was obtained and all cardiovascular medication was discontinued with the exception of glyceryl trinitrate. An oral placebo (mannitol, 225 mg) was administered for 6 weeks. Platelet aggregation studies were performed and exercise testing on a bicycle ergometer was carried out as described below. After the 6-week placebo period, subjects with angina pectoris were randomized into placebo ($n = 10$) and propranolol ($n = 10$) treatment groups. The placebo group remained on the same placebo regimen, while the active treatment group was started on 160 mg daily of oral propranolol in four divided doses. Neither the patient nor the physician knew whether placebo on the active substance was given. All patients continued taking glyceryl trinitrate as needed. After 16 and again after 50 weeks of therapy, serum propranolol levels were determined and platelet aggregation studies and exercise tolerance tests were repeated. At this time, both placebo and propranolol therapy was abruptly stopped. In the propranolol-treated group, five patients were withdrawn and given placebo and five received no further medication whatsoever. Final propranolol blood levels, platelet aggregation studies, and exercise tolerance tests were repeated 48 hours after cessation of the study medications.

Platelet Aggregation Studies. Blood was obtained after a 12-hour fast. After an initial resting period of 30 minutes, a 19-gauge needle was inserted, without the use of a tourniquet, into an antecubital vein and a slow infusion of physiologic saline begun. After 15 minutes of rest, with the patient relaxed, blood was sampled by free flow into plastic tubes containing 10 volume percent acid citrate dextrose (ACD). The blood specimens were then immediately processed for analysis. The specimens were coded so that those performing the aggregation studies had no knowledge of the patient, the diagnosis, or type of drug therapy.

Platelet aggregation studies were performed using the turbidometric method of Born,[14] as described above. In this study, the aggregating agents used were ADP and epinephrine. The ADP concentrations producing irreversible aggregation in untreated patients and healthy subjects were 0.5, 1, 2, 5, 10, 20, and 100 μmol; comparable epinephrine concentrations for aggregation were in the range of 0.05 to 5500 μmol. As described above, the lowest concentration producing a full biphasic response was recorded as the threshold dose; the threshold concentration of ADP and epinephrine was assessed without extrapolation between different concentrations. In repeated ADP and epinephrine determinations using coded samples, reproducibility was within 10 percent of mean.

Exercise Testing. Bicycle ergometer testing was performed by another examiner who had no knowledge of the subject's drug status during the study. Multistage graded exercise was performed utilizing a bicycle ergometer (Schwinn ergometric exerciser) as the patient pedaled against a predetermined load. After blood had been obtained for platelet studies, patients were started at a work load of 150 kpm per minute, which was increased by 150 kpm every 3 minutes until chest pain, fatigue, or a heart rate of 150/beats per minute occurred. An abnormal ECG response was defined as a flat or down-sloping ST-segment depression of at least 1 mm persisting for at least 0.08 seconds after the termination of the QRS complex with the P–Ta segment as the baseline of reference.

Blood pressure in the brachial artery was recorded by sphygmo-manometer before and immediately after exercise. The heart rate–blood pressure product, an indirect assessment of myocardial oxygen consumption,[18] was calculated from measurements obtained immediately after cessation of exercise.

Propranolol Blood Levels. Assay of the level of propranolol in blood was performed on coded samples obtained at least 2 hours after the last tablet of propranolol or placebo was ingested and just prior to exercise testing. The serum levels were measured in double-blind fashion, using the fluorometric methods of Black et al.,[19] as modified by Coltart and Shand.[20]

Statistical Analysis. In this study, for all variables except platelet aggregation data, arithmetical means with the standard error are presented and Student's *t* tests for paired and unpaired data were employed. For aggregation data, geometric means are presented. Geometric means are preferred since the concentrations of ADP and epinephrine used were essentially geometric dilutions. The Wilcoxon Rank Sum Test was used for tests of significance comparing platelet aggregability of healthy subjects, untreated angina patients, and treated angina patients. Comparison of aggregation data from the same patient group treated with various experimental protocols were done with the Wilcoxon Signed Rank Test and the Sign Test.

RESULTS

In Vitro Studies with Normal Platelets

Platelet Aggregation Studies. Propranolol, 0.1–1 μmol, raised the ADP threshold for second-phase platelet aggregation in PRP (Fig. 1) when the threshold was low (less than 2×10^{-6} mol). Propranolol altered both the rate and extent of the second phase and promoted disaggregation without affecting primary aggregation. The inhibition produced by a given concentration of propranolol depended upon the ADP threshold of the platelet suspension (Table 1), platelets with lower thresholds being more easily inhibited. The primary phase of aggregation induced by threshold ADP was abolished only by propranolol concentrations greater than 2×10^{-4} mol.

Platelet aggregation by epinephrine, collagen and thrombin was also altered by propranolol (Table 1). Second-phase aggregation induced by

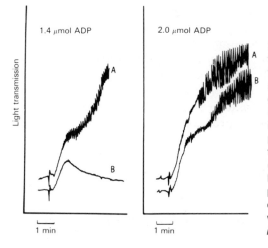

Figure 1. Alteration in platelet threshold for ADP-induced aggregation in PRP by a low concentration of propranolol. Left-hand panel: aggregation response to threshold ADP (1.4×10^{-6} mol). A, no propranolol; B, in presence of 0.1×10^{-6} mol propranolol. Right-hand panel: aggregation response to suprathreshold ADP (2.0×10^{-6} mol). A, no propranolol; B, in presence of 0.1×10^{-6} mol propranolol. (Although full aggregation occurred in B, the second phrase was slowed). *(Reprinted with permission from ref. 12.)*

threshold epinephrine was delayed and inhibited by 2×10^{-5} mol propranolol, whereas the primary phase was not altered (represented by 9 percent aggregation in the presence of 10^{-4} mol propranolol). The rate and extent of collagen-induced aggregation were inhibited by propranolol and the lag phase was markedly prolonged. Similarly, thrombin-induced aggregation (of washed platelets) was both slowed and diminished by the drug at concentrations of 10^{-5} mol or more.

TABLE 1. EFFECT OF PROPRANOLOL ON PLATELET AGGREGATION BY THRESHOLD CONCENTRATIONS OF AGGREGATING AGENTS

Threshold Aggregating Agent*†	Propranolol Concentrations (%) ($\times 10^{-6}$ mol)				
	0	10	20	50	100
ADP (1.5×10^{-6} mol)	100	60	50	33	27
ADP (5.0×10^{-6} mol)	100	98	—	61	47
Epinephrine (0.5×10^{-6} mol)	100	98	37	18	9
Collagen (50 μg/ml)	100	63	—	30	13
Thrombin (0.025 units/ml)	100	91	68	43	12

*Values are percentages of control aggregation. Each figure represents the mean value from three to five experiments using platelets from different healthy donors. In each experiment, the extent of aggregation in the presence of propranolol, as maximum change in light transmission after addition of aggregant, was expressed as percent of that achieved in the absence of propranolol.

†*Minimum concentration which produced complete aggregation, as defined in Materials and Methods, in PRP, except for experiments with thrombin, which were performed with washed platelets. *(Reprinted with permission from Ref. 12.)*

Propranolol inhibited platelet aggregation immediately and preincubation of platelets with drug did not increase the inhibitory effect. When added to platelets after an aggregating agent but before the onset of the second wave, propranolol blocked further aggregation by epinephrine (Fig. 2A, B) or ADP (not shown). Adding the drug after the second wave had begun halted or reversed further aggregation (Fig. 2C), depending upon the drug concentration. Shape change induced by aggregating agents was not inhibited by propranolol.

Effect of Propranolol on the Platelet Release Reaction. The release of ^{14}C-serotonin from platelets was inhibited by propranolol pretreatment when platelets were subsequently stimulated by any of the aggregating agents used above. There was a parallel inhibition of both aggregation and ^{14}C-serotonin release from propranolol-treated platelets after collagen stimulation. Both processes were inhibited by 5×10^{-6} to 10^{-4} mol propranolol, whereas higher concentrations produced a nonspecific loss of both serotonin and ^{3}H-adenine nucleotides in the absence of aggregation, suggesting platelet membrane damage. The release of ^{14}C-serotonin from platelets during ADP- or epinephrine-mediated aggregation was inhibited by even lower concentrations of propranolol. Inhibition of serotonin release from thrombin-stimulated platelets, however, required 5×10^{-5} mol drug or more.

Platelets stimulated with small amounts of epinephrine and ADP,

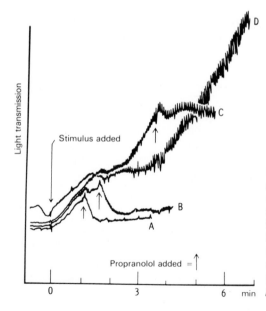

Figure 2. Inhibition of platelet aggregation by propranolol introduced after the aggregating stimulus, epinephrine (0.9×10^{-6} mol), added at time 0. Propranolol (10^{-4} mol) added at A, 1 minute; B, 1.5 minute; C, 3 minutes; D, no propranolol added. Additions indicated by arrows. Experiment performed in PRP. *(Reprinted with permission from ref. 12.)*

each at a concentration too low to produce a threshold aggregation response, undergo full aggregation accompanied by an augmented release of serotonin. Propranolol inhibited such potentiation of platelet aggregation and ^{14}C-serotonin release (Table 2). The inhibition in the potentiated system required less propranolol than was needed to inhibit platelet aggregation by the threshold ADP alone.

Effects of Propranolol on Platelet Responses to the Ionophore A23187. The divalent cation ionophore A23187 induced platelet aggregation and the release reaction,[21-24] as depicted in Figure 3. Propranolol, added prior to ionophore, inhibited the aggregation and release of ^{14}C-serotonin (latter not shown). Added after ionophore, propranolol did not alter the platelet response to A23187 and did not reverse aggregation.

Low concentrations of ionophore which caused neither aggregation nor serotonin release ($0.5 - 2 \times 10^{-6}$ mol in PRP, less than 10^{-6} mol in washed platelets) potentiated the effects of sub-threshold ADP and collagen (Table 3) and epinephrine (not shown). The potentiation of aggregation and serotonin release was also blocked by propranolol (Table 3).

The ionophore A23187 has previously been shown to promote the uptake of ^{45}CaCl$_2$ by platelets. The uptake of ^{45}CaCl$_2$ by washed platelets was enhanced 2.5-fold by 0.5×10^{-6} mol ionophore, a concentration which did not induce platelet aggregation or serotonin release. Since the volume of trapped medium in the platelet pellet, measured with ^{3}H-inulin, did not differ between ionophore-containing and control samples, the uptake of ^{45}CaCl$_2$ represented increased cell-bound calcium. Propranolol ($2.5 - 5 \times 10^{-5}$ mol) inhibited the ionophore-induced enhancement of calcium uptake by platelets.

TABLE 2. EFFECT OF PROPRANOLOL ON PLATELET AGGREGATION PRODUCED BY A COMBINATION OF SUBTHRESHOLD EPINEPHRINE AND ADP.

Propranolol Concentration ($\times 10^{-6}$ mol)	Platelet Aggregation (%)	Serotonin Release (% of control)
0	100	100
10	68.6	52
20	40.5	11.3
40	38	5.5

*Mean of four experiments, done in duplicate, using platelets from different donors. Platelet aggregation was induced by a combination of epinephrine (1/10 threshold concentration) and ADP (1/4 threshold concentration). Threshold values were determined for each donor. All experiments performed in PRP. *(Reprinted with Permission from Ref 12.)*

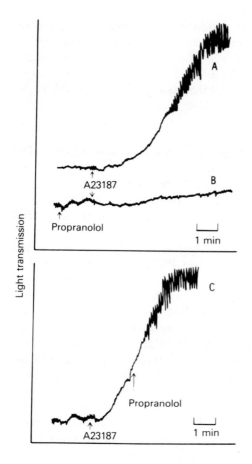

Figure 3. Propranolol inhibition of platelet aggregation induced by the ionophore A23187. Top panel: A, aggregation produced by 2×10^{-6} mol ionophore in platelet-rich plasma, B, inhibition of aggregation by ionophore in platelets pretreated with 5×10^{-5} mol propranolol. Bottom panel: C, lack of inhibition when propranolol was added after ionophore. *(Reprinted with permission from ref. 12.)*

TABLE 3. INHIBITION BY PROPRANOLOL OF IONOPHORE-POTENTIATED PLATELET AGGREGATION AND RELEASE.

Agents Added to Platelets	Aggregation (%)	Release of ^{14}C-Serotonin (%)
Ionophore A23187	5.3	0.6
Collagen	0	0.4
Ionophore + collagen	93.7	39.2
Propranolol (10^{-6} mol) + ionophore + collagen	14.9	3.4
ADP	9.8	0.5
Ionophore + ADP	86.5	27.8
Propranolol (10^{-6} mol) + ionophore + ADP	11.0	1.2

*Representative experiment in PRP. Collagen 50 μg/ml, ionophore 3×10^{-6} mol (this concentration alone did not aggregate the platelets). ADP 0.6×10^{-6} mol.
(Reprinted with permission from Ref. 12)

Comparison of Propranolol Isomers. The propranolol used to inhibit platelet aggregation and serotonin release in the above studies was a racemic mixture of $d(+)$ and $l(-)$ isomers (the clinical form of the drug). The separate $d(+)$ and $l(-)$ isomers of propranolol were then compared: $d(+)$ propranolol and $l(-)$ propranolol were equipotent as inhibitors of platelet aggregation by ADP, and their effects did not significantly differ from the effect of racemic propranolol (Fig. 4). Both isomers also produced equal inhibition of platelet aggregation and release induced by the other aggregating agents discussed above.

In contrast, another β-adrenergic blocking drug, practolol, did not affect platelet aggregation even at ten times the highest concentrations of propranolol tested (1 mmol practolol) (Fig. 5). Furthermore, practolol did not alter the inhibitory effect of the propranolol on platelet responses.

Uptake of Propranolol by Platelets. At plasma concentrations of 10^{-7} to 10^{-5} mol propranolol, the cells accumulated 10 to 30 times the plasma levels of drug, the binding increasing with the drug concentrations (Table 4). Uptake occurred equally well at 0°C as at 25° or 37°C and was rapid, reaching the maximum in 1 minute. The bound drug exchanged

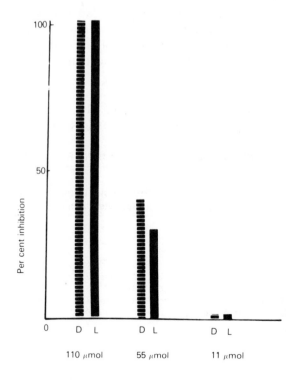

Figure 4. Effects of $d(+)$ and $l(-)$ isomers of propranolol on platelet aggregability. The two isomers, in similar concentrations, were equipotent as inhibitors of platelet aggregation by ADP, and their effects did not significantly differ from the effect of racemic propranolol.

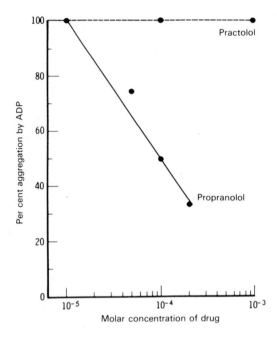

Figure 5. Comparison of practolol and propranolol on ADP-induced platelet aggregability. Practolol, which lacks membrane-stabilizing properties and has low lipid solubility, does not inhibit platelet aggregation even at 10 times the highest concentration of propranolol.

easily with unlabeled propranolol. When platelets labeled with ^{14}C-propranolol were fractionated, the membrane fraction showed highest drug-specific activity, although granules and cytosol were also labeled. The ease of exchange of labeled drug may account for its presence in all subcellular fractions.

Effect of Propranolol on Platelet Adhesion to Collagen. The effect of propranolol on the adhesion of ^{14}C-serotonin-labeled platelets to colla-

TABLE 4. ACCUMULATION OF ^{14}C-PROPRANOLOL BY PLATELETS IN PRP.

Concentration of Propranolol in Plasma ($\times 10^{-6}$ mol) (1 mg/ml)	Ratio of Propranolol Concentration in Platelets/Plasma*
0.1	11.1 ± 2.6[†]
1.0	13.6 ± 2.2[†]
5.0	22.1 ± 2.7[†]
10.0	25.6 ± 5.7[†]

*PRP (300,000 platelets/μl) incubated 10 minutes at 37°C with 0.1 to 10×10^{-6} mol ^{14}C-propranolol and ^{3}H-inulin; platelets separated by centrifugation through silicone oil for two minutes at 8000 g.
[†]Mean $\pm$ SD.
(Reprinted with Permission from Ref. 12.)

gen-coated tubes was measured and was compared to the effect of acetylsalicylic acid. Platelet adhesion to collagen was inhibited by concentrations of propranolol from 10^{-7} to 10^{-5} mol, as shown in Figure 6. The inhibitory effect of racemic *d,l*-propranolol was similar in magnitude to that produced by either the *d*(+) or *l*(−) isomer alone, the two isomers having roughly equal inhibitory effects.

Propranolol was a more potent inhibitor of platelet adhesion to collagen than acetylsalicylic acid in this test system (Table 5). The two drugs used together decreased platelet adhesion to collagen only slightly more than propranolol alone. The lack of additive effect was observed at all concentrations of drugs tested.

Effects of Propranolol on Platelet Factor 3 Availability. The Stypven time in PRP incubated with Celite to induce maximum availability of platelet factor 3 was not altered by propranolol (5 to 500×10^{-6} mol). Shortening of the Stypven time of PRP activated by ADP or collagen, which are weaker activators of factor 3, was decreased 43 and 71 percent respectively, by 7.5×10^{-5} mol propranolol, but not by lower drug concentrations.

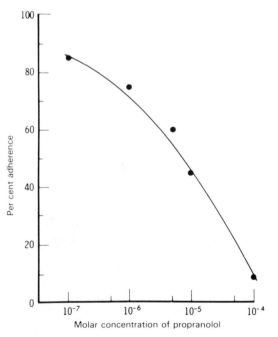

Figure 6. Propranolol inhibition of platelet adherence to collagen. Mean values from five experiments using washed platelet suspensions. *(Reprinted with permission from ref. 12.)*

TABLE 5. EFFECTS OF ACETYLSALICYLIC ACID AND PROPRANOLOL ON PLATELET ADHERENCE TO COLLAGEN-LOCATED TUBES.

Agent tested	Adherence in Presence of Drug (% of control)		
	1×10^{-6} mol	5×10^{-6} mol	1×10^{-5} mol
Acetylsalicylic acid	91.8	71.3	61.0
Propranolol	72.1	66.3	30.0
Acetylsalicylic acid + propranolol*	70.3	59.3	25.2

*Values are means of quadruplicate determinations in three experiments using washed platelets. *(Reprinted with permission from Ref. 12.)*

Studies in Patients with Angina Pectoris

Platelet Aggregation Studies. Before propranolol therapy, patients with angina pectoris demonstrated increased platelet sensitivity to aggregating concentrations of both ADP and epinephrine when compared with healthy subjects. The mean concentration of ADP necessary for the biphasic threshold response and maximum aggregation was 1.55 μmol in patients and 3.72 μmol in healthy subjects ($p < 0.01$); mean epinephrine concentration for maximum aggregation was 1.26 μmol in patients and 6.46 μmol in healthy subjects ($p < 0.01$) (Fig. 7).

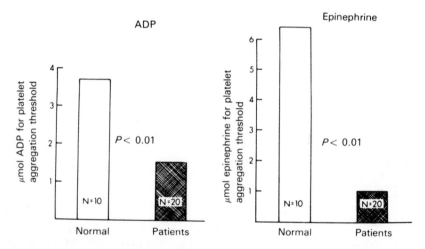

Figure 7. Comparison of ADP- and epinephrine-induced platelet aggregability in normal subjects and patients with angina pectoris. Platelets of normal subjects require significantly higher concentrations of ADP (left panel) and epinephrine (right panel) to attain aggregation threshold than do patients with angina pectoris. *(Reprinted with permission from ref. 11.)*

Serial studies performed on the patients receiving placebo showed no change in the increased platelet sensitivity to either ADP or epinephrine. Following abrupt placebo withdrawal, no change in platelet aggregation threshold was observed (Table 6).

Administration of propranolol in a dose of 160 mg per day had a dramatic effect in reducing platelet sensitivity to ADP and epinephrine in patients with angina pectoris. After 16 weeks of propranolol therapy, a mean of 3.43 μmol ADP was required to produce a biphasic aggregation response compared to 1.32 μmol before therapy (p <0.001). With epinephrine, 12.9 μmol was required after propranolol therapy, in contrast to 1.02 μmol before therapy (p <0.01). No additional changes were noted in ADP or epinephrine platelet aggregation threshold after 50 weeks of propranolol therapy (Figs. 8, 9, Table 6).

Following abrupt propranolol withdrawal, harvested platelets demonstrated marked increase in sensitivity to aggregating agents. Only 1.0 μmol ADP was now required to aggregate platelets and only 0.57 μmol epinephrine, threshold values significantly lower than the aggregating

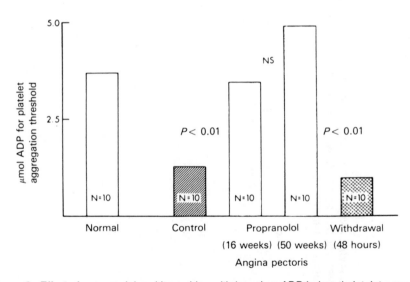

Figure 8. Effect of propranolol and its sudden withdrawal on ADP-induced platelet aggregability in patients with angina pectoris. After propranolol, platelets of treated patients are less sensitive to ADP (geometric mean) compared to before treatment, and not significantly different from normal. Forty-eight hours following abrupt propranolol withdrawal, platelets of patients have returned to their pretreatment hyperresponsiveness to ADP. *(Reprinted with permission from ref. 11.)*

TABLE 6. WITHDRAWAL AND GROUP MEAN (GEOMETRIC MEAN) CONCENTRATIONS OF ADP- AND EPINEPHRINE (EPI)-INDUCED PLATELET AGGREGATION IN PATIENTS WITH ANGINA PECTORIS TREATED WITH PROPRANOLOL AND PLACEBO AND FOLLOWING ABRUPT TREATMENT WITHDRAWAL.

Angina Placebo-Treated	Age	Control		Placebo (16 weeks)		Placebo (50 Weeks)		Withdrawal	
		ADP (μmol)*	EPI (μmol)*	ADP (μmol)	EPI (μmol)	ADP (μmol)	EPI (μmol)	ADP (μmol)	EPI (μmol)
1	54	2	5.5	2	5.5	1	5.5	1	5.5
2	60	2	5.5	2	0.5	2	0.5	2	0.5
3	48	2	0.5	2	0.5	5	5.5	2	5.5
4	38	5	0.5	2	5.5	2	0.5	5	0.5
5	54	2	5.5	5	0.5	1	5.5	1	27.5
6	55	2	5.5	1	5.5	2	0.5	0.5	5.5
7	40	2	0.5	2	5.5	2	0.5	2	0.5
8	59	2	0.5	2	5.5	1	0.5	2	0.5
9	57	1	5.5	1	0.5	2	5.5	1	5.5
10	53	0.5	0.5	1	0.5	0.5	5.5	2	0.5
		1.78	1.4	1.78	1.4	1.55	1.4	1.55	1.32

TABLE 6. *(continued)*

Angina Propranolol-Treated	Age	Control		Propranolol 160 mg/day (16 weeks)		Propranolol 160 mg/day (50 weeks)		Withdrawal	
		ADP (μmol)	EPI (μmol)	ADP (μmol)	EPI (μmol)	ADP (μmol)	EPI (μmol)	ADP (μmol)	EPI (μmol)
1	57	0.5	0.5	5	5.5	5	27.5	0.5	0.5
2	60	0.5	0.5	5	5.5	5	5.5	0.5	0.05
3	34	2	0.5	2	5.5	5	5.5	1	0.05
4	48	2	5.5	5	55.0	2	55.0	1	0.5
5	54	2	0.5	2	5.5	5	27.5	2	0.5
6	57	2	5.5	5	55.0	5	27.5	2	0.5
7	48	2	0.5	5	27.5	10	27.5	2	0.5
8	50	2	5.5	5	27.5	5	55.0	1	5.5
9	59	1	0.5	5	5.5	5	5.5	1	0.5
10	57	1	0.5	2	5.5	5	27.5	0.5	0.5
		1.32	1.02	3.43†	12.9†	4.9‡	13.2‡	1.0§	0.5§

*Geometric mean.

†Values different from control value at $p < 0.01$ confidence level.

‡No significant difference compared to values at 16 weeks.

§Values different from 50 weeks at $p < 0.01$ confidence level; no difference compared to control value. *(Reprinted with permission from Ref. 11.)*

concentrations required during propranolol therapy (Figs 8, 9, Table 6). In six of 10 patients, the platelets were even more hyperaggregable than in the control state before initiation of propranolol therapy.

The mean serum concentration of propranolol was 47 ± 9 ng/ml (range 25 to 120 ng/ml) at a dose level of 160 mg/day and 1 ± 8 ng/ml 48 hours after treatment withdrawal.

There were no significant changes from control in the mean levels of blood glucose, cholesterol, triglycerides, haematocrit or platelet count during the serial sampling periods or after abrupt propranolol withdrawal.

Exercise Tests. During the control period, all 20 patients with angina pectoris had a positive ECG response to exercise. Administration of propranolol was followed by significant increase in exercise tolerance in the patients with angina pectoris. In the ten patients who received propranolol (160 mg/day), total work increased by 130 percent from a control of 765 ± 125 kpm to $1,790 \pm 285$ kpm after propranolol ($p < 0.01$). This

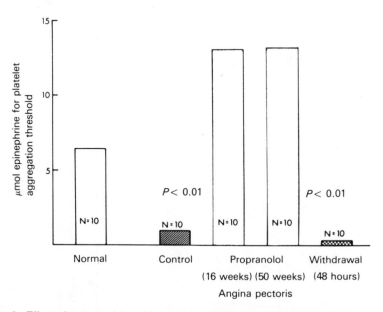

Figure 9. Effect of propranolol and its sudden withdrawal on epinephrine-induced platelet aggregability in patients with angina pectoris. After propranolol, platelets of treated patients are less sensitive to epinephrine (geometric mean) compared to before treatment, and not significantly different from normal. Forty-eight hours following abrupt propranolol withdrawal, platelets of patients have returned to their pretreatment hyperresponsiveness to epinephrine. *(Reprinted with permission from ref. 11.)*

beneficial effect on work performance was associated with a significant drop in the heart rate–blood pressure product from $16,800 \pm 1540$ to $12,000 \pm 885$ after propranolol ($p < 0.01$). In ten patients on propranolol, typical anginal pain still was the endpoint.

Forty-eight hours after abrupt propranolol withdrawal, all patients returned to their pretreatment exercise tolerance level. In some instances, performance was less than during the control state. After 50 weeks of propranolol therapy, just prior to drug withdrawal, mean work level was $1,690 \pm 200$ kpm, but fell 63 percent to 630 ± 170 kpm ($p < 0.01$) 48 hours after propranolol cessation (Fig. 10, Table 7). The product of heart rate and blood pressure ($HR \times BP$) was $11,200 \pm 1,300$ after 50 weeks of propranolol therapy, and increased to $15,500 \pm 513$ following drug withdrawal ($p < 0.01$) (Fig. 11, Table 7). The decline in work performance was similar whether propranolol-treated patients were withdrawn onto placebo or from all treatment. There were no significant differences in work performance or $HR \times BP$ in placebo-treated patients when comparing values obtained during the control period, during placebo therapy, and after withdrawal of placebo.

All patients withdrawn from propranolol noted increased frequency of anginal pains; however, no myocardial infarctions or arrhythmias occurred. Propranolol therapy was quickly reinstituted in all patients following completion of studies. No changes in frequency of angina were observed in placebo-treated patients after withdrawal from placebo.

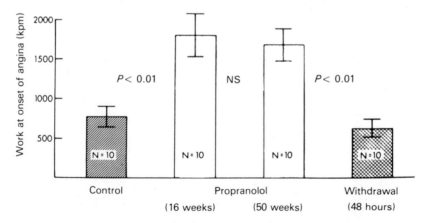

Figure 10. Effects of propranolol therapy and its sudden withdrawal on work performance in patients with angina pectoris. A significant mean increase in work performance occurs with propranolol therapy. Following abrupt cessation of propranolol, mean work performance returned to pretreatment levels. Work is measured in kilopond meters (kpm). *(Reprinted with permission from ref. 11.)*

TABLE 7. EFFECTS OF PLACEBO AND PROPRANOLOL THERAPY AND ABRUPT TREATMENT WITHDRAWAL IN PATIENTS WITH ANGINA PECTORIS.

	Patients			Propranolol Blood Levels (ng/ml)	Exercise		Platelet Aggregation	
	No.	Mean Age (Years)	Sex		Total work (kpm)	HR × BP	ADP (mmol)*	EPI (mmol)*
Placebo								
Control	10	52	6♂	0	866 ± 122	16,000 ± 467	1.78	1.40
16 weeks	10			0	933 ± 136	16,333 ± 416	1.78	1.40
50 weeks	10		4♀	0	883 ± 113	16,344 ± 383	1.55	1.40
Withdrawal	10			0	840 ± 136	15,700 ± 484	1.55	1.32
Propranolol								
Control	10	54	6♂	0	765 ± 125	16,800 ± 1540	1.32	1.02
16 weeks	10			54.8 ± 9.2	1790 ± 285	12,000 ± 885	3.43	12.90
50 weeks	10		4♀	47.6 ± 8.4	1690 ± 200	11,200 ± 1300	4.90	13.20
Withdrawal	10			1 ± 8	630 ± 117	15,500 ± 513	1.00	0.57

*Geometric mean. (Reprinted with permission from Ref. 11.)

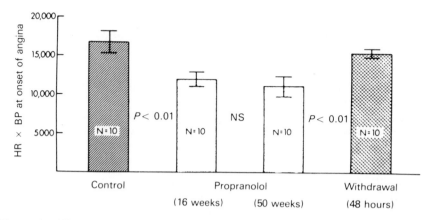

Figure 11. Effects of propranolol therapy and its sudden withdrawal on the heart rate–blood pressure product (HR × BP) in patients with angina pectoris. A significant decrease in the HR × BP at the onset of angina, even though exercise level was higher after treatment, is demonstrated after propranolol therapy. Following abrupt propranolol withdrawal, the HR × BP increases to pretreatment levels. *(Reprinted with permission from ref. 11.)*

DISCUSSION

Propranolol, added to normal platelets in vitro, inhibited platelet aggregation induced by ADP, epinephrine, collagen, thrombin, and the ionophore A23187. Propranolol inhibited mainly the secondary phase of aggregation and serotonin release, and had little effect upon primary aggregation. Platelet adhesion to collagen and availability of platelet factor 3 were also inhibited by the drug.

The use of propranolol is becoming widespread in clinical settings ranging from angina pectoris to migraine headache.[25] It was therefore of interest to ascertain whether this drug altered platelet functions at concentrations achieved in clinical practice. The low thresholds for platelet aggregation by ADP and epinephrine present in the patients with severe angina pectoris became normal (i.e., the platelets were less responsive to these aggregating substances) during chronic therapy with oral propranolol using dosages sufficient to improve exercise tolerance.[9,11] After propranolol withdrawal, the initial low aggregation thresholds were again observed, and in some instances platelets were more hyperaggregable compared to pretreatment levels.[11] The question arose whether this change in platelet function could be a direct effect of propranolol on platelets.

Peak plasma levels of propranolol following usual clinical doses range from 20 to 200 ng/ml (10^{-7} to 10^{-6} mol)[26]. Propranolol, added in vitro to normal platelets, altered platelet aggregability, serotonin release, and adhesion to collagen at similar concentrations. Inhibition of aggregation by 10^{-7} to 10^{-6} mol of propranolol was only observed in platelets with low thresholds for aggregation by ADP. Platelets from healthy donors with less sensitive thresholds required more than 10^{-5} mol of the drug for inhibition in vitro. Although the ADP threshold phenomenon (i.e., ADP-induced second phase aggregation of serotonin release) results from the low concentration of ionized calcium in citrated plasma,[27] it correlates well with other measurements of platelet reactivity. Propranolol may reset the threshold of platelet responsiveness, but in a clinical context the effect is limited to platelets that have shown increased sensitivity to aggregating stimuli. Such "sensitive" platelets have been observed in patients with hypercholesterolemia, diabetes mellitus, hypertension, recent stroke or myocardial infarction, and chronic angina pectoris.[5,7-9,28-30]

In patients with angina pectoris, at propranolol plasma levels ranging from 25 to 120 ng/ml, ADP- and epinephrine-induced platelet aggregability were normalized compared to pretreatment levels and exercise tolerance improved. Forty-eight hours after abrupt propranolol withdrawal at a plasma level of 1 ± 8 ng/ml, the platelet aggregability thresholds had returned to their pretreatment abnormal levels and exercise tolerance deteriorated.

We have also shown that platelets accumulate ^{14}C-propranolol in vitro 10- to 30-fold over plasma concentrations. Preferential accumulation of the drug by platelets in vivo may relate to its high degree of lipid solubility,[31] thus accounting for altered platelet responsiveness at the plasma propranolol concentrations measured in vivo.

Several lines of evidence suggest that propranolol alters platelet behavior by mechanisms other than β-adrenergic blockade. Propranolol is known to have a "local anesthetic" or membrane-stabilizing effect.[31-33] This effect has been shown in red blood cells,[33] nerve,[34] and skeletal[33] and cardiac muscle,[34,35] and has previously been suggested as the mechanism of inhibition of epinephrine-induced platelet aggregation.[36,37] Concentrations of propranolol needed for a membrane effect are higher (10^{-6} to 10^{-4} mol) than for β-adrenergic blockade (10^{-9} to 10^{-8} mol). Also, the membrane-stabilizing effect is not stereospecific, unlike β-blockade. Thus d($\pm$) and l($-$) propranolol have similar membrane effects, whereas the d($+$) isomer has only 1 percent of the β-blocking capacity of the l($-$) isomer.[31,38] The concentration of propranolol required to inhibit platelet function in vitro (10^{-7} to 10^{-4} mol) is high, suggesting a membrane effect. This conclusion is supported by the finding that d($+$) and l($-$) forms are equipotent inhibitors of platelet aggregation, serotonin release and platelet adhesion to collagen. Other β-adrenoceptor blocking drugs having similar membrane-stabilizing effects (pindolol and oxprenolol[39] have similar effects as propranolol on platelets. Furthermore, practolol, a potent β-adrenergic blocking drug that is not lipid-soluble and lacks membrane-stabilizing activity,[31] has no effect upon platelet function. Thus, the membrane effect and not β-adrenergic blockade appears crucial for the action of propranolol on platelets.

Like other membrane-stabilizing substances, the main effect of propranolol was to inhibit the second phase of platelet aggregation and serotonin release. Shape change was not inhibited by propranolol, suggesting that the drug did not interfere with the initial contact or binding of aggregants with the platelet surface. All platelet functions affected by propranolol are calcium-dependent, whereas platelet shape change,[40] which is independent of divalent cations, was not affected.

Propranolol may alter platelet function by affecting the availability of calcium within platelets. The drug displaces calcium from membrane sites[41] and inhibits lipid-facilitated transport of calcium.[42] Both platelet aggregation and the release reaction involve the transport of calcium ions into the platelet cytoplasm from other sites—either the dense tubular system in the platelet[24] or the external medium.[43] Platelet-dense tubular membranes, like the sarcoplasmic reticulum of muscle, sequester calcium.[44] Ionophores such as A23187 can transport extracellular calcium ions into cells and can shift intracellular calcium from physiologically sequestered locations into the cytoplasm, as has been shown for muscle.[45]

Propranolol inhibited ionophore-mediated potentiation of platelet aggregation by subthreshold amounts of ADP and collagen and inhibited uptake of $CaCl_2$ induced by A23187. The effects were observed only when the propranolol was induced prior to the ionophore, suggesting that propranolol may act to inhibit the access of ionophore to calcium at critical intracellular sites. Although inhibition of ADP-induced platelet aggregation in citrated PRP might reflect the low plasma concentration of ionized calcium, we also found that propranolol was inhibitory to washed platelets suspended at physiologic calcium ion concentrations. Therefore low external calcium concentration was not crucial to demonstrate a propranolol effect.

From the in vitro platelet studies in normal subjects we conclude that propranolol is bound by platelets and renders the platelet membrane less sensitive to the action of aggregant substances. At clinically achieved levels of drug, propranolol affects platelet function much less than does acetylsalicylic acid. The modulation of platelet membrane function by propranolol does not involve β-adrenergic blockade; the drug may alter platelet reactivity by interfering with internal shifts of calcium ions at intracellular sites. Whether or not the new calcium-channel-inhibiting drugs will show the same effects on platelets has yet to be determined.

From the studies in patients with angina pectoris we conclude that propranolol had definite effects on platelet function. Heightened platelet aggregability is normalized with therapeutic doses of the drug. Following abrupt treatment withdrawal, platelets returned to their pretreatment hyperaggregable state. Whether the beneficial actions of propranolol in angina pectoris, myocardial infarction, and migraine headache are related in part to this platelet effect has not been elucidated. The role of heightened platelet activity in the propranolol "withdrawal syndrome" must also be explained. Studies are needed to determine platelet behavior with gradual withdrawal of propranolol as well as the clinical and rheologic implications of adding agents such as acetylsalicylic acid to inhibit platelet aggregability in this situation.

REFERENCES

1. Haft J: Role of blood platelets in coronary artery disease. Am J Cardiol 43, 1197, 1979.
2. Ross R, Glomset J, Kariya B, Harker L: A platelet dependent serum factor that stimulates the proliferation of arterial smooth muscle cells in vitro. Proc Nat Acad Sci USA 71, 1207, 1974.
3. Jorgensen L, Hovig T, Rowsell HC, Mustard JF: Adenosine diphosphate induced platelet aggregation and vascular injury in swine and rabbits. Am J Pathol 61, 161, 1970.
4. Murphy EA, Mustard JF: Coagulation tests and platelet economy in atherosclerotic and control subjects. Circulation 25, 114, 1962.
5. Steele PP, Weily HS, Davies H, Genton E: Platelet function in coronary artery disease. Circulation 48, 1194.
6. Harker LA, Slichter S: Platelet and fibrinogen consumption in man. N Engl J Med 287, 999, 1972.
7. Carvalho CA, Colman RW, Lees RS: Platelet function in hyperlipoproteinemia. N Engl J Med 290, 434, 1974.
8. Sagel J, Colwell JA, Crook L, Laimins M: Increased platelet aggregation in early diabetes mellitus. Ann Intern Med 82, 733, 1975.
9. Frishman WH, Weksler B, Christodoulou JP, et al: Reversal of abnormal platelet aggregability and change in exercise tolerance in patients with angina pectoris following oral propranolol. Circulation 50, 887, 1974.
10. Frishman WH, Christodoulou J, Weksler B, et al: Aspirin therapy in angina pectoris: effects on platelet aggregation, exercise tolerance, and electrocardiographic manifestations of ischemia. Am Heart J 92, 1, 1976.

11. Frishman WH, Christodoulou J, Weksler B, et al: Abrupt propranolol withdrawal in angina pectoris: effects on platelet aggregation and exercise tolerance. Am Heart J 95, 169, 1978.

12. Weksler BB, Gillick M, Pink J: Effect of propranolol on platelet function. Blood 49, 185, 1977.

13. Mustard JF, Perry DW, Ardlie NG, Packham MA: Preparation of suspensions of washed platelets from humans. Br J Haematol 22, 193, 1972.

14. Born GVR: Aggregation of blood platelets by adenosine and its reversal. Nature 194, 927, 1962.

15. Marcus A, Zucker-Franklin D, Safier L, Ullman H: Studies on human platelet granules and membranes. J Clin Invest 45, 14, 1966.

16. Cazenave JP, Packham MA, Mustard JF: Adherence of platelets to a collagen-coated surface: Development of a quantitative method. J Lab Clin Med 82, 978, 1973.

17. Spaet TH, Cintron J: Studies on platelet factor-3 availability. Br J Haematol 11, 269, 1965.

18. Robinson BF: Relation of heart rate and systolic blood pressure to the onset of pain in angina pectoris. Circulation 35, 1073, 1967.

19. Black JW, Duncan WAM, Shanks RG: Comparison of some properties of pronethalol and propranolol. Br J Pharmacol 25, 577, 1965.

20. Coltart DJ, Shand DG: Plasma propranolol levels in the qualitative assessment of beta-adrenergic blockade in man. Br Med J 3, 731, 1970.

21. Mürer EH, Stewart G, Rausch M, Day HJ: Calcium ionophore A23187: effect on platelet function, structure and metabolism. Thromb Diath Haemorrh 34, 72, 1975.

22. Feinman RD, Detwiler TC: Platelet secretion induced by divalent cation ionophores. Nature 249, 172, 1974.

23. Massini P, Lüscher EF: Some effects of ionophores for divalent cations on blood platelets: comparison with the effects of thrombin. Biochim Biophys Acta 372, 109, 1974.

24. White JG, Rao GH, Gerrard JM: Effects of the ionophore A23187 on blood platelets. I. Influence on aggregation and secretion. Am J Pathol 77, 135, 1974.

25. Frishman W, Silverman R: Clinical pharmacology of the new beta-adrenergic blocking drugs. Part 3. Comparative clinical experiments and new therapeutic applications. Am Heart J 98, 119, 1979.

26. Shand DG, Nuckolls EM, Oates JA: Plasma propranolol levels in adults. Clin Pharmacol Ther 11, 112, 1970.

27. Mustard JF, Perry DW, Kinlough-Rathbone RI, Packham MA: Factors responsible for ADP-induced release reaction of human platelets. Am J Physiol 228, 1757, 1975.

28. Danta G: Second phase platelet aggregation induced by adenosine diphosphate in patients with cerebral vascular disease and in control subjects. Thromb Diath Haemorrh 23, 159, 1970.

29. Salky N, Dugdale M: Platelet abnormalities in ischemic heart disease. Am J Cardiol 50, 612, 1973.

30. Vlachakis ND, Aledort L: Hypertension and propranolol therapy effect on blood pressure, plasma catecholamines and platelet aggregation. Am J Cardiol 45, 321, 1980.

31. Frishman W: Clinical pharmacology of the new beta-adrenergic blocking drugs. Part I. Pharmacodynamic and pharmacokinetic properties. Am Heart J 97, 663, 1979.

32. Grobecker H, Lemmer B, Hellenbrecht D, Wiethold G: Inhibition by antiarrhythmic and β-sympatholytic drugs of serotonin uptake by human platelets. Experiments in vitro and vivo. Eur J Clin Pharmacol 5, 145, 1977.

33. Langslet A: Membrane stabilization and cardiac effects of d,1-propranolol, d-propranolol and chlorpromazine. Eur J Clin Pharmacol 13, 6, 1970.

34. Lucchesi BR, Iwami T: The antiarrhythmic properties of ICI 46037, a quaternary analog of propranolol. J Pharmacol Exp Ther 162, 49, 1968.

35. Manninen W: Movements of sodium and potassium ions and their tracers in propranolol treated red cells and diaphragmatic muscle. Acta Physiol Scand (Sup.) 335, I 76, 1970.

36. Mills DCB, Roberts GCK: Effects of adrenaline on human blood platelets. J Physiol 193, 443, 1967.

37. Bygdeman S, Johnsen 0: Studies on the effect of adrenergic blocking drugs on catecholamine-induced platelet aggregation and uptake of noradrenaline and 5-hydroxytryptamine. Acta Physiol Scand 75, 129, 1969.

38. Howe R, Shanks RG: Optical isomers of propranolol. Nature 210, 1336, 1966.

39. Frishman W, Silverman R: Clinical pharmacology of the new beta-adrenergic blocking drugs. Part 2. Physiologic and metabolic effects. Am Heart J 97, 797, 1979.

40. Born GVR: Observations on the change in shape of blood platelets brought about by the adenosine disphosphate. J Physiol 209, 487, 1970.

41. Seeman P: Membrane stabilization by drugs: tranquilizers, steroids and anesthetics. Int Rev Neurobiol 9, 145, 1966.

42. Nayler WG: The effect of pronethalol and propranolol on lipid facilitated transport of calcium ions. J Pharmacol Exp Ther 153, 479, 1966.

43. Robblee LS, Sherpo D, Belamarich FA, Towle C: Platelet calcium flux and the release reaction. Ser Haematol 6, 311, 1973.

44. Statland BE, Heagen BM, White JG: Uptake of calcium by platelet relaxing factor. Nature 233, 521, 1969.

45. Scarpa A, Baldassare J, Inesi G: The effect of calcium ionophores on fragmented sarcoplasmic reticulum. J Gen Physiol 60, 735, 1972.

CHAPTER 10

β-Adrenergic Blockade in Patients with Myocardial Infarction: Treatment and Prevention

William H. Frishman, Shlomo Charlap, Heschi H. Rotmensch, and Curt D. Furberg

β-Adrenoceptor antagonists have been shown to be safe and effective in the treatment of patients with systemic hypertension, arrhythmia, angina pectoris, hypertrophic cardiomyopathy, thyrotoxicosis, open-angle glaucoma, and for migraine headache prophylaxis.[1] β-Blockers have also been suggested for the prevention of myocardial infarction and mortality in patients with stable angina pectoris and systemic hypertension, but their protective effects in these conditions remain questionable.[2,3] More controversial has been the role of β-adrenergic blockade in preventing myocardial infarction and death in patients with preinfarction angina syndrome and for reducing myocardial infarction size and mortality during the hyperacute phases of myocardial infarction. Although no definitive evidence exists for any primary prophylactic benefit of β-adrenoceptor blocking drugs against myocardial infarction and mortality, the results of many recent long-term clinical trials have demonstrated that some of these agents are effective in reducing the risk of death and nonfatal reinfarction in survivors of an acute myocardial infarction.[4-6] The United States FDA has already approved two β-blockers, propranolol and timolol, for this prophylaxis indication.

In this chapter, the use of β-blockers in the prevention and treatment of myocardial infarction is reviewed. First, the theoretical and practical considerations for using β-adrenoceptor blocking drugs as prophylactic therapy for preventing the first myocardial infarction in high-risk patients is explored. Second, the experimental and clinical experiences with these drugs as protective therapies in preinfarction angina and during the hyperacute phase of myocardial infarction are discussed. Finally, the clinical experiences with β-adrenergic blockade as a long-term intervention for reducing the risk of mortality in survivors of an acute myocardial infarction are assessed.

PREVENTION OF MYOCARDIAL INFARCTION AND DEATH IN PATIENTS WITH STABLE ANGINA PECTORIS AND SYSTEMIC HYPERTENSION

Although β-adrenoceptor blockade does not directly affect the progression of coronary atheroma, it does reduce myocardial oxygen requirements.[7,8] This, in turn, enables the cardiac muscle to tolerate for a while what would otherwise be an inadequate supply of oxygen. The reduction of myocardial oxygen requirements is due to a decreased heart rate and blood pressure, and a reduction in myocardial contractility.[7,8] β-Adrenergic blockade may also increase coronary perfusion by slowing the heart rate and lengthening cardiac diastole.[9] In experimental studies, the drugs have been shown to improve distribution of blood flow in the ischemic myocardium, as well as improving the utilization of myocardial substrate.[10] The drugs are potent antiarrhythmic agents,[11] and some are known to inhibit platelet aggregation (see Chapter 9).[12]

In patients with angina pectoris, these agents have been useful in reducing pain and improving exercise tolerance.[1] An adequate degree of β-adrenoceptor blockade can provide marked pain relief in 80 percent of patients. This success rate can be improved upon by selecting the best tolerated β-blocker in combination with nitrates and/or calcium-channel blockers. Thus, the quality of life can be improved in patients with angina pectoris.

A major unresolved question in clinical medicine is whether the β-adrenoceptor blockers can influence the natural history of patients with stable angina pectoris and arterial hypertension by prolonging life expectancy and reducing the risk of the first myocardial infarction. There are multiple subgroups of patients with angina pectoris classified by differences in symptomatology (stable or unstable), coronary anatomy, left ventricular function, and stress test results. These multiple patient variables make a proper study design in patients with angina pectoris almost untenable. The results of a few poorly designed trials have not demonstrated any marked reduction in the annual mortality rate of patients with stable angina pectoris treated with β-blockers when compared to the findings of larger epidemiologic studies in untreated patients.[3] There is, however, indirect evidence to suggest that β-blockers may be having a favorable impact on mortality in patients with angina pectoris. The recent Coronary Artery Surgery study revealed a 1.6 percent annual mortality in patients receiving medical therapy that included β-blockers, a rate much lower than predicted.[13]

Patients with systemic hypertension also have an increased risk for myocardial infarction and cardiovascular death. β-Adrenergic blockers, which are proven effective in therapy of patients with hypertension,[13] have been suggested as a treatment for the primary prevention of myocardial infarction and death in these patients. At present, only the results of retrospective studies, which by nature of their design were not free of bias, and which were made in a relatively small number of patients, are available.[14–16]

Stewart,[14] in a 5-years' retrospective review, observed a 24 percent reduction in first myocardial infarctions in 121 hypertensive patients receiving propranolol when compared to 48 patients whose antihypertensive drug regimen did not include a β-blocker. In this study, the relatively high incidence of coronary events in the group not receiving β-blockers may have included patients at a rather high cardiac risk. Berglund et al.[15] found a significant reduction in the cumulative incidence of myocardial infarction and cardiac death when 635 middle-aged male patients, whose antihypertensive therapy was mainly β-blockers, were compared to a control group of 391 nontreated hypertensives over a period of 72 months. Although there was no random allocation to the two patient groups, cardiovascular risk factors were distributed equally, but entry blood pressure was slightly higher in the β-blocker-treated patients.

Similar findings were described by Beevers et al.[16] who reported on the results of a retrospective open-clinic study of 920 consecutive patients below the age of 65 years who were receiving antihypertensive therapy. Vascular complications had developed prior to treatment in 242 patients. β-Blocking drugs, mainly oxprenolol or propranolol, were used alone or in combination with other antihypertensive drugs in 416 patients; 504 patients never received β-blockers. There was a tendency both for males and females who had received β-blockers to suffer fewer myocardial infarctions and strokes than those patients receiving other therapies. This trend was found in patients presenting initially with and without vascular complications, and was observed in patients aged 40 to 50 years and 55 to 64 years. There were no significant differences in the blood pressure levels before therapy was begun in the two treatment sub-groups, and no difference in the average blood pressures during treatment. In this study, diuretic therapy was also found to be safe and effective.

In essence, these studies suggest that in hypertensive patients, β-blocker therapy, even when started before the clinical manifestation of coronary heart disease, may lower cardiovascular morbidity and mortality. These studies also demonstrate the problems of interpreting the results, problems that inevitably arise in retrospective analyses without a random allocation design. Moreover, it appears that the number of patients studied was too small for providing a conclusive answer to the problem of primary prevention of myocardial infarction.

In order to demonstrate this alleged benefit with β-blockers, prospective studies with either randomized or double-blind patient allocation will have to be conducted, in which the incidence of cardiac events in patients on a β-blocker-containing regimen is compared with the incidence in patients on traditional antihypertensive treatment without β-blockers. To be proven statistically, a 25 to 50 percent reduction in events should be achieved. Given these assumptions, the sample size required can be estimated to total about 15,000 patient treatment-years, taking into account a 5 percent annual dropout rate. It is obvious that such numbers of patients can be collected only by a major collaborative effort.

The Medical Research Council (MRC) Hypertension Trial should go some way toward accomplishing this goal.[17] In the MRC trial now in progress, patients are randomly allocated to either placebo or active treatment. The active treatment group is then sub-divided; one subgroup receives a thiazide alone, and the second subgroup a β-blocker alone. The results of this study are being awaited with great interest.

At present, as is the case with lipid-lowering drugs and platelet-inhibiting agents, only theoretical considerations suggest employing β-adrenergic blockers as a primary prophylactic treatment against myocardial infarction and death. Nonetheless, β-blockers are now a treatment of choice for the long-term relief of angina pectoris and for treatment of unstable angina. In patients without evidence of symptomatic coronary artery disease, there are no conclusive data as yet supporting the use of β-blockers as a first-line antihypertensive regimen based only on their cardioprotective effects. Although no definitive proof exists for the primary prophylactic benefits of β-adrenoceptor blocking drugs against myocardial infarction and death, recent studies have demonstrated that some of these agents are useful for reducing the long-term risk of nonfatal reinfarction and cardiovascular death in survivors of a myocardial infarction.[4-6]

β-ADRENOCEPTOR BLOCKADE IN THE EARLY
PHASE OF ACUTE MYOCARDIAL INFARCTION

In patients with acute myocardial infarction, the presence of severe pain, tissue injury, and circulatory disturbances provides important physiologic stresses that trigger an increased catecholamines discharge.[18] This observation is based on evidence derived from several clinical studies, where measurements of urinary-free catecholamine excretion[19] and plasma catecholamine levels were elevated.[20]

An increase in "sympathetic tone" following myocardial infarction may play an important supportive role in maintaining contractile function in ischemic areas of the myocardium, as well as enhancing the function of residual nonischemic areas.[3,7] However, there are two potentially deleterious consequences from an increase in sympathetic nervous activity. First, increased sympathoadrenal discharge may be the cause of serious cardiac arrhythmias after myocardial infarction.[18,21] Second, the positive inotropic and chronotropic effects of catecholamines lead to an increase in total cardiac work and myocardial oxygen consumption by causing increments in heart rate, blood pressure, and contractility.[22] This action may be critical in areas of the heart that are receiving very limited coronary blood flow, an effect that could extend necrosis.[23,24] In animal experiments, isoproterenol has been shown to impair both contractile performance and metabolism of the ischemic myocardial tissue, observations that suggest that enhanced adrenergic activity may be harmful in human beings.[24]

β-Adrenergic blockers have been considered for use as standard therapy in patients with acute myocardial infarction to prevent the undesirable consequences of increased sympathoadrenal discharge: arrhythmogenesis and extension of myocardial injury.[3,7,25,26] The drugs can alter those factors that determine increases in myocardial oxygen consumption, and may augment coronary blood flow by increasing diastolic perfusion time.[9,23,24] They may also reduce the incidence of ventricular fibrillation. On the other hand, β-adrenergic blockade can have unfavorable consequences in some cases of fresh infarction. Cardiac impulse formation may be greatly impaired and conduction diminished to a degree that causes cardiac arrest.[1] Furthermore, exacerbation of congestive heart failure in patients dependent on the positive inotropic effects of catecholamines is a well-recognized sequelae of β-blockade.[27]

Antiarrhythmic Effects of β-Blockers in Acute Myocardial Infarction

The arrhythmogenic actions of catecholamines have been recognized for over 70 years. The occurrence of ventricular arrhythmias in experimental myocardial infarctions is associated with increased plasma levels of catecholamines.[28] It has been observed that the removal of sympathetic influences to the heart, regardless of the means, will lead to a reduced incidence of arrhythmias following experimental coronary occlusion in animals.[29]

The exposure of ischemic tissue to high levels of catecholamines favors the appearance of multiple reentry pathways and the development of ventricular fibrillation.[30] These experimental data suggest that β-blockade would be particularly effective in preventing or aborting ventricular arrhythmias that occur in acute myocardial infarction. Experimental studies in dogs with myocardial infarction have demonstrated that pretreatment with β-adrenoceptor blockers elevated the threshold for ventricular fibrillation and prevented or reduced the incidence of malignant ventricular tachyarrhythmias.[31] The antiarrhythmic effects of the different β-adrenoceptor blocking agents are similar and appear to be related to their common β_1-adrenergic blocking properties, not to membrane-stabilizing activity or intrinsic sympathomimetic activity.[13]

For preventing primary ventricular fibrillation in patients during acute myocardial infarction, there are now data from different controlled clinical studies suggesting that β-blockers have a favorable effect on the incidence of in-hospital ventricular fibrillation.[32,33] Whether or not β-blockers are more effective than other antiarrhythmic agents in preventing ventricular fibrillation has yet to be determined.

For the elective therapy of cardiac arrhythmias during an acute infarction, Lemberg et al.[34] reported favorably on the use of propranolol in 34 patients with 43 episodes of tachyarrhythmias complicated by mild to moderate heart failure. The dosage of propranolol employed in the studies was 0.5 to 0.75 mg intravenously given at 2-minute intervals, until sinus rhythm returned or the ventricular rate slowed down to 80 beats per minute. The arrhythmias included atrial fibrillation, atrial flutter, supraventricular tachycardia, and ventricular tachycardia, all with ventricular rates over 100 beats per minute. A majority of patients responded to a total intravenous dose of less than 5 mg of propranolol.

β-Blocking drugs may be used adjunctively with other antiarrhythmic agents and dc electrocardioversion.[18] When using β-blockers for the rapid treatment of arrhythmia, the drug should always be administered intravenously (propranolol is the only intravenous drug available) since adequate blood levels of the agent may not be reached following acute oral administration due to interpatient variability in gastrointestinal absorption and first-pass hepatic metabolism.[1,35]

The therapeutic efficacy of β-blockade as an antiarrhythmic intervention is now well accepted (see Chapters 3, 4).[35–38] However, potential side effects must be considered when employing these drugs as antiarrhythmic agents in acute myocardial infarction because, as mentioned earlier, these drugs can cause or potentiate congestive heart failure, hypotension, atrioventricular conduction delay, and airways obstruction.[1] Routine administration of β-blockers to all patients with acute myocardial infarction may, thus, not be justified as yet.[39] When using β-blockers as antiarrhythmic agents in acute myocardial infarction, the deleterious effects of tachyarrhythmias in hemodynamic terms and the benefits of reversion to sinus rhythm or slowing of the rapid ventricular rate must be balanced against the possible cardiovascular depression produced by the drugs themselves. Whether or not β-adrenoceptor blocking drugs with intrinsic sympathomimetic activity, such as pindolol or oxprenolol, will provide safer antiarrhythmic alternatives to propranolol, has yet to be proven.

Reduction or Containment of Myocardial Infarction

The size of an acute myocardial infarction, which can vary in size from a few grams to 40 percent or more of the left ventricular mass, depends on a critical balance between oxygen supply and demand for a portion of the myocardium. The extent of injury is determined primarily by the size of the supply territory of the coronary vessel that is narrowed or occluded, and the adequacy of the collateral circulation.[23,25,40] Experimental studies suggest that myocardial ischemia progresses increasingly to infarction if the period of myocardial oxygen and substrate deprivation is prolonged beyond 4 to 6 hours.[41] If coronary blood flow is restored after 3 hours, however, some of the ischemic tissue will not undergo necrosis.[23,42]

The anatomic lesions in the coronary circulation are not the sole determinants of infarct size, as shown by a large body of experimental evidence: from these data it appears that infarct size after a standardized arterial ligation can be modified by early interventions.[23,43] It has been shown in many experimental studies that there is an ischemic region around the initially infarcted area that may not necrose until several hours have elapsed. It has also been demonstrated that reduction of myocardial oxygen requirements or increasing coronary blood flow can decrease the final size of an infarct from what would have been predicted, and that an elevation in myocardial oxygen demands or a reduction in coronary blood flow will increase the infarct size.[23,25,44] Since myocardial infarction size has important prognostic implications as far as pump failure and fatal arrhythmogenesis are concerned, the question has arisen whether a reduction in the extent of the ischemic injury following coronary artery occlusion may improve the long-term mortality and morbidity resulting from acute myocardial infarction.

Of all the many interventions that are possible for decreasing or containing the size of a myocardial infarct, β-adrenergic blockade is probably the most physiologically attractive (Table 1).[23,41,45] β-adrenergic blocking drugs lower myocardial oxygen demands by reducing heart rate, blood pressure, and myocardial contractility, and may augment

TABLE 1. POSSIBLE MECHANISMS BY WHICH β-BLOCKERS PROTECT THE ISCHEMIC MYOCARDIUM[7,8]

1. Reduction in myocardial oxygen consumption.
   a. Reduction in heart rate, blood pressure, and myocardial contractility.
2. Augmentation of coronary blood flow.
   a. Increase in diastolic perfusion time by reducing heart rate.
   b. Augmentation of collateral blood flow.
   c. Redistribution of blood flow to ischemic areas.
3. Alterations in myocardial substrate utilization.
4. Decrease in microvascular damage.
5. Stabilization of cell and lysosomal membranes.
6. Shift of oxyhemoglobin dissociation curve to the right.
7. Inhibition of platelet aggregation.

coronary blood flow by increasing diastolic perfusion time (see Chapter 8).[44] Another proposed mechanism for the beneficial action of β-adrenergic blockade is its ability to alter substrate utilization of the heart.[44,46] During myocardial infarction, adrenergic activity stimulates lipolysis, resulting in increased circulating free fatty acids.[10,46] This in turn may augment free fatty acid uptake by the heart, a metabolic effect that can increase myocardial oxygen consumption, infarct size and the risk of arrhythmogenesis. By blocking β-adrenergic receptors in experimental myocardial infarction, a decrease in lipolysis and myocardial free fatty acid uptake occurs, with a shift in myocardial substrate utilization towards glucose.[10] The β-adrenergic blocking drugs may also increase collateral blood flow and favorably redistribute blood flow to the ischemic myocardium.[47,48] Some β-blockers have antiplatelet actions that may have beneficial effects on the coronary microvasculature (see Chapter 9).[12] Favorable effects on the oxygen hemoglobin dissociation curve have also been demonstrated.[12,49] Cardiac lysosomal membranes can be stabilized with β-adrenergic blockade during experimental myocardial anoxia.[50]

Experimental Interventions. With experimental occlusion of coronary arteries in dogs, propranolol has been demonstrated to reverse epicardial ST-segment elevations on the electrocardiogram and to favorably alter the creatine phosphokinase release curve, changes that may reflect a reduction in the predicted size of a myocardial infarction.[23,44,51] Similar experimental observations have been made with practolol[52] and timolol.[53] Exogenous catecholamines have been found to have the reverse effect.[22,44] The majority of animal studies using β-blockers in acute myocardial infarction are disappointing from the standpoint of a practical study design. They are directed not at survival, but at prevention of arrhythmias or necrosis during the acute phase of infarction, the animals usually dying or being killed within 24 hours of the experimental infarction. The most important finding from these studies is that β-blockade must be instituted as soon as possible after the onset of coronary occlusion in order to have a favorable impact on infarction size; administration of β-blockers more than 6 hours after the acute phase of myocardial infarction appears to have no effect.

The results of experimental studies seem to indicate that β-blockade may improve myocardial blood flow, lessen the risk of acute arrhythmias, and limit experimental infarct size. However, the studies have failed to identify which pharmacologic effect of β-blockade is responsible for improvement in myocardial ischemia, nor have they shown that any such changes correlate with any reduction in morbidity and mortality. In view of these deficiencies, it would seem rather futile to try to extrapolate any of the conclusions of animal studies to the clinical myocardial infarction situation.

Clinical Investigations. One of the major problems hampering clinical research in the reduction or containment of myocardial infarction has been the lack of techniques to precisely quantify the amount of myocardium that undergoes necrosis during an evolving myocardial infarction in human beings. Measures, such as electrocardiographic ST-segment elevations and thallium-201 myocardial imaging, reflect primarily the extent and severity of myocardial ischemia—that is, the area at risk of necrosis—not the actual infarct size. Others, including measurements of left ventricular filling pressure, and radionuclide ventriculography, reflect global or regional myocardial dysfunction but cannot separate disturbances due to infarction from those caused by ischemia. They also do not distinguish between the effects of prior and recent infarction.[44]

Readily available measurements most directly related to infarct size are electrocardiographic quantification of Q-wave development and R-wave loss, and serologic estimation of the quantity of creatine kinase (CK) released from necrotic myocardium.[44] Clinical analysis of the patient's course and prognosis after infarction can provide important evidence supporting a net favorable treatment effect. However, this approach lacks specificity because results are influenced by numerous factors other than infarct size, and extremely large numbers of patients are usually required to demonstrate treatment effects.

Because no single technique for infarct quantification is highly accurate in multiple subsets of patients with acute myocardial infarction, investigators seeking to obtain widely generalizable results in intervention trials must employ multiple measurement techniques in relatively unselected patients. Clinical trials organized on the basis of favorable preliminary results from pilot studies must employ (1) modern techniques of experimental design, including randomization of eligible patients to treatment and placebo–control groups, (2) blinding of patient and investigator to avoid biases in nonexperimental therapy or patient attitude, and (3) data monitoring during the trial by uninvolved parties to identify beneficial or adverse effects of therapy.

The results of experimental studies have shown that the time interval between the onset of ischemia and the initiation of the intervention is a critical determinant of the efficacy of tested agents in reducing infarct size.[41,42] The necessity for early intervention creates a major logistic difficulty for those who attempt to conduct proper clinical trials, which require obtaining pretreatment informed consent, and collection of baseline data—such as ECG maps, hemodynamic measurements, thallium-201 scintigrams, or gated radionuclide scan.

Early clinical studies (prior to the 1970s) in patients with myocardial infarction revealed no clinical benefit when oral propranolol was employed as the intervention agent.[54-57] These early clinical trials ignored the short time span during which pathophysiologic changes in infarction could be modified, as well as the kinetics of propranolol absorption and metabolism by the liver.[1] Moreover, they did not consider the possibility that a beneficial effect of β-blockers on infarct size might still occur in the absence of a demonstrable reduction in acute mortality rate.

In humans, Pelides et al. demonstrated that practolol given intravenously within 72 hours of an infarct reduced the degree of precordial ST-segment elevation.[58] The safety of intravenous propranolol, the most widely used agent in this class, was demonstrated by Mueller et al.[59] After administering propranolol within the first 12 hours of infarction, these investigators showed a reduction in myocardial hypoxia estimated by an increased lactate uptake. In this study, there was no deterioration in clinical left ventricular function observed with treatment. Reductions in cardiac contractility, cardiac index, and myocardial oxygen consumption were associated with improved myocardial metabolism and bioenergetics. Despite these favorable hemodynamic and metabolic findings, the investigators could not demonstrate an absolute decrease in infarct size or an increase in ultimate survival.

Gold et al. demonstrated a reduction in ischemic injury, defined by a reduction in ST-segment elevation on the ECG, when intravenous propranolol was given during acute myocardial infarction.[60] This effect on the ECG was less marked, however, in patients with total coronary occlusions. These investigators suggested that (1) propranolol may be more effective in subendocardial wall infarction, where coronary blood flow is not completely compromised and where ischemia may be a more important component of the injury than necrosis, and (2) propranolol may be less effective in transmural myocardial infarction, which has more complete cessation of effective flow and where necrosis may greatly overshadow reversible ischemia.

Clinical studies with propranolol,[61] atenolol,[33] and metoprolol,[62,63] β1-selective agents, and pindolol,[64] a β-blocker with intrinsic sympthomimetic activity, used intravenously in acute myocardial infarction, have shown decreased precordial ST-segment deviation and release of ischemic chest pain.

Peter et al.[61] measured total creatine kinase appearance and peak levels in a randomized trial of 95 patients seen within 12 hours of onset of an uncomplicated myocardial infarction that appeared to be transmural by electrocardiographic criteria. Although no objective clinical benefit could be demonstrated from propranolol in this group of uncomplicated patients, there were no serious side effects from the drug, and enzyme (CPK) levels were some 30 percent lower on average in patients who were treated within 4 hours of the onset than in control patients. If treatment were delayed beyond 4 hours, there was no significant difference between enzyme levels in the treated and control patients. In a subsequent study of patients with a typical history of recent prolonged chest pain but no diagnostic ECG changes, the same research group was able to show that fewer completed infarcts occurred in treated patients than in control.[65]

Yusuf et al.[33] found a significant decrease in CPK-MB release and enhanced R-wave preservation in a placebo-controlled study of 477 patients with impending or early myocardial infarction using intravenous atenolol within 12 hours of symptom onset. In this study, atenolol reduced the incidence of completed infarction in patients with threatened infarction, and may have influenced infarct size in patients with definite infarcts at entry by reducing ECG changes and CPK enzyme measurements. In addition, fewer treated patients than control patients suffered subsequent heart failure, atrial fibrillation, in-hospital cardiac arrests, or death. In a double-blind controlled study of 1395 patients, Hjalmarson et al.[62] showed that intravenous metoprolol could reduce LDH isoenzyme levels in the plasma compared to placebo treatment. A reduced incidence of ventricular fibrillation was also seen with metoprolol therapy (see Table 2).

TABLE 2. RANDOMIZED TRIALS ATTEMPTING TO REDUCE INFARCT SIZE WITH β-BLOCKERS IN HUMANS[62]

Study	Drug	Duration of Treatment
Peter et al.[61] (open study)	Propranolol 0.1 mg/kg IV 320 mg/27 hr po	27 hr
Yusuf et al.[33] (open study)	Atenolol 5 mg IV 100 mg/day po	10 days
Hjalmarson et al.[62] (placebo-controlled)	Metoprolol 15 mg IV 200 mg/day po	90 days
McIlmoyle et al.[63] (placebo-controlled)	Metoprolol 15 mg IV 200 mg/day po	90 days
Muller et al. (MILIS)[68] (placebo-controlled)	Propranolol 0.1 mg/kg IV 20–200 mg/day po	9 days
Sederholm et al.[69] (placebo-controlled)	Timolol IV/24 hr 20 mg/day po	10 days

*Effects on enzyme release with β-blocker treatment versus placebo.

If β-blockers given early and at adequate dosage can indeed restrict infarct size in human beings, the benefit-to-risk ratio must be calculated for each patient prior to the use of this therapy in the acute phase of myocardial infarction. There are inherent problems with this therapy that must be considered: (1) β-Blockers may increase left ventricular volume and end-diastolic pressure by their negative chronotropic and inotropic effects, especially in severely damaged hearts.[1,3,66] By this mechanism they may increase the oxygen demands of ischemic myocardial tissue. At the same time the drugs may increase left ventricular end-diastolic pressure and limit an already compromised subendocardial blood flow.[3] These risk factors could easily offset the beneficial reduction in heart rate and blood pressure with β-adrenoceptor blockade. (2) Since patients have varying degrees of "sympathetic tone," there is no established β-adrenoceptor blocking dose with any agent. One might require a dose four times that of another patient to achieve the same β-blocking effect.[1] The drugs should also be given intravenously in acute myocardial infarction to achieve their immediate effects,[3] and this might precipitate sudden bradyarrhythmias or conduction abnormalities.[18] One should avoid using long-acting oral preparations in this condition.[67] (3) Despite the adverse effects of isoproterenol recently defined in experimental animals with myocardial infarction, heightened sympathetic tone may not be deleterious for all patients.[3,22] Patients with a considerable amount of frank necrosis and little ongoing ischemia may need their

Enzyme	Start of Treatment	No. of Pts.	Results*
CK	<4 hr	37	Lower level with propranolol
	4–12 hr	58	No difference
CK-MB	<12 hr	477	Lower level with atenolol
LDH 1+2	≤12 hr	952	Lower level with metoprolol
	>12 hr	427	No difference
CK-MB	<6 hr	391	Lower level with metoprolol
CK-MB	<18 hr	269	No difference
CK-MB	<4 hr	144	Lower level with timolol

sympathetic tone to preserve pump function. β-Adrenoceptor blockade could actually worsen cardiac failure in these patients.

β-Adrenoceptor blocking drugs are indicated with nitrates and/or calcium-entry blocking drugs as immediate postinfarction therapy if new symptoms of angina pectoris develop in patients after acute myocardial infarction, and for a subgroup of patients with hyperkinetic circulatory response to their infarcts (e.g., hypertension, tachycardia) without evidence of left ventricular dysfunction.[3]

The FDA has not yet approved the concept of intravenous β-blockade for reducing the size of an acute myocardial infarction. Long-term clinical studies are now in progress, both in the United States and Europe, to address this question.[67]

Preliminary results from one of these trials, the Multicenter Investigation of Limitation of Infarct Size (MILIS), revealed no effects with propranolol therapy started within 18 hours of chest pain. In this study, sponsored by the National Institutes of Health, 269 patients with acute myocardial infarction were randomized to receive either placebo or propranolol (0.1 mg/kg IV followed by a 9-day oral regimen). Patients were treated, on average, 9 hours after pain started. There were no significant differences between placebo and propranolol on CK-MB release, the incidence of myocardial infarction, ECG R wave loss, change in left ventricular ejection fraction, pyrophosphate images, or mortality.[68]

These findings contrast with those of another recent controlled study which compared intravenous timolol to placebo and their effects on patients with acute myocardial infarction. In this study the β-blocker was shown to reduce the CPK-MB and improve the ECG manifestations of ischemia. However, no differences in mortality were reported.[69]

THE USE OF β-ADRENERGIC BLOCKADE IN UNSTABLE ANGINA AND PREINFARCTION SYNDROMES

When severe reversible myocardial ischemia rather than frank necrosis is the cause of prolonged chest pain, β-blockade is recommended, along with nitrates and/or calcium-entry blockers, especially in those patients with preinfarction states ("intermediate syndrome").[69] By decreasing[70] heart rate, blood pressure, and contractility, and/or by increasing coronary blood flow, β-adrenoceptor blockade can reduce ischemia and relieve pain.[3,44,70] Left ventricular function, which may be transiently depressed in acute ischemia, generally improves as the injury is lessened.[52] Once the situation is stabilized with medical treatment, more definitive measures, including coronary angiography and, when appropriate, coronary artery reconstructive procedures, may be considered.

The potentially protective properties of propranolol, metoprolol, and atenolol for prolonged myocardial ischemia in the absence of infarction have been reported by several groups of investigators.[71,72] In a randomized, double-blind study of 68 patients with unstable angina, the propranolol-treated patients experienced fewer coronary events than placebo-treated patients.[71] In patients admitted to a coronary care unit because of prolonged ischemic chest pain in another study, myocardial infarctions developed less frequently in patients treated with propranolol: 30 to 90 patients experienced infarction, in contrast to 62 to 90 patients who did not receive the drug.[72]

Yusuf et al. also observed that fewer patients with preinfarction angina went on to develop frank infarctions when administered intravenous and oral atenolol rather than placebo.[33]

Implications
The results of experimental and clinical investigations suggest that β-adrenoceptor blockers may be an important protective therapy for patients with acute myocardial infarction and preinfarction angina. β-Adrenergic blockade can decrease cardiac work and improve perfusion and metabolism of the ischemic myocardium. However, the effectiveness of β-adrenoceptor blocking agents in treating myocardial ischemia depends on the functional state of the heart. The more left ventricular performance is determined by the mechanical and contractile properties of ischemic areas, the more likely it is that β-adrenoceptor blockade

will improve functioning of the jeopardized myocardium. However, a deleterious effect can be anticipated when impaired ventricular performance is primarily determined by frank myocardial necrosis. With careful evaluation of the benefit-to-risk potential in individual patients, β-adrenoceptor blockade can be a potentially useful therapeutic intervention for preserving ischemic myocardium and prolonging life.

The value of early β-adrenoceptor blocking therapy within 6 to 18 hours of a myocardial infarction in humans is now being readdressed in four cooperative acute-phase trials being carried out in Europe and the United States. One of these studies, using propranolol, is The Multicenter Investigation of Limitation of Infarct Size (preliminary results are shown in Table 2).[67-68] Another is the International Study of Infarct Survival (ISIS), which will test atenolol eventually in 18,000 patients.[67]

LONG-TERM REDUCTION OF CARDIOVASCULAR MORTALITY RISK IN SURVIVORS OF ACUTE MYOCARDIAL INFARCTION

On discharge from the hospital, survivors of an acute myocardial infarction remain in an unstable state.[73-78] For patients under 70 years of age, there is a 10 percent mortality rate during the first posthospital year after myocardial infarction and a 4 percent annual mortality rate for the subsequent 2 or 3 years. The mortality rate is highest in the first 3 months after hospital discharge, with a progressive decline thereafter.[79] Approximately 50 percent of the posthospital deaths are sudden, the primary mechanism being ventricular fibrillation, and these arrhythmic deaths are distributed uniformly throughout the postinfarction period.

Risk stratification studies in survivors of an acute myocardial infarction have identified subsets of patients with high, intermediate, and low mortality rates. However, clinical criteria are not available that can distinguish patients likely to die of sudden cardiovascular death from those whose death is likely to be nonsudden. The high-risk subset (20 to 55 percent mortality in the first postinfarction year) makes up 20 percent of the postinfarction population. This group is characterized by (1) clinical evidence of left ventricular dysfunction by physical exam and nuclear imaging studies during the acute hospitalization, (2) electrocardiographic evidence for ongoing ischemic heart disease with a limited submaximal exercise test prior to hospital discharge, and (3) complex ventricular premature contractions on a Holter ECG recording obtained prior to discharge.[24,77,79] The more of these factors that are present, the higher the patient risk. Patients with second and third infarctions who have these characteristics have an even higher mortality. A low-risk subset (2 percent mortality in the year after a myocardial infarction) makes up 25 percent of the postinfarction population. This subset is characterized by (1) no prior infarction before the index coronary event, (2) the absence of both high-grade ventricular ectopy and congestive heart failure during the acute phase of hospitalization, and (3) a negative submaximal exercise test performed just prior to discharge.[24,80] In between these two subgroups are the remaining 55 percent of the postinfarction population. This intermediate subgroup has one or two of the high-risk subset characteristics, and a first year mortality rate of approximately 10 percent. Patients with subendocardial infarction or recurrent angina pectoris are at greater risk of reinfarction and/or cardiac death compared to those without these clinical features.

A desirable therapeutic goal would be to reduce the long-term morbidity and mortality in survivors of a myocardial infarction. A variety of therapeutic approaches have been examined, ranging from general measures (dietary modification, weight reduction, cessation of cigarette smoking, physical exercise), to coronary reconstructive surgery, to specific drug treatment. Specific pharmacologic interventions have included anticoagulants,[81] agents that inhibit platelet aggregation,[82] lipid-lowering agents,[83] calcium-entry blockers,[84] and antiarrhythmic drugs.[79] Among the interventions evaluated to date, only β-adrenergic blockade has been clearly demonstrated to be effective.[4-6]

LONG-TERM β-ADRENERGIC BLOCKADE IN THE POSTINFARCTION PERIOD

The risk factors that are operative during the postinfarction period include ongoing myocardial ischemia, cardiac arrhythmia, and mechanical left ventricular dysfunction.[72-78] At least two of the factors are influenced by the degree of sympathetic drive, since the incidence of arrhythmias[21] and the work done by the ventricles are both increased by catecholamines.[22] In animals, denervation of the heart by stellate ganglionectomy has been shown to reduce arrhythmias and improve survival after coronary ligation.[29] The synthesis of β-blockers offered the possibility that they might modify the natural history of myocardial infarction by preventing the undesirable consequences of enhanced sympathoadrenal discharge.[3]

Since the clinical introduction of propranolol in 1963, β-blockers have been used in human beings for the treatment of arrhythmias and angina pectoris.[11] As these conditions are commonly observed in many patients following acute myocardial infarction, β-blockers were considered by early investigators as a possible postinfarction intervention for reducing the risk of cardiovascular death and reinfarction.[3] However, since these drugs could also depress left ventricular function in patients dependent on the positive inotropic actions of catecholamines, which is the other factor contributing to mortality risk, they were avoided initially in the postinfarction state for fear of precipitating symptomatic heart failure.

In 1965, Snow observed in a small nonblinded study that moderate doses of oral propranolol, when given to patients within 24 hours of acute myocardial infarction, reduced mortality without serious complication.[85] Snow's initial findings prompted the start-up of other postinfarction trials that sought to demonstrate whether his results were repeatable, whether other β-blockers demonstrated such a beneficial effect, and by what mechanisms β-blockers might be reducing postinfarct mortality. Unfortunately, the results reported by Snow were not easy to reproduce. Only in recent years have studies with more sophisticated and rigid clinical trial designs provided the persuasive evidence that β-blockers have a beneficial therapeutic effect in therapy of many postinfarction patients.

The β-Blocker Postinfarction Trials—Study Design

Since 1965, over 20 long-term β-blocker postinfarction trials employing various experimental designs have been completed.[4-6,54-57,85-100] These long-term studies have investigated over 17,000 survivors of acute myocardial infarction in an attempt to document a reduction in total mortality, sudden death, and reinfarction with an oral β-blocker treatment intervention. Nine different β-blockers have been evaluated at different

TABLE 3. PHARMACOLOGICAL PROPERTIES OF THE β-ADRENOCEPTOR BLOCKING DRUGS TESTED IN LONG-TERM TRIALS

	Relative β₁-Selectivity	Intrinsic Sympathomimetic Activity	Membrane-Stabilizing Activity
Alprenolol*	0	+	+
Atenolol	+	0	0
Metoprolol†	+	0	0
Oxprenolol*	0	+	+
Pindolol	0	+ +	0
Practolol*	+	+	+
Propranolol	0	0	+ +
Sotalol*	0	0	0
Timolol	0	0	0

*Not available for clinical use in the United States.
†Results of some studies not available.

dose levels (alprenolol, atenolol, metoprolol, oxprenolol, pindolol, practolol, propranolol, sotalol, and timolol) (Table 3). A long-term trial evaluating metoprolol is complete but the results are not available as yet.[67]

The results of the long-term postinfarction β-blocker trials are difficult to compare because they were derived from studies using different protocol designs and study populations, with time since last infarction ranging from a few hours to 7 years or more and extent of clinical follow-up ranging from 3 weeks to 7 years. Considering the 1-year post discharge mortality rate in infarct survivors of 10 percent, it has been estimated that a properly designed placebo-controlled double-blind randomized trial would need to follow over 2000 subjects to demonstrate conclusively that a pharmacologic intervention caused a 30 percent reduction in death over a 2-year treatment period.[101] Only three completed β-blocker trials, using the drug practolol,[88,89] propranolol,[6] and timolol,[4] have fulfilled this population criterion. Clinical trials that are based on insufficient numbers of subjects cannot detect small differences in outcome between treated and untreated patients, a major weakness of the earlier propranolol trials.[54-57]

In all but one of the long-term postinfarction trials, only one β-blocking drug was evaluated against placebo. Therefore, it is not known whether any single β-blocking compound has advantages over another when used as postinfarction therapy. Some investigators argue that any favorable effect these drugs have in the postinfarct state is related to their common β_1-adrenergic blocking property. Others argue that specific pharmacodynamic and pharmacokinetic differences manifested by these drugs (intrinsic sympathomimetic activity, β_1-selectivity, membrane-stabilizing properties, lipid solubility, protein binding) may be important, so that these drugs would not be interchangeable.[102]

There is also a marked variability in the statistical methodologies employed in evaluating the results of the different β-blocker postinfarction studies. Trials of drugs that have easily measured effects—for example, the reduction of blood pressure—are reasonably straightforward, but when the drug's mode of action is in doubt, only very definite end points of the trial are useful. If β-blockers are to be used for the reduction of mortality in survivors of acute myocardial infarction, the only relevant end point is death itself. Reinfarction is difficult to define and different modes of death—by reinfarction or sudden death—are often impossible to distinguish and therefore make unsatisfactory trial end points. Less firm clinical end points, such as an alteration in some indirect measurement of infarct size, are at present not helpful to the clinician who wishes to know whether to give an individual patient a β-blocker. In many of the long-term β-blocker trials, there were no significant effects on total mortality demonstrated when comparing placebo and β-blocker treatments. The investigators often divided the treatment groups by the patient characteristics of their choice, (e.g., age, presence of various risk factors on admission, mode of death), reanalyzed the data from these smaller groups, and obtained significant results.[103] However, this type of statistical analysis increases the risk of a Type I statistical error, thus limiting the value of the results. Also, in many of the early trials, the investigators failed to include in their final morbidity and mortality analyses data from those patients who were withdrawn from the study after randomization. The inclusion of these data in the final study analysis is important, because when physicians institute treatment with any drug, they must know whether patients will tolerate the medication or whether some apparent side effect will lead to its being discontinued. It can be argued that when a drug is withdrawn, it does not have much chance of being proven effective; clinical trials should nevertheless by analyzed on an "intention to treat" basis. This implies that in the final data analysis of a trial, all patients should be retained in the group to which they were originally assigned. The "intention to treat" analysis also demonstrates the fatality rate among patients whom a physician might have decided to treat with the active drug, and it also shows the fatality rate among untreated patients. This is important, for if the mortality rate among patients given placebo differs from what might have been expected, a comparison with the active treatment group may be meaningless.

In analyzing and comparing the findings of the different β-blocker secondary prevention trials, there are certain characteristics to look for in a study that was properly designed and analyzed. First, the trial must be placebo-controlled and double-blind (despite the difficulty of doing this latter accurately when β-blockers lower heart rate). Second, an adequate number of subjects should be randomly entered into the study with a suitable time for follow-up provided. Third, study end points should be clearly defined at the onset of the trial and findings analyzed on an "intention to treat" basis. The designs of the 14 long-term trials which fulfill these criteria are shown in Table 4.

Results of Long-Term Prevention Trials
The results of the 13 major long-term β-blocker trials in infarct survivors are shown in Table 5. The individual studies using different β-blockers are discussed below.

Alprenolol. Alprenolol, a nonselective β-blocker with membrane and partial agonist activities, is not available for clinical use in the United States. It was used in the first long-term (greater than 6 months) post infarction study.[86] In this small, double-blind, randomized study, there

TABLE 4. DESIGN OF LONG-TERM β-BLOCKER TRIALS IN SURVIVORS OF ACUTE MYOCARDIAL INFARCTION

Trial	Patients Randomized	β-Blocker	Daily Dose (mg)	Mean Entry Time after MI (days)	Mean Length of Follow up (mo)
Wilhelmsson et al.[87]	230	Alprenolol	400	7–21 after discharge	24
Ahlmark et al.[91]	393	Alprenolol	400	14 after diagnosis	24
Barber et al.[90]	500	Practolol	600	<1.0	24
Multicentre International Study[88,89]	3053	Practolol	400	13.2	14
Andersen et al.[92]	480	Alprenolol	400	<1.0	12
Baber et al.[95]	720	Propranolol	120	8.5	9
Norwegian Multicenter Study[4]	1884	Timolol	20	11.5	17
BHAT[6]	3738	Propranolol	180–240	13.8	25
Hansteen et al.[96]	560	Propranolol	160	4–6	12
Julian et al.[98]	1456	Sotalol	320	8.3	12
Taylor et al.[97]	1103	Oxprenolol	80	14 mo*	48
Pindolol Study Group[99]	529	Pindolol	15	1–21	24
European Infarction Study[100]	1741	Oxprenolol	160–320	14–36	12
Lopressor Intervention Study[67]	2397†	Metoprolol	200	5–14	12

*Time between infarction and entry into trial ranged from under 1 month to 7 and one-half years.
†Study complete, recruitment curtailed for various reasons; results not available.

TABLE 5. RESULTS OF LONG-TERM β-BLOCKER TRIALS (>9 MO) IN SURVIVORS OF ACUTE MYOCARDIAL INFARCTION

Trial	Patients Control	Randomized Intervention	Mortality (%) Control	Mortality (%) Intervention	p Value*
Wilhelmsson et al.[87]	116	114	12.1	6.1	0.18
Ahlmark et al.[91,†]	93	69	11.8	7.2	0.48
Barber et al.[90,†,‡]	147	151	31.3	27.2	0.51
Multicentre International Study[88,89]	1520	1533	8.2	6.3	0.051
Andersen et al.[92,‡]	242	238	26.2	25.2	0.92
Baber et al.[95]	365	355	7.4	7.9	0.91
Norwegian Multicenter Study[4]	939	945	16.2	10.4	0.0003
BHAT[6]	1921	1916	9.8	7.2	0.005
Hansteen et al.[96]	282	278	13.1	9.0	0.16
Julian et al.[98]	583	873	8.9	7.3	0.32
Taylor et al.[97]	471	632	10.2	9.5	0.78
Pindolol Study Group[99]	266	263	17.7	17.1	0.36
European Infarction Study[100]	880	861	5.1	6.6	0.14

*p values computed for chi-square test comparing the proportion of deaths in each group.
†Incomplete reporting.
‡Mortality rates include all in-hospital deaths

319

were no differences in total mortality seen after 1 year of treatment with either placebo or alprenolol 400 mg/day.[86]

In two subsequent trials using oral alprenolol, some benefit in the post infarction state was seen.[87,91] The first was a double-blind, placebo-controlled study in 230 patients that showed a significant reduction in sudden death.[87] The second, an open study in 162 patients, not only confirmed a reduction in sudden death but also showed a reduction in nonfatal reinfarction.[91] In both of these studies, treatment was begun 2 to 4 weeks after infarction and was continued for 2 years. When the data were reanalyzed, the site of infarct was not found to be a significant factor.

Andersen et al.[92] reported the results of a double-blind study of alprenolol versus placebo in a total of 480 patients starting with an intravenous dose on hospital admission and continuing with oral treatment for 1 year. Total mortality for the study was about equal in treatment and placebo groups (61 versus 64), but when the population was split and analyzed by age, there was a significant reduction in mortality with alprenolol in those patients 65 years of age and under, while there was a nonsignificant increase in mortality for patients over 65. The harmful effect in the elderly was attributed to the administration of intravenous β-blockade on the first day of infarction to patients with hypotension or congestive heart failure. This observation regarding a possible age-related benefit of β-blockade was not confirmed by the larger long-term β-blocker trials.[4-6]

Atenolol. Atenolol is β_1-selective, with no membrane or partial agonist activity, and has been approved by the FDA for the treatment of systemic hypertension. In a randomized double-blind postinfarction trial in 388 patients, the effects on total mortality of oral atenolol (50 mg twice daily), propranolol (40 mg three times daily), and placebo were compared.[93] Using an analysis based on an "intention to treat" there were no differences in total mortality observed among the groups after 1 year of treatment.

An acute intervention trial using intravenous and oral atenolol showed a favorable trend on in-hospital mortality, a reduction of repetitive ventricular arrhythmias, and a reduction in CPK-MB levels compared to placebo treatment.[33] Despite these favorable findings, however, no significant difference in the long-term mortality (up to 2 years of follow-up) was shown between placebo and atenolol therapy.[33]

Metoprolol. Metoprolol is β_1-selective, with no membrane or partial agonist activity, and has been approved by the FDA for the treatment of hypertension. Recently, Hjalmarson et al. reported on the findings of a large double-blind study from Sweden comparing the effects of placebo and metoprolol on total mortality in patients with acute myocardial infarction.[5] Over 2600 patients fulfilled the entry criteria for suspected myocardial infarction. Fourteen percent of these were excluded because a contraindication to β-blocker therapy was present. Ten percent were excluded from randomization because of a need for β-blocker therapy. Twenty-three percent were excluded for other reasons. A total of 1395 patients were eventually randomized to metoprolol or placebo—698 to metoprolol and 697 to placebo.

Patients between the ages of 40 and 74 were studied. Although all patients met the criteria for suspected myocardial infarction at entry, not all went on to evolve a definite myocardial infarction. Criteria for definite and probable myocardial infarction were applied retrospectively according to the protocol for the purpose of subgroup analysis. Eight hundred and nine of the 1395 patients fell into the definite myocardial infarction category, 162 into the probable myocardial infarction category, and the remaining 424 into neither. Most of those remaining 424 patients did have ischemic heart disease and probably had simple angina pectoris when admitted to the hospital.

Metoprolol or matching placebo was given as three intravenous boluses of 5 mg each at 2-minute intervals. More than 98 percent of patients tolerated the full intravenous dose and oral therapy was started with 50 mg orally every 6 hours for 48 hours, then 100 mg twice daily. If less than the full intravenous dose was tolerated, the patient was started initially on 25 mg every 6 hours prior to receiving the full oral metoprolol dose. In the study, the first injection of study medication was given to patients on an average of 11.3 hours after the onset of chest pain, and the mean intervention time was the same for patients in both the treatment and control groups. Over 90 percent of the patients were started on treatment within 24 hours after the onset of their symptoms. All patients were followed for 90 days.

Approximately 19 percent of patients were withdrawn from treatment in each group. The withdrawal pattern was quite similar to that found in other studies.[4,6] A significantly larger number of patients were withdrawn from the metoprolol group for bradycardia and hypotension, whereas more patients were withdrawn from the placebo group for a condition requiring β-blocker therapy. In that the follow-up period was much shorter in the metoprolol study, and that the clinical condition of patients in the metoprolol study was somewhat different than that reported in the timolol and Beta-Blocker Heart Attack trials,[4,6] the absolute percentage withdrawal rates in the three studies are not strictly comparable. In these studies, conduction abnormalities and heart failure did not appear to be important side effects of the three drugs, indicating that they were relatively well tolerated.[4-6]

During the 90-day follow-up period (using an "intention to treat" analysis), there were 40 deaths in the metoprolol group (5.7 percent) and 62 deaths in the placebo group (8.9 percent). This 36 percent reduction in total mortality was statistically significant compared to placebo. The investigators also observed a reduction in LDH isoenzymes in patients treated within 12 hours of infarction, and a reduction in the frequency of ventricular fibrillation.[32,62] Mortality was the same whether the treatment was started before or after 12 hours, suggesting that infarct size reduction was not contributing to the benefit. Judging from the mortality curves, which did not start to diverge until after 5 to 7 days of therapy, the benefit seen with metoprolol may have been related to the 90-day oral maintenance regimen rather than intravenous treatment intervention.

Most deaths occurred among patients who evolved a definite myocardial infarction at study entry. When the group of patients who did not have definite myocardial infarctions were reexamined, it was seen that there were equal numbers of death in the two treatment groups; however, the numbers were so small that no statistically valid conclusions could be made. Unfortunately, the double-blind study was not extended further, but it did suggest the feasibility of treating hemodynamically stable patients with β-blockers during the hyperacute stage of an acute myocardial infarction.

A large multicenter double-blind trial in the United States [American Lopressor Intervention Trial (LIT)] has now been completed. This study compared oral metoprolol to placebo and analyzed their effects on long-term survival and sudden death.[67] Recruitment for the study was terminated prematurely for various reasons. Two smaller European trials comparing metoprolol to placebo have completed their recruitment, but these studies are still ongoing.[67]

Oxprenolol. Oxprenolol, a nonselective β-blocker with partial agonist activity and no membrane activity, is not available for use in the United States. The effect on total mortality of this β-blocking drug was compared to that of disopyramide phosphate, an antiarrhythmic drug, and placebo in a randomized double-blind study of 473 patients conducted in Europe.[94] Therapy was started during the first hours of myocardial infarction and treatment was continued for 6 weeks. There were no significant differences in total mortality with oxprenolol (40 mg three times daily), disopyramide (150 mg three times daily), and placebo treatment.

Oxprenolol was evaluated by Taylor et al. in low-risk male patients with uncomplicated myocardial infarction.[97] This trial entered patients from 1 month to 7½ years after infarction, and provided the longest time for patient follow-up. Overall, there was no significant difference in the mortality and nonfatal reinfarction rate between placebo and oxprenolol treatment groups. Retrospective subgroup analysis suggested that the effect of treatment was influenced by time of treatment. Patients in whom oxprenolol treatment was started within 4 months of infarction had low total mortality compared to the placebo group. There was no long-term benefit in mortality seen when treatment was started beyond 4 months.

The European Infarction study group evaluated 1741 patients who survived an acute myocardial infarction.[100] In this multicenter double-blind randomized study, the effects of oxprenolol (160 mg twice daily) on survival and nonfatal reinfarction were compared to placebo. The patients were entered 14 to 36 days after myocardial infarction and were followed for 1 year. The results of this study showed a strongly unfavorable mortality trend with the β-blocker compared to placebo (6.6 percent versus 5.1 percent). Subgroup analyses revealed that low-risk patients did worse with oxprenolol therapy than high-risk patients (previous myocardial infarction or heart failure at randomization).

Pindolol. Pinodolol is a nonselective β-blocker with partial agonist activity and no membrane-stabilizing activity. Pindolol 15 mg daily was compared to placebo in high-risk patients who had electrical and/or mechanical complications after an acute myocardial infarction.[99] This Swedish–Australian trial entered patients 1 to 21 days after infarction, with follow-up up to 2 years. Overall, there was no significant difference in mortality, sudden death, and nonfatal reinfarction rates between the pindolol and placebo treatment groups. Retrospective subgroup analyses suggested that patients administered pindolol later than 5 days postinfarction had a better response than the patients receiving drug treatment earlier. Pindolol is approved by the FDA for the treatment of systemic hypertension.[99]

Practolol. Practolol is β_1-selective, with partial agonist activity and no membrane activity. Prior to the completion of the BHAT, the largest reported β-blocker postinfarction study was the International Multicentre Trial using practolol, an agent no longer available because of a drug-induced oculomucocutaneous syndrome.[88,89] In this study, 3053 patients were randomly allocated either to practolol (200 mg twice daily) or placebo treatment, starting 1 to 4 weeks after the established diagnosis of acute myocardial infarction; patients were then followed for periods ranging between 1 and 3 years. In the practolol group, there was a significant reduction in both total mortality and sudden death compared to placebo. Furthermore, a nonsignificant trend in favor of practolol was found with respect to nonfatal reinfarctions. In addition, significant reductions of angina pectoris and cardiac arrhythmias were noted in the practolol group when compared with patients taking placebo.

When deaths in patients still on treatment are analyzed or when a further subgrouping not allowed for in the initial trial design is done, the investigators conclude that patients with previous anterior infarction who continued on treatment were especially helped. The dangers of such retrospective analyses as opposed to prospective allocation on the basis of predetermined entry criteria must be emphasized, however.

In another randomized, double-blind postinfarction study, practolol (200 mg twice daily) was compared to placebo in 298 patients.[90] Patients were started on therapy immediately upon admission to the coronary care unit and followed for 2 years. The overall mortality was in favor of practolol, but not significantly so, except in those patients who had entry heart rates in excess of 100 beats per minute. Again, the retrospective subgrouping in the final data analysis raises the possibility of a Type I statistical error.

Propranolol. Propranolol is nonselective, with membrane activity, and no partial agonist activity. It is approved for the treatment of hypertension, arrhythmia, and angina pectoris, and is now approved for reducing the risk of mortality in survivors of a myocardial infarction.

In a European multicenter trial reported on by Baber et al.[95] that compared placebo to oral propranolol, 720 patients with previous anterior wall myocardial infarctions (a design to detect a 50 percent reduction in mortality) were enrolled 2 to 14 days after their infarct. In this randomized, double-blind study, patients were followed for up to 9 months. At 3 months, there was no difference in mortality between the placebo and propranolol (120 mg daily) treatment groups, nor any difference in nonfatal reinfarctions. The investigators suggested that a small difference could have been missed that a study in a larger patient population might have demonstrated.

The National Institutes of Health recently curtailed one of its major clinical trials, the β-Adrenoceptor Blocker Heart Attack Trial (BHAT), which evaluated the effect of long-term propranolol therapy on total mortality in survivors of an acute myocardial infarction.[6,104] BHAT was a large multicenter randomized, double-blind trial comparing propranolol to placebo in assessing their effects on survival in patients enrolled 5 to 21 days after the onset of infarction. The study was designed to avoid the methodologic problems of previous trials. From June 1978 to October 1980, 3837 men and women aged 30 to 69 years with documented myocardial infarction (representing 23 percent of age-eligible patients) were enrolled and randomized to one of the two study groups (1916 to propranolol and 1921 to placebo). Baseline demographic comparability between the patient groups was excellent. The average time from infarction to treatment randomization was 13.8 days.[6]

All patients were initially assigned to receive 40 mg of propranolol or placebo three times daily before hospital discharge. Depending on serum propranolol levels, a maintenance dose of 60 or 80 mg three times daily was then prescribed and patients were followed on an average for 2 years. Although the treatment intervention was originally scheduled to end in June 1982, the results were so favorable with propranolol that an independent monitoring board stopped the study in October, 1981. After a mean follow-up time of 25 months, a total mortality rate of 9.8 percent was observed in the placebo group versus a 7.2 percent rate in the propranolol group, a 26 percent reduction in mortality. Propranolol also caused reductions in total cardiovascular mortality (26 percent), sudden cardiac death (28 percent), and nonfatal reinfarction (16 percent).[6,104,105] Twenty-four percent of the patients in each group were withdrawn from the randomized treatment for various reasons but are included in the final data analysis. The propranolol regimen was well tolerated, and treated patients had a slightly increased frequency of congestive heart failure compared to placebo. In this study, propranolol was beneficial for all age groups, males and females, blacks and whites, and for patients in different cardiovascular risk strata. The site of previous myocardial infarct had no impact on the efficacy of propranolol. The BHAT results indicated that the beneficial effects of propranolol occurred primarily in the first 12 to 18 months after myocardial infarction. There are no data from BHAT addressing the possible benefits of starting β-blocker therapy at a time remote from the infarction, or at what time point treatment should be discontinued. As a result of this study, the FDA has recently approved propranolol at a dose range of 180 to 240 mg daily in two or three divided oral doses, to be started 5 to 21 days after the acute phase of myocardial infarction for reducing the risk of patient mortality except in those situations where the drug is contraindicated.

The results of a prospective, randomized, double-blind trial from Norway were reported on by Hansteen et al., in which the effect of propranolol and placebo on the incidence of sudden death were compared in a high-risk group of patients who survived the acute phase of myocardial infarction.[96] Altogether, 4929 patients with definite acute myocardial infarction were screened for inclusion—574 (11.6 percent) died before randomization and 3795 (77 percent) were excluded, including all low-risk patients. Five hundred and sixty patients aged 35 to 70 years were stratified into two high-risk groups and randomly assigned treatment with propranolol 40 mg four times daily or placebo. Group I consisted of patients who had been treated for ventricular fibrillation, asystole, or prolonged ventricular tachycardia in the Intensive Care Unit. Group II consisted of patients with one or more of the following complications during the acute phase of myocardial infarction: ventricular tachycardia of short duration, complicated ventricular premature beats, atrial fibrillation or flutter not previously diagnosed, sinus tachycardia exceeding 120 beats per minute for more than 3 hours, and left ventricular failure. Patients with severe heart failure—i.e., cardiogenic shock or pulmonary edema—and patients who still presented with signs of heart failure at the time of randomization were excluded.[96]

Treatment was started 4 to 6 days after the infarction. By 1 year, there had been 11 sudden deaths in the propranolol group and 23 in the placebo group, a significant difference. All together, there were 25 deaths in the propranolol group and 37 in the placebo group, with 16 and 21 nonfatal reinfarctions observed, respectively. Withdrawal because of heart failure during the first 2 weeks of treatment was significantly more common among propranolol-treated patients than among the controls, but thereafter the withdrawal rate was the same.[96]

The mechanism of propranolol's benefit in reducing the risk of cardiovascular mortality in survivors of an acute myocardial infarction is not known. In a study by Koppes et al., patients with premature ventricular complexes (PVCs) were selected for propranolol treatment 2 months after the acute infarction.[106] The dosage of propranolol was increased stepwise over a period of time until the PVCs were completely suppressed (average dose 160 mg daily). The study was small (32 patients) and not controlled. There were no sudden deaths during the 6-month follow-up period. These results suggest an antiarrhythmic effect of propranolol for its prophylactic actions, and the possible need to use varied dosing regimens in therapeutic trials to achieve adequate β-blockade.[106]

In BHAT, 24-hour ambulatory ECG monitoring was performed in patients at baseline and in the subgroup of patients after 6 weeks of therapy. In the placebo group, an increased incidence in ventricular arrhythmias was seen at 6 weeks compared to baseline. This increase was blunted by propranolol therapy.[107] Whether or not this finding contributed to the observed benefit in this trial on cardiovascular mortality in sudden death is not known.

Sotalol. Sotalol, a nonselective β-blocker without membrane or partial agonist activity, is not approved for clinical use in the United States. It is a β-blocker that also possesses Class III antiarrhythmic properties. The drug was evaluated by Julian et al.[98] in a randomized, double-blind trial that demonstrated a nonsignificant favorable trend (18 percent) for total mortality with sotalol compared to placebo. From the combined end point, fatal and nonfatal myocardial infarction, there was a significant difference in 41 percent between the sotalol and placebo groups.[98]

Timolol. Timolol, a nonselective, orally active β-blocker with no partial agonist or membrane activity, has received FDA approval for the treatment of systemic hypertension and for reducing the risk of mortality and nonfatal reinfarction in survivors of an acute myocardial infarction. The latter approval was based on the results of a large multicenter trial from Norway,[4,108] where the effects of timolol in fixed doses (10 mg twice daily) were compared with that of placebo in patients surviving an acute myocardial infarction. The primary objective of this study was to determine whether long-term administration of timolol in this population, stratified for risk, would result in a significant reduction in total mortality, sudden death, and reinfarction over the follow-up period. The trial was initiated, designed, and directed by the academic hospital sector of Norway, with financial support provided by industry. Treatment was started seven to 28 days after infarction in 1884 patients (945 taking timolol, and 939 placebo) who represented 52 percent of those evaluated for entry; the patients were followed for 12 to 33 months (mean 17 months). The trial was kept double-blind as far as is possible with a β-blocker. The groups were well balanced at entry, and statistical adjustment for minor differences did not alter the conclusions materially. Twenty-three percent of control patients and 29 percent of the timolol group were withdrawn from randomized treatment, the difference being due mainly to the usual side effects of a nonselective β-blocker. Withdrawn patients were followed for survival and for reinfarction.

The trial was terminated when the last patients to enter had been followed for 12 months. At this time, 98 patients (10.4 percent) randomized to timolol had died, compared with 152 (16.2 percent) of the control group, a significant reduction in total mortality of 36 percent analyzed on an "intention to treat" basis. The benefit of timolol was evident regardless of patient age and size of infarct.[109] The first-year placebo mortality rate of 11.3 percent in the timolol study[4] was about twice that seen in BHAT,[6] which suggests that a high-risk population was studied in Norway. In spite of this difference in study population, treatment effect was similar, with reductions in the first-year mortality rate of approximately 33 percent with timolol, and 39 percent in BHAT (in both trials patients were followed for a minimum of 1 year).

Nonfatal reinfarction was reported in 88 patients randomized to timolol compared to 141 among controls, an apparent reduction of 34 percent in the rate. This result, however, is more open to question than the similar benefit seen for death, because diagnostic bias cannot be wholly excluded. Similar to the results of BHAT, the Norwegian timolol study demonstrated beyond a reasonable doubt that in these randomized patients, timolol achieved a major reduction in deaths and in nonfatal reinfarction. Based on the results of the Norwegian timolol trial, the FDA has approved the drug for hemodynamically stable survivors of an acute myocardial infarction in the fixed dose of 10 mg twice daily, starting 7 to 28 days after the acute infarction, except in those patients with contraindications to β-blockade.

Trial Interpretation

Most of the long-term β-blocker trials showed a lower mortality rate in the β-blocker treatment group compared to placebo (Table 5).[4–6,87–92,96–99,110] To enable a comparison of the different major trials while taking into account differences in control group mortality rates, the effect of intervention has for each study been estimated by the relative difference (control mortality minus intervention mortality divided by control mortality times 100). For each estimate, the approximately 95 percent confidence limits are also given (Fig. 1).[97,99,111] They allow one to conclude reasonably that the true effect of an intervention in any particular trial lies somewhere within the bounds of the confidence limits. The overall conclusion from the studies is that β-blockers have a benefit on long-term

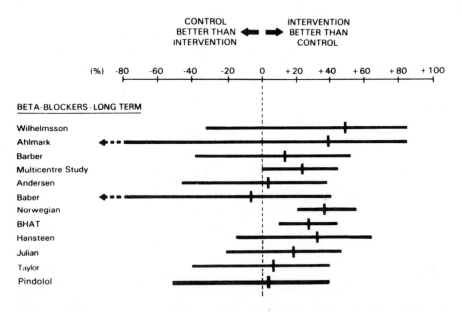

Figure 1. Estimates with approximate 95 percent confidence limits of the relative differences in total mortality between control and intervention in 32 long-term trials of β-blockers after myocardial infarction.[4–6,87–92,95–99] [Reprinted from Circulation 67 (Suppl I):I-48, 1983, with permission from The American Heart Association, Inc.[111]]

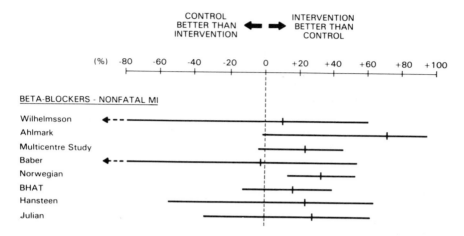

Figure 2. Estimates with approximate 95 percent confidence limits of the relative differences in nonfatal myocardial infarction between control and intervention in 8 long-term trials of β-blockers after myocardial infarction.[4,87,89,91,95–98,105] [Reprinted from Circulation 67 (Suppl I):I-84, 1983 with permission from The American Heart Association, Inc.[105]]

survival in postinfarction patients. The pooled estimate of benefit for β-blockers is 22 percent.

Eight of the nine trials reporting on the incidence of nonfatal reinfarction found lower rates in the β-blocker treatment group (Fig. 2).[99,105] When one pools the results, one finds a reduction in nonfatal reinfarction of 22 percent, a benefit identical to that of overall mortality.[105,110]

In the seven trials that reported on sudden death,[4,6,87–89,91,96,98,110] pooled data revealed a 28 percent reduction in total mortality compared to placebo, and a 33 percent reduction in sudden cardiac death. It appears that β-blockers are effective in reducing total mortality, nonfatal myocardial reinfarction, and sudden death.

CLINICAL APPLICATION OF β-ADRENERGIC BLOCKADE IN SURVIVORS OF MYOCARDIAL INFARCTION

There is now a substantial body of data obtained from carefully constructed and analyzed clinical trials to substantiate the claim that some orally active β-adrenergic blockers are efficacious in reducing the risk of death in many survivors of an acute myocardial infarction.[4–6,111] Should all postinfarction patients be treated with β-blockers? There are obvious contraindications to the use of β-blockers, such as advanced congestive heart failure, Raynaud's phenomenon, a tendency to bronchial asthma, significant disorders or atrioventricular and sinus node function, and vasospastic angina. These conditions restrict the postinfarction population in whom β-blocker therapy can be administered. Furthermore, in the major postinfarction β-blocker studies, approximately 50 percent of the eligible patients (including many high-risk individuals) were excluded.[4-6,96] Therefore, similar patient selection should be utilized if comparable mortality reduction is to be achieved in standard clinical practice. It would appear from the findings of recent studies that the greatest benefit from β-blocker therapy is found in those patients who are over 60 years of age, and in the medium- to high-risk postinfarction groups.[109,112,113] There is a serious question whether the low-risk postinfarction patients (first infarct, no left ventricular dysfunction, normal predischarge exercise test, and absence of complex ventricular arrhythmias), who have a 1-year posthospital discharge mortality of 2 percent, require prophylactic treatment with β-blockers.[114] It is also not known whether β-blockers should be used as long-term prophylactic therapy in patients who have undergone successful coronary bypass surgery.[110] Certainly, postinfarction patients with angina pectoris, hypertension, supraventricular arrhythmias, and strongly positive stress electrocardiograms should be considered for treatment with β-blockers as soon as these indications arise.[110]

Is one β-adrenergic blocker superior to another in survivors of an acute myocardial infarction, or is there a common protective effect seen with all the drugs in this class? Trials investigating seven different β-blockers found favorable mortality trends that seem to indicate that the benefit is conferred by the drug class rather than by a specific β-blocker. However, differences in efficacy may be seen among the β-blockers, since the results of three recent trials with partial agonist β-blocker have shown little or no benefit.[97,99,100]

When should treatment be initiated with β-blockers, by what route, and at what dose, and for how long? It would appear from the Swedish metoprolol study that β-adrenergic treatment can be initiated early and safely in hemodynamically stable patients.[5] However, the β-blocking drugs have not yet received FDA approval for early intravenous use in acute myocardial infarction. Half of the previous studies with intravenous and/or oral treatment did not reveal favorable effects on survival with an early drug intervention (Fig. 3).[5,54-57,63,68,90,92-94,115-121] In contrast, timolol was the first orally active β-blocker approved by the FDA as a long-term prophylactic agent in survivors of an acute myocardial infarction, at a fixed daily dose of 20 mg (in two divided doses) to be started 7 to 28 days after the acute myocardial infarction. Propranolol was recently approved for this use, based on the findings of BHAT at a range

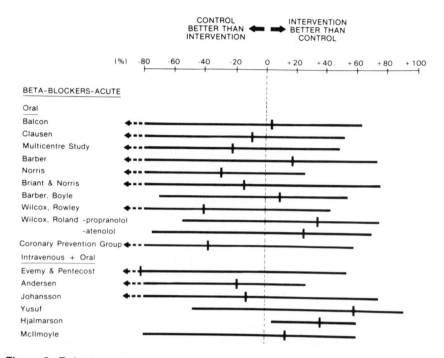

Figure 3. Estimates with approximate 95 percent confidence limits of the relative differences in total mortality between control and intervention in 16 β-blocker trials in the acute phase of myocardial infarction.[5,54–57,63,90,92–94,115–120] [Reprinted from Circulation 67 (Suppl I): I-24, 1983, with permission from The American Heart Association, Inc.[121]]

of 180 to 240 mg daily in two to three divided doses to be started 5 to 21 days after the onset of infarction. Whether or not the sustained release form of propranolol will be effective as a postinfarction treatment, needs to be determined.[122] It is also not yet clear which dose regimen is preferable—a fixed dose or titration of the dose until clinical β-adrenergic blockade is achieved.

No conclusive data are available regarding a benefit on long-term survival in β-blocker therapy if it is begun months to years after acute infarction. Nonetheless, it is reasonable to assume that a beneficial effect on mortality and morbidity would occur if treatment were initiated within a few months after hospitalization. Support of this view arose from retrospective subgroup analyses from the CPRG oxprenolol trial, which suggested a beneficial effect on survival if treatment was started within 4 months, and no benefit if therapy were initiated 4 months or later after myocardial infarction.[97]

The findings of these studies suggest that the major beneficial effects of β-blockers accrue in the first 12 to 18 months postinfarction, and that the incremental benefit thereafter is small.[4,6] The limited information available from the trial shows more deaths from the placebo treatment group than in the β-blocker groups as far out as 48 months.[4,6,97] This would suggest that there is a sustained benefit from continued therapy. If one is concerned with the extended use of these drugs in the general postinfarction population, patients in the intermediate and high-risk subsets, who substantially benefit the most from β-blocker therapy, might be a group for longer courses of therapy. An argument for stopping β-blocker treatment after a fixed time period is the recent observation that some β-blockers can lower plasma-HDL cholesterol and raise triglycerides, potentially increasing the risk of atherogenesis.[123–125] Whether this should be a concern in patients who already have advanced heart disease is debatable. Finally, in the long-term trials, there was no evidence of a β-blocker "withdrawal reaction" in those patients who discontinued active treatment, an early concern with the drugs that has not been observed in the postinfarction population.[126] Patients who require continued β-blocker treatment for other reasons (angina pectoris, hypertension, migraine, and arrhythmia) should be maintained on this treatment regimen as needed.[110]

How will postinfarction β-blocker therapy effect utilization of coronary reconstructive procedures in this population? Coronary artery reconstructive surgery appears to be of benefit in patients with significant angina and angiographically documented severe left main or three-vessel coronary artery disease. Therapy with β-blockers should reduce the frequency and severity of angina, and therefore may diminish clinical indications for coronary angiography and bypass surgery. In addition, since there is a documented reduction in 1-year postinfarction mortality with β-blockers, risk–benefit considerations may now favor continued medical therapy in many patients rather than surgical intervention.

Is there a difference in the postinfarction safety profiles of the different β-blockers? Severe side effects from β-adrenergic blocking drugs were infrequent in the postinfarction trials. Compared to placebo, there appeared to be a higher incidence of symptomatic congestive heart failure, sinus bradycardia, hypotension, bronchial obstruction, fatigue, and mental depression with the β-blockers.[127] Caution should still be exercised, however, when using β-blockers in high-risk patients whose myocardial function may be dependent on stimulation from the sympathetic nervous system. The different β-blockers used in these trials appeared to demonstrate comparable safety profiles, except for practolol, which caused a unique series of side effects, leading to its withdrawal from the world market.[88,89,127]

How are the β-blockers acting to protect certain patients with previous myocardial infarction from death and reinfarction (see Chapter 8)? By virtue of their basic pharmacologic actions, the drugs as a group can attenuate sympathetic cardiac stimulation and perhaps the potential for reentrant ventricular arrhythmia and sudden death.[13,46,128] The drugs inhibit lipolysis and can reduce stress-induced increases in free fatty acids that can induce arrhythmia.[10] All β-blockers have been found to exert a powerful suppressive effect on plasma renin.[11] Owing to the concomitant aldosterone-lowering effect, β-blockers might also be protecting patients from the dangers of hypokalemia. The platelet inhibiting actions of some β-blockers (see Chapter 9) probably do not contribute to their benefit in infarct survivors since this effect is related to nonspecific membrane stabilization and not to β-adrenergic blockade (timolol lacks this membrane-stabilizing property).[12] Other less probable mechanisms for benefit include favorable effects on the oxygen dissociation curve,[49,129] and reduction in transmembrane myocardial calcium fluxes.[10]

Whatever the mechanisms, it is clear that the appropriate use of β-blockers in postinfarction patients should improve the outcome of many patients. In addition, in view of the high incidence of myocardial infarction in Western societies, the widespread use of β-blockers in postinfarction patients should produce a measurable reduction in the overall mortality rate from coronary heart disease. The decline in cardiovascular mortality, which has been evident in the epidemiologic data of several Western countries for the past 15 years, should become more widespread with the greater use of β-blockers in survivors of an acute myocardial infarction who have no contraindications to their use.

REFERENCES

1. Frishman WH: β-Adrenoceptor antagonists—new drugs and new indications. N Engl J Med 305:500, 1981.
2. Braunwald E: Treatment of the patient after myocardial infarction. N Engl J Med 302:290, 1981.
3. Frishman WH: Clinical pharmacology of the new β-adrenoceptor blocking drugs. Part 12. Beta-adrenoceptor blockade in myocardial infarction: The continuing controversy. Am Heart J 99:529, 1980.
4. The Norwegian Multicenter Study Group. Timolol-induced reduction in mortality and reinfarction in patients surviving acute myocardial infarction. N Engl J Med 304:801, 1981.
5. Hjalmarson Å, Emfeldt D, Herlitz J, et al: Effect on mortality of metoprolol in acute myocardial infarction. Lancet ii:823, 1981.
6. β-Blocker Heart Attack Trial Research Group. A randomized trial of propranolol in patients with acute myocardial infarction. 1. Mortality results. JAMA 247:1107, 1982.

7. Braunwald E, Muller JE, Kloner RA, Maroko PR: Role of beta-adrenergic blockade in the therapy of patients with myocardial infarction. Am J Med 74:113, 1983.

8. Frishman WH: Multifactorial actions of β-adrenergic blocking drugs in ischemic heart disease: current concepts. Circulation 67 (Suppl I):I-11, 1983.

9. Boudoulas H, Lewis RP, Rittgers SE, et al: Increased diastolic time: A possible important factor in the beneficial effect of propranolol in patients with coronary artery disease. J Cardiovasc Pharmacol 1:503, 1979.

10. Opie LH: Myocardial infarct size. Part 2. Comparison of anti-infarct effects of beta-blockade, glucose-insulin, potassium, nitrates, and hyaluronidase. Am Heart J 100:531, 1980.

11. Frishman W, Silverman R: Clinical pharmacology of the new beta-adrenergic blocking drugs. Part 2. Physiologic and metabolic effects. Am Heart J 97:797, 1979.

12. Frishman WH, Weksler BB: Effects of β-adrenoceptor blocking drugs on platelet function in normal subjects and patients with angina pectoris, in Roskamm H, Graefe KH (eds), Advances in β-Blocker Therapy: Proceedings of an International Symposium. Amsterdam, Excerpta Medica, 1980, p 164.

13. Braunwald E: Effects of coronary by-pass grafting on survival. New Engl J Med 309:1181, 1983.

14. Stewart McDG: Compared incidence of first myocardial infarction in hypertensive patients under treatment containing propranolol or excluding β-receptor blockade. Clin Sci 51 (Suppl):509s, 1976.

15. Berglund G, Sannerstedt R, Andersson O, et al: Coronary heart disease after treatment of hypertension. Lancet 1:1, 1978.

16. Beevers DG, Johnston JH, Larkin H, Davies P: Clinical evidence: β-Adrenoceptor blockers prevent more cardiovascular complications than other antihypertensive drugs. Drugs 25 (Suppl 2):326, 1983.

17. MRC (Medical Research Council). A randomized controlled trial for mild to moderate hypertension, design and pilot trial experience. Br Med J 1:1437, 1977.

18. Jewitt DE, Singh BN: The role of β-adrenergic blockade in myocardial infarction. Prog Cardiovasc Dis 16:421, 1974.

19. Jewitt DE, Mercer CJ, Reid D, et al: Free noradrenaline and adrenaline secretion in relation to the development of cardiac arrhythmias and heart failure in patients with acute myocardial infarction. Lancet 1:635, 1969.

20. McDonald L, Baker C, Bray C, et al: Plasma catecholamines after cardiac infarction. Lancet 2:1021, 1969.

21. Han J: Mechanisms of ventricular arrhythmia associated with myocardial infarction. Am J Cardiol 24:800, 1969.

22. Vatner SF, McRitchie RJ, Maroko PR, et al: Effects of catecholamines, exercise and nitroglycerin on the normal and ischemic myocardium in conscious dogs. J Clin Invest 54:563, 1974.

23. Maroko PR, Kjekshus JK, Sobel B, et al: Factors influencing infarct size following experimental coronary artery occlusions. Circulation 43:67, 1971.

24. Kirk ES, Sonnenblick EH: Newer concepts in the pathophysiology of is-

chemic heart disease. Am Heart J 103:756, 1982.

25. Maroko PR, Braunwald E: Modification of infarct size after coronary occlusion. Ann Intern Med 79:720, 1973.

26. Singh BN: Beta-blockers and acute myocardial infarction. Drugs 15:218, 1978.

27. Frishman W, Silverman R, Strom J, et al: Clinical pharmacology of the new beta-adrenergic blocking drugs. Part 4. Adverse effects. Choosing a β-adrenoceptor blocker. Am Heart J 98:256, 1979.

28. Ceremuzynski L, Staszewska-Barczak J, Herbaczynsha-Cedro K: Cardiac rhythm disturbances and the release of catecholamines after coronary occlusion in dogs. Cardiovasc Res 3:190, 1969.

29. Ebert PA, Vanderbeck RB, Allgood RJ, Sabiston DC: Effect of chronic cardiac denervation on arrhythmias after coronary artery ligation. Cardiovasc Res 4:141, 1970.

30. Khan MI, Hamilton JT, Manning GW: Protective effects of beta-adrenoceptor blockade in experimental coronary occlusion in conscious dogs. Am J Cardiol 30:832, 1972.

31. Hoffman BF, Singer DH: Appraisal of the effects of catecholamines on cardiac electrical activity. Ann NY Acad Sci 139:914, 1967.

32. Rydén L, Ariniego R, Arnman K, et al: A double-blind trial of metoprolol in acute myocardial infarction. N Engl J Med 308:614, 1983.

33. Yusuf S, Sleight P, Rossi P, et al: Reduction in infarct size, arrhythmias and chest pain by early intravenous beta-blockade in suspected acute myocardial infarction. Circulation 67 (Suppl I):I-32, 1983.

34. Lemberg L, Castellanos A, Aroebal AG: The use of propranolol in arrhythmias complicating acute myocardial infarction. Am Heart J 80:479, 1970.

35. Nies AS, Shand DG: Clinical pharmacology of propranolol. Circulation 52:6, 1975.

36. Lichstein E, Morganroth J, Harrist R, Hubble E: Antiarrhythmic effects of beta-blockers: Preliminary data from the Beta-Blocker Heart Attack Trial for the BHAT study group. Circulation 67 (Suppl I):I-5, 1983.

37. Koppes GM, Beckmann CH, Jones FG: Propranolol therapy for ventricular arrhythmias 2 months after myocardial infarction. Am J Cardiol 46:322, 1980.

38. von der Lippe G, Lund-Johansen P, Kjekshus J: Effects of timolol on late ventricular arrhythmias after acute myocardial infarction. Acta Med Scand 651 (Suppl I):253, 1981.

39. Frishman WH, Sonnenblick EH: Propranolol therapy in acute myocardial infarction. Cardiovasc Med 2:311, 1977.

40. Norris RM: Beta-adrenoceptor blockade in acute myocardial infarction. Am Heart J 99:683, 1980.

41. Miura M, Thomas R, Ganz W, et al: The effect of delay in propranolol administration on reduction of myocardial infarct size after experimental coronary occlusion in dogs. Circulation 59:1148, 1979.

42. Reimer KA, Lowe JE, Rasmussen MM, Jennings RB: The wave front of phenomenon of ischemic cell death. 1. Myocardial infarct size versus du-

ration of coronary occlusion in dogs. Circulation 56:786, 1977.

43. Maroko PR, Libby P, Ginks WR, et al: Coronary artery reperfusion. 1. Early effects on local myocardial function and the extent of myocardial necrosis. J Clin Invest 51:2710, 1972.

44. Hillis LD, Braunwald E: Myocardial ischemia. N Engl J Med 296:971, 1034, 1093, 1977.

45. Reimer KA, Rasmussen MM, Jennings RB: Reduction by propranolol of myocardial necrosis following temporary coronary occlusion in dogs. Circ Res 33:353, 1973.

46. Opie LH: Myocardial infarct size. Part 1. Basic considerations. Am Heart J 100:355, 1980.

47. Vatner SF, Baig H, Manders WT, et al: Effects of propranolol on regional myocardial function, electrograms, and blood flow in conscious dogs with myocardial ischemia. J Clin Invest 60:353, 1977.

48. Kloner RA, Fishbein MC, Cotran RS, et al: The effect of propranolol on microvascular injury in acute myocardial ischemia. Circulation 55:872, 1977.

49. Schrumph J, Sheps DS, Wolfson S, et al: Alterted hemoglobin-oxygen affinity with long-term propranolol therapy in patients with coronary artery disease. Am J Cardiol 40:76, 1977.

50. Welman E, Fox KM, Selwyn AP, Carroll BJ: The effect of established β-adrenoreceptor blocking therapy on the release of cytoscolic and lysosomal enzymes after acute myocardial infarction in man. Clin Sci Mol Med 55:549, 1978.

51. Pierce WS, Carter DR, McGavran MH, Waldhausen JA: Modification of myocardial infarct volume. Arch Surg 107:682, 1973.

52. Libby P, Maroko PR, Covell J, et al: Effect of practolol on the extent of myocardial ischemic injury after experimental coronary occlusion and its effects on ventricular function in the normal and ischaemic heart. Cardiovas Res 7:167, 1973.

53. Lefer AM, Cohn JR, Osman GH: Protective action of timolol in acute myocardial ischemia. Eur J Clin Pharmacol 41:379, 1977.

54. Balcon R, Jewitt DE, Davies JPH, Oram S: A controlled trial of propranolol in acute myocardial infarction. Lancet 2:919, 1966.

55. Clausen J, Felsby M, Schonau Jorgensen F, et al: Absence of prophylactic effect of propranolol in myocardial infarction. Lancet 2:920, 1966.

56. Multicentre Trial. Propranolol in acute myocardial infarction. Lancet 2:1435, 1966.

57. Norris RM, Caughey DE, Scot PJ: Trial of propranolol in acute myocardial infarction. Br Med J 2:398, 1968.

58. Pelides LJ, Reid DS, Thomas R, Shillingford JP: Inhibition by β-blockade of the ST segment elevation after acute myocardial infarction in man. Cardiovasc Res 6:295, 1972.

59. Mueller HS, Ayres SM, Religa A, Evans RG: Propranolol in the treatment of acute myocardial infarction. Circulation 49:1078, 1974.

60. Gold HK, Leinbach RC, Maroko PR: Propranolol-induced reduction of

signs of ischemic injury during acute myocardial infarction. Am J Cardiol 38:689, 1976.

61. Peter T, Norris RM, Clarke ED, et al: Reduction of enzyme levels by propranolol after acute myocardial infarction. Circulation 57:1091, 1978.

62. Hjalmarson Å, Herlitz J: Limitation of infarct size by beta-blockers and its potential role for prognosis. Circulation 67 (Suppl I):I-68, 1983.

63. McIlmoyle, Evans A, McBoyle D, et al: Early intervention in myocardial ischemia (Abstr). Proceedings of the British Cardiac Society. Br Heart J 47:189, 1982.

64. Heikkila J, Nieminen MS: Protection of ischemic myocardium with intravenous pindolol in acute myocardial infarction (Abstr). Am J Cardiol 45:484, 1980.

65. Norris RM, Clarke ED, Sammel NL, et al: Protective effect of propranolol in threatened myocardial infarction. Lancet 2:907, 1978.

66. Frishman W, Smithen C, Belfer B, et al: Noninvasive assessment of clinical response to oral propranolol. Am J Cardiol 35:635, 1975.

67. Cutler JA: A review of on-going trials of beta-blockers in the secondary prevention of coronary heart disease. Circulation 67 (Suppl I):I-62, 1983.

68. Muller J, Roberts R, Stone P, et al: Failure of propranolol administration to limit infarct size in patients with acute myocardial infarction (Abstr). Circulation (Suppl III): III-294, 1983.

69. Sederholm M, Richardson P, Kjekshus J, et al: Intravenous timolol in the early management of acute myocardial infarction (Abstr). Circulation (Suppl III) III-294, 1983.

70. Frishman WH: Beta-adrenergic blockade in the treatment of coronary artery disease, in Hurst JW (ed), Clinical Essays on the Heart. New York, McGraw-Hill, 1983, vol II, pp 25–63.

71. Davies RO, Mizgala HF, Tinmouth AL, et al: Prospective controlled trial of long-term propranolol on acute coronary events in patients with unstable coronary artery disease (Abstr). Clin Pharmacol Ther 17:232, 1975.

72. Fox KM, Chopra MP, Portal RW, Aber CP: Long-term beta-blockade possible protection from myocardial infarction. Br Med J 1:117, 1975.

73. Coronary Drug Project Research Group. Factors influencing long-term prognosis after recovery from myocardial infarction. J Chronic Dis 27:267, 1974.

74. Vedin A, Wilhelmsen L, Wedel H, et al: Prediction of cardiovascular deaths and non-fatal reinfarction after myocardial infarction. Acta Med Scand 201:309, 1977.

75. Luria MH, Knoke JA, Wacks JS, Luria MA: Survival after recovery from myocardial infarction: two and five year prognostic indices. Am J Med 67:7, 1979.

76. Moss AJ, Davis HT, DeCamilla J, Bayer LW: Ventricular ectopic beats and their relation to sudden and nonsudden cardiac death after myocardial infarction. Circulation 60:998, 1979.

77. Davis HT, DeCamilla J, Bayer LW, Moss AJ: Survivorship patterns in the posthospital phase of myocardial infarction. Circulation 60:1252, 1979.

78. The Multicenter Post-Infarction Research Group. Risk stratification after myocardial infarction. N Engl J Med 309:331, 1983.
79. May GS, Eberlein KA, Furberg CD, et al: Secondary prevention after myocardial infarction: a review of long-term trials. Prog Cardiovasc Dis 24:331, 1982.
80. Fein SA, Klein NA, Frishnian WH: Exercise testing soon after uncomplicated myocardial infarction. Prognostic value and safety. JAMA 245:1863, 1981.
81. Frishman WH, Ribner H: Anticoagulation in myocardial infarction. A modern approach to an old problem. Am J Cardiol 43:1207, 1979.
82. Persantine-Aspirin Reinfarction Study Research Group. Persantine and aspirin in coronary artery disease. Circulation 62:449, 1980.
83. Oliver MF, Heady JA, Morris JN, Cooper J: A cooperative trial in the primary prevention of ischaemic heart disease using clofibrate. Br Heart J 40:1069, 1978.
84. Myocardial Infarction Study Group. Secondary prevention of ischemic heart disease: a long-term controlled lidoflazine study. Acta Cardiol 24 (Suppl):7, 1979.
85. Snow PJD: Effect of propranolol in myocardial infarction. Lancet 2:551, 1965.
86. Reynolds JL, Whitlock RML: Effects of beta-adrenergic receptor blocker in myocardial infarction treated for one year from onset. Br Heart J 34:252, 1972.
87. Wilhelmsson C, Vedin JA, Wilhelmsen L, et al: Reduction of sudden deaths after myocardial infarction by treatment with alprenolol: preliminary results. Lancet 2:1157, 1974.
88. Multicentre International Study. Improvement in prognosis of myocardial infarction by long-term beta-adrenoreceptor blockade using practolol: A multicentre international study. Br Med J 3:735, 1975.
89. Multicentre International Study. Reduction in mortality with long-term beta-adrenoceptor blockade: a multicentre international study. Br Med J 2:49, 1977.
90. Barber JM, Boyle D McC, Chaturvedi NC, et al: Practolol in acute myocardial infarction. Acta Med Scand 587 (Suppl):213, 1976.
91. Ahlmark G, Saetre H: Long-term treatment with β-blockers after myocardial infarction. Eur J Clin Pharmacol 10:77, 1976.
92. Andersen MP, Bechsgaard P, Frederiksen J, et al: Effect of alprenolol on mortality among patients with definite or suspected acute myocardial infarction: preliminary results. Lancet 2:865, 1979.
93. Wilcox RG, Roland JM, Banks DC, et al: Randomized trial comparing propranolol with atenolol in immediate treatment of suspected myocardial infarction. Br Med J 280:885, 1980.
94. Wilcox RG, Rowley JM, Hampton JR, et al: Randomized placebo-controlled trial comparing oxprenolol with disopyramide phosphase in immediate treatment of suspected myocardial infarction. Lancet 2:765, 1980.
95. Baber NS, Wainwright Evans D, Howitt G, et al: Multicentre post-infarc-

tion trial of propranolol in 49 hospitals in the United Kingdom, Italy and Yugoslavia. Br Heart J 44:96, 1980.

96. Hansteen V, Moinichen E, Lorentsen E, et al: One year's treatment with propranolol after myocardial infarction: preliminary report of Norwegian Multicentre Trial. Br Med J 284:155, 1982.

97. Taylor SH, Silke B, Ebbutt A, et al: A long-term prevention study with oxprenolol in coronary heart disease. N Engl J Med 307:1293, 1982.

98. Julian DG, Prescott RJ, Jackson FS, Szekely P: A controlled trial of sotalol for one year after myocardial infarction. Lancet 1:1142, 1982.

99. Australian and Swedish Pindolol Study Group. The effect of pindolol on the two years mortality after complicated myocardial infarction. Eur Heart J 4:367, 1983.

100. European Infarction Study Group. European Infarction Study (E.I.S.)—A secondary beta-blocker prevention trial after myocardial infarction (Abstr). Circulation 68 (Suppl III):III-294, 1983.

101. Hampton JR: The use of beta-blockers for the reduction of mortality after myocardial infarction. Eur Heart J 2:254, 1981.

102. Editorial. Beta-blockers after myocardial infarction. Lancet 2:873, 1981.

103. Hampton JR: Presentation and analysis of the results of clinical trials in cardiovascular disease. Br Med J 282:1371, 1981.

104. Goldstein S: Propranolol therapy in patients with acute myocardial infarction: the Beta-Blocker Heart Attack Trial. Circulation 67 (Suppl I):I-53, 1983.

105. Furberg CD, Bell RL: Effect of beta-blocker therapy on recurrent non-fatal myocardial infarction. Circulation 67 (Suppl I):I-83, 1983.

106. Koppes GM, Beckmann CH, Jones FG: Propranolol therapy for ventricular arrhythmias 2 months after myocardial infarction. Am J Cardiol 46:322, 1980.

107. Lichstein E, Morganroth J, Harrist R, Hubble E: Antiarrhythmic effects of beta-blockers: Preliminary data from the Beta-Blocker Heart Attack Trial for the BHAT Study Group. Circulation 67 (Suppl I):I-5, 1983.

108. Pedersen TR: The Norwegian Multicenter Study of timolol after myocardial infarction. Circulation 67 (Suppl I):I-49, 1983.

109. Rodda BE: The Timolol Myocardial Infarction Study: An evaluation of selected variables. Circulation 67 (Suppl I):I-101, 1983.

110. Turi ZG, Braunwald E: Use of β-blockers after myocardial infarction. JAMA 249;2512, 1983.

111. May GS: A review of long-term beta-blocker trials in survivors of myocardial infarction. Circulation 67 (Suppl I):I-46, 1983.

112. Hawkins CM, Richardson DW, Vokonas PS: Effect of propranolol in reducing mortality in old myocardial infarction patients: The Beta-Blocker Heart Attack Trial Experience. Circulation 67 (Suppl I):I-94, 1983.

113. Furberg CD, Byington RP: What do subgroup analyses reveal about differential response to beta-blocker therapy? Circulation 67 (Suppl I):I-98, 1983.

114. Griggs TR, Wagner GS, Gettes LS: Beta-adrenergic blocking agents after

myocardial infarction: an undocumented need in patients at lowest risk. J Am Coll Cardiol 1:1530, 1983.

115. Barber JM, Murphy FM, Merrett JD: Clinical trial of propranolol in acute myocardial infarction. Ulster Med J 36:127, 1967.

116. Briant RB, Norris RM: Alprenolol in acute myocardial infarction: double-blind trial. N Z Med J 71:135, 1970.

117. Coronary Prevention Research Group. An early intervention, secondary prevention study with oxprenolol following myocardial infarction. Eur Heart J 2:389, 1981.

118. Evemy KL, Pentecost BL: Intravenous and oral practolol in the acute stages of myocardial infarction. Eur J Cardiol 7:391, 1978.

119. Johansson BW: A comparative study of cardioselective beta-blockade and diazepam in patients with acute myocardial infarction and tachycardia. Acta Med Scand 207:47, 1980.

120. Yusuf S, Ramsdale D, Peto R, et al: Early intravenous atenolol treatment in suspected acute myocardial infarction. Lancet 2:273, 1980.

121. May GS: A review of acute-phase beta-blocker trials in patients with myocardial infarction. Circulation 67 (Suppl I):I-21, 1983.

122. Leahey WJ, Neill JD, Varma MPS, Shanks RG: Comparison of the efficacy and pharmacokinetics of conventional propranolol and a long-acting preparation of propranolol. Br J Clin Pharm 9:33, 1980.

123. Leren P, Helgeland A, Holme I, et al: Effect of propranolol and prazosin on blood lipids. The Oslo Study. Lancet 2:4, 1980.

124. Shulman RS, Herbert PN, Capone RJ, et al: Effects of propranolol on blood lipids and lipoproteins in myocardial infarction. Circulation 67 (Suppl I):I-19, 1983.

125. Johnson BF: The emerging problem of plasma lipid changes during antihypertensive therapy. J Cardiovasc Pharm 4 (Suppl 2):213s, 1982.

126. Baber NS, Lewis JA: Beta-adrenoceptor blockade and myocardial infarction: When should treatment start and for how long should it continue? Circulation 67 (Suppl I):I-71, 1983.

127. Friedman LM: How do the various beta-blockers compare in type, frequency and severity of their adverse effects? Circulation 67 (Suppl I):I-89, 1983.

128. Anderson JL, Rodier HE, Green LS: Comparative effects of beta-adrenergic blocking drugs on experimental ventricular fibrillation threshold. Am J Cardiol 51:1196, 1983.

129. Frishman W, Wilner G, Smithen C, et al: Effects of exercise and propranolol on hemoglobin oxygen affinity in patients with angina pectoris. Clin Res 24:614, 1976.

CHAPTER 11

Labetalol Therapy in Patients with Systemic Hypertension and Angina Pectoris: Effects of Combined α- and β-Adrenoceptor Blockade

William H. Frishman, Joel A. Strom, Marc Kirschner, Marcia P. Poland, Edmund H. Sonnenblick, and Neal Klein

β-Adrenoceptor blocking drugs are widely accepted for the treatment of arrhythmias, hypertension, and angina pectoris.[1,2] Labetalol is an adrenergic blocking agent that, like propranolol, blocks both β_1- and β_2-vascular and bronchial adrenoreceptors.[3,4] However, labetalol is unique in that it also has both α-adrenergic blocking properties and direct vasodilatory activity.[3,5]

For the treatment of hypertension and angina pectoris, α-adrenergic blocking drugs have had limited application compared with β-adrenoceptor blocking drugs. This observation with β-blockers may in part be due to the unwanted effects of reflex tachycardia and orthostatic hypotension,[6] which can aggravate symptomatic coronary artery disease. In selected patients with variant angina, α-blocking agents have been used as adjunctive therapy.[7] Patients with coronary artery disease manifest increased coronary vascular resistance following the cold pressor test.[8] Phentolamine, an α-adrenoreceptor blockade, has been shown to reverse this effect. This latter finding raises the possibility that α-adrenoceptor blockade could play a role in the treatment and prevention of myocardial ischemia.[8,9]

Labetalol has been shown to be a potent antihypertensive drug (see Chapters 13 and 14).[4,10–18] Its hemodynamic profile also suggested its pos-

From the American Journal of Cardiology, Volume 48, November 1981, pp 917–928, with permission.

sible use in patients with hypertension and angina pectoris (see Chapter 7).[4,10] Intravenous administration of labetalol in patients with angina pectoris was shown to result in a marked increment in exercise tolerance.[19] In the present study, the efficacy and safety of oral labetalol treatment were assessed in hypertensive patients with angina pectoris.[20] The effects of labetalol on plasma renin activity, platelet function, and noninvasive indexes of left ventricular function were also evaluated.

METHODS

Patient Selection

Ten men with stable angina pectoris and systemic hypertension were entered into the study after written and informed consent was obtained. The mean patient age was 59.4 years (range 48 to 68). The diagnosis of angina pectoris was established by clinical history (at least 5 attacks per week of angina on effort for 1 month with no evidence of an accelerated course), response to nitroglycerin, and the development of typical symptoms with exercise testing. In addition, all patients demonstrated at least 1 mm of ischemic electrocardiographic ST-segment depression with exercise. The diagnosis of coronary artery disease was made on the basis of coronary angiography (75 percent luminal narrowing of at least one major coronary vessel) in six patients and an ischemic electrocardiographic response to exercise in the other four patients. No patient had previous coronary arterial bypass surgery. Systemic hypertension was documented in all patients by an average 3-minute standing diastolic pressure of 90 to 115 mm Hg (using Korotkoff phase V) on at least two separate outpatient visits while untreated.

Patients with the following conditions were excluded from the study: coexistent valvular heart disease, congestive heart failure, anemia, bronchial asthma, hyperlipidemia, severe bradycardia (resting heart rate less than 50 beats per minute), intermittent claudication or myocardial infarction within 3 months. Throughout the trial, patients took no medication (including aspirin) except sublingual nitroglycerin for anginal attacks and the study capsules.

Experimental Design

The study was divided into three phases. In the 3-week baseline phase, patients received a placebo (Schering–Plough Inc., Bloomfield, NJ) three times daily; this was followed by a 4-week labetalol treatment phase and a 1-week withdrawal phase. Both placebo and labetalol were supplied in identical maroon opaque capsules. The dose of oral labetalol was titrated weekly (100 to 400 mg three times daily) to achieve a reduction in blood pressure and lessening of the patient's anginal symptoms. The optimal antihypertensive effect was defined as an average 3-minute standing diastolic blood pressure of less than 90 mm Hg that has also been reduced by at least 10 mm Hg from placebo baseline. Lessening of angina pectoris was defined as a significant decrease in the subjective frequency of anginal attacks and a significant increment in measured exercise duration. If the antihypertensive goal was achieved at a lower dose than maximum, but angina did not lessen, the dose of labetalol was increased. However, this dose increase was made only if the patient could tolerate it without manifesting clinical signs of hypotension. At the end of this 4-week therapeutic period, the dose of labetalol was tapered rapidly over a 2-day interval. The patients were reassessed 1 week after cessation of treatment.

Methods of Observation

All patients kept a detailed daily record of the anginal attacks they experienced, the number of nitroglycerin tablets taken, and an estimation of the physical activity for that day. Every week, patients were evaluated with a detailed history and cardiopulmonary examination that included measurements of supine and standing (3 minute) heart rate and blood pressure. Blood pressure and heart rate determinations were always made at the same time of day, 2 hours after ingestion of placebo or oral labetalol, which is the time for the drug's peak pharmacologic effect.[21] All data reported for comparisons reflect the peak effect of the drug. Patients also underwent multistage treadmill exercise tests each week. At the end of the placebo and labetalol treatment phase, resting M-mode echocardiograms were obtained, and systolic time interval determinations were made from simultaneous high-frequency phonocardiograms, electrocardiograms, and external carotid pulse tracings. In addition, blood was obtained for platelet aggregation studies, plasma renin activity, and plama aldosterone levels.

At the end of the placebo treatment, labetalol treatment, and labetalol withdrawal periods, blood specimens were obtained for complete blood count, platelet counts, tests of clotting function (prothrombin and partial thromboplastin time), and biochemical screening [total protein, albumin, calcium, phosphate, cholesterol, triglycerides, uric acid, urea nitrogen, glucose, sodium, potassium, creatine, carbon dioxide, chloride, total bilirubin, alkaline phosphatase, glutamic pyruvic transaminase (SGPT), lactic dehydrogenase (LDH), glutamic oxaloacetic transaminase (SGOT), and creatine kinase (CK)]. Chest roentgenograms, routine urinalyses, and resting electrocardiograms were performed.

Blood for plasma labetalol levels was obtained at weekly intervals during the placebo, labetalol treatment, and withdrawal periods.

Twenty-four hour urinary collections were obtained for total volume, sodium, chloride, potassium, and creatinine. These collections were obtained at the time of the plasma renin and plasma aldosterone determinations.

Exercise Tests

Multistage treadmill exercise testing employing the Bruce protocol[22] was performed weekly. The blood pressure was measured every 3 minutes during exercise by the auscultatory method and lead V_5 was continuously monitored on the oscilloscope. The electrocardiogram was recorded every minute during the exercise and recovery periods. The end point of exercise was severe angina pectoris or electrocardiographic evidence of myocardial ischemia, or both. An abnormal electrocardiographic response was defined as a flat or a 0.08-second long downsloping ST segment depression of 1 mm after the terminus of the QRS complex with the P–Ta segment as the baseline of reference.

Measurements of heart rate, systolic and diastolic blood pressure, ST segment displacement, arrhythmia, and rate–pressure product (systolic blood pressure times heart rate) were measured at the last minute of each stage of exercise. At the end point of exercise, each test was also analyzed for the maximal heart rate, systolic blood pressure and rate-pressure product achieved, peak stage of exercise, total exercise duration (seconds), ST segment displacement (mm), and reason for exercise limitation. The exercise work, expressed in kilopond-meters (kpm), was calculated from the formula: work (kpm) = sin $\alpha \times$ speed (m/sec) $\times$ body weight (kg) $\times$ exercise time (seconds) divided by 10^3, where α is the angle of inclination of the treadmill.

Echocardiographic Methods

Serial M-mode echocardiograms were performed in the supine position in each patient. A Picker echocardiograph (model 80C) was employed, using a 2.25-MHz, 13-mm-diameter transducer in all studies. The transducer location and examination position were kept constant in all patients allowing for serial comparisons.

End-diastolic left ventricular dimension, septal wall thickness, and posterior wall thickness were measured at the beginning of the Q wave of the electrocardiogram. Care was taken not to assess these indexes at the maximal left ventricular dimension recorded and in a consistent relation to mitral valve landmarks. End-systolic left ventricular wall dimension, septal wall thickness, and posterior wall thickness were identified at the time of minimal left ventricular diameter. Dimensional data were averaged over five to ten cycles per recording. Left ventricular ejection time was taken as the interval from the Q wave to left ventricular end-shortening minus 50 milliseconds. Left ventricular volumes were calculated according to the method of Teichholz et al.[23] Ejection fraction was obtained by subtracting end-systolic from end-diastolic volume and by dividing this value by the end-diastolic volume. Other derived indexes of left ventricular function were calculated with standard methods and included the velocity of circumferential fiber shortening $(V_{cf}) = (LV_d - LV_s) \div (LV_d \times LV$ ejection time), where LV = left ventricular and LV_d and LV_s = left ventricular end-diastolic and systolic wall dimension, respectively.

Systolic Time Intervals
Simultaneous high-frequency phonocardiogram, electrocardiogram, and external carotid pulse tracing were recorded at a paper speed of 100 mm per second. All recordings were obtained with the patient in a semi-supine position with approximately 30 degree elevation of the head and trunk. All studies were performed in the early morning with the patient in the postabsorptive state.

Systolic time intervals were measured according to standard technique as previously described by our laboratory.[24-26] In all instances, five cardiac cycles were analyzed and mean values calculated. The resulting mean systolic time intervals were corrected for heart rate using the linear regression equations of Weissler et al.[24] All subsequent references to preejection period and left ventricular ejection time refer to their rate-corrected values.

Plasma Renin Activity and Aldosterone
Peripheral blood was obtained after an overnight fast from patients through an indwelling peripheral catheter after the patient was upright for 2 hours. The samples were withdrawn into a chilled tube of ethylenediamine tetraacetic acid (EDTA). Plasma renin activity was determined by radioimmunoassay using the angiotensin I Immutope kit (Squibb). Plasma aldosterone levels were determined by radioimmunoassay using the aldosterone radioimmunoassay kit (International CIS).

Platelet Aggregation Studies
These studies were performed according to the turbidometric method of Born,[27] as modified by Mustard et al.,[28] and previously reported from this laboratory.[29] The aggregating agents used were adenosine diphosphate (ADP) and epinephrine. The ADP concentrations producing irreversible aggregation in untreated patients and normal subjects were 0.5, 1, 2, 5, 10, 20, and 100 μM; comparable epinephrine concentrations for aggregation were in the range of 0.5 to 5500 μM. The lowest concentra-

tion producing a full biphasic response was recorded as the threshold dose; the threshold concentration of ADP or epinephrine was assessed without extrapolation between different concentrations. In repeated ADP and epinephrine determinations using coded samples, reproducibility was within 10 percent of the mean.

Labetalol Levels
The concentrations of labetalol were measured in plasma by the spectrofluorometric method of Martin et al.[30]

Statistical Analysis
Group means are presented with the standard error of the mean as the index of dispersion. Differences from baseline were analyzed using Student's two-tailed t test except for frequency of anginal attacks, which was analyzed using the Wilcoxon one-tailed, matched-pairs signed-ranks test. All significant differences were reported at the probability level of 0.05 or less. Plasma levels of labetalol were compared with the administered oral dose using a linear regression analysis.

RESULTS

Effects on Resting Blood Pressure and Heart Rate (Table 1, Figure 1)
Labetalol treatment at all dose levels (300 to 1200 mg daily) caused a significant reduction in mean supine and standing systolic and diastolic blood pressures. The maximal mean effect was seen at the 900 mg per

TABLE 1. EFFECTS OF PLACEBO AND LABETALOL ON RESTING HEART RATE AND BLOOD PRESSURE (BP) IN PATIENTS WITH BOTH ANGINA PECTORIS AND HYPERTENSION

	Baseline (Placebo)	Labetalol (Mean Dose 1050 mg)	Difference	p value
Supine				
Heart rate (beats/min)	80.8 ± 4.6	65.6 ± 2.3	− 15.2 ± 3.0	<0.01
Systolic BP (mm Hg)	166.5 ± 6.3	142.2 ± 4.9	− 24.3 ± 7.1	<0.01
Diastolic BP (mm Hg)	102.7 ± 2.6	87.7 ± 1.5	− 15.0 ± 3.2	<0.01
3-Minute standing				
Heart rate (beats/min)	81.5 ± 4.9	69.0 ± 2.8	− 12.5 ± 3.7	<0.01
Systolic BP (mm Hg)	156.8 ± 4.2	127.5 ± 3.0	− 29.3 ± 5.1	<0.01
Diastolic BP (mm Hg)	101.4 ± 2.3	83.9 ± 3.0	− 18.5 ± 3.5	<0.01

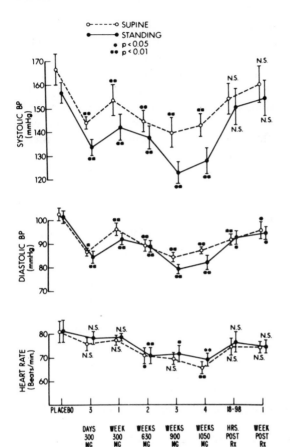

Figure 1. Supine and standing resting blood pressure (BP) and heart rate before, during and after treatment with increasing doses of oral labetalol. Values are mean ± standard error of the mean. N.S. = not significant; p = probability; Rx = treatment.

day dose level. One week after labetalol treatment was stopped, systolic blood pressure returned to placebo baseline levels, whereas diastolic blood pressure, although higher on labetalol treatment, remained significantly below the placebo baseline, $p<0.05$. The mean heart rate was significantly reduced after 600 mg of labetalol in both the supine and standing positions. In three patients, the heart rate was 60 beats per minute or less during labetalol therapy. One patient had a placebo baseline heart rate of 59 beats per minute that decreased to 55 beats per minute at the 900 mg per day dose level. The other 2 patients had a baseline heart rate of 73 and 78 beats per minute that decreased to 56 and 60 beats per minute, respectively, after 900 and 1200 mg per day of labetalol.

In this study, normalization of blood pressure was defined as a standing diastolic blood pressure of less than 90 mm Hg that was also reduced by at least 10 mm Hg from the baseline value. Mean diastolic pressure was reduced well below 90 mm Hg in the standing position with labetalol treatment, an 18.5 ± 3.5 mm Hg decrease ($p<0.01$). The blood pressure of nine of ten patients was normalized during labetalol therapy—two receiving 300 mg, four receiving 600 mg, and three receiving 900 mg daily. In these patients, control was achieved with a mean labetalol dose of 764 mg per day. The one patient whose pressure was not normalized had an 18 mm Hg decrease in diastolic blood pressure to 95 mm Hg with 1200 mg of labetalol.

Effects on Angina Pectoris (Table 2)

After 4 weeks of labetalol treatment (mean dose 1050 mg), there was a significant reduction in the frequency of angina pectoris attacks per week. Labetalol in a dose of 300 mg per day had no effect on the frequency of anginal attacks. However, all patients responded to larger doses of labetalol. The quality of life of the patients was enhanced; they reported an increased ability to perform activities of daily living. All patients were in functional class III (New York Heart Association Criteria[31]) upon entering the study and showed improvement to class II after 4 weeks of labetalol treatment.

Effects on Exercise Variables

Heart rate, systolic blood pressure, and rate-pressure product (Table 2, Fig. 2 and 3): Just before exercise, there was a significant reduction ($p<0.05$) in resting heart rate, systolic blood pressure, and rate–pressure product at a mean labetalol dose of 900 mg daily compared with values during placebo administration (Fig. 2). During exercise, there was a significant reduction in all of these variables (measured at the end of Stage I and Stage II) with labetalol (300 to 1200 mg per day) compared with placebo baseline values. One week after active treatment was stopped, heart rate and rate–pressure product values with exercise were not significantly different from placebo baseline values. However, systolic pressure at Stage II of exercise remained lower than at placebo baseline ($p<0.05$) but was still significantly higher than after 3 and 4 weeks of labetalol treatment (mean daily dose 900 and 1050 mg). After 4 weeks of labetalol treatment (mean daily dose 1050 mg), peak systolic and diastolic pressures, heart rate, and rate–pressure product at maximal exercise were reduced significantly from placebo baseline values (Table 2).

In addition to the effects of labetalol on resting and exercise-induced values of blood pressure, the changes in systolic blood pressure

TABLE 2 EFFECTS OF LABETALOL ON FREQUENCY OF ANGINAL ATTACKS, EXERCISE TOLERANCE AND DETERMINANTS OF MYOCARDIAL OXYGEN CONSUMPTION IN TEN SUBJECTS (MEAN VALUES ± STANDARD ERROR OF THE MEAN)

	Baseline (Placebo)	Labetalol (Mean Dose 1050 mg)	Difference	p
Frequency of Angina (attacks/week)	7.6 ± 1.6	2.1 ± 0.8	−5.5 ± 1.8	<0.005
Stress test results				
Exercise duration (sec)	351.6 ± 56.2	463.2 ± 45.2	+111.6 ± 25.4	<0.01
Exercise work (kpm/10_3)	3.5 ± 0.9	4.9 ± 1.0	+1.4 ± 0.6	<0.01
Peak Systolic BP (mm Hg)	192.8 ± 11.0	147.4 ± 9.9	−45.4 ± 9.9	<0.01
Peak Diastolic BP (mm Hg)	102.7 ± 3.3	83.9 ± 3.0	−18.8 ± 2.4	<0.01
Peak Heart Rate (beats/min)	138.0 ± 8.6	125.1 ± 5.2	−12.9 ± 4.9	<0.03
Peak rate–pressure product (HR × SBP/10^2)beats-mm Hg/min	250.4 ± 28.4	163.2 ± 17.0	−87.2 ± 19.8	<0.01
Inhibition of heart rate increment (beats/min)				
Change from rest to stage 1	36.9 ± 5.1	30.7 ± 4.1	−6.2 ± 3.4	NS*
Change from rest to stage II ($n = 8$)	49.4 ± 6.4	42.9 ± 5.2	−6.5 ± 4.1	NS
Inhibition of systolic BP increment (mm Hg)				
Change from rest to stage 1	26.7 ± 6.8	2.2 ± 4.6	−24.5 ± 7.7	<0.02
Change from rest to stage II ($n = 8$)	47.7 ± 8.4	17.0 ± 5.5	−30.7 ± 11.6	<0.001

*NS = not significant

349

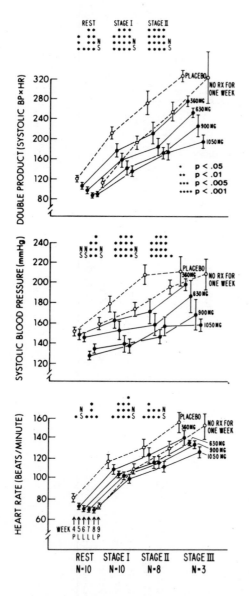

Figure 2. Comparative effects of placebo, increasing doses of oral labetalol, and withdrawal of labetalol treatment on resting and exercise-induced measurements of systolic blood pressure (BP), heart rate (HR), and rate–pressure product. Measurements were made at rest with patients in the standing position just before exercise, and during exercise at the end of stages I, II, and III (Bruce protocol). The number of patients who reached each exercise interval on both placebo and labetalol therapy are listed under the horizontal axis. Values are mean ± standard error of the mean.

with exercise were attenuated. The exercise-induced increments in systolic blood pressure seen at Stages I and II with placebo were reduced with labetalol—at Stage II with all doses, at Stage I with 600 and 1200 mg per day (Figs. 2 and 3, Table 2). There was a 92 percent inhibition of the systolic blood pressure increment at Stage I with labetalol (1050 mg) and a 64 percent inhibition at Stage II.

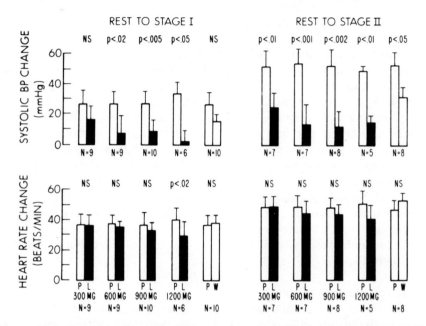

Figure 3. Comparative effects of placebo, increasing doses of oral labetalol and withdrawal of labetalol treatment on the exercise-induced changes in heart rate and systolic blood pressure from resting values. Measurements of resting blood pressure and heart rate were made just before exercise with patients in the standing position. The exercise-induced changes were measured at the end of stages I and II of exercise (Bruce protocol). The number of patients who reached each exercise stage on both placebo and labetalol therapy is listed below the horizontal axis, with the daily labetalol dose these patients were receiving. L = labetalol treatment; P = placebo treatment; W = treatment withdrawal. Values are mean values ± standard error of the mean.

Although resting and exercise-induced values of heart rate were reduced with labetalol compared with placebo baseline values, the increment in heart rate with exercise was not significantly attenuated. After treatment with labetalol, there was a slight but insignificant reduction in the heart rate increments seen at Stages I and II with placebo. Only at the 1200 mg daily dose level was the heart rate increment at Stage I significantly inhibited.

Effects on the Stress Electrocardiogram (ST-Segment Changes and Arrhythmias)

In the placebo baseline studies, all patients manifested ST-segment depression with exercise, which occurred in six of ten patients at Stage I. After 4 weeks of labetalol treatment two of these six patients had no ST-segment depression at Stage I and two had a reduction in the magnitude of ST-segment depression; the remaining two demonstrated no change from the placebo study.

Four patients manifested arrhythmias during the placebo baseline stress test; one patient had unifocal premature ventricular complexes that were eliminated with exercise at all dose levels of labetalol; one patient had premature ventricular complexes and ventricular bigeminy in the placebo baseline study, a rare premature ventricular complex while receiving 300 mg per day of labetalol and no such complexes at the higher dose levels; one patient had premature ventricular complexes and short runs of ventricular tachycardia that persisted during treatment with 300 mg per day but disappeared at the higher dose levels; one patient had frequent unifocal premature ventricular complexes and periods of ventricular bigeminy in the placebo baseline test that were eliminated completely with labetalol treatment. No patient manifested new arrhythmias, or enhanced ventricular arrhythmia while receiving labetalol treatment.

Exercise Tolerance (Table 2)
Similar to the observations made on frequency of anginal attacks, there were no significant effects on exercise tolerance with 300 mg per day of labetalol. However, significant increases in total exercise time and exercise work on the treadmill were seen with larger doses. Indeed, after 4 weeks of labetalol treatment (mean dose 1050 mg per day), there was a 32 percent increase in treadmill time compared with the placebo baseline study, ($p < 0.01$), and a 40 percent increase in total exercise work ($p < 0.01$). The significant increases in treadmill time and exercise work with labetalol were accompanied by a significant decrease in myocardial oxygen demands as estimated from the calculation of the peak heart rate–blood pressure product at the end point of exercise (Fig. 4, Table 2). Although a mean labetalol dose of 764 mg per day normalized blood pressure in nine patients, the maximal improvement in exercise tolerance in these patients was not observed until a mean labetalol dose of 1050 mg per day was reached.

Effects of Labetalol Withdrawal (Fig. 2 and 3)
One week after labetalol treatment was stopped, there was an increase in the frequency of anginal attacks to near baseline levels, and exercise tolerance returned to baseline levels (351.6 ± 56.2 seconds with placebo compared with 378 ± 40.2 seconds after withdrawal). The withdrawal of labetalol resulted in a rapid return to baseline levels of angina and exercise variables without evidence for further deterioration in patient status. No patient manifested unstable angina or an acute myocardial infarction during the 1-week withdrawal period.

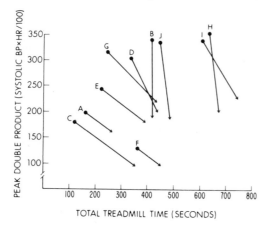

Figure 4. Effects of placebo and maximal labetalol dose on the duration of treadmill exercise and peak heart rate–blood pressure product at the end point of exercise. Compared with placebo baseline measurements (closed circles), exercise time increases and peak rate–pressure product decreases with labetalol (arrows). A to H = Patients 1 to 10, respectively.

There was no evidence of a labetalol withdrawal "rebound" effect. One week after treatment with labetalol, there was a return of the resting and exercise-induced values of blood pressure, heart rate, and rate–pressure product toward the placebo values. Although not significant for all variables, the mean values of blood pressure and heart rate were actually lower than placebo baseline values; however, they were still higher than during labetalol treatment.

Plasma Blood Levels (Fig. 5)
The plasma blood levels of labetalol were obtained 1.5 hours after the last dose and just before treadmill testing. There was a linear relation between plasma level and drug dose ($r = 0.728$, $p < 0.001$). The concentra-

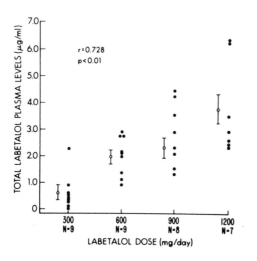

Figure 5. Correlation between the changes in plasma labetalol levels and orally administered labetalol dose. The number of patients who were administered each dose level are listed below the horizontal axis.

tions found after 300, 600, 900, and 1200 mg of labetalol per day were 0.70 ± 0.23, 2.08 ± 0.24, 2.39 ± 0.43, and 3.81 ± 0.66 $\mu g/ml$, respectively. There appeared to be no definite relation between plasma drug level and clinical response to the drug (blood pressure and heart rate lowering effects).

Effects on Noninvasive Indexes of Left Ventricular Function (Table 3)
When compared with placebo, there were no effects of labetalol (mean dose 1050 mg daily) on noninvasive indexes of resting left ventricular function, using systolic time interval measurements and echocardiographic determinations (end-diastolic volume index, ejection fraction, V_{cf}). Echocardiographic measurements of septal wall thickness (diastolic) were 11.0 ± 1.3 mm in the placebo period and 11.0 ± 0.8 mm after 4 weeks of labetalol therapy; posterior wall thickness was 10.0 ± 0.8 mm with placebo, and 10.3 ± 0.8 mm with labetalol.

Clotting Function
There were no effects of labetalol (mean dose 1050 mg daily) on platelet count, prothrombin time, partial thromboplastin time, or ADP- and epinephrine-induced platelet aggregability when compared with placebo baseline values.

Plasma Renin and Aldosterone Levels (Fig. 6)
Mean plasma renin activity was reduced, but not significantly, with labetalol (72.8 ± 38.5 ng per 100 ml per hour with placebo and 21.3 ± 8.4 ng per 100 ml per hour with labetalol). The seven patients with low plasma renin activity in the baseline period (range less than 3.0 to 30.3 ng per 100 ml per hour) had little change with labetalol. However, there were dramatic reductions in plasma renin activity in the three patients with relatively high values (range of 105.0 to 376.7 ng per 100 ml per hour). There was no relation between the reductions in plasma renin activity and the degree of blood pressure response with labetalol. There were no differences between placebo and labetalol and the concentrations of sodium, potassium, and creatinine excreted in the urine over 24 hours. Plasma aldosterone levels were not altered with labetalol compared with placebo—113.0 ± 13.2 pg/ml with placebo, 106.9 ± 11.8 pg/ml with labetalol.

Safety Variables
No changes in body weight were noted with labetalol treatment. One patient complained of dizziness that was self-limited and one patient described an episode of impotence that was also self-limited. All routine screening blood tests, urinalyses, electrocardiograms, and chest x-ray

TABLE 3. EFFECTS OF PLACEBO AND LABETALOL ON NON-INVASIVE INDEXES OF LEFT VENTRICULAR FUNCTION

Noninvasive Hemodynamic Studies	Placebo Baseline	Labetalol (1050 mg)	Difference*
Systolic Time Intervals (sec)			
Preejection period (PEP_c) (sec)	0.12 ± 0.00	0.13 ± 0.00	0.01 ± 0.01
Left ventricular ejection time ($LVET_c$) (sec)	0.42 ± 0.01	0.41 ± 0.01	0.01 ± 0.02
PEP/LVET	0.29 ± 0.01	0.30 ± 0.01	-0.02 ± 0.02
Echocardiographic variables			
End-diastolic volume index (ml/m²)	74.3 ± 8.7	67.3 ± 5.8	-8.3 ± 5.4
End-systolic volume index (ml/m²)	32.9 ± 5.1	30.7 ± 5.2	-2.0 ± 2.7
Stroke volume index (ml/m²)	41.3 ± 4.6	36.7 ± 2.4	-6.4 ± 4.6
Cardiac index (liters/min/m²)	3.3 ± 0.3	3.0 ± 0.5	-0.3 ± 0.5
Ejection fraction (%)	56.8 ± 3.2	56.6 ± 4.4	1.7 ± 3.6
Velocity of circumferential fiber shortening (V_{cf}) (circ†/sec)	1.02 ± 0.08	0.95 ± 0.09	-0.04 ± 0.01

*All differences were not significant.
†circ = circumference.

355

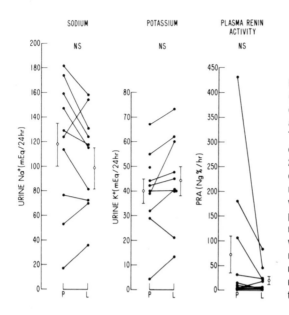

Figure 6. The effect of placebo (P) and labetalol (L) on 24-hour excretion of urinary electrolytes and plasma renin activity (PRA). There were no significant effects of labetalol treatment on mean 24-hour sodium and potassium excretion or on mean plasma renin activity. The three patients with the highest pretreatment plasma renin activity show a marked reduction in this variable with labetalol. The closed circles represent individual patient measurements, the open circles mean values ± standard error of the mean.

films remained unchanged during the study. There were no effects of labetalol on serum triglyceride and cholesterol levels.

DISCUSSION

Effects on Hypertension

The results of this study demonstrate that oral labetalol is an effective therapy for patients with both angina pectoris and hypertension. The drug significantly reduced systolic and diastolic blood pressures, both supine and standing, upon initiation of treatment (300 mg daily). An augmentation of the antihypertensive effect was seen in most patients with larger doses (600 to 1200 mg daily). Nine of 10 patients had their blood pressure controlled with 300 to 1200 mg of labetalol daily, a finding consistent with the observations of our group and other investigators who used labetalol in patients with hypertension (see Chapters 7, 13, and 14).[12,13,32,33] The effects of the drug on systolic blood pressure were more pronounced in the standing position. The differences between standing and supine blood pressure determinations after labetalol therapy may relate to the vasodilatory effects of α-adrenergic blockade, which are more pronounced in the erect position.[11,17] Symptomatic postural hypotension was not seen in this study, an adverse reaction usually described with intravenous administration of the drug or with oral doses well over 1200 mg per day.[16,34,35]

Effects on Heart Rate

Unlike pure α-adrenergic blocking drugs and hydralazine, which tend to increase the resting heart rate in hypertensive patients, labetalol reduces blood pressure without increasing the heart rate.[10,16,36,37] In this study, labetalol significantly reduced both the supine and standing resting heart rates. The effects of labetalol in reducing heart rate were slightly more marked in the supine position; however, the difference from the standing value was not significant. The doses of labetalol needed to reduce heart rate were larger than those needed to reduce blood pressure. The α-adrenergic and vasodilatory effects of the drug may predominate with smaller doses; larger doses may be necessary to achieve effective β-adrenoceptor blockade and slowing of heart rate.

Mechanism of Hypotensive Effects

The exact mechanism or mechanisms for the effects of labetalol in reducing blood pressure are not known. It has been suggested that labetalol reduces blood pressure predominantly by reducing peripheral vascular resistance while maintaining cardiac output.[10,16,37] This response is quite different from that usually seen with β-adrenoceptor blocking drugs, both selective and nonselective, which result in a more delayed antihypertensive effect, a greater reduction in heart rate, a decrease in cardiac output, and a rise or no change in vascular resistance.[38,39] In this study, the resting supine echocardiographic studies demonstrated a slight but insignificant reduction in cardiac index with antihypertensive doses of labetalol, again suggesting a predominant vasodilatory mechanism for the drug's antihypertensive effects.

It has been proposed that the renin–angiotensin system plays a role in the antihypertensive mechanism of β-blocking agents.[1] The β-blocking agents in general lead to a decrease in both plasma renin activity[1] and plasma aldosterone.[40] In contrast, vasodilating antihypertensive drugs induce a compensatory increase in plasma renin activity, and a potent vasodilatory response can even result in secondary hyperaldosteronism with edema.[41,42] The effects of labetalol on plasma renin activity and aldosterone levels have previously not been well defined. Elevated plasma renin activity, no change, and reduced plasma renin activity with labetalol have all been reported.[4,10,16,34,43–45] In this study, labetalol had no demonstrable effects on plasma renin activity in all seven patients with low pretreatment levels. However, in the three patients with high plasma renin activity, there was a dramatic reduction in this variable after therapy. This finding with labetalol is in sharp contrast to the observations made with pure vasodilators,[41,42] suggesting that in its effect on plasma renin activity, labetalol is behaving like a pure β-adrenergic blocking drug. Reports describing the effects of labetalol on plasma aldosterone levels have not been conclusive. Although some investigators[43–45] have reported that labetalol reduced elevated plasma aldosterone levels, there were no significant effects of the drug on plasma aldosterone seen in our study.

Effects on Platelet Function

Labetalol had no effect on variables of coagulative function, specifically ADP- and epinephrine-induced platelet aggregability. In contrast, propranolol definitely reduces platelet aggregability, an effect that is related to that drug's membrane stabilizing properties and not to β-adrenergic blockade.[29,46,47] Because labetalol has insignificant membrane stabilizing activity, we would not expect an effect on platelets related to this mechanism.[3] However, phentolamine, a nonselective α-adrenergic blocking agent, has definite in vitro effects on platelet aggregability related to blockade of demonstrable α-receptors in platelet membranes.[48,49] The platelet α-receptor is of the presynaptic α_2 variety and not the α_1 subtype.[50] The α_1 subtype is the classical vascular smooth muscle receptor that, when stimulated, mediates vasoconstriction.[50] The complete lack of any platelet effect with labetalol would suggest that the drug may be operating through blockade of α_1-receptors alone and not through α_2-adrenoceptor blockade. This is a receptor-blocking profile similar to that described for prazosin, a selective α_1-adrenoceptor blocking agent.[51]

It would follow that the effectiveness of labetalol in systemic hypertension and the lack of associated tachycardia may be at least partly due to the absence of α_2-adrenoceptor blocking properties of the drug. The hemodynamic effects of labetalol have been compared with those of a propranolol–hydralazine combination.[16,52] In reality, the hemodynamic profile of labetalol in hypertension may be more akin to that of a propranolol–prazosin combination.

Effects on Angina and Exercise Tolerance

There was a significant reduction in the frequency of spontaneous attacks of angina pectoris with labetalol compared with placebo, and a significant improvement in exercise tolerance. In contrast to the blood pressure–lowering effect of labetalol, which were seen with doses of 300 mg daily, the lessening of angina and improved exercise tolerance were not seen until a dose of 600 mg daily was reached. Also, the maximal improvement in exercise tolerance and relief of angina was seen at dose levels of labetalol that were higher than those that achieved optimal blood pressure control. Again, the rate-lowering effects of β-adrenergic blockade may be more important at the higher dose range.

At comparable levels of exercise (Stages I and II), labetalol reduced the heart rate, systolic blood pressure, and rate–pressure product from placebo baseline levels. The rate of increment in systolic blood pressure and rate–pressure product with exercise were also attenuated. These findings are consistent with those of other investigators[18,53,54] who demonstrated, both in hypertensive patients and in normal subjects, a greater attenuation of the blood pressure response to exercise with labetalol than with propranolol or oxprenolol.[18,53,54] Although the heart rate was reduced at rest with labetalol and at each exercise level, there was only a slight and insignificant reduction in the degree of heart rate increment with exercise. These findings are also consistent with the observations of investigators[18,54] who found a greater attenuation of the heart rate response to exercise with propranolol than with labetalol in hypertensive patients.

The peak exercise heart rate, blood pressure, and rate–pressure product were significantly reduced with labetalol, and these changes from placebo baseline values were associated with a marked increase in exercise tolerance. Labetalol also reduced the degree of electrocardiographic ST-segment depression with exercise and eliminated all exercise-induced ventricular arrhythmias. Labetalol appears to possess the characteristics of an effective drug for hypertensive patients with angina pectoris—the ability to reduce components of myocardial oxygen demand during exercise, enabling a patient to perform more external work.

Adverse Effects

There were no detrimental effects of labetalol on noninvasive measurements of left ventricular volumes and indexes of left ventricular function. A slight and insignificant reduction of left ventricular end-diastolic volume was seen with labetalol, which may relate to the vasodilatory or "unloading" effects of the drug. The noninvasive assessment of left ventricular function in patients with ischemic heart disease using systolic time interval measurements and M-mode echocardiography can be valuable, particularly when serial measurements are made in the same patient using a consistent technique.[26,55,56] The lack of an effect of labetalol on left ventricular function contrasts sharply with observations made in our laboratory using propranolol, which caused a dose-related reduction in resting left ventricular function and an increase in end-diastolic volume.[26] These differences may relate to the α-blocking property of labetalol, which may in itself improve resting left ventricular function.[57]

Lack of Rebound Phenomenon

In patients with angina pectoris, there have been reports of exacerbation of angina pectoris, and, in some cases, myocardial infarction after abrupt discontinuation of propranolol therapy.[58,59] One week after the withdrawal of labetalol treatment, no hyperadrenergic "rebound" state was demonstrable, although symptoms of angina did return to placebo baseline levels. The resting and exercise-induced heart rate and blood pressure were slightly lower than placebo baseline levels but were still higher than with labetalol treatment. This finding might reflect either a prolonged action of the drug despite its short plasma half-life,[30,60] or a patient training effect. There are no known active metabolites of the drug.[4]

Relation Between Labetalol Plasma Level and Pharmacologic Effect

Like may β-adrenergic blocking drugs, labetalol is said to demonstrate first-pass hepatic metabolism when administered in oral form to patients.[4,30,61] This means that a substantial fraction of an oral dose will undergo hepatic biotransformation during the first pass through the liver and fail to enter the systemic circulation.[4] Smaller doses may be completely metabolized, with little drug reaching the plasma, whereas larger doses can saturate this hepatic system and provide a significant plasma level.[4] In this study, there was a linear relation between increasing oral doses of labetalol and plasma levels. Similar to the pattern with other β-adrenergic blocking drugs, there was no clear-cut relation between plasma level of labetalol and pharmacologic effects in patients (heart rate or blood pressure-lowering effects).

Therapeutic Advantages of Labetalol

Beyond the improvement in tolerance and reduction in anginal attacks, there are other potential advantages in using an α- and β-adrenoceptor blocking agent in angina pectoris. Because neurogenic vasoconstrictor impulses to the coronary resistance vessels are transmitted through sympathetic nerves acting upon α-adrenergic receptors in the coronary vascular bed, there may be an important role for α-adrenergic blocking drugs in the prevention of coronary spasm and in the preservation of restricted coronary blood flow.[7-9,62-64] This was suggested in a study by Mudge et al.[8] in which phentolamine was shown to block reflex coronary vasoconstriction regularly elicited by the cold pressor test. Orlick et al.[7] demonstrated that α-adrenergic blockade was a useful adjunct in selected patients with variant angina.

Adrenergic blockade with nonselective β-blocking drugs may be detrimental in patients in whom ischemia is due to reduced oxygen delivery secondary to coronary spasm.[65,66] Nonselective β-adrenoceptor blockade may also allow the unopposed influence of coronary vasoconstrictor impulses to prevail. Coronary blood flow was found to increase after intravenous administration of labetalol in dogs.[67] Labetalol, but not propranolol, reduced the pressor response caused by immersing a hand in ice-cold water.[68] The reduced cold pressor response, which is similar to that seen with phentolamine, is attributable to the α-blocking actions of labetalol and may block reflex coronary vasoconstriction in certain patients with angina. Labetalol, with its α-adrenergic blocking properties, may increase coronary blood flow while also reducing myocardial oxygen demands in human beings. This hypothesis is supported by a recent experimental report[69] in which the protective effect of labetalol treatment was shown to be markedly higher than that of placebo and propranolol on myocardial cell necrosis after coronary occlusion in rats.

Labetalol may have applicability in situations where other β-adrenergic blocking drugs are contraindicated. Because labetalol decreases peripheral vascular resistance, it may prove to be useful in patients with angina pectoris and hypertension associated with mild congestive heart failure or peripheral vascular disease.

Implications

In this study, labetalol was shown to be a safe and effective agent for reducing spontaneous attacks of angina pectoris, improving exercise tolerance and reducing elevated blood pressure. The drug has no demonstrable effects on resting left ventricular function and may reduce elevated plasma renin activity. Studies need to be undertaken in exercising patients to assess left ventricular function. Double-blind studies must be initiated in patients with angina pectoris and hypertension comparing labetalol therapy with other known antianginal regimens. The effects of labetalol in normotensive patients with angina pectoris must also be examined. Labetalol is a pharmacologic advance that provides a new conceptual approach for managing patients with angina pectoris and hypertension: α- and β-adrenergic blockade.

REFERENCES

1. Frishman W, Silverman R: Clinical pharmacology of the new beta-adrenergic blocking drugs. Part 2. Physiologic and metabolic effects. Am Heart J 97:797, 1979.
2. Frishman W, Silverman R: Clinical pharmacology of the new beta-adrenergic blocking drugs. Part 3. Comparative clinical experience and new therapeutic applications. Am Heart J 98:119, 1979.
3. Brittain RT, Levy GP: A review of the animal pharmacology of labetalol, a combined α and β-adrenoceptor blocking drug. Br J Clin Pharmacol 3 (Suppl 3):681, 1976.
4. Frishman W, Halprin S: Clinical pharmacology of the new beta-adrenergic blocking drugs. Part 7. New horizons in beta-adrenoceptor blockade therapy: labetalol. Am Heart J 98:660, 1979.
5. Johnson GL, Prioli NA, Ehrreich SJ: Anti-hypertensive effects of labetalol. (Abstr). Fed Proc 36:1049, 1977.
6. Moyer JH, Caplovitz C: The clinical results of oral and parenteral administration of imadazoline hydrochloride (Regitine) in the treatment of hypertension and an evaluation of the cerebral hemodynamic effects. Am Heart J 45:602, 1953.
7. Orlick AE, Ricci DR, Alderman EL, et al: Effects of alpha adrenergic blockade upon coronary hemodynamics. J Clin Invest 62:459, 1978.
8. Mudge GH Jr, Grossman W, Mills RMJ, et al: Reflex increase in coronary vascular resistance in patients with ischemic heart disease. N Engl J Med 295:1333, 1976.
9. Hillis LD, Braunwald E: Coronary artery spasm. N Engl J Med 299:695, 1978.
10. Mehta J, Cohn JN: Hemodynamic effects of labetalol, an alpha and beta adrenergic blocking agent in hypertensive subjects. Circulation 55:370, 1977.
11. Koch G: Haemodynamic effects of combined α and β-adrenoceptor blockade after intravenous labetalol in hypertensive patients at rest and during exercise. Br J Clin Pharmacol 3 (Suppl 3):725, 1976.
12. Prichard BNC, Boakes AJ: Labetalol in long-term treatment of hypertension. Br J Clin Pharmacol 3 (Suppl 3): 743, 1976.
13. Bolli P, Waal-Manning HJ, Wood AJ, Simpson FO: Experience with labetalol in hypertension. Br J Clin Pharmacol 3 (Suppl 3):765, 1976.
14. Joekes AM, Thompson FD: Acute hemodynamic effects of labetalol and its subsequent use as an oral hypotensive agent. Br J Clin Pharmacol 3 (Suppl 3):789, 1976.
15. Richards DA, Prichard BNC, Boakes AJ, et al: Pharmacological basis for antihypertensive effects of intravenous labetalol. Br Heart J 39:99, 1977.
16. Brogden RN, Heel RC, Speight TM, Avery GS: Labetalol: A review of its pharmacology and therapeutic use in hypertension. Drugs 15:15, 1978.
17. Fagard R, Amery A, Reybrouch T, et al: Response of the systemic and pul-

monary circulation to alpha- and beta-receptor blockade (labetalol) at rest and during exercise in hypertensive patients. Circulation 60:1214, 1979.

18. Pugsley SJ, Armstrong BK, Nassim MA, Bellin LJ: Controlled comparison of labetalol and propranolol in the management of severe hypertension. Br J Clin Pharmacol 3 (Suppl 3):777, 1976.

19. Boakes AJ, Prichard BNC: The effect of AH 5158, pindolol, propranolol, d-propranolol on acute exercise tolerance in angina pectoris. Br J Pharmacol 47:673, 1973.

20. Frishman WH, Strom JA, Kirschner M, et al: Labetalol therapy in patients with systemic hypertension and angina pectoris: Effects of combined alpha- and beta-adrenergic blockade. Am J Cardiol 48:917, 1981.

21. Richards DA, Maconochie JG, Bland RE, et al: Relationship between plasma concentrations and pharmacological effects of labetalol. Eur J Clin Pharmacol 11:85, 1977.

22. Bruce RA: Multistage treadmill tests of submaximal and maximal exercise, in Exercise Testing and Training of Apparently Healthy Individuals: A Handbook for Physicians. New York, American Heart Association, 1972, p 32.

23. Teichholz LE, Kreulen T, Herman MV, Gorlin R: Problems in echocardiographic-angiographic correlations in the presence or absence of asynergy. Am J Cardiol 37:7, 1976.

24. Weissler AM, Harris WS, Schoenfeld CD: Bedside techniques for evaluation of left ventricular function in man. Am J Cardiol 23:577, 1969.

25. Lewis RP, Rittgers SE, Forester WF, Boudoulas H: A critical review of systolic time intervals. Circulation 56:146, 1977.

26. Frishman W, Smithen C, Befler B, et al: Noninvasive assessment of clinical response to oral propranolol therapy. Am J Cardiol 35:635, 1975.

27. Born GVR: Aggregation of blood platelets by adenosine diphosphate and its reversal. Nature 194:927, 1962.

28. Mustard JF, Hegardt B, Roswell HC, MacMillan RL: Effect of adenosine nucleotides on platelet aggregation and clotting time. J Lab Clin Med 64:548, 1964.

29. Frishman WH, Weksler B, Christodoulou JP, et al: Reversal of abnormal platelet aggregability and change in exercise tolerance in patients with angina pectoris following oral propranolol. Circulation 50:887, 1974.

30. Martin LE, Hopkins R, Bland R: Metabolism of labetalol by animals and man. Br J Clin Pharmacol 3 (Suppl 3):695, 1976.

31. Criteria Committee of the New York Heart Association. Diseases of the Heart and Blood Vessels, 6th ed. Boston, Little, Brown, 1964, p 112.

32. Frick MH, Porsti P: Combined alpha- and beta-adrenoceptor blockade with labetalol in hypertension. Br Med J 1:1046, 1976.

33. Michelson EL, Frishman WH, Sawin HS, et al: Long-term efficacy and safety of labetalol in the treatment of hypertension. (Abstr) J Am Coll Cardiol 1:611, 1983.

34. Koch G: Combined α- and β-adrenoceptor blockade with oral labetalol in

hypertensive patients with reference to haemodynamic effects at rest and during exercise. Br J Clin Pharmacol 3 (Suppl 3):729, 1976.

35. Dargie HJ, Dollery CT, Daniel J: Labetalol in resistant hypertension. Br J Clin Pharmacol 3: Suppl 3:751, 1976.

36. Andersson O, Berglund G, Hansson L: Antihypertensive action, time of onset and effects on carbohydrate metabolism of labetalol. Br J Clin Pharmacol 3 (Suppl 3):757, 1976.

37. Edwards RC, Raftery EB: Haemodynamic effects of long-term oral labetalol. Br J Clin Pharmacol 3 (Suppl 3):733, 1976.

38. Shinebourne E, Fleming J, Hamer J: Effects of beta-adrenergic blockade during exercise in hypertensive and ischemic heart disease. Lancet 2:1217, 1967.

39. Prichard BNC, Shinebourne E, Fleming J, Hamer J: Hemodynamic studies in hypertensive patients treated by oral propranolol. Br Heart J 32:236, 1970.

40. Waal-Manning HJ: Hypertension: Which beta-blocker? Drugs 12:412, 1976.

41. O'Malley K, Velasco M, Wells J, McNay JL: Control of plasma renin activity and changes in sympathetic tone as determinants of minoxidil-induced increase in plasma renin activity. J Clin Invest 55:230, 1975.

42. Pohl JEF, Thurston H, Swales JD: The antidiuretic actions of diazoxide. Clin Sci 42:145, 1972.

43. Trust PM, Rosei EA, Brown JJ, et al: Effect of blood pressure, angiotensin II and aldosterone concentrations during treatment of severe hypertension with intravenous labetalol: comparison with propranolol. Br J Clin Pharmacol 3 (Suppl 3):799, 1976.

44. Lammitausta R, Koulou M, Allonen H: Alpha- and beta-adrenoceptor blocking properties of labetalol in renin release. Int J Clin Pharmacol Biopharm 17:240, 1979.

45. Kornerup HJ, Pederson EB, Christensen NJ, Pedersen A: Labetalol in the treatment of severe essential hypertension: Relationship between arterial blood pressure, plasma catecholamines, plasma renin activity, plasma aldosterone, and body weight. Acta Med Scand Suppl 625:59, 1978.

46. Weksler BB, Gillick M, Pink J: Effect of propranolol on platelet function. Blood 49:185, 1977.

47. Frishman WH, Weksler BB: Effects of β-adrenoceptor blocking agents on platelet function in normal subjects and patients with angina pectoris, in Roskamm H, Graefe K (eds), Advances in β Blocker Therapy. Proceedings of an International Symposium, Monte Carlo, 1980. Amsterdam, Excerpta Medica 1980, p 164.

48. Inset P, Nirenberg P, Turnbull J, Shatti SJ: Relationships between membrane cholesterol, α-adrenergic receptors, and platelet function. Biochemistry 52:69, 1978.

49. Newman KD, Williams LT, Bishopric NH, Lefkowitz R: Identification of α-adrenergic receptors in human platelets by ^{3}H dihydroergocryptine binding. J Clin Invest 61:395, 1978.

50. Langer SZ: Subclassification of β-adrenoceptors in α_1 and β_2 types: Relevance to cardiovascular effects on drugs (abstr). Circulation 62 (Suppl III):III–6, 1980.
51. Cambridge D, Davey MJ, Massingham R: Prazosin, a selective antagonist of postsynaptic β-adrenoceptors. Br J Pharmacol 59:514, 1977.
52. Prichard BNC, Thompson FO, Boakes AJ, Joekes AM: Some hemodynamic effect of compound AH 5158 compared with propranolol plus hydralazine and diazoxide: The use of AH 5158 in the treatment of hypertension. Clin Sci Molec Med 48:97s, 1975.
53. Johnson BF, LaBrody J, Munro-Faure A: Comparative antihypertensive effects of labetalol and the combination of oxprenolol and phentolamine. Br J Clin Pharmacol 3 (Suppl 3):783, 1976.
54. Richards DA, Woodlings EP, Maconochie JG: Comparison of the effects of labetalol and propranolol in healthy men at rest and during exercise. Br J Clin Pharmacol 4:15, 1977.
55. Fortuin NJ, Hood WP, Craige E: Evaluation of left ventricular function by echocardiography. Circulation 46:26, 1972.
56. Pombo JF, Troy BL, Russell RO: Left ventricular volume and ejection fraction by echocardiography. Circulation 43:480, 1971.
57. Gould L, Gomprecht RF, Jaynal F: The effects of phentolamine on the duration of the phases of ventricular systole in man. Am J Med Sci 260:29, 1970.
58. Alderman EL, Coltart DJ, Wettach GE, Harrison DC: Coronary artery syndromes after sudden propranolol withdrawal. Ann Intern Med 81:925, 1974.
59. Miller RR, Olson HG, Amsterdam EA, Mason DT: Propranolol withdrawal rebound phenomenon: exacerbation of coronary events after abrupt cessation of antianginal therapy. N Engl J Med 293:416, 1975.
60. Frishman W: Clinical pharmacology of the new beta-adrenergic blocking drugs. Part 1. Pharmacodynamic and pharmacokinetic properties. Am Heart J 97:663, 1979.
61. Richards DA, Maconochie JG, Bland RE, et al: Relationship between plasma concentrations and pharmacological effects of labetalol. Eur J Clin Pharmacol 11:85, 1977.
62. Schwartz PJ, Stone HL: Tonic influence of the sympathetic nervous system on myocardial reactive hyperemia and on the coronary blood flow distribution in dogs. Circ Res 41:51, 1977.
63. Mohrman DE, Feigi EO: Competition between sympathetic vasoconstriction and metabolic vasodilation in the canine coronary circulation. Circ Res 44:79, 1978.
64. Murray PA, Vatner SF: Alpha-adrenoceptor attenuation of the coronary vascular response to severe exercise in the conscious dog. Circ Res 45:654, 1979.
65. Braunwald E: Coronary artery spasm and acute myocardial infarction—a new possibility for treatment and prevention. N Engl J Med 299:1301, 1978.
66. Gunther S, Miller J, Mudge GH, Grossman W: Therapy of coronary vaso-

constriction in patients with coronary artery disease. Am J Cardiol 47:157, 1981.

67. Maxwell GM: Effects of alpha- and beta-adrenoceptor antagonist (AH 5158) upon general and coronary hemodynamics of intact dogs. Br J Pharmacol 44:370, 1973.

68. Maconochie JG, Richards DA, Woodlings EP: Modification of pressor responses induced by "cold". Br J Pharmacol 4:389, 1977.

69. Chiariello M, Brevitti G, DeRosa G, et al: Protective effects of simultaneous alpha and beta-adrenergic receptor blockade on myocardial cell necrosis after coronary artery occlusion in rats. Am J Cardiol 46:249, 1980.

CHAPTER 12

β-Adrenoceptor Blockade and Coronary Artery Surgery

William H. Frishman, Yasu Oka, Joel A. Strom, Ronald M. Becker, and Robert W. B. Frater

β-Adrenoceptor blocking drugs are important therapeutic agents for a multitude of cardiovascular and noncardiovascular disorders.[1] With their increasing use, a great number of patients can be expected to present for surgery and general anesthesia while taking these drugs.

During the past several years, recommendations have varied widely regarding the use of propranolol and other β-blockers in patients scheduled for coronary artery bypass operations, from the complete withdrawal of therapy 2 weeks prior to surgery[2] to the continuation of therapy at the same or lesser dosage just prior to the operation.[3-6] Some clinical reports associate abrupt withdrawal of long-term propranolol therapy with an increase in angina pectoris and development of new arrhythmias, myocardial infarction, and sudden death.[7-9] These observations raise the question as to whether the risk of β-blocker withdrawal before coronary bypass surgery is greater than the risk of the purported myocardial depression attributed to the interaction between β-adrenoceptor blockade and general anesthesia.

Retrospective and prospective reports reviewing large coronary surgical experiences where propranolol therapy was not withdrawn preoperatively for medical reasons failed to identify the deleterious action between anesthesia and preoperative propranolol administration.[3-6,10-17]

Reprinted in part from The American Heart Journal, Volume 99, pp 255–269, February 1980, with permission.

367

Moreover, in animal studies, general anesthetic agents commonly used during bypass surgery have been shown not to potentiate the effects of propranolol.

A previous study from our group, in patients who underwent coronary artery bypass surgery, demonstrated a higher incidence of postoperative arrhythmias and hypertension when individuals were withdrawn from propranolol pre-operatively, when compared to a population who either never received the drug or had the drug maintained postoperatively.[18] We, therefore, undertook this prospective study to elucidate the mechanism for these phenomena. Our protocol was designed to seek answers to the following questions:

1. Are there hazards to patients associated with either preoperative maintenance or withdrawal of propranolol therapy?
2. Are there hazards related to a persistent β-blocking effect during endotrachial intubation, induction of general anesthesia, and coronary bypass surgery?
3. Does continued β-blockade lead to a poor post-operative cardiac performance?
4. Does propranolol withdrawal contribute to the high incidence of hypertension and arrhythmias observed following coronary bypass surgery? If so, what are the mechanisms?
5. How should propranolol and other β-adrenoceptor blocking drugs be utilized in the perioperative periods?

PATIENTS AND METHODS

Patients

Fifty-four consecutive patients with stable angina pectoris scheduled for elective coronary artery bypass, and receiving long-term propranolol therapy, were entered in a perspective randomized trial. They were compared with 17 patients scheduled for bypass operations who received no propranolol therapy prior to surgery (Group I). The 54 propranolol-treated patients were randomized into three treatment groups (Table 1): 17 patients had propranolol therapy abruptly withdrawn 48 hours before the operation (Group II); 18 patients had therapy abruptly withdrawn 10 hours prior to surgery (Group III); and 19 patients had their full propranolol dose until the morning of surgery, half the usual dose 2 hours prior to surgery, and postoperatively 1 mg intravenously every 4 hours for 36 to 48 hours (Group IV).

TABLE 1. PROPRANOLOL TREATMENT GROUPS IN PATIENTS UNDERGOING CORONARY ARTERY BYPASS SURGERY

Group	Preoperative Therapy	Postoperative Therapy
I	None	None
II	Drug stopped 48 hours prior to surgery	None
III	Drug stopped 10 hours prior to surgery	None
IV	Full dose until morning of surgery: one-half dose 2 hours prior to surgery	1 mg IV every 4 hours

The population characteristics of the patient groups are given in Table 2. The groups had similar resting hemodynamic function and preoperative coronary anatomy. There were no patients with ejection fractions below 0.45, ventricular aneurysms, preexisting arrhythmias, or coexisting valvular disease. Patients with resting heart rates of 55 beats per minute while on propranolol were excluded from randomization.

Anesthesia and Surgical Technique

All patients received the same preanesthetic and anesthetic medication. Premedication consisted of morphine sulfate 0.15 mg/kg and scopolamine 0.015 mg/kg, given intramuscularly 40 to 60 minutes before induction of anesthesia.

Following the intravenous administration of 3 mg d-tubocurarine or 1 mg pancuronium, patients were induced with thiopental (3 to 4 mg/kg)

TABLE 2. CHARACTERISTICS OF PATIENT GROUPS

	Group I	Group II	Group III	Group IV
Patient number	17	17	18	19
Age (yr)	59 ± 1	53 ± 2	55 ± 2	56 ± 2
Sex				
Male	11	11	12	11
Female	6	6	6	8
LVEDP (mm Hg)*	14 ± 1	14 ± 1	15 ± 2	15 ± 1
Number of grafts	2.3　0.2	2.3　0.2	2.4　0.2	2.5　0.2
Propranolol dose (mg/day)	—	154 ± 18	151 ± 15	133 ± 20
Previous myocardial infarct (% of group)	23	23	28	26
Previous hypertension (% of group)	35	41	28	32

*Obtained just prior to induction of anesthesia.

and 0.5 to 2 percent halothane in oxygen. After administration of succinylcholine (1.5 mg/kg) and topical anesthetic of the larynx (lidocaine 4 percent), the trachea was intubated with an appropriately sized endotracheal tube. Anesthesia was maintained with halothane 0.5 to 1 percent supplemented with nondepolarizing muscle relaxants.

The coronary artery bypass was performed using standard techniques. The operative procedure was accomplished with the aid of cardiopulmonary bypass, hemodilution perfusion, and moderate total body hypothermia (28° to 32° C). A single period of aortic cross-clamping was used for all distal anastomoses, with hypothermic hyperkalemic cardioplegia to protect the myocardium. Average time for each distal coronary anastomosis was 13 minutes. All patient ECGs were monitored continuously for approximately 3 days in a surgical intensive care unit.

Methods of Observation
Preoperative blood pressure and heart rate measurements were obtained 24 hours prior to surgery and in the operating room. Intravenous and intraarterial cannulas were inserted under local anesthesia. Continuous tracings of blood pressure and lead II (ECG) were recorded. Before induction of anesthesia, the presence of angina pectoris or arrhythmias was noted. During the course of anesthesia and the postoperative period, the hemodynamic parameters measured included blood pressure, heart rate, arrhythmias, and the displacement of the ECG ST-segment. The heart rate–blood pressure product (RPP) and indirect measurement of myocardial oxygen consumption were also calculated.[19,20]

For purposes of tabulation, hemodynamic observations were recorded during the following time periods: (1) 24 hours prior to surgery; (2) in operating room prior to anesthesia induction; (3) intubation; (4) 1 hour of anesthesia; (5) 15 minutes postoperatively (intensive care unit); (6) 1 to 2 hours postoperatively; and (7) 24 hours postoperatively. Also noted were the rate of recovery of cardiac function following cardiopulmonary bypass and the need for cardiotonic drugs.

Propranolol and Renin Levels
In measuring plasma propranolol levels, blood specimens were obtained at the time of anesthesia induction, just after cardiopulmonary bypass was complete, and immediately upon arrival in the intensive care unit. Measurements were made utilizing the modified fluorometric method of Coltart and Shand.[21] Blood specimens for determining plasma renin activity were obtained several times: in the operating room prior to induction (control); 5 minutes after intubation; and following surgery (15 min-

utes and 2 hours). Plasma renin activity was measured by the radioimmunoassy technique of Chervu et al.[22]

Statistical Analysis

In this chapter, mean data are presented with the standard error of the mean as the index of dispersion. The significance of differences between groups was determined by chi-square analysis and differences in mean data by Student's *t* test for nonpaired data.

RESULTS

Patients (Table 2)

The four patient groups were remarkably homogenous for mean characteristics such as sex, history of hypertension and previous myocardial infarction, duration of anesthesia, duration of cardiopulmonary bypass, number of coronary vessels bypassed, and ease of discontinuing cardiopulmonary bypass.

There were five perioperative infarctions (new Q waves) seen and one death. The incidence of infarction among the different groups was Group I, 6 percent (1 out of 17); Group II, 18 percent (3 out of 17); Group III, 6 percent (1 out of 18); Group IV, 0 percent (none out of 19). The one death occurred in a Group II patient, 28 hours after surgery, from low cardiac output as a consequence of infarction.

Hemodynamics

Hemodynamic results are shown in Figures 1 through 6 and Table 3. During the control period (24 hours prior to surgery), patients in Groups III and IV (both still receiving propranolol) had significantly lower mean RPP than did Groups I and II patients. Immediately prior to surgery, patients in Groups III and IV continued to manifest lower mean RPP.

With intubation, there was a dramatic increase in mean RPP in all four groups, predominantly due to a marked systolic blood pressure elevation (in some patients up to 280 mm Hg). However, the RPP increment in Group IV patients was significantly blunted compared to Groups I to III. This resulted in a mean RPP value for Group IV that was significantly lower than that seen in the other three groups. Group I patients (no propranolol) also had a lower RPP increment than Groups II and III.

After 1 hour of halothane anesthesia, the mean blood pressure and RPP had returned to near control (24 hours preoperatively) levels for all

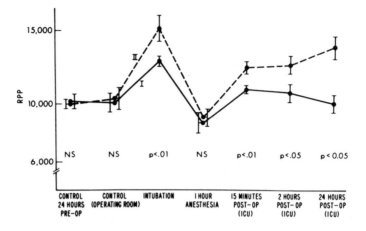

Figure 1. Mean RPP of Group I patients (no propranolol) and Group II patients (propranolol discontinued 48 hours preoperatively) before, during, and after coronary artery surgery. Group I is shown with a solid line, Group II with a broken line. Group II patients demonstrate a significant increment in mean RPP during intubation and the postoperative intervals in comparison to Group I patients. The *p* values refer to the differences between groups at the different study intervals. NS = not significant.

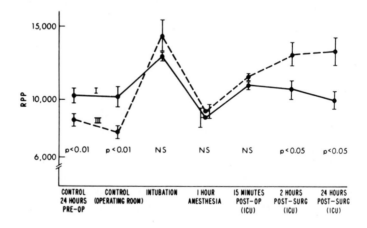

Figure 2. Mean RPP of Group I patients (no propranolol) and Group III patients (propranolol discontinued 10 hours preoperatively) before, during, and after coronary artery surgery. Group I is shown with a solid line, Group III with a broken line. Group III patients had a significantly lower mean RPP (probably due to persistence of β-adrenoceptor blocker effect) than Group I during the preoperative intervals. With intubation there is no difference between groups, however. Two hours and 24 hours postoperatively, the mean RPP is significantly higher in Group III patients compared to Group I.

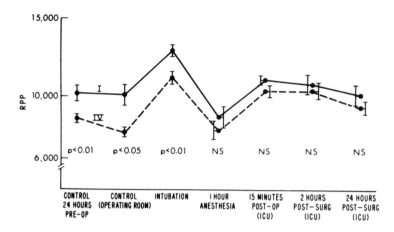

Figure 3. Mean RPP of Group I patients (no propranolol) and Group IV patients (propranolol maintained until 2 hours preoperatively, restarted immediately postoperatively) before, during, and after coronary artery surgery. Group I is shown with a solid line, Group IV with a broken line. Group IV patients had significantly lower RPP than Group I patients during the preoperative intervals. The increment in mean RPP with intubation was significantly blunted in Group IV patients. The operative and postoperative differences in mean RPP between groups were not significant.

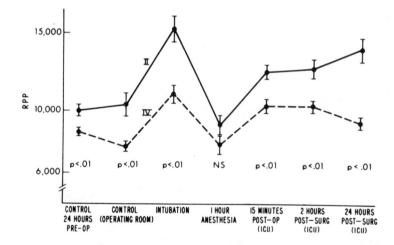

Figure 4. Mean RPP of Group II patients (propranolol discontinued 48 hours preoperatively) and Group IV patients (propranolol maintained until 2 hours preoperatively, restarted immediately postoperatively) before, during, and after coronary artery surgery. Group II is shown with a solid line, Group IV with a broken line. Group IV patients had a significantly lower mean RPP at almost every study interval compared to Group II patients.

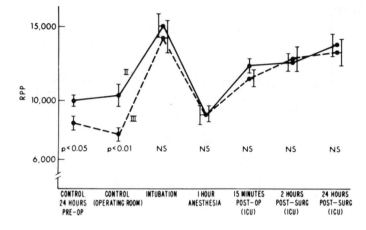

Figure 5. Mean RPP of Group II patients (propranolol discontinued 48 hours preoperatively) and Group III patients (propranolol discontinued 10 hours preoperatively) before, during, and after coronary artery surgery. Group II is shown with a solid line. Group III with a broken line. Group III patients had a significantly lower mean RPP during the preoperative periods; however, there were no differences observed between the groups during the other study intervals. A marked increment in mean RPP during intubation and the postoperative periods was seen.

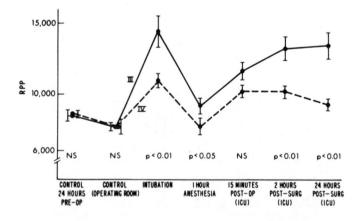

Figure 6. Mean RPP of Group III patients (propranolol discontinued 10 hours preoperatively) and Group IV patients (propranolol maintained until 2 hours preoperatively, restarted immediately postoperatively), before, during, and after coronary artery surgery. Group III is shown with a solid line, Group IV with a broken line. There were no differences between the groups during the preoperative control periods. However, there were significant increments in mean RPP during intubation and the postoperative periods in group III patients compared to Group IV patients.

groups; however, Group IV continued to manifest a significantly lower mean RPP than the other three groups.

In the ICU, 15 minutes following surgery, the mean RPP was found to rise in all four groups (though not as markedly as during intubation). Group II patients had the highest increment in both mean pulse rate and RPP compared with the other three groups. Two hours later, patients in Group III were found to have a greater increment in mean heart rate and RPP compared to 15 minutes postoperatively. At this point, Groups II and III were similar with a higher mean heart rate and RPP than Groups I and IV.

Twenty-four hours postsurgery, the mean heart rate, blood pressure, and RPP continued to climb in both Groups II and III (with the RPP approaching the level found during intubation). Blood pressure, heart rate, and RPP in Groups I and IV remained significantly lower than in Groups II and III.

Arrhythmias

There was a significant difference in the incidence of supraventricular arrhythmias among the four study groups during the immediate 24-hour postoperative period (Table 4, Fig. 7). In Group I, seven patients remained in normal sinus rhythm, and ten developed supraventricular arrhythmias (six sinus tachycardia >110, four paroxysmal supraventricular tachycardia or atrial flutter). Group II patients had the highest incidence of supraventricular arrhythmias among the four study groups. One patient remained in normal sinus rhythm and 16 developed supraventricular arrhythmias (8 sinus tachycardia >110, and 8 paroxysmal supraventricular tachycardia or atrial flutter–fibrillation). In Group III, 15 of 18 patients developed supraventricular arrhythmias (7 sinus tachycardia > 110, 8 paroxysmal supraventricular tachycardia or atrial flutter–fibrillation). In Groups IV, 14 patients were in normal sinus rhythm and 5 developed arrhythmias (3 sinus tachycardia >110 and 2 paroxysmal atrial tachycardia or atrial flutter–fibrillation). The incidence of arrhythmias was significantly higher in Groups II and III than in Groups I and IV. Patients in Group IV had fewer episodes of supraventricular arrhythmia than the other three treatment groups. In each group, all episodes of paroxysmal arrhythmia responded to intravenous propranolol (or supplementary propranolol in Group IV patients). Ventricular arrhythmias were rarely seen in the initial 24-hour postoperative period.

Plasma Renin Activity

Plasma renin activity (PRA) determinations were lower in Group IV patients than in all other groups during the control, intubation, and

TABLE 3. EFFECTS OF DIFFERENT PROPRANOLOL WITHDRAWAL REGIMENS ON HEART RATE, SYSTOLIC BLOOD PRESSURE, AND RATE PRESSURE PRODUCT IN PATIENTS UNDERGOING CORONARY ARTERY BYPASS SURGERY

Observation Period	Group I*	Group II†	Group III‡	Group IV¶
Control (24 hr preop)				
Heart rate	79 ± 3	76 ± 3	72 ± 2	70 ± 2
Blood pressure	131 ± 4	132 ± 3	122 ± 6	125 ± 3
Rate–pressure product	10,200 ± 485	10,000 ± 364	8,500 ± 436	8,600 ± 252
Control (immediate preop)				
Heart rate	78 ± 4	79 ± 3	66 ± 5	67 ± 3
Blood pressure	130 ± 6	132 ± 4	118 ± 5	114 ± 3
Rate–pressure product	10,100 ± 655	10,400 ± 752	7,700 ± 485	7,700 ± 275
Intubation				
Heart rate	71 ± 2	80 ± 2	84 ± 4	71 ± 3
Blood pressure	180 ± 7	190 ± 6	173 ± 7	154 ± 5
Rate–pressure product	13,000 ± 364	15,300 ± 846	14,500 ± 1,116	11,200 ± 458
1 hr anesthesia				
Heart rate	73 ± 4	76 ± 4	75 ± 3	66 ± 1
Blood pressure	115 ± 5	120 ± 4	125 ± 7	108 ± 4
Rate–pressure product	8,742 ± 723	9,100 ± 631	9,235 ± 543	7,817 ± 596
15 min postop (ICU)				
Heart rate	84 ± 3	97 ± 3	88 ± 2	80 ± 3
Blood pressure	132 ± 3	131 ± 4	132 ± 5	135 ± 4
Rate–pressure product	11,100 ± 242	12,600 ± 436	11,700 ± 631	10,400 ± 435
2 hr postop (ICU)				
Heart rate	84 ± 7	96 ± 4	92 ± 5	79 ± 2
Blood pressure	130 ± 4	136 ± 3	144 ± 7	136 ± 3
Rate–pressure product	10,800 ± 655	12,800 ± 582	13,300 ± 800	10,400 ± 435
24 hr postop (ICU)				
Heart rate	84 ± 2	105 ± 5	96 ± 3	77 ± 2
Blood pressure	116 ± 3	137 ± 7	140 ± 7	120 ± 4
Rate–pressure product	10,100 ± 582	14,000 ± 776	13,400 ± 946	9,300 ± 389

*Group I: No propranolol
†Group II: Propranolol stopped 48 hours preoperatively.
‡Group III: Propranolol stopped 10 hours preoperatively.
¶Group IV: Propranolol stopped 2 hours preoperatively, continued postoperatively.

TABLE 3. *(continued)*

		Statistical Significance			
Group I vs. Group II	*Group I vs. Group III*	*Group I vs. Group IV*	*Group II vs. Group III*	*Group II vs. Group IV*	*Group III vs. Group IV*
NS	NS	<0.01	NS	NS	NS
NS	NS	NS	NS	NS	NS
NS	<0.01	<0.01	<0.05	<0.01	NS
NS	<0.01	<0.01	<0.05	<0.01	NS
NS	NS	<0.01	<0.05	<0.01	NS
NS	<0.05	<0.05	<0.01	<0.01	NS
<0.01	<0.01	NS	NS	<0.05	<0.05
NS	NS	<0.05	NS	<0.01	<0.01
<0.01	NS	<0.01	NS	<0.01	<0.01
NS	NS	<0.05	NS	<0.05	<0.05
NS	NS	NS	NS	<0.05	<0.05
NS	NS	NS	NS	NS	<0.05
<0.01	NS	NS	<0.05	<0.01	<0.05
NS	NS	NS	NS	NS	NS
I<0.01	NS	NS	NS	<0.01	NS
NS	NS	NS	NS	<0.01	<0.05
NS	NS	NS	NS	NS	NS
p<0.05	p<0.05	NS	NS	<0.01	<0.01
<0.01	<0.01	<0.05	NS	<0.01	<0.01
<0.01	<0.01	NS	NS	<0.05	<0.05
<0.05	<0.05	NS	NS	<0.01	<0.01

TABLE 4. INCIDENCE OF POST-OPERATIVE (24 HOURS) SUPRAVENTRICULAR
TACHYARRHYTHMIA FOLLOWING CORONARY ARTERY BYPASS

	Group I	Group II	Group II	Group IV
No. of patients	17	17	18	19
Normal sinus rhythm	7	1	3	14
Supraventricular tachyarrhythmias	10	16	15	5
Sinus tachycardia→110	6	8	7	3
Paroxysmal atrial tachyarrhythmias*	4	8	8	2

*Paroxysmal atrial tachycardia, atrial fibrillation, atrial flutter.

post-operative periods. There were no significant differences in mean
PRA between Groups II, III, and IV during the intubation and postoperative intervals. Comparing Groups I and IV, the results were: Control
(operating room) Group I, 1.13 ± 0.04 ng–ml per hour, and Group IV,
0.96 ± 0.11 ng/ml per hour; after intubation, Group I, 1.36 ± 0.26 ng/ml
per hour, and Group IV, 0.98 ± 0.12 ng/ml per hour; 15 minutes postoperation Group I, 1.86 ± 0.10 ng/ml per hour, and Group IV, $0.95 \pm$

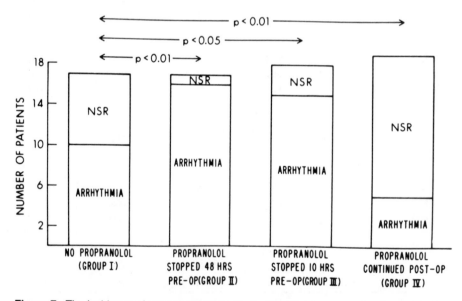

Figure 7. The incidence of supraventricular arrhythmias postcoronary artery bypass in the
different propranolol treatment groups. There was a significant increase in the frequency of
arrhythmias in Group II patients (propranolol discontinued 48 hours preoperatively) and
Group III patients (propranolol discontinued 10 hours preoperatively) compared to Group I
(no propranolol). Group IV patients (propranolol maintained postoperatively) had a significantly lower incidence of arrhythmias compared to Group I patients (no propranolol).

0.15 ng/ml per hour ($p<0.01$); 2 hours postoperation Group I, 1.66 ± 0.53 ng/ml per hour, and Group IV, 1.08 ± 0.19 ng/ml per hour.

Plasma Propranolol Levels

Propranolol plasma levels measured at the time of intubation were negligible for Group II patients, and 9.32 ± 0.82 ng/ml in Group III patients (minimal therapeutic level is 20 to 40 ng/ml). One hour after cardiopulmonary bypass, the drug level in Group III declined progressively to 3.75 ± 0.30 ng/ml, so that in the immediate postoperative period it was negligible, 2.26 ± 0.22 ng/ml. Renal clearance of propranolol was found to increase during cardiopulmonary bypass. Group IV patients had a plasma propranolol level of 39.1 ± 1.17 ng/ml at the time of induction that decreased considerably by the end of cardiopulmonary bypass to 5.2 ± 0.80 ng/ml.

DISCUSSION

Although the therapeutic value of β-blockers is well-established for angina pectoris, systemic hypertension, arrhythmias, hypertrophic obstructive cardiomyopthy, thyrotoxicosis, and pheochromocytoma,[1] the attitudes of anesthesiologists and surgeons range from frank enthusiasm to frank antagonism regarding their use just prior to anesthesia and surgery. This debate has recently extended to the anesthetic management of patients undergoing coronary bypass surgery who are receiving β-blockers for the treatment of angina pectoris. Similar to the earlier controversy with reserpine during surgery, clinical evidence for withholding β-adrenoceptor blockade for days prior to elective anesthesia and surgery is sparse and largely anecdotal. Indeed, many cardiologists are properly reluctant to withdraw a form of therapy on which their patients are highly dependent, since the consequences of withdrawal may be increased angina pectoris, myocardial infarction, and death. Thus, those who recommend abrupt withdrawal of these drugs days prior to elective coronary artery surgery should have compelling evidence that patients receiving β-blockers are at significantly more risk during anesthesia and surgery than if these agents are withdrawn. The study described in this chapter provides no such evidence. Rather, the data demonstrate that continuation of propranolol up to surgery, and its reinstitution postoperatively, protects patients with angina pectoris from the undesirable hemodynamic sequelae of laryngoscopy, endotracheal intubation, and the stresses of the early postoperative period.

The potential dangers of general anesthesia in patients taking β-blockers have been remarked upon since 1964.[24] The contention in these early reports was that β-adrenoceptor blockade would result in profound myocardial depression during general anesthesia.

Propranolol-induced myocardial depression has been implicated as a cause of the postoperative left ventricular failure occasionally seen after coronary artery bypass surgery. In 1972, Viljoen et al.[2] described five patients with advanced coronary artery disease who received propranolol (100 to 320 mg per day) to within 24 hours of surgery: four died in surgery and one had a stormy postoperative course. The authors concluded that propranolol was a major factor in these deaths, and recommended that it be discontinued 2 weeks before surgery. However, close scrutiny of Viljoen's report reveals that these five cases were complicated by other factors, making it difficult to implicate propranolol alone as the sole cause for the morbidity and mortality seen. In 1973, Faulkner et al.[25] demonstrated that the negative inotropic effect of propranolol disappeared within 48 hours. They suggested that Viljoen's recommendation for a 2-week β-blocker withdrawal period was unfounded.

In 1974, Caralps and coworkers[10] reviewed 100 cases of coronary artery bypass, including 25 patients receiving 40 to 200 mg of propranolol 24 hours or less before surgery. They found that the operative course of patients receiving propranolol, many of whom had unstable angina pectoris, was no different from that of untreated patients. In a larger review of 303 patients who underwent coronary artery surgery, the same investigators found that propranolol-treated subjects (48 hours or less prior to surgery) not only tolerated the operative procedure well, but also demonstrated a lower mortality (3.8 percent for patients receiving propranolol versus 6.6 percent for those never receiving the drug).[11]

In 1975, Kaplan and coworkers[17] reviewed the records of 169 patients undergoing coronary artery bypass, of whom 143 had been taking propranolol. They attempted to assess whether the preoperative administration of propranolol had any bearing on intraoperative or postoperative complications. The operative mortality in their study was 4 percent in patients administered propranolol within 48 hours of surgery and 6 percent in all other patients. The authors concluded that propranolol could be given safely within 12 to 48 hours of coronary artery surgery. In 1976, Kaplan and Dunbar[12] also showed that patients with angina pectoris undergoing noncardiac surgical procedures and general anesthesia could safely tolerate propranolol administration to within 24 hours of their operation.

The relative safety of maintaining propranolol just prior to surgery, established by these retrospective studies, emphasized the need for a prospective study to delineate the true clinical interaction between propranolol and general anesthesia for coronary artery operations.[9] Reports associating the abrupt withdrawal of long-term propranolol therapy with an increase in angina pectoris, and the development of new arrhythmias, myocardial infarction, and sudden death, raised the issue of whether the risk of such withdrawal before coronary artery bypass surgery was greater than the risk of purported myocardial depression.[7-9]

The mechanism for the β-blocker withdrawal reaction is unknown (see Chapter 5). Since propranolol lowers myocardial oxygen requirements, abrupt withdrawal of the drug may then raise the oxygen requirements beyond what the coronary arteries can supply, resulting in severe ischemia or myocardial infarction.[26,27] Other postulated mechanisms include increased platelet aggregability,[28] hypersensitivity to circulating catecholamines (analogous to denervation hypersensitivity),[29] and increased levels of thyroid hormone.[27]

Shand and Wood,[26] in an editorial, noted that the propranolol withdrawal syndrome, although real, was rare. Shiroff and his associates[30] found the syndrome to be infrequent in patients with angina pectoris who had their propranolol stopped abruptly prior to cardiac catheterization. The effect may have been blunted in Shiroff's series because these patients had reduced in-hospital physical activity. A rebound effect following propranolol withdrawal may be more important in the setting of surgical stress, however. There is now good evidence to show that plasma catecholamines and the level of adrenergic tone are elevated during laryngoscopy and endotracheal intubation,[31-36] and again after coronary bypass surgery is completed.[16,37-48] There are marked increments in blood pressure demonstrated during endotracheal intubation, and a marked increase in heart rate, blood pressure, and arrhythmia risk in the immediate postoperative state.[16,31-43] Patients who have their propranolol stopped abruptly may become hypersensitive to catecholamines during these periods.[27,29]

In a retrospective study by Langou et al.,[49] the risk of perioperative myocardial infarction was significantly increased by abrupt propranolol withdrawal 24 hours before coronary surgery, as compared to a gradual withdrawal regimen (32 percent infarct rate versus 7.3 percent infarct rate). Recent studies by Kirsh et al.,[5] Kopriva et al.,[14] and Boudoulas et al.[16] demonstrated the safety of propranolol administered within 1 to 5 hours of coronary artery surgery.

In a large prospective trial by Slogoff et al.,[4] chronic propranolol therapy was administered in full dosage just prior to surgery and a comparison was made to patient groups where therapy was not given or abruptly withdrawn 24 to 72 hours preoperatively. Patients abruptly withdrawn from their propranolol treatment days prior had the highest incidence of intraoperative ischemia and arrhythmias. The incidence of hypotension and bradycardia was not increased in patients who had propranolol continued. Moreover, no difference among groups was noted in the ease of discontinuation of cardiopulmonary bypass, need for cardiac stimulants, and in mortality.

In another recent prospective study, Boudoulas et al.[3] reported that propranolol maintained just prior to surgery was associated with a lower incidence of supraventricular tachyarrhythmias in the postoperative period, when compared to patients where propranolol was abruptly discontinued 24 hours prior to surgery. There were no complications related to propranolol during the intraoperative period. Left ventricular function, measured from systolic time intervals, was the same pre- and postoperatively, with both treatment regimens.

Patients with angina pectoris who had propranolol withdrawn more than 48 hours prior to surgery demonstrated a higher incidence of supraventricular arrhythmias and hypertension following coronary artery bypass, when compared to patients who had the drug maintained just prior to surgery.[18,50] We proposed a propranolol withdrawal effect as the cause for these phenomena. This study was designed, therefore, to assess the safety of different preoperative propranolol withdrawal treatment regimens in patients undergoing coronary artery surgery.

The results of this study show that propranolol can be given safely to hemodynamically stable patients about to undergo elective coronary bypass surgery. Propranolol-treated patients (Group IV–drug maintained just prior surgery and resumed postoperatively) had a significant blunting of the hypertensive reflex usually seen during intubation,[31] and demonstrated a negligible increment in the mean rate–pressure product during the postoperative period. A significant reduction in the incidence of supraventricular arrhythmias was also noted. Of concern was the finding that there were greater increments in mean systolic blood pressure and RPP during the intubation and postoperative periods in those patients where propranolol was stopped 10 to 48 hours prior to surgery (Groups II, III) than in Group I (no propranolol) and Group IV patients. There was also a significantly higher incidence of arrhythmias seen in those groups who had propranolol abruptly withdrawn 10 to 48 hours prior to surgery when compared to Group IV.

The data in this report suggest that there is a true propranolol "withdrawal effect," which becomes manifest in some patients during coronary artery surgery. This phenomenon does not appear to be mediated by the renin–angiotensin system, as was previously suggested,[51,52] but instead by a hyperadrenergic response to a stress situation.[16] Patients who never received propranolol did not demonstrate a large increment in mean rate–pressure product in the postoperative period, despite having higher serum renin activity when compared to Group IV patients (propranolol maintained). The marked increments in mean RPP (an indirect index of myocardial oxygen demand)[19,20] and the frequency of arrhythmias in the postoperative periods was a specific finding in those patients who had propranolol abruptly withdrawn. Patients who had propranolol maintained just prior to surgery (Group IV) failed to demonstrate this increment in mean RPP or in the incidence of arrhythmia. Catecholamines were not measured, so it is not known whether the postoperative RPP increments in this study are secondary to increased catecholamine levels and/or adrenoceptor hypersensitivity, as suggested by other investigators.[16,29,39]

In this study, the finding that patients being withdrawn from β-blockers just 10 hours prior to surgery were not being protected from marked increments in RPP during the surgery (intubation) and in the postoperative period was surprising, in light of the prolonged pharmacodynamic half-life of propranolol,[53,54] which contrasts to its shorter pharmacokinetic half-life.[55,56] This might be explained by the increased clearance of the drug during cardiopulmonary bypass and the heightened adrenergic state in the immediate postoperative period. Following cardiopulmonary bypass, negligible propranolol plasma levels were found in Groups III and IV, reinforcing a need to maintain propranolol intravenously during the immediate postoperative period to protect against the consequences of a postoperative hyperadrenergic state.[37–41]

There are important clinical implications of this study. First, increased myocardial oxygen demands during intubation may be more important in causing myocardial ischemia. The findings of intubation-induced hypertension and tachycardia have been demonstrated in many studies, emphasizing the need to protect patients (with β-adrenergic blockade or α-β-blockade) from this catecholamine-mediated phenomenon.[31,36] Moreover, a propranolol withdrawal effect, following abrupt premature discontinuation of the drug, may further aggravate this situation.[29] Many of the perioperative myocardial infarctions observed with coronary bypass surgery[57] may relate to the intubation-related increase in RPP, an effect that usually persists for 5 minutes.[34] In this study, five myocardial infarctions were seen in Groups II and III versus none in Group IV.

Second, there is probably no need to given propranolol during the operative period. Halothane, enflurane, and isoflurane are the general anesthetics most commonly used for coronary artery bypass surgery and, like propranolol, are myocardial depressants (agents that will lower the oxygen demand of the heart).[58] The drugs have been shown to decrease the activity of the sympathetic nervous system and to reduce the output of catecholamines by adrenergic nerve endings and the adrenal medulla. Direct effects on autonomic nerve terminals have not been demonstrated and there is no reason to believe, nor any evidence to support, the notion that halothane may act on adrenal receptors.[58] As demonstrated in this report, patients in all four groups had similar mean RPP after 1 hour of halothane anesthesia. The effects of propranolol and halothane are usually additive and not potentiated with the concentrations of halothane used in coronary artery surgery.[59]

Third, the well-documented hyperadrenergic state in the early postoperative period[37–42] may explain the high incidence of hypertension and arrhythmias reported in this study and others.[37–41] Intravenous maintenance propranolol used postoperatively appears to blunt these stress reactions,[50] whereas premature propranolol withdrawal preoperatively seems to aggravate it. The supraventricular arrhythmias appear to be catecholamine mediated since they all respond to intravenous propranolol therapy. Unlike propranolol, the efficacy of digoxin in treating postoperative arrhythmias has not been demonstrated.[60]

Maintenance of myocardial oxygen needs at relatively low levels by propranolol might be especially important in the prebypass operative period in patients undergoing complete coronary artery revascularizations. The demonstration that perioperative myocardial infarction often occurs in the period between induction of anesthesia and onset of cardiopulmonary bypass emphasizes the need for myocardial protection during this most vulnerable period.[61,62] During the postbypasss period, myocardial oxygen demands should also be controlled, especially in patients who undergo incomplete coronary revascularization procedures, where the threat of myocardial ischemia may still remain, or following noncardiac operative procedures in patients with angina pectoris, where the entire myocardium may remain at risk.

The mortality of patients with angina pectoris undergoing elective noncardiac procedures has been reported to be multiples higher than that of patients undergoing elective coronary revascularization procedures.[63] Proper anesthetic technique and careful hemodynamic monitoring are important for all patients with ischemic coronary artery disease who undergo cardiac or noncardiac operations. In our study, the perioperative myocardial infarctions occurred only in those patients who either had propranolol abruptly withdrawn or had never received the drug preoperatively.

Many of the newer β-adrenoceptor blocking agents (i.e., atenolol, metoprolol—β$_1$-selective; pindolol—intrinsic sympathomimetic activity;

labetalol—α- and β-blocking activity) have been evaluated in patients undergoing surgery and, like propranolol, have been found to be well tolerated.[33,64-69] Since many of the β-adrenoceptor blocking agents have similar effects on angina pectoris, arrhythmia, and hypertension (Chapter 4), the potential dangers of abrupt treatment withdrawal with these agents should be similar to that reported with propranolol withdrawal.[70,71]

CONCLUSIONS

1. Propranolol can safely be maintained until just prior to coronary artery surgery in hemodynamically stable patients and resumed in the immediate postoperative period with no difficulty.
2. Propranolol blunts the profound increases in myocardial oxygen demand seen during endotracheal intubation and the postoperative period. These hemodynamic changes appear to be catecholamine-mediated and unrelated to the renin–angiotensin system.
3. There is a demonstrable propranolol withdrawal effect when the drug is abruptly stopped 10 to 48 hours prior to coronary artery surgery. This early withdrawal of β-blocker treatment appears to aggravate the hyperadrenergic state seen during the intubation and postoperative periods.
4. There is an accelerated clearance of propranolol during cardiopulmonary bypass, with a rapid disappearance of the drug, demonstrating the need to temporarily restart the drug in the immediate postoperative period where adrenergic tone is high.
5. There is a high incidence of postoperative supraventricular arrhythmias seen in patients withdrawn from propranolol 10 to 48 hours prior to surgery. These arrhythmias are probably catecholamine mediated because their incidence is reduced by introducing propranolol prophylaxis,[71] and they respond readily to treatment with propranolol.
6. The recognition of a propranolol withdrawal effect in patients during cardiac surgery raises an even greater concern for patients with chronic angina pectoris undergoing noncardiac surgical procedures.

RECOMMENDATIONS

We strongly believe now that with the proper indications for its continued clinical use, chronic therapy with propranolol should be maintained in moderate doses up to the time of surgery. We recommend that half the usual dose be given orally 2 hours prior to surgery and that administration of intravenous propranolol be resumed in the immediate postoperative period. This is an empirical approach but appears not only to minimize the occurrence of complications from the patients' disease in the preoperative period, but cardiovascular stability may actually be improved by the persistence of propranolol effects during anesthesia and surgery. The lower heart rate and blood pressure with β-blockade are favorable for minimizing myocardial oxygen needs during surgery. The incidence and severity of tachycardia and dysrhythmias are probably lower in postoperative patients maintained on β-blockers up to the time of surgery.

Propranolol and other β-blockers should not be abruptly withdrawn, even as early as 10 hours prior to surgery. The question of gradual withdrawal of therapy prior to surgery has not been well resolved, but in the absence of any apparent complications with continued propranolol use in most patients, there is little justification for a gradual withdrawal regimen.

REFERENCES

1. Frishman WH: The beta-adrenoceptor blocking drugs. Int J Cardiol 2:165, 1982.
2. Viljoen JF, Estafanous FG, Kellner GA: Propranolol and cardiac surgery. J Thorac Cardiovasc Surg 64:826, 1972.
3. Boudoulas H, Lewis RP, Synder GL, et al: Beneficial effect of continuation of propranolol through coronary bypass surgery. Clin Cardiol 2:87, 1979.
4. Slogoff S, Keats AS, Ott E: Preoperative propranolol therapy and aortocoronary bypass operation. JAMA 240:1487, 1978.
5. Kirsh MM, Behrendt DM, Jackson AP, et al: Myocardial revascularization in patients receiving long-term propranolol therapy. Ann Thorac Surg 25:117, 1978.
6. Romagnoli A, Keats AS: Plasma and atrial propranolol after preoperative withdrawal. Circulation 52:1123, 1975.
7. Alderman EL, Coltart DJ, Wettach GE, Harrison DC: Coronary artery syndromes after sudden propranolol withdrawal. Ann Intern Med 81:625, 1974.
8. Miller RR, Olson HG, Amsterdam EA, Mason DT: Propranolol withdrawal rebound phenomenon. Exacerbation of coronary events after abrupt cessation of antianginal therapy. N Engl J Med 293:416, 1975.
9. Shand DG: Propranolol withdrawal. N Engl J Med 293:449, 1975.
10. Caralps JM, Mulet J, Wienke HR, et al: Results of coronary artery surgery in patients receiving propranolol. J Thorac Cardiovasc Surg 67:526, 1974.
11. Moran JM, Mulet J, Caralps JM, Pifarré R: Coronary revascularization in patients receiving propranolol. Circulation 49 + 50 (Suppl II):II–116, 1974.

12. Kaplan JA, Dunbar RW: Propranolol and surgical anesthesia. Anesth Analg 55:1, 1976.
13. Kopriva CJ, Guinazu A, Barash PG: Massive propranolol therapy and uncomplicated cardiac surgery. JAMA 239:1157, 1978.
14. Kopriva CJ, Brown ACD, Pappas G: Hemodynamics during general anesthesia in patients receiving propranolol. Anesthesiology 48:28, 1978.
15. Jones EL, Kaplan JA, Dorney ER, et al: Propranolol therapy in patients undergoing myocardial revascularization. Am J Cardiol 38:696, 1976.
16. Boudoulas H, Snyder GL, Lewis RP, et al: Safety and efficacy of continued propranolol administration through coronary bypass surgery. (Abstr). Am J Cardiol 41:359, 1978.
17. Kaplan JA, Dunbar RW, Bland JW, et al: Propranolol and cardiac surgery: a problem for the anesthesiologist. Anesth Analg 54:571, 1975.
18. Salazar C, Frishman W, Friedman S, et al: β-Blockade for supraventricular tachycardia post-coronary artery surgery: a propranolol withdrawal syndrome. Angiology 30:816, 1979.
19. Robinson BF: Relation of heart rate and systolic blood pressure to the onset of pain in angina pectoris. Circulation 35:1072, 1967.
20. Nelson RR, Gobel FL, Jorgenson CR, et al: Hemodynamic predictors of myocardial oxygen consumption during static and dynamic exercise. Circulation 50:1179, 1974.
21. Coltart DJ, Shand DG: Plasma propranolol levels in the quantitative assessment of β-adrenergic blockade in man. Br Med J 3:731, 970.
22. Chervu LR, Lory M, Liang T, et al: Determination of plasma renin activity by radioimmunoassay: Comparison of results from two commercial kits with bioassay. J Nucl Med 13:806, 1972.
23. Powell CE, Slater IH: Blocking of inhibitory adrenergic receptors by a dichloro-analog of isoproterenol. J Pharmacol Ther 122:480, 1958.
24. Johnstone M: Propranolol during halothane anesthesia. Br J Anaesth 38:516, 1966.
25. Faulkner SL, Hopkins JT, Boerth RC, et al: Time required for complete recovery from chronic propranolol therapy. N Engl J Med 289:607, 1973.
26. Shand DG, Wood AJJ: Editorial: Propranolol withdrawal syndrome—why? Circulation 58:202, 1978.
27. Prichard BNC, Walden RJ: The syndrome associated with the withdrawal of β-adrenergic receptor blocking drugs. Br J Clin Pharm 13:337s, 1982.
28. Frishman WH, Christodoulou J, Weksler B, et al: Abrupt propranolol withdrawal in angina pectoris: Effects on platelet aggregation and exercise tolerance. Am Heart J 95:169, 1978.
29. Boudoulas H, Lewis RP, Kates RE, Dalamangas G: Hypersensitivity to adrenergic stimulation after propranolol withdrawal in normal subjects. Ann Intern Med 87:433, 1977.
30. Shiroff RA, Mathis J, Zelis R, et al: Propranolol rebound—a retrospective study. Am J Cardiol 41:778, 1978.
31. Tomori Z, Widdicombe JG: Muscular bronchomotor and cardiovascular reflex elicited by mechanical stimulation of the respiratory tract. J Physiol (Lond) 200:25, 1969.

32. Prys-Roberts C, Greene LT, Melache R, Foëx P: Studies of anesthesia in relation to hypertension. II: Haemodynamic consequences of induction and endotracheal intubation. Br J Anaesth 43:531, 1971.
33. Prys-Roberts C, Foëx P, Biro GP, Roberts JG: Studies of anaesthesia in relation to hypertension. V: Adrenergic beta-receptor blockade. Br J Anaesth 45:671, 1973.
34. Stoelting RK, Peterson C: Circulatory changes in patients with coronary artery disease following thiamylal-succinylcholine and tracheal intubation. Anesth Analg 55:232, 1976.
35. DeVault M, Greifenstein FE, Harris LC: Circulatory responses to endotracheal intubation in light general anesthesia—the effect of atropine and phentolamine. Anesthesiology 21:360, 1960.
36. Bassell GM, Lin YT, Oka Y, et al: Circulatory response to tracheal intubation in patients with coronary artery disease and valvular disease. Bull NY Acad Med 54:842, 1978.
37. Boudoulas H, Lewis RP, Vasko JS, et al: Left ventricular function and adrenergic hyperactivity before and after saphenous vein bypass. Circulation 53:802, 1976.
38. Wallen JL, Kaplan JA, Jones EL: Anesthesia for coronary revascularization, in Kaplan J (ed), Cardiac Anesthesia. New York, Grune and Stratton, 1979, pp 270–271.
39. Whelton PK, Flaherty JT, MacAllister NP, et al: Hypertension following coronary artery bypass surgery: the role of preoperative propranolol therapy. (Abstr). Am J Cardiol 43:422, 1979.
40. Goldstein R, Corash L, Tallman J, et al: Decrease in platelet survival and enhancement of sympathetically mediated reflex rises in heart rate after abrupt withdrawal of propranolol. (Abstr). Am J Cardiol 43:416, 1979.
41. Bernstein V, Miyagishima RT: Rapid beta-blockade for control of atrial arrhythmias following coronary bypass surgery. (Abstr). Ann R Coll Phys Surg Can 11:33, 1979.
42. Roberts AJ, Niarchos AP, Subramanian VA, et al: Systemic hypertension associated with coronary artery bypass surgery: Predisposing factors, hemodynamic characteristics, humoral profile, and treatment. J Thorac Cardiovasc Surg 74:846, 1977.
43. Hine IP, Wood WG, Mainwaring B, et al: The adrenergic response to surgery involving cardiopulmonary bypass, as measured by plasma and urinary catecholamine concentrations. Br J Anaesth 48:355, 1976.
44. Barta E, Kuzela L, Kvetnansky R: Activity of sympathetic nerves in heart during cardiopulmonary bypass in patients. J Cardiovasc Surg 17:174, 1976.
45. Tan CK, Glisson SN, El-Etr AA, Ramakrishnaiak KB: Levels of circulating norepinephrine and epinephrine before, during and after cardiopulmonary bypass in man. J Thorac Cardiovasc Surg 71:928, 1976.
46. Pratilas V, Vlachakis ND, Litwak R: Hypertension and plasma catecholamines following aorto-coronary bypass surgery. (Abstr). Clin Res 25:244A, 1977.
47. Fouad FM, Estafanous FG, Tarazi RC: Hemodynamics of post-myocardial revascularization hypertension. Am J Cardiol 41:564, 1978.

48. Wallach R, Karp RB, Reves LG, et al: Mechanism of hypertension after saphenous vein bypass surgery. (Abstr). Circulation (Suppl III) 55, 56:III–141, 1977.
49. Langou RA, Wiles JC, Peduzzi PN, et al: Incidence and mortality of perioperative myocardial infarction in patients undergoing coronary artery bypass grafting. Circulation (Suppl II) 56:II–54, 1977.
50. Mohr R, Smolinsky A, Goor DA: Prevention of supraventricular tachyarrhythmias with low dose propranolol after coronary bypass. J Thorac Cardiovasc Surg 81:840, 1981.
51. Taylor KM, Morton IJ, Brown JJ, et al: Hypertension and the renin–angiotensin system following open heart surgery. J Thorac Cardiovasc Surg 74:839, 1977.
52. Niarchos AP, Roberts AJ, Case D, et al: Hemodynamic characteristics of hypertension after coronary bypass surgery and effects of the converting enzyme inhibitor. Am J Cardiol 43:586, 1979.
53. Wilson M, Morgan G, Morgan T: The effect of blood pressure of β-adrenoceptor blocking drugs given once daily. Clin Sci Mol Med 51:527s, 1976.
54. Boudoulas H, Beaver BM, Kates RE, Lewis RP: Pharmacodynamics of inotropic and chronotropic responses to oral therapy with propranolol. Chest 73:146, 1978.
55. Frishman W: Clinical pharmacology of the new beta-adrenergic blocking drugs. Part 1. Pharmacodynamic and pharmacokinetic properties. Am Heart J 97:663, 1979.
56. Shand DG: Pharmacokinetics of propranolol: A review. Postgrad Med J 52 (Suppl 4):22, 1976.
57. Bristow JO: A cardiologist's view of coronary bypass surgery, In Yu PN, Goodwin JF (eds), Progress in Cardiology. Philadelphia, Lea and Febiger 1977, vol 6, pp 28–29.
58. Kaplan JA, Hug CC: Anesthesia and cardiac disease, in Hurst JW (ed), The Heart. New York, McGraw-Hill, 1982, pp 1613–30.
59. Slogoff S, Keats AS, Hibbs CW, et al: Failure of general anesthesia to potentiate propranolol activity. Anesthesiology 47:504, 1977.
60. Tyras DH, Stothert JC, Kaiser GC, et al: Supraventricular tachyarrhythmias after myocardial revascularization: a randomized trial of prophylactic digitalization. J Thorac Cardiovasc Surg 77:310, 1979.
61. Isom OW, Spencer FC, Feigenbaum H, et al: Pre-bypass myocardial damage in patients undergoing coronary revascularization: an unrecognized vulnerable period. (Abstr). Circulation 52 (Suppl II):119, 1975.
62. Delva E, Maillé JG, Solymoss BC, et al: Evaluation of myocardial damage during coronary artery grafting with serial determinations of serum CPK MB isoenzyme. J Thorac Cardiovasc Surg 75:467, 1978.
63. Pritchett ELC, Orgain ES: Evaluation and management of patients with heart disease who undergo noncardiac surgery, in Hurst JW (ed), The Heart. New York, McGraw-Hill, 1982, pp 1630–36.
64. Scott DB, Buckley FP, Drummond GB, et al: Cardiovascular effects of labetalol during halothane anesthesia. Br J Clin Pharmacol 3 (Suppl 3):817s, 1976.

65. Cope DHP: Use of labetalol during halothane anesthesia. Br J Clin Pharmacol 8 (Suppl 2):223s, 1979.
66. Scott DB: The use of labetalol in anesthesia. Br J Clin Pharmacol 13 (Suppl 1):133s, 1982.
67. Yoshikawa K, Tosaki Y, Yoshiva I: Use of LB–46, a new antiarrhythmic agent during anesthesia. Med J Osaka Univ 23:189, 1972.
68. Nicholas G, Nicholas F, Rozo L: Problems posed by anesthesia in the hypertensive treated with beta-blockers. Arch Mal Coeur 69:1311, 1976.
69. Erding E, Nalbantgil E, Kiliccioglu B, et al: Prevention by pindolol of electrocardiographic changes during bronchoscopy, performed under local and general anesthesia. Ann Anesthesiol Franc 18:747, 1977.
70. Frishman W, Silverman R: Clinical pharmacology of the new beta-adrenergic blocking drugs. Part 2. Physiologic and metabolic effects. Am Heart J 97:797, 1979.
71. Silverman NA, Wright R, Levitsky S: Efficacy of low-dose propranolol in preventing post-operative supraventricular tachyarrhythmias. Ann Surg 146:194, 1982.

PART THREE

Labetalol in Hypertension

CHAPTER 13

A Multiclinic Comparison of Labetalol to Metoprolol in the Treatment of Mild to Moderate Systemic Hypertension

William H. Frishman, Eric L. Michelson, Brian F. Johnson, and Marcia P. Poland

β-Adrenoceptor blocking drugs are widely accepted for the treatment of systemic hypertension.[1] Metoprolol is a β-blocking drug that acts relatively selectively at cardiac β_1-adrenergic receptors. Unlike propranolol, a nonselective β-blocker, metoprolol in low doses does not block the β_2-receptors in the peripheral arterioles that mediate dilatation of these resistance vessels. This property might be an advantage in the treatment of hypertension with relatively low doses of metoprolol, but this possibility has not been demonstrated. β_1-Selective agents may also be safer than nonselective β-blockers in patients with obstructive pulmonary disease since bronchial β_2-receptors remain available to mediate adrenergic bronchodilatation.[2,3]

Labetalol, 5-(1-hydroxy-2-[(1-methyl-3-phenylpropyl) amino] ethyl) salicylamide, is a recently developed drug that, like propranolol and unlike metoprolol, blocks both β_1 and β_2 vascular and bronchial adrenoreceptors. However, labetalol is unique in that it also has selective peripheral α_1-adrenergic blocking properties, β_2 stimulatory actions, and direct vasodilatory activity (see Chapter 7). In human beings, the β-blocking potency of oral labetalol is 3 times that of its α-blocking potency.[4-6]

Labetalol has been shown to be a potent antihypertensive drug but its status relative to other β-blocking drugs has not been well defined.[7-11]

Reprinted from the American Journal of Medicine 75; 54–67, October 17, 1983, with permission.

It has been suggested that labetalol reduces blood pressure predominately by reducing peripheral vascular resistance while maintaining cardiac output.[12,13] In this study, the safety and antihypertensive efficacy of oral labetalol and metoprolol were compared in patients with mild-to-moderate hypertension using a randomized double-blind multicenter trial design. Considering the recent reports that have suggested adverse effects of certain β-blockers on plasma lipids and lipoproteins,[14,15] the effects of metoprolol and labetalol on these parameters were also assessed.

METHODS

Patients

This was a multicenter double-blind parallel treatment group study in patients with mild-to-moderate hypertension. One hundred eighteen patients with mild-to-moderate essential hypertension were entered in the study from three centers (Einstein, Lankenau, and the University of Massachusetts), after written and informed consent was obtained. Mild-to-moderate essential hypertension was defined as an average (three measurements, 1 minute apart, after 2 minutes standing) standing diastolic blood pressure (SDBP) of 90 to 115 mm Hg (using Korotkoff phase V) after 3 and 4 weeks of placebo. Patients of any race and of either sex between the ages of 18 and 70 years were included. Twenty-two patients did not enter the active treatment phase of the study for various reasons (e.g., SDBP <90 mm Hg or >115 mm Hg) and they are not included in the efficacy and safety analyses. An additional five patients were withdrawn during titration with active medication; their results are included in the safety analyses but not in the efficacy analyses. The demographic data of the remaining 91 patients who received active treatment are shown in Table 1. There were no significant differences between the two treatment groups with regard to their demographic profiles.

Patients with the following conditions were excluded from study entry: congestive heart failure, coexistent valvular heart disease, recent cerebrovascular accident (within 1 year) and myocardial infarction (within 6 months), anemia, heart block, sinus bradycardia (resting heart rate <50 beats per minute), angina pectoris, bronchial asthma, pregnancy, renal disease, hepatic disease, and insulin-dependent diabetes. Throughout the study patients took no medication that would effect blood pressure.

TABLE 1. DEMOGRAPHIC PROFILE OF PATIENTS INCLUDED IN THE EFFICACY ANALYSIS

	Labetalol	Metoprolol
Total number of patients	44	47
Age (years)		
Mean	51.0	52.7
Range	23–65	24–70
Sex		
Male	30	31
Female	14	16
Race		
Caucasian	38	39
Black	5	8
Oriental	1	0
Severity of hypertension		
SDBP <105 mm Hg (mild)	23	24
SDBP >105 mm Hg (moderate)	21*	18*
Duration of hypertension		
Median	5.0	5.0
Range	3 mo–30 yr	1 mo–40 yr
Previous antihypertensive treatment		
No	8	12
Yes	36	35

*Six patients in each group had a baseline SDBP >115 mm Hg to <120 mm Hg and one metoprolol patient had an SDBP of 122 mm Hg. These were above the upper limit prescribed by the protocol but were considered acceptable for all analyses.

Experimental Design

The study was divided into four phases (Fig. 1). Patients who met all the study inclusion criteria entered into a 4-week placebo period to establish that they had mild-to-moderate hypertension, i.e., a mean standing diastolic blood pressure (SDBP) of 90 to <115 mm Hg at each of the last two weekly visits. The average of these two mean SDBP was the baseline SDBP. The patients were instructed to take their medication twice daily in as close to 12-hour intervals as possible and their follow-up visits were scheduled 8 to 12 hours after a dose. At the last visit of this placebo phase, the patients were randomly assigned to the labetalol or the metoprolol group. Placebo, metoprolol, and labetalol were supplied in identical capsules by the Schering-Plough Corporation (Kennelworth, NJ) to assure double-blind conditions.

A 4-week titration began with an initial dose of 100 mg of labetalol twice daily or 50 mg of metoprolol twice daily. The dose of labetalol was

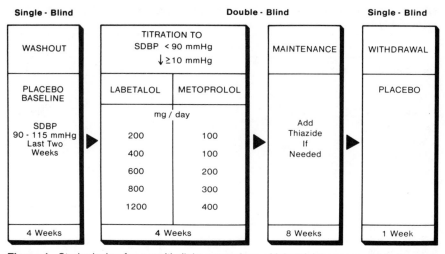

Figure 1. Study design for a multi-clinic comparison of labetalol to metoprolol in the treatment of mild-to-moderate systemic hypertension.

increased to 200 mg twice daily in 2 to 3 days and the dose of metoprolol was maintained. The dose of labetalol or metoprolol was increased at weekly intervals thereafter to achieve a SDBP that had been reduced from the baseline by $\geq$10 mm Hg to <90 mm Hg.

An 8-week maintenance phase followed during which the patients received the dosage regimen taken during the last week of the titration phase unless their SDBP goal was not maintained. In this event, the dose was increased in stepwise fashion to the maximum allowed dose of 1200 mg/day labetalol or 400 mg/day of metoprolol. If, however, the SDBP still remained $\geq$100 mm Hg, the investigator could add hydrochlorothiazide, 25 mg twice daily and concomitantly decrease the study medication one level, i.e., 1200 to 800 mg/day of labetalol or 400 to 300 mg/day of metoprolol. If necessary, to achieve the SDBP goal, the dose of study medication and hydrochlorothiazide could be increased to the maximum. However, if the SDBP still remained >100 mm Hg, the investigator could remove the patient from the study. At the end of the maintenance phase, labetalol and metoprolol were tapered over a 2- to 4-day period (depending upon their maintenance dose), after which all patients received placebo for 1 week.

Evaluation of Efficacy

Supine and standing blood pressures were recorded at each study visit. The average of three consecutive measurements after the patient was supine for 5 minutes and again after the patient was standing for 2 minutes was used for the evaluation of efficacy.

The changes from baseline in heart rate as well as the systolic and diastolic blood pressures were compared for the labetalol and metoprolol treatments after 1 week of titration and at the last visits of the titration and maintenance phases.

The antihypertensive effects of labetalol and metoprolol were rated according to the extent of the fall in the SDBP as follows: good—a fall of ≥10 mm Hg; fair—a fall of 5 to <10 mm Hg; poor—a fall of <5 mm Hg. The two treatment groups were subdivided into mild and moderate hypertension (i.e., SDBP baseline 90 to <105 and ≥105 to ≤115 mm Hg) to determine the antihypertensive response by severity of hypertension.

Evaluation of Safety

At the initial visit, the health status of each patient was assessed from a medical history and from the results of a physical examination, ophthalmologic examination, a 12-lead electrocardiogram, and a battery of laboratory tests (blood chemistries, antinuclear antibody, complete blood count, and urinalysis). All these were repeated at the end of maintenance.

The patients' heart rate, body weight, and any reports of adverse experiences were recorded at each visit. The postural blood pressure changes were determined in order to assess occurrences of orthostatic hypotension. Electrocardiograms, physical examinations of the heart and lungs, and laboratory tests were repeated at the end of the placebo, titration, and maintenance phases. The two groups were compared with respect to changes in heart rate, body weight, and postural changes in blood pressure and heart rate. Patient complaints as well as those complaints ruled drug related were also compared.

Lipids and Lipoprotein Determinations

Blood samples for lipid and lipoprotein determinations were obtained at the end of the placebo and maintenance treatment phases of the study in 70 patients (35 metoprolol, 35 labetalol) with no previous history of clinically significant lipid abnormalities. All subjects had been fasting for 10 to 12 hours, with the last drug dose ingested 8 to 12 hours prior to study. Blood was drawn from an antecubital vein into Vacutainer tubes containing 10 to 14 mg of dry EDTA per milliliter of blood. Plasma was separated immediately.

Lipid and lipoprotein determinations were done in duplicate from coded samples, with total laboratory blinding of drug dose. The laboratory was standardized according to criteria developed by the Lipid Research Clinics Program.[16] Total plasma cholesterol and triglyceride concentrations were determined by the Autoanalyzer II. Lipoprotein fractionation and quantitation were determined by preparative ultracentrifugation techniques as previously described.[17]

Statistical Analyses

Group means are presented, with the standard error of the mean as the index of dispersion. The poolability of the data from the three centers was evaluated by comparing the demographic and baseline data, and by examining the investigator-by-treatment interaction. In the absence of a consistent pattern of investigator-by-treatment differences, the data from the three investigators were pooled. The antihypertensive effect ratings of the two treatment groups after 1 week of treatment, at the end of titration, and at the end of maintenance for patients receiving monotherapy only were compared using the Two-Sample Wilcoxon Test. The effects on blood pressure and heart rate were compared using differences from baseline (average of the last two visits of the placebo phase). The two treatments were compared using analysis of variance. Treatment, investigator, and investigator-by-treatment effects were partitioned out. In addition, for the titration phase visits, the changes from baseline for each treatment group compared to zero used the two-tailed paired t-tests. For the maintenance phase visits, the changes from the end of titration were compared using two-tailed t-tests. The number of patients reporting at least one complaint during the study or a specific complaint were compared using Fisher's 2×2 Exact Test. Postural changes in blood pressure and heart rate for the two treatment groups were compared using analysis of variance.

RESULTS

The data obtained by all the investigators in this muticenter study were examined and found to be poolable.

Patients

Of the 118 patients who entered the placebo phase, 96 patients were randomly assigned to receive labetalol or metoprolol. Five patients failed to complete the titration phase and were excluded from the efficacy analyses: two from each treatment group due to adverse experiences and one labetalol-treated patient due to hospitalization for an acute viral illness (these five patients are included in the safety analyses). Forty-four patients on labetalol and 47 on metoprolol completed the titration phase, and 38 patients in each group completed the maintenance phase. The ability of the two drugs to maintain an antihypertensive effect was analyzed by comparing the blood pressure reductions achieved at the end of the titration phase with those at the end of the maintenance phase in the patients who completed both treatment phases.

Effects on Blood Pressure

The effects of labetalol and metoprolol on standing and supine blood pressure are shown in Figure 2 and Table 2. Both drugs significantly lowered the systolic and diastolic blood pressure ($p < 0.01$) compared to placebo, with no significant differences between the two treatment groups. The posttreatment placebo period shows the rapid return of the blood pressure toward baseline in both treatment groups. No significant difference between the two treatments was seen at the end of either the titration or maintenance phases. The mean reductions in the supine and standing blood pressure in the two treatment groups were similar after the first week of treatment, and at the end of the titration and maintenance phases. This was also true when the treatment groups were stratified into mild and moderate hypertension subgroups. Table 3 shows standing blood pressure. Similar results were seen for the supine blood pressure.

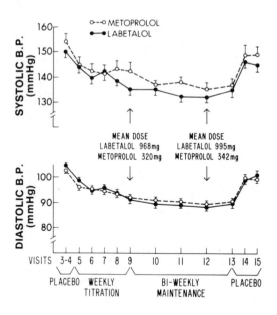

Figure 2. Standing blood pressure (BP) at rest, before, during and after treatment with oral labetalol and metoprolol. Both drugs significantly reduced blood pressure, with no differences between them. Following treatment withdrawal blood pressure returned to baseline values. Values are mean ± standard error of the mean; p = probability.

TABLE 2. STANDING AND SUPINE BLOOD PRESSURE AND HEART RATES, REDUCTIONS FROM BASELINE IN PARENTHESES AND BETWEEN GROUP DIFFERENCES

	N	Labetalol Treated Group	N	Metoprolol Treated Group	Between Group Difference (p)
Standing Blood Pressure, mm Hg (Reduction from Baseline)					
Baseline	44	149.8±2.2/104.1±1.1	47	153.4±3.3/102.4±1.1	
End week 1	43	139.6±2.5/94.8±1.5 (−10.5±2.1/−9.7±1.0)	47	142.1±3.0/95.1±1.3 (−11.3±2.1/−7.3±1.0)	+0.8/−2.4 (NS)
End titration	44	135.0±2.4/91.1±1.8 (−14.8±2.2/−13.0±1.4)	47	142.1±3.5/91.7±1.4 (−11.3±2.6/−10.8±1.3)	−3.5/−2.2 (NS)
End maintenance	38*	135.4±2.7/90.8±1.4 (−14.8±2.0/−12.5±1.3)	38	137.6±2.6/91.2±1.3 (−14.2±2.9/−10.6±1.4)†	−0.6/−1.9 (NS)
Supine Blood Pressure, mm Hg (Reduction from Baseline)					
Baseline	44	147.6±2.2/97.0±1.2	47	152.4±3.0/96.4±1.3	
End week 1	43	140.9±3.0/89.8±1.8 (−6.9±2.5/−7.5±1.3)	47	140.6±2.9/87.9±1.2 (−11.9±1.9/−8.5±1.1)	+5.0/1.0 (NS)
End titration	44	137.3±2.5/87.7±1.6 (−10.2±2.0/−9.3±1.1)	47	141.2±3.6/86.4±1.6 (−11.2±2.1/−10.0±1.3)	+1.0/+0.7 (NS)
End maintenance	38*	138.1±2.5/87.4±1.4 (−9.8±1.6/−8.7±1.0)	38	136.6±2.8/85.7±1.5 (−13.1±2.7/−9.2±1.7)†	+3.4/+0.5 (NS)
Standing Heart Rate, beats/min (Reduction from Baseline)					
Baseline	44	81.6±1.5	47	80.3±1.3	
End week 1	43	77.0±1.6 (−4.9±1.4)	47	72.7±1.4 (−7.6±1.2)	+2.7 (NS)
End titration	44	73.0±1.5 (−8.6±1.2)	47	66.1±1.4 (−14.2±1.5)	+5.6 (<0.005)
End maintenance	38	75.6±1.6 (−6.1±1.4)	38	64.7±1.3 (−15.9±1.5)	+9.8 (<0.001)
Supine Heart Rate, beats/min (Reduction from Baseline)					
Baseline	44	74.6±1.6	47	76.2±1.4	
End week 1	43	72.5±1.4 (−2.3±1.4)	47	69.2±1.3 (−7.1±1.1)	+4.8 (<0.01)
End titration	44	67.4±1.5 (−7.2±1.1)	47	62.3±1.1 (−13.9±1.4)	+6.7 (<0.001)
End maintenance	38	68.5±1.7 (−5.8±1.4)	38	61.9±1.4 (−14.4±1.5)	+8.6 (<0.001)

*Baseline for labetalol group (N=38) was 150.2±2.5/103.3±1.2 standing and 147.8±2.5/96.1±1.3 supine; baseline for metoprolol group (N=38) 151.8±3.5/101.8± 1.2 standing and 149.7±3.2/94.9±1.4 supine.
†Increase in diastolic BP from the end of titration to the end of maintenance was 2.6±1.1 (p<0.03) in the standing position and 2.5±1.3 (p<0.05) in the supine position

TABLE 3. MEAN STANDING SYSTOLIC/DIASTOLIC BLOOD PRESSURE, MEAN CHANGE IN BLOOD PRESSURE FOR MILD (SDBP <105 mm Hg) AND MODERATE (SDBP >105 mm Hg) HYPERTENSIVE PATIENTS

		Placebo Baseline		End Titration		Placebo Baseline*		End Point of Maintenance
	N	Mean ± SEM	N	Mean ± SEM	N	Mean ± SEM	N	Mean ± SEM
Mean BP								
Mild SDBP <105 mmHg								
Labetalol	23	141.9±1.9/ 97.9±0.7	23	129.9±3.5/ 85.9±1.9	21	141.5±1.9/ 97.6±0.8	21	130.0±2.0/ 87.8±1.5
Metoprolol	29	148.6±3.4/ 97.4±0.7	29	139.1±4.6/ 87.7±1.4	26	146.2±2.6/ 97.6±0.7	26	135.5±2.5/ 88.5±1.5
Moderate SDBP								
Labetalol	21	158.5±3.1/110.9±0.9	21	140.6±2.8/ 96.9±2.5	17	160.8±3.6/110.3±1.0	17	142.0±5.2/ 94.6±2.3
Metoprolol	18	161.3±6.2/110.6±1.1	18	146.9±5.5/ 98.0±2.0	12	163.8±9.0/110.8±1.5	12	141.9±6.0/ 97.1±1.5
Mean BP Reduction								
Mild								
Labetalol				−12.0±3.2/−12.1±1.7				−11.5±1.6/ −9.8±1.4
Metoprolol				−9.5±2.8/−9.7±1.6				−10.7±2.9/ −9.2±1.6
Difference				−2.5/ −2.4				−0.8/ −0.6
Moderate								
Labetalol				−17.9±3.1/−14.0±2.2				−18.8±3.8/−15.7±2.1
Metoprolol				−14.4±5.3/−12.5±2.4				−21.8±6.3/−13.7±2.5
Difference				−3.5/ −1.5				+3.1/ −2.0

*Baseline for those patients who entered the maintenance phase on labetalol or metoprolol alone.
BP = Blood pressure.
SDBP = Standing diastolic blood pressure.
SEM = Standard of mean.
N = Number of patients.

401

With labetalol, the blood pressures at the end of the maintenance phase were not significantly different from those at the end of titration. In the metoprolol-treated patients the systolic pressures at the two end points were not different either. However, in the metoprolol group the supine and standing diastolic blood pressure (DBP) was significantly higher at the end point of maintenance than at the end of titration. The supine DBP was 2.5 ± 1.3 mm Hg higher ($p < 0.05$) and the standing DBP was 2.6 ± 1.9 mm Hg higher ($p < 0.03$) than at the end of the titration phase. Heart rates were not significantly different from those at the end of titration in the metoprolol group. However, standing heart rate was 3.0 ± 1.3 beats per minute higher ($p < 0.03$) in the labetalol group. Thus, the antihypertensive effect of labetalol that was attained at the end of titration was generally maintained over the 2-month maintenance period, whereas a small but statistically significant increase occurred in the diastolic blood pressure of the metoprolol group, probably denoting some waning of the antihypertensive effect across time.

Effect of Adding Hydrochlorothiazide
Nine patients in each treatment group received hydrochlorothiazide in the maintenance period because their standing diastolic blood pressure was ≥ 100 mm Hg while on monotherapy. One additional metoprolol patient developed edema and required hydrochlorothiazide although his blood pressure was controlled. Six of the nine labetalol patients had a baseline standing diastolic blood pressure in the moderate range and three in the mild range. Two of the metoprolol-treated patients were moderate hypertensives and eight were mild. Four of 13 black patients who were enrolled in this study (three of five in the labetalol group and one of eight in the metoprolol group) required a diuretic.

Before the addition of a thiazide diuretic, poor or no response to monotherapy with labetalol or metoprolol was seen in six and seven patients, respectively. A fair response (fall of 5 to 9 mm Hg) was seen in three metoprolol-treated patients and a good response (fall of 10 to 16 mm Hg) in three labetalol-treated patients. Despite the fall of 10 to 16 mm Hg in these three labetalol-treated patients, the standing diastolic blood pressure remained over 100 mm Hg. When hydrochlorothiazide was added to the treatment, six of the nine labetalol-treated patients responded with falls of 8 to 30 mm Hg and seven of the ten metoprolol-treated patients with falls of 6 to 32 mm Hg.

Antihypertensive Effect Rating
The antihypertensive effect ratings at the end of one week of treatment, at the end of titration, and at the end point of maintenance are presented in Table 4.

TABLE 4. ANTIHYPERTENSIVE EFFECT RATING* (NUMBER OF PATIENTS WITH SDBP <90 mm Hg AND PERCENT OF TOTAL GROUP POPULATION)

	Labetalol				Metroprolol			
	Good	Fair	Poor	Total	Good	Fair	Poor	Total
After 1 week of treatment	25 (12)	10 (3)	8 (0)	43 (15; 35%)	16 (9)	18 (1)	13 (1)	47 (11; 23%)
End of titration	33 (23)	4 (1)	7 (0)	44 (24; 55%)	26 (18)	13 (6)	8 (0)	47 (24; 51%)
End point of maintenance	25 (13)	3 (2)	10 (2)	38 (17; 45%)	21 (12)	9 (3)	8 (0)	38 (15; 39%)

After 1 week of treatment, significantly more labetalol-treated patients had a good response (i.e., SDBP ≥ 10 mm Hg) than metoprolol-treated patients; no significant treatment differences were seen at the end of titration or at the end point of maintenance. However, at the end of maintenance, 66 percent (25 out of 38) of the labetalol-treated patients had a fall of ≥ 10 mm Hg compared with 55 percent (21 of 38) of the metoprolol-treated patients.

Table 5 shows the number of patients whose blood pressure was considered ''controlled'' (SDBP < 90 mm Hg), regardless of the absolute fall in blood pressure. Overall, 45 percent of the labetalol-treated patients and 39 percent of the metoprolol-treated patients had their blood pressure controlled on monotherapy. These differences are also illustrated when the patients are stratified by the severity of hypertension. At the end point of maintenance, 62 percent of the mild hypertensives and 24 percent of the moderate hypertensives were controlled by labetalol compared to 54 and 8 percent, respectively, by metoprolol.

Moreover, Table 5 shows that 82 percent (14 of 17 patients) of the moderately hypertensive patients treated with labetalol had a ≥ 10 mm Hg reduction in their standing diastolic blood pressure compared to 58 percent (7 of 12) in the metoprolol group. The antihypertensive ratings for the 13 black patients enrolled in the study were generally poor for both treatments. Only one of five labetalol-treated black patients and two of eight metoprolol-treated black patients had a good effect (i.e., ≥ 10 mm Hg fall in SDBP).

Doses Used in the Study
The study protocol allowed an increase in the labetalol dose to a maximum of 1200 mg labetalol and to 400 mg of metoprolol daily. The actual

TABLE 5. ANTIHYPERTENSIVE RATING BY SEVERITY OF HYPERTENSION*
(NUMBER OF PATIENTS WITH SDBP <90 mm Hg AND PERCENT OF TOTAL
GROUP POPULATION).

	Labetalol				Metoprolol			
	Good	Fair	Poor	Total	Good	Fair	Poor	Total
Mild (SDBP 90–<105 mm Hg)	11 (9)	3 (2)	7 (2)	21 (13; 62%)	14 (11)	7 (3)	5 (0)	26 (14; 54%)
Moderate (SDBP ≥ 105–≤115 mm Hg)	14 (4)	0 (0)	3 (0)	17 (4; 24%)	7 (1)	2 (0)	3 (0)	12 (1/ 8%)

*Ratings are the same as Table 4.

prescribed doses and the number of patients taking each dose at the end of titration and the end point of maintenance are shown in Table 6.

From the end of titration to the end of maintenance, the daily dose was increased to maintain the efficacy in 9 patients in the labetalol group and 13 in the metoprolol group. A decrease of the dose in patients who achieved the therapeutic goal was not required by the protocol. Consequently, the average daily doses were somewhat higher at the end of the maintenance phase than at the end of the titration phase (Table 6).

The majority of the increases were to the highest dose (i.e., seven labetalol patients were increased from 800 to 1200 mg and eight metoprolol patients were increased from 300 to 400 mg). During the same period, the dose was reduced because of adverse experiences in five patients in the labetalol group and two in the metoprolol group.

In general, most of the moderate hypertensive patients received the highest dose while the doses required for the mild hypertensive patients were spread over the dose range. In mild hypertension, 52 percent of the labetalol patients and 54 percent of the metoprolol patients required the highest dose at the end of the maintenance period. This contrasts with the doses in moderate hypertension, where 75 percent of the labetalol group and 90 percent of the metoprolol group required the highest dose.

Postural Changes
There were small (1.3 to 2.7 mm Hg) and clinically insignificant postural falls in the mean systolic blood pressure of the labetalol-treated patients and no change in the metoprolol-treated patients during the study (Table 7). At the end of maintenance, there were more labetalol-treated pa-

TABLE 6. NUMBER OF PATIENTS WITH MILD (SDBP <105 mm Hg) AND MODERATE (SDBP ≥105 mm Hg) HYPERTENSION TAKING EACH DOSE OF LABETALOL AND METOPROLOL

		End Titration		End Maintenance	
	Daily Dose	Mild (N = 23)	Moderate (N = 21)	Mild (N = 21)	Moderate (N = 17)
Labetalol	400 mg	2 (9%)	0 (—)	2 (10%)	0 (—)
	600 mg	6 (26%)	1 (5%)	6 (28%)	1 (6%)
	800 mg	7 (30%)	4 (19%)	2 (10%)	3 (18%)
	1200 mg	8 (35%)	16 (76%)	11 (52%)	13 (76%)
Metoprolol		(N = 28)	(N = 17)	(N = 26)	(N = 12)
	100 mg	2 (7%)	0 (—)	3 (11%)	0 (—)
	200 mg	9 (32%)	0 (—)	2 (8%)	1 (8%)
	300 mg	10 (36%)	2 (15%)	7 (27%)	0 (—)
	400 mg	7 (25%)	15 (85%)	14 (54%)	11 (92%)

TABLE 7. THE SUPINE AND STANDING BP AND THE MEAN CHANGE FROM THE SUPINE TO STANDING POSITION FOR THE LABETALOL GROUP (L) AND THE METOPROLOL GROUP (M)

	Placebo Baseline			Active Treatment		
	Supine	Standing	Postural Change	Supine	Standing	Postural Change
End 1 week Rx						
Labetalol (*N* = 43)	148/97	150/104	+2.3/+7.2	141/90	140/95	−1.3/+5.0
Metoprolol (*N* = 47)	152/96	153/102	+1.0/+6.1	141/88	142/95	−0.9/+5.3
End titration						
Labetalol (*N* = 44)	148/97	150/104	+2.3/+7.2	137/88	135/91	−2.3/+3.4
Metoprolol (*N* = 47)	152/96	153/102	+1.0/+6.1	141/86	142/92	+0.9/+5.3
End Maintenance						
Labetalol (*N* = 38)	148/96	150/103	+2.4/+7.2	138/87	135/91	−2.1/+3.5
	150/95	152/102	+2.1/+6.9	137/86	138/91	+1.0/+5.5

tients with postural falls in the systolic pressure than with metoprolol (26 versus 15 patients). The normal physiologic increase in systolic and diastolic pressure was maintained by metoprolol and inhibited by labetalol. Nine patients had falls in standing diastolic pressure with labetalol compared to five with metoprolol. Only three of the nine labetalol-treated patients had a fall in diastolic BP $\geq$ 6 mm Hg at the end of maintenance.

Heart Rate

The mean heart rates of both treatment groups at each visit in the supine and standing positions are shown in Figure 3. The mean heart rate was reduced in both treatment groups in the supine and standing positions. Metoprolol, however, lowered the supine and standing heart rate significantly more than did labetalol ($p < 0.01$). The mean heart rate reductions after the first week of treatment, at the end of titration, and at the end of maintenance are shown in Table 2.

It is noteworthy that 19 of 38 metoprolol-treated patients had a fall in their standing heart rate of > 16 beats per minute whereas only 6 of 38 labetalol-treated patients had such falls.

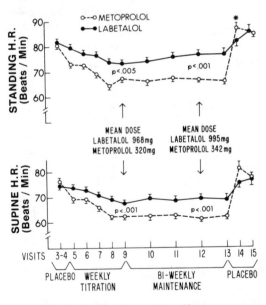

Figure 3. Standing and supine heart rate (HR) at rest, before, during, and after treatment with oral labetalol and metoprolol. Both drugs significantly reduced heart rate; however, metoprolol caused a greater reduction. Following treatment withdrawal, heart rate returned towards baseline after labetalol; following metoprolol there was a slight heart rate "overshoot" compared to baseline. Values are mean ± standard error of the mean; p = probability that the two treatments are different.

Six metroprolol-treated patients had symptomatic bradycardia (HR < 60 beats per minute in both the supine and standing positions), which precluded an increase in the metoprolol dose. There were no patients in the labetalol group who had dosage titrations limited by bradycardia. This difference between the two groups was statistically significant ($p < 0.05$).

There was no correlation between the falls in blood pressure and heart rate at the end of the maintenance phase in either group.

Adverse Experiences

Thirty-seven of 48 labetalol-treated patients and 35 of 49 metoprolol-treated patients reported at least one complaint during the double-blind portion of the study, as shown in Table 8. Twelve labetalol-treated patients and seven metoprolol-treated patients reported dizziness. This

TABLE 8. NUMBER OF PATIENTS WITH COMPLAINTS AT ANY TIME DURING THE STUDY (WITH THOSE RULED DRUG-RELATED ADVERSE EXPERIENCES BY THE INVESTIGATORS IN PARENTHESIS)

		Labetalol (N = 48)	Metoprolol (N = 49)
Complaints (drug related side effects)		37 (20)	35 (16)
Body as a whole:	Leg cramps	3 (0)	0 (0)
	Fatigue	14 (5)	15 (6)
	Headache	7 (1)	9 (1)
Cardiovascular:	Peripheral edema	2 (0)	3 (0)
Heart Rate:	Bradycardia	0 (0)	6 (6)
Central Nervous System:	Dizziness	12 (5)	7 (2)
Gastrointestinal system:	Diarrhea	2 (0)	5 (0)
	Dyspepsia	7 (4)	0 (0)
	Nausea	8 (3)	3 (1)
Musculoskeletal system:	Myalgia	3 (0)	0 (0)
Psychiatric disorders:	Paranoia	2 (1)	3 (1)
	Somnolence	3 (1)	4 (1)
Resistance mechanism:	Viral infection	3 (0)	1 (0)
Respiratory system:	Nasal stuffiness	3 (1)	0 (0)
	Dyspnea	3 (0)	2 (1)
Special senses:	Bitter pill after taste	5 (5)	0 (0)
Urinary System Disorder:	Micturition disorders	4 (0)	8 (0)

complaint was judged to be drug related in five (10 percent) labetalol- and two (4 percent) metoprolol-treated patients. In the labetalol group, dizziness was reported to be severe after the first dose in one patient who chose to discontinue, moderate in four patients and mild in seven. Dizziness generally occurred 30 minutes to 2 hours after a dose. Its association to postural blood pressure changes was not evaluated in most cases. The severity was usually mild, the effects transient, often not recurrent, and patients usually did not return for evaluation until 8 to 12 hours after dosing. However, associated orthostatic changes were confirmed in individual patients.

Seven patients in the labetalol group and none in the metoprolol group had dyspepsia ($p < 0.01$). Dyspepsia was reported at only one visit in four of these seven patients; this symptom disappeared when labetalol was taken with food. Eight labetalol-treated patients and four metoprolol-treated patients reported nausea. Two labetalol-treated patients reported changes in their normal dream pattern. One of these patients reported vivid, unpleasant dreams and the other reported nightmares. One labetalol patient reported ejaculatory failure and one labetalol and one metoprolol-treated patient reported impotence.

No clinical signs or symptoms of drug-induced lupus erythematosus were seen. No significant changes in the physical examinations were found at the end of the study.

Early Terminations From the Study. Seven labetalol-treated patients and five metoprolol-treated patients terminated the study early due to adverse experiences. Three of the seven labetalol-treated patients were terminated because of edema, two of whom had been treated with a diuretic prior to entry into the study. One patient developed exertional dyspnea and one had epigastric distress; the remaining two discontinued because of fatigue; one of these two had complained of dizziness and fatigue after the first dose. Two of the five metoprolol-treated patients were terminated because of sinus bradycardia, accompanied by sinus arrhythmia in one patient and syncope in the other; the third patient terminated because of severe nightmares and fatigue and a fourth for dyspnea, fatigue, and orthostatic dizziness; the fifth patient complained of grittiness in the eyes with photophobia and an occasional "halo" effect in his central vision together with a general lethargy.

Body Weight. There were no clinically significant increases in the mean body weights of the labetalol or metoprolol treatment groups. However, two patients in each group were reported to have weight gains of 3 to 6 pounds; and one patient from the labetalol group had 1+ ankle edema and lethargy in association with a six pound weight gain.

Electrocardiograms. There were no serious ECG abnormalities secondary to labetalol or metoprolol treatment other than the metoprolol induced sinus bradycardia detailed above.

Ophthalmologic Examination. There were no clinically significant changes attributable to labetalol or metoprolol on the ophthalmologic examination. The Keith–Wagener Grading of Retinopathy was essentially unchanged, with the exception of the following: one labetalol-treated patient improved from Grade II to 0, two changed from Grade 0 to I, and one from Grade 0 to II; five metoprolol-treated patients who had no retinopathy at baseline developed a Grade I narrowing at the end of maintenance and one deteriorated from Grade I to Grade II.
from Grade I to Grade II.

Laboratory Studies. Two metoprolol-treated patients had a transient decrease in their total white blood cell counts. No other clinically significant changes were seen in the complete blood counts. There were no clinically significant changes in urinalysis, blood glucose, BUN, or creatinine.

Six labetalol and two metoprolol-treated patients had elevations in their transaminase levels to greater than twice top normal at the end of the study. One additional metoprolol-treated patient had a transient greater than three times top normal elevation at the end of titration that returned toward normal at the end of the study. Of the six labetalol-treated patients, four had baseline transaminase levels above top normal but less than twice top normal. In none were there elevations in alkaline phosphatase or bilirubin and there were no clinical signs of drug-induced hepatitis. These elevations returned toward normal when repeat studies were done off therapy.

Plasma Lipids and Lipoproteins. The effects of labetalol and metoprolol on plasma triglycerides, cholesterol, and very low-density lipoprotein cholesterol, and of high-density lipoprotein-cholesterol are shown in Table 9. There were no effects of either drug or the addition of thiazide on plasma lipids and lipoprotein fractions except for a small but significant ($p < 0.01$) reduction in total cholesterol and low density lipoproteins in the metoprolol-treated group.

TABLE 9. COMPARATIVE EFFECTS OF LABETALOL AND METOPROLOL ON PLASMA LIPIDS

	Placebo (N = 35)	Labetalol (Maintenance Dose)	Placebo (N = 35)	Metoprolol (Maintenance Dose)
Lipid fraction				
Triglycerides (mg/dl)	135.7± 9.4	136.6± 8.2	156.7±14.1	174.3±12.4
Total cholesterol (mg/dl)	217.7± 6.2	217.8± 6.4	215.5± 6.1	201.3± 5.5*
Low-density lipoprotein cholesterol (mg/dl)	135.9± 6.3	136.8± 6.4	137.5± 5.3	128.1± 4.3*
High-density lipoprotein cholesterol (mg/dl)	48.2± 2.9	47.8± 2.5	46.7± 2.3	43.8± 1.8
High-density lipoprotein cholesterol				
Low-density lipoprotein-cholesterol	0.23±0.02	0.23±0.02	0.22±0.02	0.22±0.01

*Significant ($p<0.01$) change from placebo baseline and significantly different from labetalol ($p<0.01$).

Drug Withdrawal. Two to four days after the last tapered dose of the study medication (Visit 14) the mean blood pressure of both treatment groups rose towards the pretreatment levels and became significantly higher than at the end of the maintenance period ($p<0.005$). One week later (Visit 15), the systolic blood pressure returned to baseline levels but the standing diastolic blood pressure in both treatment groups was still somewhat lower than at baseline ($p<0.07$).

Two metoprolol-treated patients (but no labetalol-treated patients) were reported to have symptomatic "rebound hypertension" approximately 24 hours after discontinuation of treatment. The blood pressure of these patients rose 28/16 and 33/40 mm Hg, repectively, in the 24-hour period. This rapid rise exceeded their baseline by 7/5 and 10/20 mm Hg, respectively.

Two to four days after the last tapered dose, the mean heart rate rose to baseline levels in the labetalol-treated group, and exceeded ($p<0.03$) the baseline in the metoprolol-treated group (Table 10). The mean post treatment increase in heart rate from the end of the maintenance phase was significantly higher in the metoprolol-treated group.

TABLE 10. HEART RATES AT BASELINE COMPARED TO 2 TO 4 DAYS POSTTREATMENT

	Baseline	Posttreatment	Difference	Probable Difference
Supine				
Labetalol	75.1 ± 2.1	74.3 ± 2.3	−0.8 ± 1.6	NS
Metoprolol	75.4 ± 2.2	80.7 ± 2.7	5.3 ± 2.2	<0.03
Standing				
Labetalol	82.6 ± 2.1	81.2 ± 2.6	−1.4 ± 1.8	NS
Metoprolol	80.5 ± 2.0	86.1 ± 2.1	5.6 ± 1.7	<0.005

DISCUSSION

Effects on Hypertension

This double-blind comparison study shows that labetalol and metoprolol are effective and safe agents for the treatment of patients with mild-to-moderate systemic hypertension. The two drugs were, in general, equally effective in lowering the blood pressure, with labetalol exerting a somewhat greater effect on the standing blood pressure and metoprolol on the supine. That the β-blocker labetalol is more efficacious in lowering the standing than the supine blood pressure is consistent with its ancillary α-adrenergic blocking and direct vasodilatory actions, as well as with the findings of previous investigators.[18,19] It is noteworthy that the described effects were achieved with doses of labetalol of up to 1200 mg daily, which are less than the maximum daily doses of this drug currently used abroad (2400 mg).[20] Symptomatic postural hypotension was not a significant limiting factor in this study with either drug.

Approximately 40 percent of patients treated with either labetalol or metoprolol achieved the study's therapeutic goal of a standing diastolic blood pressure of less than 90 mm Hg that had also been decreased by ≥10 mm Hg. In the subgroup of patients with moderate hypertension,[24] percent responded to labetalol with decreases of standing diastolic blood pressure to less than 90 mm Hg compared to 8 percent after metoprolol treatment.

Both drugs reduced blood pressure upon initiation of treatment (metoprolol 100 mg daily, labetalol 200 mg daily). An augmentation of the antihypertensive effect of both drugs was seen in most patients with larger doses (metoprolol 200 to 400 mg/day, labetalol 600 to 1200 mg/day). The β-blocking potency of the labetalol doses used in this study was approximately equivalent to that of the metoprolol dose.[21] That the average daily doses of labetalol and metoprolol were slightly higher at the end of maintenance than after completion of titration, should be carefully interpreted. The protocol required increasing the dose if the effect was not maintained at any one visit but did not provide for a decrease of the dose if the effect was well maintained. Under these circumstances, the known variability in blood pressure and its measurement could be expected to cause a tendency towards the minimal dose increases observed.

Similar numbers of patients in this study required the addition of hydrochlorothiazide to their regimen of labetalol and metoprolol, resulting in additional effects in the two treatment groups. The antihypertensive ratings for the 13 black patients enrolled in the study were generally poor for both groups. Only one of five labetalol-treated black patients and two of eight metoprolol-treated black patients had a good monotherapy effect.

Mechanisms of Hypotensive Effect

The exact mechanism or mechanisms for the effects of labetalol in reducing blood pressure are not known. It has been suggested that labetalol reduces blood pressure predominantly by reducing peripheral vascular resistance while maintaining cardiac output.[12,13,22] This response is quite different from that usually seen with most β-adrenoceptor blocking drugs, both selective and nonselective, which result in a more delayed antihypertensive effect, a greater reduction in heart rate, a decrease in cardiac output, and a rise or no change in vascular resistance.[22,23]

It has been suggested that the renin–angiotensin system plays an important role in the antihypertensive mechanism of β-blocking agents.[24] The β-blocking agents in general lead to a decrease in both plasma renin activity and plasma aldosterone.[24,25] In contrast, vasodilating antihypertensive drugs induce a compensatory increase in plasma renin activity and a potent vasodilatory response can even result in secondary hyperaldosteronism with edema.[26,27] Although plasma renin activity was not measured in this study, our group demonstrated previously that labetalol has no demonstrable effects in hypertensive patients with low pretreatment levels of plasma renin.[9] However, in patients with high plasma renin activity, there is a dramatic reduction in this parameter with labetalol therapy.[9] This finding with labetalol contrasts sharply with the observations made with pure vasodilators,[26,27] suggesting that in its effect on plasma renin activity, labetalol is behaving like a pure β-adrenergic blocking agent. The effects of labetalol on plasma aldosterone are still not well defined.[28,29]

Heart Rate

Unlike pure α-adrenergic blocking drugs and vasodilators such as hydralazine, which tend to increase the resting heart rate in hypertensive patients, labetalol reduces blood pressure without increasing the heart rate.[8,9,22,30] In this study, labetalol slightly reduced the supine and standing resting heart rates without a postural difference. Metoprolol caused a much greater reduction in heart rate compared to labetalol at similar β-blocking and antihypertensive doses. In this study, treatment with metoprolol resulted in pronounced heart rate decrements with significant bradycardia in six patients, compared to no patients treated with labetalol. Bradycardia precluded increases of metoprolol to efficacious levels in these six patients.

Effects on Plasma Lipids

There are recent data that suggest that certain medications used to treat hypertension may affect plasma lipids.[15] Thiazides, chlorthalidone, and probable furosomide increase plasma triglycerides and total cholesterol.[15] However, there is probably no adverse effect on cholesterol lipoprotein fractions; the ratio between low-density lipoprotein cholesterol and high-density lipoprotein cholesterol is probably unchanged.[15] Prazosin, an α-adrenergic blocker has been associated with reductions in total cholesterol levels.[14,15] It appears that β-adrenoceptor blockade leads to an increase in plasma triglycerides but has little effect on total cholesterol.[15,31] Although there have been few studies examining lipoprotein fractions with beta blockade, evidence is accumulating that propranolol can reduce high-density lipoprotein cholesterol.[15,31] There is some concern that the observed lipid changes induced by diuretics and β-blockers may be detrimental in accelerating the arterosclerotic process.

In the present comparative study, neither metoprolol nor labetalol had potentially adverse effects on the levels of triglycerides, cholesterol, and lipoprotein fractions. The observed reduction in total cholesterol in patients receiving metoprolol was unexpected and was related entirely to a reduction in low-density lipoprotein cholesterol. Previous studies with metoprolol have shown increases in mean triglycerides ranging from 9 to 41 percent, but often without statistical significance.[15] However, ours is the first study to demonstrate a reduction in total cholesterol with metoprolol, and the reason for these differing findings is not obvious.

It is tempting to suggest that the reported differences between our observations with metoprolol and labetalol on lipids and those seen with propranolol are related to the pharmacologic differences between drugs. However, labetalol, like propranolol, is a nonselective β-blocker, and the high doses of metoprolol utilized in this study were consistent with nonselective β-blockade. Some of the variations in our results from those seen with other β-blockers may reflect different experimental conditions in relation to diet, levels of exertion, preexisting abnormalities of plasma glucose or lipids, and doses and duration of treatment. There is evidence that plasma lipid determinations are highly dependent on methodology. Further, there is considerable physiologic variability within subjects, which is most noted for triglycerides. A further unknown relates to the high-density lipoprotein-2 subfraction, as this appears to carry with it the vascular protective capacity of high-density lipoproteins.[32] This lipoprotein subfraction was not measured in our study.

Safety Parameters

The findings in the safety parameters are consistent with the pharmacologic profiles of the two drugs except for the clearly more frequent occurrence of gastrointestinal system symptoms (dyspepsia, nausea), and dizziness in the labetalol-treated patients. Bradycardia was more predominant in the metoprolol treatment group.

Withdrawal Effects

At the end of the study, the doses of both drugs were tapered over approximately 2 to 4 days. At the end of this period the blood pressures returned to the baseline levels in both treatment groups, but the heart rates in patients treated with metoprolol exceeded the baseline. In addition, two of the metoprolol-treated patients experienced a symptomatic rebound in their hypertension requiring treatment as compared to none of the patients who were treated with labetalol. This suggests a potential safety advantage of labetalol. In patients with hypertension and angina pectoris, we recently reported no adverse withdrawal effects after labetalol discontinuation.[9]

Clinical Implications

It appears from this study that both labetalol and metoprolol were safe and effective drugs for treating patients with mild-to-moderate hypertension. For comparable blood pressure–lowering effects, there was less bradycardia with labetalol. The combined α- and β-adrenergic blocking property of labetalol is a pharmacologic advance that provides a new conceptual approach for managing patients with hypertension.

REFERENCES

1. Frishman WH, Silverman R: Clinical pharmacology of the new beta adrenergic blocking drugs. Part 3. Comparative clinical experience and new therapeutic applications. Am Heart J 98:119, 1979.
2. Koch-Weser J: Metoprolol. N Engl J Med 301:698, 1979.
3. Frishman WH: β-Adrenoceptor antagonists: new drugs and new indications. N Engl J Med 305:500, 1981.
4. Apperley, GH, Daly MJ, Levy GP: Selectivity of β-adrenoceptor antagonists on bronchial, skeletal, vascular and cardiac muscle in the anaesthetised cat. Br J Pharmacol 57:235, 1976.
5. Frishman WH, Halprin S: Clinical pharmacology of the new beta-adrenergic blocking drugs. Part 7. New horizons in beta-adrenoceptor blockade therapy: labetalol. Am Heart J 98:660, 1979.
6. Richards DA, Tuckman J, Prichard BNC: Assessment of alpha and beta adrenoceptor blocking actions of labetalol. Br J Clin Pharmacol 3:849, 1976.
7. Dargie HJ, Dollery CT, Daniel J: Labetalol in resistant hypertension. Br J Clin Pharmacol 3 (Suppl 3):751, 1976.
8. Brogden RN, Heel RC, Speight TM, Avery G: Labetalol: A review of its pharmacology and therapeutic uses in hypertension. Drugs 15:251, 1978.
9. Frishman WH, Strom JA, Kirschner M, et al: Labetalol therapy in patients with systemic hypertension and angina pectoris: effects of combined alpha and beta adrenoceptor blockade. Am J Cardiol 48:917, 1981.
10. Prichard BNC, Richards DA: Comparison of labetalol with other antihypertensive drugs. Br J Clin Pharmacol 13 (Suppl 1):41s, 1982.
11. Waal-Manning HJ, Simpson FO: Review of long term treatment with labetalol. Br J Clin Pharmacol 13 (Suppl 1):65s, 1982.
12. Svendsen TL, Rasmussen S, Hartling OJ: Sequential hemodynamic effects of labetalol at rest and during exercise in essential hypertension. Postgrad Med 56 (Suppl 2):21, 1980.
13. Koch G: Hemodynamic changes after acute and long-term combined alpha-beta adrenoceptor blockade with labetalol as compared with beta-receptor blockade. J Cardiovasc Pharmacol 3 (Suppl 1):30s, 1981.
14. Leren P, Helgeland A, Holme I, et al: Effects of propranolol and prazosin on blood lipids. The Oslo Study. Lancet 2:4, 1980.
15. Johnson B: The emerging problem of plasma lipid changes during anti-hypertensive therapy. J Cardiovasc Pharmacol 4 (Suppl 2):213s, 1982.
16. Manual of Laboratory Operations, Lipid Research Clinics Program. Lipid and lipoprotein analysis. 1974 DHEW Publication No. (NIH) 75–628.
17. Gidez LI, Miller GJ, Burstein M, et al: Separation and quantitation of subclasses of human plasma high density lipoprotein by a simple precipitation procedure. J Lipid Res 23:1206, 1982.
18. Fagard R, Amery A, Reybrouch T, et al: Response of the systemic and pulmonary circulation to alpha- and beta-receptor blockade (labetalol) at rest and during exercise in hypertensive patients. Circulation 60:1214, 1979.

19. Prichard BNC, Boakes AJ: Labetalol in long-term treatment of hypertension. Br J Clin Pharmacol 3(Suppl 3):743, 1976.
20. Pugsley SJ, Armstrong BK, Nassim MA, Bellin LJ: Controlled comparison of labetalol and propranolol in the management of severe hypertension. Br J Clin Pharmacol 3 (Suppl 3):777, 1976.
21. Frishman WH: The beta-adrenoceptor blocking drugs. Int J Cardiol 2:165, 1982.
22. Mehta J, Cohn JN: Hemodynamic effects of labetalol, an alpha and beta adrenergic blocking agent in hypertensive subjects. Circulation 55:370, 1977.
23. Shinebourne E, Fleming J, Hamer J: Effects of beta-adrenergic blockade during exercise in hypertensive and ischemic heart disease. Lancet 2:1217, 1967.
24. Frishman WH, Silverman R: Clinical pharmacology of the new beta-adrenergic blocking drugs. Part 2. Physiologic and metabolic effects. Am Heart J 97:797, 1979.
25. Waal-Manning HJ: Hypertension: Which beta-blocker? Drugs 12:412, 1976.
26. O'Malley K, Velasco M, Wells J, McNay JL. Control of plasma renin activity and changes in sympathetic tone as determinants of minoxidil-induced increase in plasma renin activity. J Clin Invest 55:230, 1975.
27. Pohl JEF, Thurston H, Swales JD: The antidiuretic actions of diazoxide. Clin Sci 42:145, 1972.
28. Trust PM, Rosei EA, Brown JJ, et al: Effect of blood pressure, angiotensin II and aldosterone concentrations during treatment of severe hypertension with intravenous labetalol: comparison with propranolol. Br J Clin Pharmacol 3 (Suppl 3):799, 1976.
29. Kornerup HJ, Pederson EB, Christensen NJ, Pedersen A: Labetalol in the treatment of severe essential hypertension: relationship between arterial blood pressure, plasma catecholamines, plasma renin activity, plasma aldosterone and body weight. Acta Med Scand Suppl 625:59, 1978.
30. Edwards RC, Raftery EB: Haemodynamic effects of long-term oral labetalol. Br J Clin Pharmacol 3 (Suppl 3):733, 1976.
31. Shulman RS, Herbert PN, Capone RJ, et al: Effects of blood lipids and lipoproteins in myocardial infarction (Abstr). Circulation 67 (Suppl I):I-19, 1983.
32. Eder HA, Gidex LI: The clinical significance of the plasma high density lipoproteins. Med Clin N Amer 66:431, 1982.

CHAPTER 14

Multicenter Clinical Evaluation of the Long-Term Efficacy and Safety of Labetalol in the Treatment of Hypertension

Eric L. Michelson, William H. Frishman, James E. Lewis,
Winston T. Edwards, William J. Flanigan, Saul S. Bloomfield,
Brian F. Johnson, Charles Lucas, Edward D. Freis, Frank A. Finnerty,
Henry S. Sawin, and Marcia P. Poland

β-Adrenoceptor blocking agents are effective adjunctive antihypertensive agents in the majority of hypertensive patients and effective monotherapy in many patients, particularly younger, Caucasian, and often "hyperkinetic" hypertensives.[1] β-Blockers reduce both systolic and diastolic blood pressures at rest, supine, standing, with "stress," and with dynamic exertion.[1-3]

However, β-blockers are generally ineffective in reducing peripheral vascular resistance.[1] Presumably, an increase in peripheral vascular resistance is one of the primary pathophysiologic mediators of progressive hypertensive disease, thereby limiting the utility of β-blockers as monotherapy in many patients, and as adjunctive therapy in others. Conversely, vasodilators and particularly α-blockers are effective in reducing peripheral vascular resistance but have only limited clinical applicability as primary therapy because of their potential side effects, including reflex tachycardia and orthostatic hypotension.[1] For this reason the practice of combining β-blocker and vasodilator therapy has become more popular, particularly in patients with more moderate or severe hy-

Reprinted with modifications from the American Journal of Medicine 75; 68–80, October 17, 1983, with permission.

pertension, and this combination is often prescribed in conjunction with a diuretic.

Labetalol is a recently developed β-blocking agent with ancillary α-blocking properties,[1,3-9] and therefore has particularly intriguing therapeutic possibilities.[10,11] Labetalol is a competitive, nonselective antagonist of both β_2 and β_2 adrenoceptors, and administered orally has approximately one-fourth to one-sixth the β-blocking potency of propranolol.[3-8] Labetalol is also a competitive, selective antagonist of post synaptic α_1-receptors, with approximately one-sixth to one-tenth the potency of phentolamine.[3-8] In the usual range of clinical doses oral labetalol is 4 to 6 times more potent a β-blocker than α-blocker. In addition, labetalol may also have further vasodilating properties, possibly mediated via β_2-agonist activity.[9,12-14]

Pharmacologically,[3,7,8] labetalol is rapidly and well absorbed, undergoes "first-pass" hepatic metabolism and its inactive metabolites are cleared via both the kidneys and bile. Labetalol is only weakly lipophilic, has no significant intrinsic β_1-adrenoceptor mediated sympathomimetic activity, and has minimal membrane-stabilizing activity at the usual therapeutic dosages.[3,7,8,13]

Clinically, the efficacy of labetalol (both oral and intravenous forms) in treating hypertension has been demonstrated in several small series of selected patients,[3,15-18] the majority short-term in duration, and a few long-term studies.[19-22] Efficacy has been shown for mild, moderate, severe, and refractory hypertension, hypertensive crises, toxemia of pregnancy, renovascular hypertension, pheochromocytoma and for maintaining hypotension during halothane anesthesia.[15-22] In addition, evaluation of labetalol's antianginal,[3,11] antiarrhythmic,[23,24] and other potential therapeutic effects are areas of ongoing investigative interest.[25,26]

The present report details the findings of the largest United States experience to date with labetalol, a recently completed multicenter clinical evaluation of the long-term efficacy and safety of labetalol in the treatment of hypertension. Included were 337 patients treated with labetalol ($N = 193$) alone or in combination therapy ($N = 144$) for a mean of 9 ± 4 Standard Deviation (SD) months, 186 of whom were treated for at least 1 year.

METHODS

Study Design

This was a long-term (≥ 1 year) ten-clinic multicenter open-label study involving a total of 337 patients: 179 who had recently completed participation in one of three short-term (3 or 4 months) double-blind comparative studies (mild hypertension, $N=86$; mild to moderate hypertension, $N=52$; and moderate to moderately severe hypertension, $N=41$) as well as 158 new patients recruited to the open-label continuation of these three protocols. In addition to differences in the degree of hypertension, the three protocols also differed in the length of placebo baseline (1 to 4 weeks), the titration schedule and maximum allowable dose (600 mg twice daily for mild, 1200 mg twice daily for moderate and severe hypertension), and the inclusion of a "back-titration" option for mild and moderate hypertensives. Patient enrollment began July, 1980, and all three protocols were terminated by the study sponsors February 1982 in preparation for submission to the Food and Drug Administration to request drug approval. Patients were followed for a range of 1 to 20 (mean 9 ± 4 SD) months, with a median of 12 months. The study design is summarized in Figure 1.

All three protocols were conducted in four phases: Phase I: 1 to 4 weeks placebo baseline; Phase II: 1 to 5 weeks labetalol titration; Phase III: ≥48 weeks labetalol maintenance; and Phase IV: 1 week labetalol or placebo withdrawal. For patients just completing one of the double-blind labetalol protocols, the final placebo week of the previous study served as Phase I of the open-label trial.

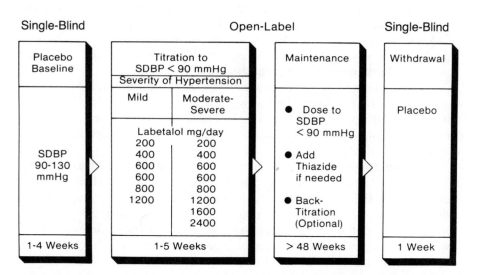

Figure 1. Summary of the study design. The study was conducted in four phases: single-blind placebo baseline, titration to achieve a standing diastolic blood pressure (SDBP) <90 mm Hg, long-term maintenance, and a single-blind placebo withdrawal period. See text for details.

For the purpose of this study the following definitions were used: mild hypertension—standing diastolic blood pressure (SDBP) of ≥ 90 to < 105 mm Hg; moderate hypertension—SDBP of ≥ 105 to <115 mm Hg; and moderately severe to severe hypertension—SDBP ≥ 115 mm Hg. By mutual agreement between investigator and sponsor selected patients with SDBP of up to 130 mm Hg were included. Routinely, blood pressure determinations were made by the same observer using the same arm by sphygmomanometry after 5 minutes in the supine position, times three, and after 2 minutes standing, times three, with the average blood pressure in each position recorded. Blood pressures were generally measured 8 to 12 hours postdose.

Labetalol dosage was titrated every 2 to 10 days to achieve a SDBP of <90 mm Hg. For patients with mild hypertension the titration schedule was twice daily administration of 100, 200, 300, 400, and 600 mg; for other patients two additional dosage levels were also included—800 and 1200 mg twice daily. Any time the SDBP reached <90 mm Hg patients were entered into the maintenance phase. If the maximum allowable labetalol dose failed to reduce SDBP to <90 mm Hg, hydrochlorothiazide (50 to 100 mg daily) could be added; it was recommended that concomitantly the labetalol dose be decreased from 600 to 400 mg twice daily in mild hypertensives and from 1200 to 600 mg twice daily in others to avoid excessive blood pressure reduction. The labetalol dose was subsequently increased and potassium supplementation given as indicated. In individual patients an alternative diuretic was used. In patients with moderate to severe hypertension not controlled with labetalol plus diuretic, a third agent (e.g., hydralazine) could be added.

During long-term maintenance (Phase III) patients received the dosage regimen taken during the last week of titration (Phase II). However, if their SDBP rose to ≥ 90 mm Hg, labetalol was titrated up to the maximal allowable dose, and a diuretic or third agent added as detailed above, as indicated.

At the termination of the maintenance phase, labetalol was abruptly discontinued and placebo was administered for 1 week (Phase IV) to evaluate for the occurrence of withdrawal signs and symptoms, and to determine whether the blood pressure returned to hypertensive levels. At the discretion of the investigator, individual patients, including some with a history of chest pain and/or significant electrocardiographic abnormalities, had their labetalol dose tapered or were placed directly on alternative active therapy.

At four of the ten centers, protocols (two mild, two mild to moderate) were amended to allow for back-titration of labetalol during Phase III. After at least 3 months of maintenance therapy, if the SDBP was

<90 mm Hg the labetalol dose was decreased weekly by one or two dosage levels, including placebo. If the SDBP rose to 90 mm Hg the dose of labetalol was again titrated upward to an effective level.

Evaluation of Efficacy

Supine and standing blood pressures were recorded at each study visit as detailed above. Visits were weekly during Phases I, II, and IV, at 1 month, and then every 3 months thereafter during Phase III. Changes from baseline in the systolic and diastolic blood pressures were analyzed at the last visit of the following treatment intervals: (1) 1 to <4 weeks, (2) 4 to <12 weeks, (3) 12 to <24 weeks, (4) 24 to <36 weeks, (5) 36 to <48 weeks, and (6) ≥48 weeks. For this analysis patients were further stratified into those receiving labetalol monotherapy and those receiving combination therapy at any time during the treatment period.

The changes from baseline in supine and standing blood pressures were also analyzed for each of the following subgroups: (1) males and females, 2) blacks and whites, (3) elderly (> 60 years of age) and younger patients, and (4) mild hypertensives and others.

The antihypertensive effects of labetalol were rated according to the extent of the fall in SDBP as follows: (1) good—a fall of ≥10 mm Hg; (2) fair—a fall of 5 to 9 mm Hg; or (3) poor—a fall of <5 mm Hg. In addition, at the last study visit each investigator provided a clinical judgment of the overall therapeutic effect of labetalol, with or without a concomitant diuretic, for each patient.

Evaluation of Safety

At the last placebo baseline visit the health status of each patient was assessed from a complete medical history, physical and ophthalmologic examinations, 12-lead electrocardiogram, and a battery of laboratory tests including blood chemistries (SMA 12 and 6), complete blood count with differential, and urinalysis. For patients completing a double-blind study with labetalol and who had a hiatus of less than 2 weeks, end-study determinations for the double-blind study were accepted as baseline for the open-label protocol.

Each patient's heart rate, body weight, and any reports of adverse experiences were recorded at each visit. Cardiopulmonary examinations, laboratory tests, and electrocardiograms were repeated at end-titration and every 3 months thereafter.

The number of patients reporting any complaint and the number reporting the most common complaints were tabulated across time (i.e., monthly for 6 months and then at 3-month intervals). To assess whether the most common complaints were dose related they were also tabulated by dose (i.e., the lowest dose at which the maximum severity of an adverse experience occurrred). If a symptom was considered possibly drug related at any visit, this determination was tabulated.

In reporting subjective adverse experiences patients were encouraged to report all symptoms, even if mild, but were only asked specifically about those symptoms reported spontaneously at that visit or the immediately previous visit. Attribution of a symptom to labetalol treatment was made for each complaint.

Patient Population

Inclusion and exclusion criteria: Adults of any race and of either sex between the ages of 18 (or consent) and 75 years with SDBP ≥90 after 1 week on placebo were eligible. Exclusion criteria included: secondary hypertension (including estrogen dependent), Grade III or IV retinopathy, guanethidine or rauwolfia agents taken within 2 weeks prior to study entry, cerebrovascular accident within 1 year or acute myocardial infarction within 6 months of entry, sinus bradycardia (≤50 beats per minute), congestive heart failure requiring therapy, angina pectoris requiring therapy, heart block greater than first degree, known hepatic (enzymes greater than twice top normal) or hematologic disease, serum creatinine >2.5 mg percent, diabetes mellitus requiring insulin, chronic obstructive pulmonary disease on therapy, bronchial asthma, seizure disorder, pregnancy or lactation, and a documented or suspected serious drug reaction or idiosyncrasy to β-blocking drugs in general or labetalol in particular. In addition, no other antihypertensive agents or potentially confounding drugs, such as imipramine, were allowed.

A total of 390 patients were recruited and enrolled for participation in this study; however, 53 patients were excluded for several reasons: SDBP too low ($N = 23$), SDBP too high ($N = 7$) consent withdrawn ($N = 9$), intercurrent medical problems ($N = 5$), or judged unreliable ($N = 9$).

A total of 337 patients received labetalol therapy. Three of these patients discontinued therapy prior to assessment of blood pressure, heart rate and body weight, so they were excluded from these analysis, but were included in the analysis of adverse experiences (reported by two of the three patients).

The demographic profile of the 337 patients is detailed in Table 1. The median age was 52 years and 70 (21 percent) patients were >60 years of age. There were 205 (59 percent) males, 219 (65 percent) Caucasians, 219 (65 percent) mild hypertensives, 85 (25 percent) moderate hypertensives and 33 (10 percent) moderately severe to severe hypertensives. A number of patients had concomitant diagnoses for which they took non-study medications. Most commonly used medications included aspirin,

TABLE 1. DEMOGRAPHIC PROFILE OF THE 337 LABETALOL-TREATED PATIENTS

Demographic Profile	Monotherapy (Labetalol Alone) n = 193	Combination Treatment (Labetalol ± Diuretic*) n = 144	Total n = 337
Age (Years)			
21–30	4	2	6
31–40	30	20	50
41–50	45	47	92
51–60	63	56	119
61–70	51	18	69
>70	0	1	1
Sex			
Male	116	89	205
Female	77	55	132
Color			
White	163	56	219
Black	30	88	118
Severity of Hypertension			
Mild (SDBP <105 mm Hg)	158	61	219
Moderate (SDBP 105 to < 115 mm Hg)	28	57	85
Severe (SDBP ≥115 mm Hg)	7	26	33
Duration of Hypertension (Years)			
Median	6	7.5	7
Range	< 1–40	<1–46	<1–46

*This includes 13 patients who received a third antihypertensive agent.
SDBP = Standing diastolic blood pressure

acetaminophen, nonsteroidal antiinflammatory agents, uricosuric agents, estrogens, thyroid replacement, and antiarrhythmics. Twenty-six (8 percent) patients had a history of diabetes mellitus and eight of these patients were receiving oral hypoglycemic drugs.

Statistical Methods

The data obtained by all investigators under the three protocols were pooled for this analysis. The changes from baseline to the end of monotherapy and to the end of the study (where appropriate) were analyzed using Student's t test for matched pairs. In addition, an analysis of variance was used. The model included four factors and their first-order interactions; second- and third-order interactions were not considered since the sample sizes in some of the cells were less than three. The four factors were color (black, white), sex (male, female), age ($\leq$ 60 years, >60 years), and baseline severity of hypertension (SDBP $\leq$

100, SDBP > 100). A standing diastolic BP (SDBP) of 100 mm Hg was chosen as the criteria for severity of hypertension since, for patients with baseline SDBPs >100, achieving the therapeutic goal was equivalent to having a good effect (i.e., 10 mm Hg reduction). The analysis was performed using the Type IV sum of squares from the GLM procedures in the Statistical Analysis System (SAS). The least-square means were associated with the probabilities determined from this analysis. However, the data presented in the text and tables represent the means of the raw, unadjusted data.

RESULTS

Of the 337 patients treated with labetalol, 186 (55 percent) completed at least 1 year of study participation (i.e., ≥48 weeks on labetalol) at the time of study discontinuation. Of the remainder, 54 (16 percent) patients were still on maintenance labetalol therapy, 32 (9.5 percent) terminated prematurely due to adverse experiences, 17 (5 percent) were found to be noncompliant (unreliable) or were lost to follow-up, 13 (4 percent) had unrelated personal reasons for discontinuation (e.g., moving, new employment), 11 (3 percent) were terminated for lack of efficacy, 18 (5 percent) had intercurrent medical problems, and 6 (2 percent) were normotensive on placebo after "back-titration."

Efficacy of Labetalol
Of the 337 patients, 329 were evaluable for efficacy on labetalol monotherapy; 3 were terminated before their first evaluation and 5 patients with severe hypertension were on diuretic therapy throughout the study. At the monotherapy end point (last visit on labetalol alone) the mean blood pressure of these 329 patients was 138/92 standing and 145/91 supine, a mean reduction from baseline of 13/10 and 5/7 mm Hg respectively, (each p <0.01). Similar reactions were seen in the 190 (58 percent) evaluable patients receiving labetalol monotherapy throughout the study: 13/11 standing and 6/7 mm Hg supine. At their last monotherapy visit, 137 (42 percent) patients were controlled at a SDBP <90 mm Hg and 172 (52 percent) were normotensive supine. In addition, 167 (51 percent) patients had ≥10 mm Hg reductions in SDBP and 122 (37 percent) ≥10 mm Hg reductions in supine diastolic blood pressure.

As detailed in Figure 2, in the 190 patients treated with labetalol alone throughout the study both the standing and supine blood pressures were lowered (p <0.01) within 4 weeks of treatment and this effect was maintained for the duration of therapy. Table 2 details both the mean

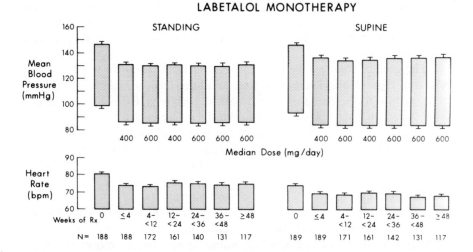

Figure 2. Effect of labetalol monotherapy on systolic and diastolic blood pressure and heart rate compared to placebo baseline for both supine and standing positions evaluated over time. The median daily dose of labetalol is also displayed, as well as the number *(N)* of patients included in each determination. As shown, labetalol's antihypertensive effects were evident within 4 weeks ($p < 0.01$) and efficacy was maintained thereafter ($p < 0.01$). Heart rate reductions were also maintained ($p < 0.01$). Data represent means ± the standard error of the mean; bpm, beats per minute; Rx, treatment.

TABLE 2. MEAN BLOOD PRESSURES AND MEAN REDUCTIONS FROM BASELINE AT EACH TIME INTERVAL FOR PATIENTS ON LONG-TERM LABETALOL MONOTHERAPY

Time Interval in Weeks	n*	Standing BP	Reduction†		n*	Supine BP	Reduction†
Baseline	188	148/99	—		190	147/93	—
<4	188	132/86	16/13		189	136/84	11/10
4 to <12	172	130/85	17/14		171	135/84	12/10
12 to <24	161	131/86	16/12		161	135/84	10/9
24 to <36	140	130/85	16/13		142	136/84	9/9
36 to <48	131	131/86	16/13		131	137/84	9/8
≥48	117	131/86	14/12		117	138/84	6/8
End point‡	187	135/88	13/11		190	141/86	6/7

*The sample sizes *(n)* differ because of early terminations and because not all patients had a visit during each time interval. The baseline blood pressure (BP) at the various time intervals varied with sample size by approximately 2 mm Hg.

†BP reductions were significant ($p<0.01$) at each time interval.

‡The last visit for all patients who received labetalol regardless of how many weeks they were treated

blood pressures and the mean reductions from baseline; it is further evident that the mean reductions in standing blood pressures on labetalol monotherapy were somewhat greater than supine blood pressure reductions.

The goal of therapy was to reduce the SDBP to normotensive levels (<90 mm Hg). Of the 190 patients treated long-term with labetalol monotherapy, 116 (62 percent) were maintained with a SDBP <90 mm Hg and 131 (69 percent) with a supine diastolic blood pressure <90 mm Hg. In addition, 102 (54 percent) of these 190 patients maintained a ≥10 mm Hg reduction in SDBP and 95 (50 percent) patients maintained a ≥10 mm Hg reduction in supine diastolic blood pressure.

Combination Therapy

The addition of a diuretic was required in 144 (43 percent) patients, including 13 (4 percent) patients also requiring a third agent (usually hydralazine). In these 144 patients the standing and supine blood pressures were 142/98 and 151/97 at the monotherapy end point, representing reductions from baseline of 12/10 and 3/6 mm Hg, respectively. As shown in Figure 3, labetalol in combination therapy lowered both the supine

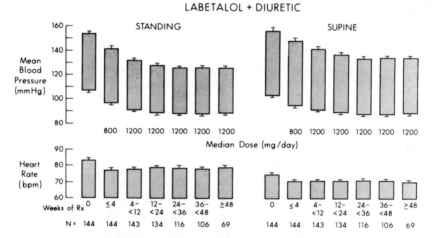

Figure 3. Effect of combination therapy with labetalol plus diuretic (plus a third agent, usually hydralazine, in 13 patients) on systolic and diastolic blood pressure and heart rate compared to placebo baseline for both supine and standing positions evaluated over time. The median daily dose of labetalol (mg) is also displayed, as well as the number (N) of patients included in each determination. As shown, the antihypertensive effects of combination therapy were evident within 4 to 12 weeks of titration (p <0.01) and efficacy was maintained thereafter (p <0.01). Heart rate reductions were also maintained (p <0.01). Data represent mean ± the standard error of the mean; bpm, beats per minute; Rx, treatment.

and standing blood pressures (p <0.01); after an initial 4- to 12-week titration period these reductions were maintained for the duration of therapy. At end study mean reductions were 25/16 mm Hg standing and 18/13 mm Hg supine, and blood pressures were 130/91 and 138/90 mm Hg respectively. Table 3 details both the mean blood pressures and the mean reductions from baseline on combination therapy. These reductions were somewhat greater (p <0.001) than for labetalol monotherapy but also required a higher daily labetalol dose (median 1200 versus 600 mg).

The goal for combination therapy was a SDBP <90 mm Hg. Of the 144 patients, 74 (51 percent) had a SDBP <90 mm Hg on therapy. Similary, 68 (47 percent) patients had their supine diastolic blood pressure controlled at <90 mm Hg. In addition, of the 144 patients, 104 (72 percent) had a ≥10 mm Hg reduction in SDBP and 85 (59 percent) patients had a ≥10 mm Hg reduction in supine diastolic blood pressure.

Patients Completing 1 Year of Therapy
One hundred eighty-six patients were treated for 1 year or longer, including 117 (63 percent) patients on labetalol alone. As shown in Figure 2 and Table 2, both supine and standing blood pressures were reduced after approximately 4 weeks of therapy (p <0.01) and this reduction was maintained thereafter; the reduction in standing blood pressure was somewhat greater than the reduction in supine blood pressure.

TABLE 3. MEAN BLOOD PRESSURES AND MEAN REDUCTION FROM BASELINE AT EACH TIME INTERVAL ON COMBINATION THERAPY

Time Interval in Weeks	n^*	Standing		n^*	Supine	
		BP	Reduction†		BP	Reduction‡
Baseline	144	155/107	—	144	156/103	—
< 4	144	142/ 97	12/11	144	148/ 95	8/ 8
4 to <12	143	132/ 91	23/16	143	142/ 91	14/11
12 to <24	134	128/ 89	27/18	134	137/ 89	19/14
24 to <36	116	126/ 88	29/19	116	133/ 87	22/15
36 to <48	106	126/ 87	30/20	106	134/ 87	23/16
≥48	69	126/ 88	28/19	69	133/ 88	21/16
End point‡	144	130/ 91	25/16	144	138/ 90	18/13

*The sample sizes (n) differ at each time interval because not all patients had a visit during each time interval as well as the fact that there were early terminations. The baseline blood pressure at the various time intervals varied with sample size by approximately 3 mmHg.
†Blood pressure (BP) reduction was significant (p <0.01) at each time interval.
‡The last visit for all patients who received labetalol regardless of how many weeks they were treated.

Similar results were observed for the 69 patients treated with combination therapy for 1 year or longer. The effect achieved after the addition of diuretic was maintained for the duration of therapy, and both supine and standing blood pressures were significantly reduced from baseline (p <0.01). Moreover, at the end of 1 year, the mean blood pressure reductions for combination therapy were 28/19 mm Hg standing and 21/16 mm Hg supine, compared to 14/12 mm Hg standing and 6/8 mm Hg supine in the monotherapy patients, although final blood pressures in both groups were comparable: 131/86 on monotherapy versus 126/88 on combination therapy standing, and 138/84 on monotherapy versus 133/88 mm Hg on combination therapy supine.

A number of demographic differences were evident in the requirement for the addition of a diuretic to labetalol. Diuretic therapy was required in only 19/70 (27 percent) elderly versus 123/265 (46 percent) younger patients (p <0.01), 56/219 (26 percent) Caucasians versus 88/118 (75 percent) Blacks (p <0.01), 43 percent of men versus 42 percent of women (p = not significant) and 61/219 (28 percent) mild hypertensive versus 83/118 (70 percent) of moderate and severe hypertensives (p <0.01). However, it appeared that racial differences in the need for diuretic reflected instead the severity of baseline hypertension. For example, 93/114 (82 percent) of Black patients had baseline diastolic blood pressures >100 mm Hg versus 86/215 (40 percent) of Caucasians. In comparison, elderly patients responded to monotherapy more often than younger patients (p = 0.05) even after accounting for differences in baseline blood pressures. In addition, as shown in Figures 2 and 3, patients requiring diuretic also required a larger median daily dose of labetalol than patients receiving monotherapy (1200 mg versus 600 mg, respectively).

Rating of Antihypertensive Effect
Overall, 206 (62 percent) of the 331 patients evaluated had a good response (≥10 mm Hg reduction in SDBP) and 184 (56 percent) of patients had a SDBP <90 mm Hg at end study. In addition, 61 percent of mild and 46 percent of moderate and severe hypertensives were normotensive (SDBP <90 mm Hg) at the end of the study. One hundred eighty-six patients were treated for 1 year or longer including 117 (63 percent) on labetalol alone. Overall, 128/186 (69 percent) patients had a good response and 121 patients (65 percent) were normotensive at the end of the study.

A total of 323 patients were evaluated by the investigators for overall clinical efficacy, taking into consideration baseline blood pressure, level of reduction, and blood pressure on therapy, not only at the end-visit, but also for the general level of control during maintenance. Of 180 ⁻ patients evaluated on labetalol monotherapy 136 (76 percent) were judged to have either a good or excellent response (i.e., ≥10 mm Hg reduction in SDBP and/ or SDBP <90 mm Hg on therapy), and similarly, 106/143 (76 percent) patients on combination therapy were judged to have a good or excellent response. Overall, the median monotherapy labetalol dose acquired to achieve a SDBP <90 mm Hg was 600 mg, with 59 percent of patients requiring 400 to 800 mg daily and only 20 percent able to be controlled with 200 mg daily. In comparison, for patients not adequately controlled with labetalol alone, the median daily dose of labetalol required for control in combination with a diuretic was 1200 mg.

Back-Titration
Back-titration of labetalol by one or two dose levels was attempted in 81 patients with SDBP controlled at <90 mm Hg for at least 3 months; 8 had moderate and 73 mild hypertension. In 25/81 (31 percent) patients back-titration was accomplished successfully with the SDBP maintained at <90 mm Hg on a reduced dose for the remainder of the study. Seven (9 percent) patients were back-titrated successfully to placebo, but the need for continued active antihypertensive therapy was confirmed in the remaining 91 percent of patients evaluated in this way.

Safety and Tolerance of Labetalol
Overall, 56 (16.6 percent) of 337 patients terminated the study prematurely due to either adverse experiences (32 patients, 9.5 percent) or intercurrent medical problems (24 patients, 7.1 percent). The most common reason for early termination was genitourinary symptoms in men (17/205; 8.3 percent); this included ejaculation failure in 9 (4.3 percent) men, impotence in 5 (2.4 percent), and decreased libido in 1 (<0.5 percent) man. Difficulty with and/or frequency of voiding was the sole complaint in 2 (1 percent) men and occurred in concert with sexual dysfunction in 2 (1 percent) others. Gastrointestinal disorders were the next most frequent reason for termination, in 12 (5 percent) patients, including dyspepsia and nausea, and 5 (2.4 percent) patients with asymptomatic abnormal hepatic enzymes, as further detailed below. Ten patients were terminated from the study when cardiovascular events occurred, including intercurrent myocardial infarctions in 3 (1.5 percent), chest pain syndromes in 2 (1 percent), and transient ischemic attacks in 2 (1 percent), including one patient referred for carotid endarterectomy and one patient with an incipient cerebrovascular accident. An additional patient had syncope, in part attributed to severe dietary restriction. Five (2.4 percent) patients were terminated for rash or pruritus, and one pa-

tient for a lichen planus eruption after 9 months on 2400 mg labetalol daily. Two weeks after labetalol was discontinued the lesions faded.

Other reasons for early termination included fatigue or weakness in 5 (2.4 percent) patients and miscellaneous causes in 6 (2.9 percent) patients, including nasal stuffiness and headache. There were no differences in early termination related to age, sex or race.

In total, 254 of 331 (77 percent) patients complained of at least one symptom during treatment with labetalol alone and 108 of 144 (75 percent) patients while on combination therapy. Table 4 details those complaints reported by at least 5 percent of the total population. Six complaints were reported by ≥10 percent of patients: dizziness, headache, fatigue, nausea, nasal stuffiness, and male sexual dysfunction (including ejaculation failure, impotence, and/or decreased libido). Except for sexual dysfunction, the majority of these complaints were reported at only a single visit, and only infrequently were symptoms persistent (e.g., nasal stuffiness) or recurrent, and usually in only a small number of patients. In general, symptoms were reported more frequently at the earlier study visits, and more frequently on labetalol dosages greater than 800 mg daily. As detailed previously, these symptoms were only infrequently more than mild, were each ruled unrelated to study medication in many instances by the investigators, and each led to early termination in only a few cases (<5). Overall, symptoms were reported with comparable frequency by patients on monotherapy and combination therapy; for this reason Table 4 details only the summary of complaints.

Other clinically significant adverse experiences included hypotension and postural hypotension. Twelve (4 percent) patients had symptomatic, exaggerated blood pressure reductions and 16 others had asymptomatic systolic blood pressure reductions to <100 mm Hg; typically, hypotension occurred at only one visit, and occasionally two visits. Chest pain was reported at least (and usually only) once by 19 (6 percent) patients and in no case was attributed directly to labetalol therapy; underlying ischemic heart disease was documented in several patients. One side effect, mild and occasionally moderate tingling of the scalp, and less frequently over the extremities or trunk (formication), appeared peculiar to labetalol. Another patient complained of vague muscoloskeletal discomfort during the study and had an associated ANA titer positive 1:80. Similar complaints had been present prestudy as well as at least one positive ANA; after a negative "collagen-vascular" work-up, labetalol was restarted and continued for 11 months without adverse experiences. No other patients developed symptoms or signs to suggest a collagen-vascular syndrome.

TABLE 4. COMPLAINTS REPORTED BY AT LEAST 5 PERCENT OF THE TOTAL 337 PATIENTS, WITH THE NUMBER (AND PROPORTION) OF TREATED PATIENTS WITH EACH SYMPTOM PRESENTED

Symptom	Reported/Judged Related	Reason For Early Termination*
General		
Asthenia	18(5%)/ 9(3%)	2(<1%)
Chest pain	20(6%)/ 1(<1%)	1(<1%)
Edema	22(6%)/ 6(2%)	0
Fatigue	74(22%)/46(14%)	3(<1%)
Headache	86(26%)/14(4%)	1(<1%)
Weight increase	18(5%)/ 4(1%)	0
Autonomic nervous system		
Dry mouth	17(5%)/14(4%)	1(<1%)
Increased sweating	16(5%)/ 2(<1%)	0
Central and peripheral nervous system		
Dizziness	99(29%)/42(12%)	2(<1%)
Scalp tingling†	32(9%)/22(6%)	2(<1%)
(Formication)†		
Gastrointestinal		
Abdominal pain	18(5%)/ 3(< 196)	0
Diarrhea	28(8%)/ 8(2%)	0
Dyspepsia	30(9%)/14(4%)	1(<1%)
Flatulence	16(5%)/12(3%)	0
Nausea	65(19%)/36(11%)	5(2%)
Vomiting	18(5%)/ 6(2%)	2(<1%)
Genitourinary		
Sexual dysfunction	38(19%)‡129(14%)‡	15(7%)‡
Respiratory system		
Dyspnea	22(7%)/ 6(2%)	0
Nasal stuffiness	45(13%)/26(8%)	2(<1%)
Special Senses		
Bitter aftertaste	18(5%)/17(5%)	0

*Not mutually exclusive.
‡Percentage calculated on total of 205 male patients.

†Twenty-three of the 32 reported tingling and/or itching of the scalp.

Other Effects. A small (<7 beats per minute, *p* <0.01) decrease in both supine and standing heart rates occurred initially and persisted for the duration of therapy, but the normal physiologic increase in heart rate observed upon arising from the supine to standing position was maintained
at 7 beats per minute on labetalol, compared to 8 beats per minute at
baseline. Twenty-two (7 percent) of the patients had a supine heart rate
≤50 per minute observed at least (and usually only) once during the
study, but only 2 (<1 percent) patients had labetalol-induced bradycardia
not present at baseline. Other than these changes in heart rate, and the
previously detailed unrelated, intercurrent ischemic episodes in isolated
patients, electrocardiographic changes were limited to sporadic observations of premature ventricular beats in nine patients, transient right
bundle branch block in two patients, and mild QT prolongation in two
patients. Drug relation was not demonstrated in any of these cases.
Also, as noted previously, many patients used nonstudy medications
concomitantly, at times during the study, including nonsteroidal antiinflammatory drugs. However, there was no apparent evidence of adverse
drug interactions with the study medications or effect on antihypertensive efficacy.

Physical Examinations

There were no pathologic changes in either physical, cardiopulmonary,
or ophthalmologic examinations attributable to drug therapy. No patients manifested new or worsened bronchospasm. Seventeen patients
had borderline abnormal intraocular pressures (20 to 25 mm Hg) at baseline, and in all cases a 2 to 6 mm Hg decrease was observed at the 6 or
12 month follow-up visit.

Laboratory

Blood Counts. A mild asymptomatic leukopenia was observed in nine
patients; seven were black males, and five were on diuretics; isolated
transient values were as low as 2300 and 2600, with associated mild neu-
tropenia. These resolved spontaneously on continued therapy in one patient and were not considered drug related, and were only observed at
end study in the others. There were no associated changes in either
hemoglobin or platelet counts.

Urinalyses. On isolated occasions 16 (5 percent) patients had 1+ to 2+
proteinuria (by "dipstick") with no concomitant changes in renal function and otherwise benign urinalyses, and in no case considered to be
drug related or clinically significant.

Blood Chemistries. Clinically significant creatinine level elevations with and without BUN changes were seen in 13 patients; 8 were also receiving a diuretic. There were no clinically significant changes in serum glucose, total protein, cholesterol, or triglyceride levels. With the exception of diuretic-induced hypokalemia and hyperuricemia in some patients, there were no clinically significant changes attributable to labetalol.

Asymptomatic transient elevations of liver transaminase (SGOT and/or SGPT) levels to twice top normal or greater were seen in 17 (5 percent) of 320 patients evaluated, including 13 (4 percent) patients with levels above twice top normal limits and 8 (3 percent) of these with levels in excess of three times top normal limits. All abnormalities reverted to normal on continued labetalol therapy, although four patients had their labetalol dose decreased for other reasons. In one patient transaminase levels became elevated and then normalized in association with starting and stopping hydralazine. Several of these patients were known to use alcohol, and some at least sporadically to excess.

In addition 22 (7 percent) patients had asymptomatic transminase elevations at their end study determinations, including 5 patients for which this was the reason for their study termination. In 8 of the 22 patients elevations were less than or equal to twice normal and in 14 (4 percent), elevations were greater than twice normal [including 7 (2 percent) patients greater than three times normal]. In all patients in which this was evaluated, gamma glutamyl transpeptidase (GGT) levels were similarly increased. In none of the total of 27 (8 percent) patients with transaminase levels increased to greater than twice normal either during (13 patients) or at end study (14 patients) was there an associated bilirubin increase, and in only one patient was there a concomitant transient elevation in alkaline phosphatase elevation.

Transaminase elevations were always asymptomatic, occurred on doses ranging from 200 to 2400 mg daily, after durations of therapy ranging from 38 to 411 days, in patients with both normal and borderline elevated baseline transaminase levels, patients known to use alcohol and those abstaining, and in each case these changes resolved spontaneously over periods ranging from 1 week to 6 months. In a total of five patients labetalol therapy was discontinued because of transaminase elevations. Levels were increased 10 to 15 times normal in three of these patients. Of the five patients discontinued, three were rechallenged; in each case mild to moderate transaminase elevations recurred weeks thereafter, which again resolved off labetalol therapy.

Of note, there were 42 patients with borderline elevated hepatic enzyme levels at baseline (less than twice top normal). In only 7 (17 percent) of these patients transaminase values rose to greater than twice normal during labetalol therapy.

Post-treatment Effects

Labetalol was abruptly discontinued in 223 patients and placebo administered for 1 week. The mean supine and standing systolic and diastolic blood pressures and heart rates after 1 week of placebo were significantly higher (p <0.01) than at the end of labetalol therapy. The mean supine and standing diastolic blood pressures, standing systolic blood pressure, and supine heart rate at the end of the post-treatment placebo week were not different (p >0.10) than placebo baseline values; mean supine systolic blood pressure and standing heart rate were increased minimally (by 2 mm Hg and 2 beats per minute), respectively; p <0.05) compared to baseline.

One week after abrupt discontinuation of labetalol the mean standing blood pressure rose by an average of 19/13 mm Hg and supine blood pressure by 15/10 mm Hg. There were 16 patients whose SDBP rose by 10 to <15 mm Hg above baseline, 10 patients by 15 to <20 mm Hg and one patient by 20 mm Hg above baseline.

There was a mean rise in heart rate of 7 beats per minute in the standing position and 6 beats per minute in the supine position comparing the end of labetalol therapy to placebo 1 week later. Nine patients had an increase of ≥ 20 beats per minute in the supine position and 32 patients in the standing position, including 6 patients with increases in both positions. In addition, in 17 (8 percent) of 223 patients evaluated, the post-treatment placebo heart rate was also ≥20 beats per minute higher than the placebo baseline.

Post-treatment Adverse Experiences

Fifty-four (24 percent) of 223 patients in whom therapy was abruptly discontinued reported at least one symptom, most frequently headache (15 patients; 7 percent), persistent nasal stuffiness (8 patients; 4 percent) and fatigue (6 patients, 3 percent). In one extremely obese, chronically edematous female both labetalol and diuretic were abruptly discontinued, and she suffered pulmonary edema 1 week later. Two patients had chest pain, including one patient who also had chest pain while on labetalol therapy; and the other had prolonged and recurrent chest pain associated with a rapid rise in blood pressure from normal to severe levels, slightly higher than baseline.

DISCUSSION

Efficacy of Labetalol

The results of this long-term open label multicenter trial indicate that labetalol alone and in combination with a diuretic is an effective, safe, and generally well-tolerated antihypertensive agent. The study included 337 patients with predominately mild and moderate hypertension, and included both young and elderly (>60 years of age) patients, males and females, whites and blacks. Many patients had previously been intolerant or inadequately controlled on conventional antihypertensive therapy. Efficacy was usually evident within 4 weeks of gradual upward titration of labetalol monotherapy (median dose 300 mg twice daily) or within 4 to 12 weeks of labetalol (median dose 600 mg twice daily) in combination with diuretic.

Labetalol was equally effective in both males and females, but elderly patients required a diuretic somewhat less often than younger patients. Patients with moderate to severe hypertension required a diuretic more often than mild hypertensives to achieve a SDBP <90 mm Hg. Racial differences in the need for diuretic (more often in blacks) were accounted for by differences in baseline blood pressures (also greater in blacks).

These findings demonstrating the potential efficacy of labetalol for a broad spectrum of hypertensive patients confirms the findings of several previous studies, the majority relatively short-term in duration and involving fewer patients.[14–21] Importantly, in the present study, efficacy evident at the end of titration was maintained for the duration of long-term labetalol therapy. In addition, labetalol was effective monotherapy in several patients not adequately controlled previously with other β-blockers devoid of α-blocking and vasodilating properties. Moreover, in patients not responding adequately to labetalol monotherapy, the combination of labetalol and a diuretic was particularly effective, especially for more moderately severe and severe hypertensives, several of whom were poorly controlled on conventional multidrug regimens.

To further demonstrate that blood pressure reductions maintained over time were due to efficacy of the therapeutic regimen rather than regression to the mean, 81 patients with predominantly mild hypertension had their labetalol dose back-titrated by a maximum of two dosage levels; in 73 (91 percent) patients the need for continued antihypertensive therapy was documented. Undoubtedly, had more of the moderately or severely hypertensive patients been back-titrated this percentage would have been smaller; conversely, if dosages had been reduced by more than two levels, the percentage may have been higher. In addition we noted that several patients with long-standing, confirmed hypertension enrolled in the double-blind short-term labetalol protocols remained normotensive for at least several months following discontinuation of labetalol therapy, precluding their enrollment in the open-label study. This suggests that additional salutary treatment-related mechanisms may facilitate back-titration.[27]

Safety and Tolerance of Labetalol

Overall, 254 (77 percent) of 331 evaluable patients complained of at least one symptom potentially attributable to drug while on labetalol alone and 108/144 (75 percent) patients while on combination therapy. Complaints were more common early in the study, and less frequent over time. Most of these were mild in severity, transient, reported only once or sporadically, and only occasionally required dosage changes. In addition, many of the side effects reflected the known pharmacology of labetalol: a combination of β-blocking, selective α-blocking, plus possible additional vasodilating properties.[3,5–8,10] Labetalol is also only weakly lipophilic and is devoid of significant intrinsic β₁-receptor mediated sympathomimetic activity at the dosages used in this study.

Notably, although labetalol is a relatively nonselective β-blocker, several side effects reported to be more common with other nonselective β-blockers and those devoid of intrinsic sympathomimetic activity were seen only rarely or not at all in this study; these included: sinus bradycardia (< 1 percent), heart block, bronchospasm, Raynaud's phenomonon, cold extremities or peripheral vascular complaints, increases in cholesterol or triglyceride levels, exacerbation of diabetes or hypoglycemic complications, precipitation of heart failure, or exertional dyspnea (< 1 percent). In general, fluid retention was not a problem, even with labetalol monotherapy, although in individual patients (<2 percent) edema was noted. In addition, sleep disorders, nightmares and depression were also reported only rarely.

Several complaints were reported relatively frequently during the study, and six symptoms were each reported by at least 10 percent of patients: dizziness, headache, fatigue, nausea, nasal stuffiness, and male sexual dysfunction. To put these numbers in perspective, several similar complaints were reported in the recently completed Beta-Blocker Heart Attack Trial[28] with the following frequencies by patients on propranolol: faintness 29 percent, blacking-out 9 percent, and tiredness 67 percent; and similarly by patients on placebo: 27 percent, 10 percent and 62 percent, respectively. In a recent report of the British Medical Research Council Working Party on Mild to Moderate Hypertension,[29] several symptoms were also reported by at least 10 percent of patients on placebo including dizziness, muscle pain, exertional dyspnea, headaches, cold extremities, paresthesias, dry mouth, blocked or running nose, and impotence, although each of these lead to study discontinuation only infrequently. These previous studies as well as the present data indicate that symptoms are reported frequently by carefully monitored cardiovascular and hypertensive patients, many of which occur with comparable frequency on placebo and β-blocker therapy.

Specific symptoms require further comment. It should be emphasized that labetalol is a potent antihypertensive agent with both α- and β-blocking and possible vasodilating properties, and is capable of rapidly reducing the blood pressure, and to a more marked extent than conventional β-blockers. Therefore, it is important to initiate therapy with low doses, titrate upward slowly, and decrease the dosage when adding a diuretic. This will help to avoid excessive blood pressure reductions, and, potentially, transient orthostatic hypotension, with attendant dizziness and lightheadedness. For these same reasons, labetalol should be used more cautiously in patients suspected of compliance problems.

Headache was a relatively frequent (26 percent), nonspecific complaint but was only occasionally (4 percent) considered drug related. When drug related, the headache often resembled either a vascular or sinus headache, and was often prefrontal or supraorbital, and usually subsided with continued dosing. Presumably this symptom was related to vasodilation.

Nausea was also reported relatively frequently (19 percent; 11 percent drug related) on labetalol. This was also a dose-related phenomenon, the etiology of which has not been elucidated; the bitter aftertaste of labetalol may be contributory, as well as the effects of α- plus β-blockade on gastrointestinal motility. Nasal stuffiness was seen in 13 percent of patients (8 percent related) on labetalol. This was also a dose-related symptom, and was presumably related to labetalol's α-blocking–vasodilating properties.

Some of the more common, bothersome complaints were related to male genitourinary dysfunction, including ejaculation failure, retrograde ejaculation, impotence, decreased libido, and micturition difficulties. Occasional patients were symptomatic even at the lowest dosages, and symptoms were sufficiently bothersome to result in early discontinuation in 15 (7 percent) males. Labetalol-related changes in ejaculation and voiding function were possibly related in part to α-blockade, possibly in conjunction with β-blockade, although the mechanisms have not yet been fully elucidated. In comparison, 43 percent of all patients complained of reduced sexual activity on propranolol and 42 percent on placebo in the Beta-Blocker Heart Attack Trial.[28] Moreover, in at least one series of untreated hypertensives, 17 percent reported impotence, compared to 7 percent of normal men.[30] Bulpitt et al. also reported that 32 percent of men treated with a diuretic developed impotence and 14 percent had ejaculation failure.[31] In the Medical Research Council Report,[29] after 2 years of therapy, impotence was reported by 23 percent of men on thiazide diuretic and 13 percent on propranolol, compared to 10 percent on placebo, and lead to early discontinuation of therapy in 19, 5, and 1 male patient per 1000 patient years, respectively.

Finally, increases in hepatic enzyme levels (SGOT and/or SGPT, plus GGT levels) were also seen relatively frequently with labetalol. A total of 27 (8 percent) of patients developed reversible, asymptomatic transaminanse elevations to greater than twice normal noted either during or at end study. However, in half (13; 4 percent) of these patients liver test alterations resolved on continued therapy. Elevations persisted and were presumably drug related in 14 (4 percent) patients, including 5 (2 percent) patients whose marked elevations (3 to 10 times normal) led to early study discontinuation. Cholestatic changes were not observed, and patients never developed fever or symptoms of hepatitis or other systemic syndromes.

One other symptom relatively specific for labetalol (32 patients; 10 percent) was as sensation of scalp tingling, occasionally involving the face, extremities, or least commonly, the trunk. This was usually mild, often self-limited and of unclear etiology, possibly cutaneous vasodilation. In comparison, "paresthesia" was reported by as many as 18 percent of women on placebo, 25 percent on propranolol, and 29 percent on thiazide, and somewhat less frequently by men (12 to 15 percent), in the recent Medical Research Council Report.[29]

Of further note, in a recent review of labetalol therapy in general practice in England,[32] Kane reported a similar profile of efficacy and safety in 8573 hypertensive patients treated for periods ranging from 1 month to 5 years. However, in contrast to the present study, male sexual dysfunction and hepatic transaminase elevations attributable to drug were only rare occurrences.

Finally, β-blocker and antihypertensive medication "withdrawal syndromes" are of considerable interest. When it is necessary to withdraw such therapy it is undoubtedly prudent to do so gradually, and in concert with the known pharmacology of the drug, the level of hypertension pretherapy, and the patient's underlying cardiovascular status. In the great majority of the 223 patients in whom therapy was abruptly discontinued in the present study, both standing and supine blood pressures and heart rates were back to their pretreatment baseline values 1 week later. It appears that return to baseline blood pressure levels and heart rate is predictable in the week following discontinuation of labetalol. Quite possibly, because labetalol has less effect on heart rate than other β-blockers, and its antihypertensive effects are not solely dependent on β-blockade, withdrawal-related adverse experiences are also relatively infrequent.

SUMMARY

Labetalol is a novel β-blocker, with additional α-blocking and possibly β$_2$-agonist mediated vasodilating properties. This pharmacologic profile has suggested a role for labetalol in both the primary and adjunctive therapy of mild, moderate, and severe hypertension. The present long-term open-label multicenter experience with labetalol used alone and in combination with diuretic, in a wide spectrum of hypertensive patients, indicates that labetalol is potentially efficacious, safe, and relatively well tolerated in the long-term treatment of hypertension.

REFERENCES

1. Koch G: Hemodynamic changes after acute and long-term combined alpha-beta-adrenoceptor blockade with labetalol as compared with beta-receptor blockade. J Cardiovasc Pharmacol 3 (Suppl 1):530, 1981.
2. Heidbreder E, Pagel G, Rockel A, Heidland A: Beta-adrenergic blockade in stress protection. Limited effect of metoprolol in psychological stress reaction. Eur J Clin Pharmacol 14:391, 1978.
3. Frishman WH: Clinical Pharmacology of the Beta-Adrenoceptor Blocking Drugs. New York, Appleton-Century Crofts, 1980, pp 171–181, 183–197.
4. Maxwell GM: Effects of alpha- and beta-adrenoceptor antagonist (AH 5158) upon general and coronary haemodynamics of intact dogs. Br J Pharmacol 44:370, 1973.
5. Richards DA: Pharmacological effects of labetalol in man. Br J Clin Pharmacol 3:721, 1976.
6. Mehta J, Cohn JN: Hemodynamic effects of labetalol, an alpha and beta adrenergic blocking agent in hypertensive subjects. Circulation 55:370, 1977.
7. Frishman W, Halprin S: Clinical pharmacology of the new beta adrenergic blocking drugs. Part 7. New horizons in beta-adrenoceptor blockade therapy: Labetalol. Am Heart J 98:660, 1979.
8. Brittain RT, Harris DM, Jack D, Richards DA: Labetalol, in Goldberg ME (ed), Pharmacological and Biochemical Properties of Drug Substances. Vol. 2, Am Pharm Assoc Acad Pharm Sci, 1979, pp 229–254.
9. Dage RC, Hsieh CP: Direct vasodilatation by labetalol in anaesthetised dogs. Br J Pharmacol 70:287, 1980.
10. Prichard BNC, Richards DA: Labetalol, an alpha- and beta-adrenoceptor-blocking agent: its use in therapeutics. J Clin Pharmacol 8:2395, 1979.
11. Taylor SH, Silke B, Nelson GIG, et al: Haemodynamic advantages of combined alpha-blockade and beta-blockade over beta-blockade alone in patients with coronary heart disease. Br Med J 285:325, 1982.
12. Carey B, Whalley ET: Labetalol possesses beta-adrenoceptor agonist action on the rat isolated uterus. J Pharm Pharmacol 31:791, 1979.
13. Levy GP, Richards DA: Labetalol, in Scriabine A (ed), Pharmacology of Antihypertensive Drugs. New York, Raven, 1980, pp 325–347.
14. Baum T, Sybertz EJ: Antihypertension actions of an isomer of labetalol and other vasodilator–β-adrenoceptor blockers. Federation Proc 42:176, 1983.
15. Dargie HJ, Dollery CT, Daniel J: Labetalol in resistant hypertension. Br J Clin Pharmacol 3 (Suppl 3):751, 1976.

16. Pugsley DJ, Armstrong BK, Nassim MA, Beilin LJ: Controlled comparison of labetalol and propranolol in the management of severe hypertension. Br J Clin Pharmacol 3 (Suppl 3):777, 1976.

17. Rosei EA, Brown JJ, Lever AF, et al: Treatment of phaeochromocytoma and of clonidine withdrawal hypertension with labetalol. Br J Clin Pharmacol 3 (Suppl 3):809, 1976.

18. Lamming D, Symonds EM: Use of labetalol and methyldopa in pregnancy-induced hypertension. J Clin Pharmacol 8:217S, 1979.

19. Prichard BNC, Boakes AJ: Labetalol in long-term treatment of hypertension. Br J Clin Pharmacol 3 (Suppl 3):743, 1976.

20. Lund-Johansen P, Bakke OM: Haemodynamic effects and plasma concentrations of labetalol during long-term treatment of essential hypertension. Br J Clin Pharmacol 7:169, 1979.

21. New Zealand Hypertension Study Group: A multicentre study of labetalol in hypertension. NZ Med J 93:215, 1981.

22. Stern N, Teicher A, Rosenthal T: The treatment of hypertension by labetalol—a new alpha- and beta-adrenoceptor blocking agent. Clin Cardiol 5:125, 1982.

23. Harley A, Coverdale HA: The electrophysiological effects of intravenous labetalol in man. Eur J Clin Pharmacol 20:241, 1981.

24. Romano S, Orfei S, Pozzoni L, et al: Preliminary clinical trial on hypotensive and antiarrhythmic effect of labetalol. Drugs Exp Clin Res VII(1):65, 1981.

25. Fagard R, Amery A, Reybrouck T, et al: Response of the systemic and pulmonary circulation to alpha- and beta-receptor blockade (labetalol) at rest and during exercise in hypertensive patients. Circulation 60:1214, 1979.

26. Nelson GIC, Ahuja RC, Hussain M, et al: Alpha- and beta-blockade with labetalol in acute myocardial infarction. J Cardiovasc Pharmacol 4:921, 1982.

27. Levinson PD, Khatri IM, Freis ED: Persistence of normal BP after withdrawal of drug treatment in mild hypertension. Arch Intern Med 142:2265, 1982.

28. Beta-Blocker Heart Attack Trial Research Group: A randomized trial of propranolol in patients with acute myocardial infarction: 1. Mortality Results. JAMA 247:1707, 1982.

29. Report of Medical Research Council Working Party on Mild to Moderate Hypertension: Adverse reactions to bendrofluazide and propranolol for the treatment of mild hypertension. Lancet 2:539, 1981.

30. Bulpitt CJ, Dollery CT: Side effects of hypotensive agents evaluated by a self-administered questionnaire. Br Med J 3:485, 1973.

31. Bulpitt CJ, Dollery CT, Carnes A: Symptoms questionnaire for hypertensive patients. J Chron Dis 27:309, 1974.

32. Kane JA: Labetalol in general practice: A review. Br J Clin Pharm 13(Suppl 1):595, 1982.

PART FOUR

Special Topics

CHAPTER 15

The Use of β-Adrenergic Blocking Agents During Pregnancy

William H. Frishman, Heschi H. Rotmensch, Shlomo Charlap, Uri Elkayam, and Neal Klein

β-Adrenergic blocking drugs have proven efficacy in the treatment of hypertension, arrhythmias, hypertrophic cardiomyopathy, hyperthyroidism, and migraine.[1] All of these conditions may manifest themselves during the reproductive years of the female patient (Table 1). Although widely used in Europe, particularly for the treatment of essential and pregnancy-associated hypertension, β-blockers are not currently approved for use during pregnancy in the United States. Any decision to treat a pregnant woman with a β-blocker must balance the potential benefit to the mother and indirectly to the fetus by maintaining maternal health versus the known and unknown potential risks to the fetus. In this chapter we will review (1) general principles regarding maternal–fetal physiology, (2) clinical experiences with β-blocker treatment during pregnancy, and (3) current recommendations concerning β-blocker use during pregnancy.

MATERNAL–FETAL PHYSIOLOGY

Pharmacotherapeutic research in humans during pregnancy is limited by ethical and practical considerations. Information is incomplete regarding the effects of β-blockers on the fetus and the potential changes in therapeutic response of the gravid woman. Thus, awareness of general phar-

445

TABLE 1. CLINICAL USE OF β-ADRENERGIC BLOCKING DRUGS IN PREGNANCY

Hypertension
Arrhythmias
    Supraventricular
    Ventricular
Hypertrophic cardiomyopathy
Throtoxicosis
Migraine headache
Dysfunctional labor
Fetal tachycardia

macokinetic principles and good clinical judgement are of utmost importance when considering β-blocker use in pregnant women.

Drug Disposition During Pregnancy
The progressively changing maternal and fetal physiology during pregnancy may have a complex influence on drug disposition and maternal therapeutic responses. Decreased motility of the gastrointestinal tract associated with pregnancy might reduce the rate or extent of absorption of β-blockers due to delayed gastric emptying.[2] On the other hand, the slowed passage of drugs along the alimentary tract might increase the total absorption of the drugs.[3] The expansion of the maternal intra- and extravascular fluid volumes as well as tissue volume due to growth of the uterus, placenta, and fetus are other factors that may affect drug disposition.[4]

The distribution of drugs into a larger physiologic volume implies that acute administration of a single dose of a drug is likely to result in lower serum concentrations in the pregnant versus the nonpregnant woman. Therefore, higher loading doses may be required in the pregnant female. Steady-state plasma concentrations of the drug resulting from chronic administration would not be expected to change significantly, unless the pregnant state alters drug clearance from the body.[4]

As plasma volume increases progressively by 50 percent at the eighth month of pregnancy, plasma protein concentrations tend to fall and may in part account for the considerable reduction in the extent of drug protein binding during pregnancy.[5-7] This reduction in the extent of protein binding will decrease total drug concentration, increase the tissue to plasma distribution of the drug, and, for some β-blockers, i.e., propranolol and alprenolol, which are highly protein bound, may lead to increased drug clearance from the body (Chapter 2).[8]

Renal blood flow and glomerular filtration rate also rise rapidly during pregnancy, increasing 50 percent by the fourth month of gestation.[9]

Therefore, β-blockers, i.e., nadolol, sotalol, and atenolol, which are eliminated primarily by renal excretion, are likely to be cleared more rapidly, leading to the possibility of subtherapeutic drug levels with normal dosage regimens.[8,10] Another factor potentially causing reduced maternal drug concentrations relative to dose is enhanced metabolic clearance of certain drugs due to progesterone-activated increases in hepatic metabolizing enzyme activity.[4,11] There is also the possibility that some drug biotransformation might occur in the placenta and the fetal liver.[12] Since the relative contribution of the above factors to the dispositional changes in pregnancy may vary considerably from one patient to another, it is generally impossible to predict whether or not a clinically important alteration of pharmacologic response during pregnancy will occur in a given individual. As a general rule, β-blocker administration during pregnancy should be based on clinical response rather than any specific dosage regimen.

Placental Drug Transfer
Sensitive analytic methods for the measurement of drug concentrations in body fluids and tissues have demonstrated that virtually all drugs can be transferred across the placenta.[12,13] The rate of diffusion across the placental barrier is directly proportional to the maternal–fetal concentration gradient and the surface area of the placenta, inversely proportional to the thickness of placental membrane,[14,15] and is increased by the drug's high degree of lipid solubility, low degree of ionization, and low molecular weight, factors favoring passage through membranes.[16] Drugs with molecular weights of less than 600 (which compromise the majority of drugs used therapeutically) cross the placenta fairly easily, whereas those with molecular weights over 1000 may be restricted by their size. Plasma binding of drugs in maternal blood may also serve to limit the degree of placental transfer. Since only the unbound (free) fraction of a drug is subject to placental transfer, the more a drug is bound to maternal plasma proteins, the less it is available for crossing to the fetus.

It has been shown that the various β-blockers cross the placental barrier and reach a significant level in the fetal serum, i.e., propranolol,[17,18] oxprenolol,[17] atenolol,[19,20] metoprolol,[21] sotalol,[22] nadolol,[23] and labetalol.[24] At delivery, maternal and fetal cord blood concentrations of these drugs are comparable,[18,22,25] though lower fetal than maternal concentrations have also be described.[26]

Potential Drug Effects on the Fetus and Newborn
During the initial 14 days following conception, the embryo is relatively resistant to exogenous toxicity. If damage does occur during this time, it may result in abortion. Congenital malformations grossly visible at

birth may result from drug exposure during the first trimester of pregnancy, and depend on the nature of the drug, its accessibility to the fetus, the duration of fetal exposure, and the genetic susceptibility of the fetus.[27] Fetal protein binding is one parameter that will determine the degree of fetal exposure to the drug, as it affects the distribution, elimination, and pharmacologic activity of the drug in the fetus. There is at present, however, no possibility of obtaining such data in the young fetus, i.e., during the period when drugs are most likely to cause birth defects. Therefore, drug administration, particularly during the first trimester of pregnancy, should be avoided whenever possible. In the second and third trimester, interference by drugs with normal fetal growth and development are the major problems encountered.[28]

In addition, one must consider the potential problems of a mother needing drug therapy who wants to breast feed her child. Many drugs taken by the mother will be found in human milk. The level in milk depends on the physiochemical properties of the drug, the degree of plasma protein binding, and the serum concentrations attained in the mother. Most β-blocking agents have been shown to be secreted in breast milk, with average steady-state concentrations in milk that are approximately five times higher than that in maternal plasma.[20,22,29-31] This finding has been said to be caused by "ion trapping" in the milk. Because the pH of milk is less than that of blood, milk can act as an "ion trap" for weak bases, such as most β-blocking agents.[32] However, in light of the relatively low daily quantity of milk ingested, the presence of a β-blocker in breast milk has not been associated with any signs of β-blockade in the infant who has normal hepatic and renal function.[30,31]

Adrenergic Influences on Maternal–Fetal Physiology

β-Adrenergic activity during pregnancy assumes physiologic importance because of the direct effects the sympathetic nervous system has on umbilical blood flow and uterine tone and contractility. Since there is difficulty in studying humans and a need to separate direct from indirect effects of β-blockers, most experimental work on umbilical blood flow has been conducted in the pregnant ewe. Oakes et al.[33] studied the effects of propranolol and isoproterenol in nonlaboring anesthetized pregnant sheep that were near term. During fetal or maternal infusion of the β-blocker, there was a significant decrease in umbilical blood flow and in the maternal and fetal heart rate. Uterine blood flow and systemic blood pressure remained unchanged. With isoproterenol infusion, there was an increase in umbilical blood flow and only a small increment in fetal heart rate. It may, therefore, be concluded that β-adrenergic tone affects basal umbilical blood flow, with a disturbance in sympathetic inputs being potentially harmful to the developing fetus.

α-Agonists influence umbilical blood flow indirectly through their action on uterine blood vessels. When a low dose of norepinephrine was infused directly into a uterine artery, a profound reduction in utero–placental blood flow developed.[34] A direct action of norepinephrine on the umbilical circulation has not been demonstrated.[35,36]

In the myometrium, there are adrenergic receptors of the α- and β-types (Table 2). Stimulation of the β-receptor results in myometrial relaxation, whereas increased α-adrenergic stimulation potentiates contractility.[37] In animal studies, propranolol has been shown to reverse the myometrial depressant action of β-stimulation.[38] Barden and associates[39] also demonstrated this effect of propranolol in pregnant humans. In their study, pregnant women at term were selected for elective induction of labor. Maternal and fetal heart rates, maternal blood pressure, and intrauterine pressure were measured in all patients. After an infusion of oxytocin to eight patients, epinephrine was administered and caused a consistent inhibition of uterine activity while accelerating maternal heart rate. These effects were completely reversed by prior propranolol treatment. Norepinephrine infusion potentiated uterine activity while decreasing maternal heart rate and increasing blood pressure. Prior propranolol treatment had no effect, whereas the α-adrenergic blocker phentolamine significantly attenuated the actions of norepinephrine. After these studies, all the subjects had normal term vaginal deliveries.

The influence of the autonomic nervous system on normal fetal circulation has also been studied in the fetal lamb preparation. In a report by Joelson and Barton,[40] isoproterenol administered to the fetus caused an increase in heart rate and a decrease in blood pressure, whereas propranolol alone caused only a slight drop in heart rate. All of the isoproterenol effects could be blocked by previous propranolol treatment.

TABLE 2. ADRENERGIC INFLUENCES ON MATERNAL–FETAL PHYSIOLOGY

	Stimulation		Blockade	
	α-Receptor	β-Receptor	α-Receptor	β-Receptor
Fetal heart rate	↔	↑	↔	↔ ↓
Maternal heart rate	↔	↑	↔	↓
Umbilical blood flow	↔	↑	↔	↓
Myometrial activity	↑	↓	↓	↑

↔no effect, ↑ increases, ↓ decreases.

When the fetus was stressed by cord occlusions, propranolol completely abolished the increase in heart rate which is usually seen. It was apparent that the effects of β-adrenergic blockade on the unstressed and undisturbed fetus were minimal. However, when the fetus is stressed, stimulation of the β-receptor may provide an important reserve for neonatal adaptation. Thus, maternal treatment with β-blockers may impair the response to fetal distress.

CLINICAL EXPERIENCE

Propranolol

Propranolol, the oldest of the available nonselective β-blockers, was the first such agent to have wide application in pregnant patients. Since its early use in the late 1960s, many favorable reports have accumulated. The drug has been employed successfully in the treatment of gestational hypertension,[41] maternal thyrotoxicosis,[42] obstructive cardiomyopathy,[43] paroxysmal atrial tachycardia,[44] dysfunctional uterine activity,[45] and fetal tachycardia.[25] To date, there have been no reports implicating propranolol in fetal malformation.[46] At least two studies included women who had been receiving propranolol before conception, and no fetal abnormalities were found.[41,47]

Despite the encouraging experience in therapy, adverse fetal effects have also been described (Table 3). In a retrospective study, Pruyn et al.[48] reported that 10 of 11 babies exposed to long-term propranolol in utero had weights and head circumferences below the 50th percentile. They suggested that the experimental data of decreased umbilical blood flow in the ewes after propranolol administration could explain their findings. A decrease in umbilical blood flow could deprive the growing fetus of needed nutrients and thus impair growth.

In contrast to the findings by Pruyn et al.,[48] in five prospective stud-

TABLE 3. REPORTED ADVERSE REACTIONS OF USE OF β-ADRENERGIC BLOCKING DRUGS IN PREGNANCY

Maternal	Fetal/Neonate
Bradycardia	Intrauterine growth retardation
Premature labor	Delayed neonatal breathing
Prolonged labor	Bradycardia
	Hypoglycemia
	Hyperbilirubinemia

ies with propranolol and oxprenolol the incidence of retardation of uterine growth in 94 pregnancies was approximately 4 percent.[41,47,49–51] In addition, two of the four mothers whose babies were small for gestational age had normal-sized babies in subsequent pregnancies despite continued propranolol therapy.[51] It would, therefore, seem inappropriate to conclude that β-adrenergic blockade during pregnancy is commonly associated with retardation of intrauterine growth.[52]

Turnstall[53] found that, in three cases, the administration of propranolol 1 mg intravenously prior to cesarean section led to a 5 to 6 minute delay in the onset of spontaneous respiration in all babies, requiring intubation in two. A subsequent randomized double-blind study by the same investigator found this complication in all neonates whose mothers received preoperative propranolol.[53]

Children of mothers who have received propranolol for various reasons in dosages of 160 mg daily were born with normal Apgar scores but had bradycardia and hypoglycemia up to 72 hours after delivery.[18,54–56] Other reported adverse effects in the fetus include hyperbilirubinemia,[48] polycythemia,[54] and prolonged labor.[55] It would appear that in the presence of hypoxia or other stresses, β-blockade would be especially counterproductive in its blocking activation of the sympathetic nervous system.[40] On the other hand, babies born in uncomplicated deliveries to mothers treated with propranolol would not be expected to have any serious cardiac alterations attributable to β-blockade.

Metoprolol

Metoprolol, a β_1-selective blocking agent, is similar in its effectiveness to other, nonselective β-adrenoceptor blocking drugs used in the treatment of angina pectoris or essential hypertension.[1] However, because of its primary β_1-selective properties, the drug would theoretically not interfere with β_2-mediated peripheral vasodilatation or β_2-effects on uterine tone.

In a large-scale, prospective clinical study in Sweden, the outcome of 184 hypertensive gravidae treated with either metoprolol and a thiazide diuretic or metoprolol in combination with hydralazine were compared to that of 97 similar patients receiving hydralazine and a thiazide.[21,28] Perinatal mortality was lower in the metoprolol-treated groups. There were no differences in the average lengths and weights of the newborns in the three groups, and no significant adverse effects were reported in the fetus attributable to metoprolol. Furthermore, it was shown that metoprolol crosses the placenta, and the drug concentration in the umbilical venous blood was about the same as in the maternal venous blood.

Atenolol

Atenolol a β_1-selective blocker, was recently approved for the treatment of hypertension in the United States.[57] In contrast to propranolol and metoprolol, which are lipophilic, the use of atenolol, a hydrophilic agent, has been associated with less central nervous system side effects, such as nightmares and hallucinations. In clinical trials in hypertensive pregnant women, atenolol, frequently used as monotherapy, has been shown to normalize blood pressure without causing obstetric or neonatal complications.[58-61] In this regard, the study by Rubin[62] is of particular interest. In this prospective, double-blind randomized trial involving 120 pregnant women with hypertension that developed in their last trimester, patients received either atenolol, 100–200 mg per day, or placebo. The results showed that atenolol effectively lowered blood pressure and improved the outcome of pregnancy. Proteinuria developed in all placebo patients compared to only four patients taking atenolol. Apgar scores and birth weights of newborn infants were virtually the same for both groups. Five infants of mothers taking placebo and two of mothers taking atenolol had hypoglycemia; two intrauterine deaths occurred in the control group and one in the atenolol group. Respiratory distress developed in three neonates of control mothers, but in none of those exposed to atenolol. However, bradycardia, defined as a heart rate of less than 120 beats per minute, occurred in more infants from the atenolol-treated mothers ($n = 22$) than from the placebo group ($n = 6$); all episodes lasted less than 10 minutes, however, and no intervention was necessary.

Oxprenolol

Oxprenolol, a noncardioselective β-blocker with intrinsic sympathetic activity, has also been used during gestational hypertension and it appears to be safe and effective. Methyldopa, up to 1 g per day, was compared to oxprenolol, up to 200 mg per day, given to 27 and 26 pregnant, hypertensive women, respectively.[50] The women receiving oxprenolol showed greater placental and fetal growth; there was no difference in the Apgar scores of the two groups.

Sotalol

Sotalol, a noncardioselective β-blocker with a low lipid solubility, has also been given to pregnant patients. The results did not reveal tetratogenicity or any significant adverse effects with this agent.[22] However, the long biologic half-life of sotalol might prove to be disadvantageous in the treatment of the pregnant patient.

Labetalol

Labetalol is a recently developed drug that, like propranolol, blocks both β_1- and β_2-adrenoceptors. However, labetalol is unique in that it also has both α_1-adrenergic blocking properties and direct vasodilating activity.[63] The clinical pharmacology of labetalol is detailed in Chapter 7. There have been a number of favorable reports describing the safe use of labetalol in the treatment of hypertension in pregnancy.[24,64–67] Clinically significant fetal hypoglycemia, bradycardia, or respiratory depression was not usually associated with maternal labetalol therapy. Michael[24] treated 85 women with severe hypertension complicating pregnancy using oral labetalol as single drug therapy. Effective control of the blood pressure was achieved in all but six patients using a maximum dose of 1200 mg per day labetalol. Perinatal mortality was 4.4 percent, and there were no congenital malformations in any of the infants delivered. In studies comparing labetalol to methyldopa in the treatment of hypertension in pregnancy, labetalol has been shown to be as effective as,[66] and possibly superior[67] to, methyldopa in obtaining good blood pressure control.

Labetalol has also been shown to be efficacious when administered intravenously in those situations where rapid reduction of blood pressure in pregnancy is required, such as in severe preeclampsia or eclampsia.[68–71] In a recent comparative study with intravenous dihydralazine, labetalol infusion appeared to offer significant advantages in the management of severe hypertension in pregnancy.[72]

RECOMMENDATIONS

At present, the evidence to support the safe use of β-blocking agents in pregnancy is inconclusive.[73] Therefore, it appears preferable to utilize other classes of effective drugs proven safe during pregnancy prior to using β-blockers. If a β-blocker must be used, it may be advisable to follow certain guidelines.

1. Include the pregnant woman and her fetus in the high-risk group to receive special care both during pregnancy and labor.
2. Avoid, whenever possible, the use of β-blocker therapy during the first trimester of pregnancy.
3. Use the lowest possible therapeutic dose. Combination of low doses of β-blockers and low doses of other agents might provide optimal drug therapy.
4. If possible, discontinue β-blocker therapy at least 2 to 3 days prior to delivery, both as a way of limiting the effects of β-block-

ers on uterine contractility and for preventing possible neonatal complications secondary to β-blockade.

5. Use of β-blockers with β_1-selectivity, intrinsic sympathetic activity, or α-blocking activity may be preferable in that these agents would be less likely to interfere with β_2-mediated uterine relaxation and peripheral vasodilation.

A comprehensive recommendation regarding β-blocker use in pregnancy is extremely difficult to make. This difficulty arises from the lack of any large-scale clinical experience with these agents in pregnant patients. More studies are still needed to better define β-blocker pharmacokinetics in the mother and fetus. Also, studies are warranted during pregnancy to assess the safety and efficacy of β-blockers with existing cardiovascular therapies. Hopefully, future clinical experiences will help clarify the role β-blocker agents should play in the treatment of maternal diseases.

REFERENCES

1. Frishman W, Silverman R: Clinical pharmacology of the new beta-adrenergic blocking drugs. Part 3. Comparative clinical experience and new therapeutic applications. Am Heart J 98:119, 1979.
2. Parry E, Shields R, Turnbull AC: Transit time in the small intestine in pregnancy. J Obstet Gynecol Br Comm 77:900, 1970.
3. Eadie MJ, Lander CM, Tyrer JH: Plasma drug level monitoring in pregnancy. Clin Pharmacokin 2:427, 1977.
4. Krauer B, Krauer F: Drug kinetics in pregnancy. Pharmacokin 2:167, 1977.
5. Dean M, Stock B, Patterson RJ, Levy G: Serum protein binding of drugs during and after pregnancy in humans. Clin Pharmacol Ther 28:253, 1980.
6. Stock B, Dean M, Levy G: Serum protein binding of drugs during and after pregnancy in rats. J Pharmacol Exp Ther 212:264, 1980.
7. Perucca E, Ruprah M, Richens A: Altered drug binding to serum proteins in pregnant women: therapeutic revelance. J Soc Med 74:422, 1981.
8. Frishman W: Clinical pharmacology of the new beta-adrenergic blocking drugs. Part 1. Pharmacodynamic and pharmacokinetic properties. Am Heart J 97:663, 1979.
9. Sims EAH, Krantz KE: Serial studies of renal function during pregnancy and the puerperium in normal women. J Clin Invest 37:1764, 1958.
10. Stock BH: Drug disposition in pregnancy. Pharm Internat (March) 2:60, 1981.
11. Fever G: Action of pregnancy and various progesterones on hepatic microsomal activities. Drug Metab Rev 9:147, 1979.

12. Levy G: Pharmacokinetics of fetal and neonatal exposure to drugs. Obstet Gynecol 58 (Suppl):9s, 1981.
13. Moya F, Thorndike V: Passage of drugs across the placenta. Am J Obstet Gynecol 84:1778, 1962.
14. Aherne W, Dunnill MS: Morphometry of the human placenta. Br Med Bull 22:5, 1966.
15. Abouleish E: The placenta and placental transfer of drugs at term. Penn Med 78:56, 68, 1975.
16. Schanker LS: Passage of drugs across body membranes. Pharmacol Rev 14:501, 1962.
17. Truelove JF, van Petten GR, Willes RF: Action of severe adrenoceptor blocking drugs in the pregnant sheep and foetus. Br J Pharmacol 47:161, 1973.
18. Cottrill CM, McAllister RG, Gettes L, Noonan JA: Propranolol therapy during pregnancy, labor and delivery; evidence for transplacental drug transfer and impaired neonatal drug disposition. J Pediatr 91:812, 1977.
19. Lundborg P: Fetal effects of antihypertensive drugs. Acta Med Scand 628 (Suppl):95, 1979.
20. Melander A, Niklasson B, Ingemarsson I, et al: Transplacental passage of atenolol in man. Eur J Clin Pharmacol 14:93, 1978.
21. Sandstrom B: Antihypertensive treatment with the adrenergic beta receptor blocker metoprolol during pregnancy. Gynecol Obset Invest 19:195, 1978.
22. O'Hare MF, Murnaghan GA, Russel CJ, et al: Sotalol as hypotensive agent in pregnancy. Br J Obstet Gynaecol 87:814, 1980.
23. Heel RC, Brogden RN, Pakes GE, et al: Nadolol: A review of its phramacological properties and therapeutic efficacy in hypertension and angina pectoris. Drugs 20:1, 1980.
24. Michael CA: The evaluation of labetalol in the treatment of hypertension complicating pregnancy. Br J Clin Pharmacol 13 (Suppl I):127s, 1982.
25. Sabom MB, Curry RC Jr, Wise DE: Propranolol therapy during pregnancy in a patient with idiopathic hypertrophic subaortic stenosis. Is it safe? South Med J 71:328, 1978.
26. Teuscher A, Bossi E, Imhof P, et al: Effect of propranolol on fetal tachycardia in diabetic pregnancy. Am J Cardiol 42:304, 1978.
27. Erikson M, Catz CS, Jaffe SJ: Drugs and pregnancy. Clin Obstet Gynecol 16:199, 1973.
28. Howard FM, Hill JM: Drugs in pregnancy. Ob Gyn Surv 34:643, 1979.
29. Sandstrom B: Adrenergic beta-receptor blockers in hypertension of pregnancy. Clin Exper Hyper B1:127, 1982.
30. Liedholm H, Melander A, Bitzen PO, et al: Accumulation of atenolol and metoprolol in human breast milk. Eur J Clin Pharmacol 20:229, 1971.
31. Devlin RG, Duchin KL, Fleiss PM: Nadolol in human serum and breast milk. Br J Clin Pharmacol 12:393, 1981.
32. Rotmensch HH, Elkayam U, Frishman W: Antiarrhythmic drug therapy during pregnancy. Ann Int Med 98:487, 1983.

33. Oakes GK, Walker AD, Ehrenkranz RA, Chez RA: Effect of propranolol infusion on the umbilical and uterine circulations of pregnant sheep. Am J Obstet Gynecol 126:1038, 1976.

34. Ladner E, Brinkman CR, Weston P, Assali NS: Dynamics of uterine circulation in pregnant and non-pregnant sheep. Am J Physiol 218:257, 1970.

35. Adams FH, Assali NS, Cushman M, Westersten A: Interrelationships of maternal and fetal circulations. 1. Flow-pressure responses to vasoactive drugs in sheep. Pediatrics 27:627, 1961.

36. Chez RA, Ehrenkranz RA, Oakes GK, et al: Effects of adrenergic agents on bovine umbilical and uterine blood flows, in Longo L, Reneau DD (eds), Fetal and Newborn Cardiovascular Physiology. New York, Garland, 1978, vol 2, pp 1–16.

37. Maughan GB, Shabanah EH, Toth A: Experiments with pharmacologic sympatholysis in the gravid. Am J Obstet Gynecol 97:764, 1967.

38. Wansbrough H, Nakanishi H, Wood C: Effect of epinephrine on human uterine activity in vitro and in vivo. Obstet Gynecol 30:779, 1967.

39. Barden TP, Stander RW: Effects of adrenergic blocking agents and catecholamines in human pregnancy. Am J Obstet Gynecol 102:226, 1968.

40. Joelson I, Barton MD: The effect of blockade on the beta-receptors of the sympathetic nervous system of the fetus. Acta Obstet Gynecol Scand 3 (Suppl) 38:75, 1969.

41. Eliahou HE, Silverberg DS, Reisin E, et al: Propranolol for the treatment of hypertension in pregnancy. Br J Obstet Gynaecol 85:431, 1978.

42. Bullock JL, Harris RE, Young R: Treatment of thyrotoxicosis during pregnancy and propranolol. Am J Obstet Gynecol 121:242, 1975.

43. Turner GM, Oakley CM, Dixon HG: Management of pregnancy complicated by hypertrophic obstructive cardiomyopathy. Br Med J 4:281, 1968.

44. Schroeder JS, Harrison DC: Repeated cardioversion during pregnancy: treatment of refractory paroxysmal atrial tachycardia during three successive pregnancies. Am J Cardiol 27:445, 1971.

45. Mitrani A, Oettinger M, Abinader EG, et al: Use of propranolol in dysfunctional labour. Br J Obstet Gynecol 82:651, 1975.

46. Shepard TH: Catalogue of Teratogenic Agents, 2nd ed. Baltimore: Johns Hopkins University Press, 1976.

47. Bott-Kanner G, Schweitzer A, Reisner SH, et al: Propranolol and hydralazine in the management of essential hypertension in pregnancy. Br J Obstet Gynaecol 87:110, 1980.

48. Pruyn SC, Phelan JP, Buchanan GC: Long-term propranolol therapy in pregnancy: Maternal and fetal outcome. Am J Obstet Gynecol 135:485, 1979.

49. Tcherdakoff PH, Colliard M, Berrard E, et al: Propranolol in hypertension during pregnancy. Br Med J 2:670, 1978.

50. Gallery EDM, Saunders DM, Hunyer SN, Gyory AZ: Randomized comparison of methyldopa and oxprenolol for treatment of hypertension in pregnancy. Br Med J 1:1591, 1979.

51. Oakley GDG, McGarry K, Limb DG, Oakley CM: Management of pregnancy in patients with hypertrophic cardiomyopathy. Br Med J 1:1749, 1979.
52. Rubin PC: Beta-blockers in pregnancy. N Engl J Med 305:1323, 1981.
53. Turnstall MB: The effect of propranolol on the onset of breathing at birth. Br J Anesthesiol 41:792, 1969.
54. Gladstone GR, Hordof AH, Gersony WM: Propranolol administration during pregnancy. Effects on the fetus. J Pediatr 86:962, 1975.
55. Habib A, McCarthy JS: Effect on the neonate of propranolol administration during pregnancy. J Pediatr 91:808, 1977.
56. Fiddler GI: Propranolol and pregnancy. Lancet 2:722, 1974.
57. Frishman WH: Atenolol and timolol, two new systemic β-adrenoreceptor antagonists. N Engl J Med 306:1456, 1982.
58. Lunell NO, Persson B, Aragon G, et al: Circulatory and metabolic effects of acute beta$_1$ blockade in severe pre-eclampsia. Acta Obstet Gynecol Scand 58:443, 1979.
59. Thorley KJ, McAinsh J, Cruikshank JM: Atenolol in the treatment of pregnancy-induced hypertension. Br J Clin Pharmacol 12:725, 1981.
60. Dubois D, Petitcolas J, Temperville B, et al: Treatment of hypertension in pregnancy with β-adrenoceptor antagonists. Br J Clin Pharmac 13:375s, 1982.
61. Fuerst M: β-Blockers may have role in pre-eclampsia. JAMA 3248:516, 1982.
62. Rubin PC, Butters L, Low RA, Reid JL: Atenolol in the treatment of essential hypertension during pregnancy. Br J Clin Pharmacol 14:279, 1982.
63. Frishman Wk, Halprin S: Clinical pharmacology of the new beta-adrenergic blocking drugs. Part 7. New horizons in beta-adrenoceptor blockade therapy. Am Heart J 98:660, 1979.
64. Mehta J, Cohn JN: Hemodynamic effects of labetalol, an alpha and beta adrenergic blocking agent, in hypertensive subject. Circulation 55:370, 1977.
65. Prichard BNC, Boakes AJ: Labetalol in long-term treatment of hypertension. Br J Clin Pharmacol 3 (Suppl 3):743, 1976.
66. Redman CWG: A randomized comparison of methyldopa (Aldomet) and labetalol (Trandate) for the treatment of severe hypertension in pregnancy. (Abstr). Clin Exp Hypertens B1:345, 1982.
67. Lamming GD, Symonds EB: Use of labetalol and methyldopa in pregnancy-induced hypertension. Br J Clin Pharmacol 8 (Suppl 2):217s, 1979.
68. Lamming GD, Broughton Pipkin F, Symonds EM: Comparison of the alpha- and beta-blocking drug, labetalol, and methyldopa in the treatment of moderate and severe pregnancy-induced hypertension. Clin Exp Hypertens 2:865, 1980.
69. Jorge CS: Labetalol in the hypertensive states of pregnancy. Emergency treatment of severe hypertension in a pregnant patient. The European Society of Cardiology. Drug Symposium on Labetalol 131, 1979.
70. Lilford RJ: Letter. Br Med J 281:1635, 1980.

71. Lunell NO, Hjemdahl P, Fredholm BB, et al: Circulatory and metabolic effects of a combined α- and β-adrenoceptor blocker (labetalol) in hypertension of pregnancy. Br J Clin Pharmacol 12:345, 1981.
72. Garden A, Davey DA, Dommisse J: Intravenous labetalol and dihydralazine in severe hypertension in pregnancy. Clin Exp Hypertens B1:371, 1981.
73. Klein NA, Frishman WH: Use of beta adrenergic blocking agents in pregnancy. In Elkayam U, Gleicher N (eds.) Cardiac Problems in Pregnancy, New York, Alan R. Liss, Inc. 1982, pp 221–225.

CHAPTER 16

β-Adrenergic Blockade and the Gastrointestinal System

Harold Jacob, William H. Frishman, Paul Farkas, and Lawrence J. Brandt

β-Adrenergic antagonists are being used with increasing frequency for a growing list of medical indications, including angina pectoris, systemic hypertension, migraine headaches, open-angle glaucoma, thyrotoxicosis, hypertrophic cardiomyopathy, myocardial infarction, and recently, for the prevention of recurrent bleeding from esophageal varices.

Gastrointestinal side effects have been reported with some frequency in patients receiving β-blocker treatment. In this chapter, the effects of the sympathetic nervous system and β-blocker treatment on the gastrointestinal system will be reviewed (Table 1). The potential benefits of β-blocker therapy for various gastrointestinal disorders will also be addressed.

GASTROINTESTINAL MOTILITY

In 1948, it was demonstrated that a quantitative relationship existed in vitro between catecholamine concentrations and certain physiologic responses. Ahlquist called the active tissue sites mediating these actions

From the American Journal of Medicine, Volume 74, pp 1042–1051, June 1983, with permission.

TABLE 1. PHARMACOLOGIC EFFECTS OF CATECHOLAMINE STIMULATION OF ADRENERGIC RECEPTORS IN THE GASTROINTESTINAL TRACT

Organ	Function	α-Agonists	β-Agonists
Esophagus	Peristalsis	↑	↓
	Lower esophageal sphincter	↑	↓
Stomach	Gastric emptying		↓
	Acid secretion	↓ (?)	↓ (?)
Small intestine	Motility	↓	↓
	Transport	↑ (ions)	↑ (ions & amino acids)
	Cell turnover	↑	↓
Large intestine	Motility	↑	↓
Mesenteric vasculature	Blood flow	Vasoconstriction	Vasodilatation
Bile duct	Motility	↑	↓
Pancreas	Exocrine secretion	?	↓

receptors, and proposed the existence of two distinct types, which he designated alpha and beta. The α-receptor is mainly associated with excitatory effects such as vasoconstriction, uterine contraction, and ureteral and pupillary smooth muscle relaxation; one important inhibitory function regulated by an α-receptor is intestinal relaxation. The β-receptor is associated with inhibitory functions and also one excitatory function, i.e., myocardial stimulation.[1]

Recent studies of adrenergic mediation of small intestinal relaxation have suggested both α- and β-receptors may be involved. In one of those studies, McMurphy and Boreus used human fetal ileum obtained from second trimester abortuses and showed that isoproterenol, adrenaline, noradrenalline, and methoxamine all had the potential to induce complete relaxation of acetylcholine stimulated contraction. The order of potency with which this inhibition was effected was isoproterenol > epinephrine-norepinephrine >>> methoxamine. Methoxamine, a relatively pure α-adrenergic activator, was one-twentieth to one-thirtieth as potent in relaxing fetal intestinal smooth muscle. These observations indicated that the ability to relax intestinal smooth muscle cells was primarily related to the β-stimulating activity of the catecholamine. The mechanism by which methoxamine relaxed intestinal muscle was felt to be a nonspecific action of the drug, as this was achieved only in doses much higher than could be achieved in vivo.[2] Moreover, small doses of β-blocking agents could fully block the relaxation induced by isoproterenol, epinephrine, and norepinephrine, which indicated that these drugs exert their final effects via a sensitive β-receptor. Phenoxybenzamine, an α-antagonist, could not inhibit the acetylcholine-stimulated contraction. Conflicting data are reported by Hart, whose studies of intestinal receptors used fetal small intestine obtained between 8 and 26 weeks of gestation. In this model propranolol consistently inhibited the relaxation response of norepinephrine; however, phenylephrine-induced relaxation was inhibited by phentolamine, supporting the role for an α-receptor.[3] Reddy and Moran, working with rabbit intestine, provided further evidence that small intestinal inhibitory responses are mediated by both α- and β-adrenergic receptors. Two important issues were also raised by the latter investigators, i.e., the loci of these receptors and the physiologic importance of the receptors relative to each other.[4]

The issue of intestinal receptor location was addressed by Van Rossum and Mujic, who proposed that the α-receptors are components of the intramural ganglion cells.[5] Support for this hypothesis can be found from the work of a number of investigators, including Norberg, who utilized fluorescent histochemical techniques for catecholamines and found that the fluorescent-staining nerves (i.e., catecholamine containing) terminated around blood vessels and intramural ganglion cells but not on smooth muscle cells. No fluorescent ganglion cells were observed. Thus, the adrenergic system appeared to be localized to the intramural neuronal preganglionic network, which suggests that adrenoreceptors are located on the ganglion cells.[6] Further evidence that the α-receptors are part of the ganglion cells comes from the observations that cold storage interferes with the function of nerve tissue in the intestine,[7–11] and that segments of rabbit jejunum stored in the cold for 1 to 3 days lost their responsiveness to the α-agents (phenylephrine and methoxamine) but not to the β-agents (epinephrine, norepinephrine, and isoproterenol). Furthermore, phentolamine, an α-blocker, did not modify the intestinal relaxation produced by epinephrine in cold-stored segments of jejunum, but in fresh segments it reduced the response. Pronethalol, a β-blocker, blocked the inhibitory responses to epinephrine, norepinephrine, and isoproterenol in cold storage and fresh preparations. Thus, responses characterized as α-adrenergic were reduced or abolished by cold storage, but those characterized as β-adrenergic were not affected; the evidence suggests, therefore, that only α-receptors are part of the neuronal structure.

One can speculate as to the location of the α- and β-receptor within the cell based on the nature of the response to α and β stimuli. α-Mediated stimuli occur rapidly, possibly due to a receptor on the cell surface with rapid changes in ganglion cell membrane polarity. Slow β-mediated responses could be due to an intracellular site or a slow reduction in contractile activity related to a metabolic alteration in the cell.[12]

Once a cell is stimulated by β-adrenoreceptors, the adenyl cyclase system is activated. This activation results in production of cyclic adenosine monophosphate (cAMP), which is believed to be the intracellular mediator of catecholamine action. Using an adenyl cyclase preparation from frog erythrocytes, Rosen et al. showed that the structural requirements for activation or inhibition of the enzyme by selected adrenoreceptor agonists and antagonists resembled the structural requirements for β-receptor activity on intact tissue preparations.[13] Ruoff also demonstrated that the stimulatory action of epinephrine on gastric mucosal cAMP in rats was mediated via beta-adrenoreceptors.[14] The association of the adenyl cyclase system and β-adrenoreceptors was further strengthened by the demonstration that the effects of β-adrenoreceptor agonists and antagonists on various tissues in the rat ($β_1$–$β_2$) correspond closely to the adenyl cyclase activities in those tissues.[15] Although most work on motility and receptors has been performed using small intestine, catecholamines (epinephrine, norepinephrine, and isoproterenol) have been shown to induce relaxation of the isolated rat colon.[16] Also, it has been shown in the rat and in humans that β-blockade reverses the epinephrine- or norepinephrine-mediated relaxation of isolated colonic strips and results in muscle contraction.[16,17] Thus, it is suggested that β-blockade has the property of unmasking α-receptors responsible for epinephrine-mediated excitation of isolated strips of colon. Hart and Mir, studying human fetal colon, have also provided evidence that the colon contains contractile α-adrenoreceptors.[18]

In striking contrast to the extensive literature that has been generated on the physiologic effects of β-blockers on intestinal motility, little is known about their effect on motility in the clinical setting. Based on evidence implicating a role for the sympathetic nervous system in postoperative ileus, Smith et al. explored the potential use of propranolol and phentolamine in the treatment of post-operative ileus induced in dogs undergoing celiotomy. Although phentolamine and propranolol prevented the inhibition of bursts of gastric action potentials associated with surgery, neither the inhibition of the small intestine action potentials nor gastrointestinal transit time as measured by sphere technique was altered.[19]

Hyperthyroidism is one situation in which laboratory and clinical data would suggest a paradoxic effect of propranolol on motility. Staslewicz et al. observed that propranolol inhibited the transit time of the small intestine in mice pretreated with thyroxine for 7 days, whereas the peristalsis of control mice was increased by propranolol.[20] Thomas et al. showed administration of propranolol resulted in a significant decrease in fat excretion and in the number of bowel movements of two patients with hyperthyroidism and steatorrhea. Roentgenographic studies of the small bowel while these patients were receiving propranolol showed that transit time was significantly prolonged compared with the initial transit times. This lengthening of transit time observed in patients with hyperthyroidism on propranolol therapy suggests that the effect of propranolol in this entity is not purely dependent on β-receptor blockade.[21] Rachmilewitz and colleagues obtained data in rats that suggested that prostaglandin E_2 mediates the effect of high doses of thyroxine on intestinal water transport either directly or via stimulation of adenylate cyclase activity.[22] It is, therefore, possible that the salutory effect of propranolol on the diarrhea observed in patients with thyrotoxicosis may be secondary to interference with the adenylate cyclase system or prostaglandins; there are no data either to support or refute this hypothesis.

The Esophagus
In a recent study of β-blockade on the esophagus in man, intravenous propranolol (2 mg) was shown to induce a significant increase in lower sphincter pressure and a rise in the amplitude and duration of esophageal peristalsis.[23]

Gastric Emptying
The effect of β-adrenoreceptor agonists and antagonists on the gastric emptying of a solid meal labeled with indium-113 was examined by Rees et al. in healthy volunteers and patients with hypertension.[24] Isoproterenol given sublingually 30 minutes before the meal prolonged the gastric emptying time. This effect of isoproterenol was blocked by propranolol in a dosage of 40 mg four times daily, administered for 1 week prior to testing. Moreover, ten subjects given only propranolol 40 mg four times daily for 1 week were shown to have significantly shortened gastric emptying times. These data suggest that normal gastric emptying may depend to some degree on adrenergic stimulation.

GASTRIC ACID SECRETION AND GASTRIN

Numerous studies on the existence of adrenergic gastric receptors and their role in the regulation of acid secretion have been reported, albeit with varying results. Bass and Patterson reported that α- and β-agonists and antagonists reduce gastric secretion in the pylorus-ligated rat model.

The inhibitory effect of α-antagonists on acid secretion was attributed to a catecholamine release phenomenon while the similar effect of the β-receptor antagonists was ascribed to the sympathomimetic effects (partial agonism) possessed by the latter, e.g., dichloroisoproterenol and pronethalol. The mechanisms whereby α- and β-agonists effect their inhibitory actions are unknown, although alterations of the synthesis, storage, release, metabolism, or uptake of body catecholamines by a systemic means or by a local mechanism restricted to the gastric mucosa have been postulated.[25] Misher et al. studied the effects of various adrenergic agonists and antagonists on gastric secretion in rats with chronic gastric cannulae. Isoproterenol markedly reduced secretory volume and acid output for 2 hours after its administration. Phenylephrine produced a biphasic response with an increase in volume and acid output in the first hour after drug administration and a decrease during the second hour. Propranolol, in doses that blocked the β-receptors, did not significantly alter basal gastric secretion, suggesting that the β-adrenergic receptor does not have a role in regulating basal secretion in the rat.[26] Conflicting data were reported by Danhof and Geume in pylorus and cardiac ligated rats where propranolol significantly inhibited the gastric acid secretion and also protected the rats against formation of gastric ulceration.[27] In further contrast, Curwain et al. demonstrated that propranolol enhanced gastric acid secretion in response to pentagastrin in the dog.[28] The discrepancies seen in these studies may be secondary to species difference, drug dosage, route of drug administration, or variations in experimental techniques.

The effect of β-adrenergic blockade upon gastric acid secretion and gastrin secretion has been studied in humans by Kronborg et al., who in evaluating 29 patients with insulin-induced hypoglycemia before and after vagotomy found that propranolol slightly decreased insulin-stimulated acid secretion before and 2 to 3 months after vagotomy. Serum levels of gastrin following the administration of insulin were lower after propranolol than those levels following placebo, but the difference achieved statistical significance only in the fasting state and 45 minutes after the administration of insulin. The inhibition of insulin-stimulated acid secretion was preceded by a decrease in serum gastrin level, suggesting that the effect on acid secretion is mediated via gastrin.[29] It is also possible that the depression of serum gastrin levels by propranolol may be due to inhibition of beta-adrenergic stimulation of the antrum. This latter concept is supported by experiments demonstrating a relationship between catecholamines and gastrin. In one such report, plasma gastrin levels were found to be elevated in two patients with pheochromocytoma.[30] This led investigators to measure plasma gastrin levels in dogs during an infusion of epinephrine, an experiment that demonstrated that gastrin levels rose.[31] Stadil and Rehfeld showed that, in man, small doses of adrenaline resulted in a significant rise in both serum gastrin concentration and gastric acid secretion while prior β-blockade suppressed these effects.[32] The physiologic role that β-adrenergic receptors play in secretion of gastrin was studied by Bransborg et al., who compared secretion of gastrin in response to β-adrenergic receptor stimulation (isoproterenol) and a test meal in normal subjects and duodenal ulcer patients. These investigators demonstrated an exaggerated response of gastrin secretion to beta-adrenergic receptor stimulation in patients with duodenal ulcer disease as compared to normal subjects. This increase response of gastrin was not specific for β-adrenergic receptor stimulation because meal-stimulated gastrin secretion was also increased in the same patients. It was also apparent that the mechanisms for hyperresponsiveness of gastrin in the patients with duodenal ulcer differed with the stimulus—propanolol completely inhibited isoproterenol-stimulated gastrin secretion but had significantly less of an effect on meal-stimulated gastrin secretion.[33] Although it is probable that β-receptors play a physiologic role in the regulation of gastric acid secretion, at present there is no evidence that beta-adrenergic receptor stimulation plays an important part in the hypersecretion of gastrin that may be seen in patients with duodenal ulcer.

POSTGASTRECTOMY HYPOGLYCEMIA

Leichter and Permutt studied the effects of phenylephrine and propranolol administration in 10 patients with postgastrectomy hypoglycemia. Oral administration of phenylephrine elixir (15 mg) 30 minutes before an oral glucose tolerance test significantly raised plasma glucose levels when compared to the glucose levels seen without the phenylephrine elixir; there was no accompanying effect, however, on either early or late symptoms of hypoglycemia and thus, any statements regarding the clinical relevance of these observations must await further study.

In contrast, propranolol (10 mg) raised the lowest plasma glucose from 37.5 ± 2.8 to 57 ± 5.2 mg/dl and prevented the occurrence of early and late symptoms of hypoglycemia. Insulin levels were unaffected by either phenylephrine or propranolol. Any statements regarding the clinical relevance of these observations must await studies that examine the feasibility of long-term propranolol for postgastrectomy hypoglycemia.[34]

SMALL BOWEL SECRETION

The effect of propranolol on various models for the study of intestinal secretion is being evaluated with increasing interest but with disparate results. Taub et al. studied the ability of commercially available propranolol (*d,l*-propranolol) to inhibit cholera enterotoxin (choleragen)-stimulated secretion of the rabbit jejunum and were unable to show any influence of propranolol pretreatment on the resultant secretion.[35] In the rat, however, Donowitz and Charney were able to show a significant reduction in choleragen-induced ileal water and electrolyte secretion when the rats were pretreated with *d,l*-propranolol, a preparation with a thousandfold greater pharmacologic potency than *d*-propranolol (a membrane-active isomer without β-adrenergic properties); pretreatment with *d*-propranolol did not affect choleragen-induced ileal net water secretion. Treatment with *d,l*-propranolol did not alter the choleragen-induced increase in adenylate cyclase activity or cyclic AMP, which suggests that this action of propranolol is stereospecific and related to its β-receptor blocking properties but not associated with inhibition of adenylate cyclase or increase in cAMP content in the choleragen model. It has been suggested that propranolol may involve the intestinal secretory process after activation of adenylate cyclase.[36] Side effects, including bradycardia and hypotension, which would almost certainly accompany the dose of *d,l*-propranolol needed to inhibit intestinal secretion suggest that it will not be a clinically useful antisecretory agent. Further work on the relationship of β-blockers and intestinal secretion is obviously warranted.

LARGE BOWEL SECRETION

Increases in colonic secretion have been documented when the colon is exposed to high concentrations of bile acids (cholorrheic enteropathy) or fatty acids (fatty acid diarrhea). Studies in the rat, rabbit, and human strongly suggest that diarrhea stimulated by bile acid and fatty acid is mediated by the cAMP system via adenylate cyclase.[37-40] Propranolol has been shown to prevent the stimulation of adenyl cyclase by deoxycholic acid and 9' 10-hydroxystearic acid[38] in histologically normal human colonic mucosa obtained from patients undergoing left hemicolectomy. In the rabbit, propranolol was also demonstrated to be an effective inhibitor of net colonic secretion. However, the actions of propranolol on the deoxycholic acid-induced adenyl cyclase stimulation was not reversible by catecholamines, suggesting that the stimulation of secretion by the bile acids and fatty acids was independent of catechol-amine influence.[39]

The ability of propranolol to block cholera toxin stimulated colonic secretion in the rat was evaluated by Donowitz et al., who showed that, as in the ileum, pretreatment with d, l-propranolol completely prevented the choleragen-induced secretion.[36]

Thus, propranolol is an inhibitor of cAMP-induced secretion regardless of the stimulus causing increased cAMP activity. Further studies to elucidate the potential clinical application of this observation are needed before propranolol can be utilized in states such as bile acid–induced diarrhea.[41]

ABSORPTION

The pharmacodynamic properties of the β-adrenergic blocking agents have been reviewed before; however, a few aspects are worth emphasizing from the gastrointestinal viewpoint.[1]

The beta-adrenergic nervous system has been shown to play a role in the intestinal transport of electrolytes and amino acids. In vitro studies by Kinzie et al. using rat jejunum showed that epinephrine and isoproterenol stimulated the uptake of amino acids and that this stimulation was blocked by propranolol. They also provided evidence that this β-adrenergic stimulated uptake of amino acids is cAMP mediated and a function of the cells at the intestinal villus tip.[41]

Morris and Turnberg used a triple lumen perfusion technique in humans to demonstrate that intravenous isoproterenol significantly increased jejunal and ileal absorption of sodium chloride and water, and increased ileal absorption of potassium. β-Blockade with intravenous propranolol significantly reduced jejunal electrolye absorption and induced secretion of ileal water and sodium. The observed change in absorption induced by propranolol was not accompanied by any obvious change in small bowel motility.[42]

Intriguing work by Parsons on the absorption of oral propranolol in patients with celiac disease has suggested that increased plasma levels of this agent occur in this malabsorptive disease. In 13 patients with celiac disease, an increased mean plasma propranolol concentration was found in all when compared to control patients. The highest levels of propranolol were seen in those patients not on a gluten-free diet, whereas those on a gluten-free diet had levels not significantly different from controls.[43] Schneider et al. studied propranolol absorption in Crohn's disease as well as in celiac disease.[44] Eight patients with celiac disease in remission on a gluten-free diet and 10 patients with Crohn's disease were each given 40 mg of propranolol orally. Blood samples were taken before the test, every half hour afterwards for 2 hours and at 4 and 6 hours after administration of the drug. Mean plasma propranolol levels in the treated celiac patients were higher than in controls during the first 4 hours, but actually lower at 6 hours. The difference in plasma propranolol concentration was significant only at 1 hour after drug administration. The authors felt this difference was due to the peak levels being reached earlier in the patients than in the controls; there was no statistically significant difference between the peak levels of the patients with celiac disease and the controls. In patients with Crohn's disease, after the first hour of propranolol administration, plasma levels of that drug were significantly raised compared to controls. The higher values seemed to correlate with an increased activity of disease as judged by an elevated erythrocyte sedimentation rate. The relevance of these observations to the usual multiple dosing regimens used with the drug remains to be clinically tested in both celiac and Crohn's disease.[44]

PANCREATICOBILIARY SYSTEM

Studies of the effects of a pure β-adrenergic receptor stimulant, isoproterenol, on pancreatic secretion have helped provide evidence for the presence and significance of the β-receptor in the pancreas. Isoproterenol has been shown to be an effective inhibitor of basal- and cholecystokinin (CCK)-stimulated pancreatic electrolyte and enzyme secretion in dogs.[45] Propranolol blocks the inhibitory action of isoproterenol, suggesting that isoproterenol inhibition of CCK-stimulated pancreatic secretion is mediated through a β-adrenergic mechanism.[46] However, the importance of species variation in such experiments is demonstrated by a study using isoproterenol to stimulate β-pancreatic receptors in the rat; there isoproterenol-induced pancreatic secretion was only slightly inhibited by propranolol.[47]

Crema et al., by utilizing a new method that permits the separate evaluation of the behavior of the choledochus and duodenum, have confirmed the existence of α- and β-receptors within the terminal bile duct of the guinea pig; the former receptor causes choledochal constriction and the latter choledochal dilatation. With the increasing use of endoscopic retrograde pancreaticobiliary tract manometry, the effects of β-blockers on the motility of the pancreaticobiliary system will certainly be studied in a more satisfactory manner.[48]

INTESTINAL VASCULAR ADRENERGIC RECEPTORS

β-Adrenergic receptors have been demonstrated in the intestinal vasculature of the rat, cat, dog, and man.[49-52] The human splanchnic circulation is influenced both by α-receptors, which mediate vasoconstriction, and β-receptors, which mediate vasodilatation.[52] Intraarterial infusion of epinephrine produces splanchnic vascular constriction, which is the net result of both its vasoconstrictive (α) and vasodilatory (β) properties. Wilson and coworkers postulated that if the vasodilatory properties were eliminated by the administration of a β-antagonist such as propranolol, the vasoconstrictive effect of epinephrine should be enhanced.[53] In support of this hypothesis, superior mesenteric artery (SMA) flow was reduced to 50 percent of control flow with an infusion of 0.475 mg/kg per minute of epinephrine, and to a maximum reduction in flow of 18.2 percent of the control flow with 1.9 mg/kg per minute of epinephrine. Following propranolol injection, the effect of epinephrine infusion of SMA blood flow was markedly enhanced. Thus, β-blockade produced a 50 percent decrease in SMA flow at an epinephrine infusion rate of only 0.075 mg/kg per minute, and a maximum reduction to 9.9 percent of the base flow was obtained with an infusion rate of 0.830 mg/kg per minute. Without β-blockade, 3.5 times more epinephrine was required to achieve an 80 percent reduction of base SMA flow. The authors concluded that SMA infusion of epinephrine following β-adrenergic blockade with propranolol is an effective pharmacologic means of reducing splanchnic blood flow. Rosch et al. have successfully used a selective intraarterial infusion of propranolol and epinephrine to treat six patients with acute gastrointestinal bleeding which could be demonstrated angiographically. Bleeding was secondary to diverticulosis in three patients, telangiectasias in two, and granulomatous colitis in one. In all six patients, bleeding was successfully controlled.[54]

Right hepatic artery infusion of epinephrine and propranolol has been successfully used to treat a patient with hemobilia secondary to a percutaneous liver biopsy.[55] Although propranolol in combination with epinephrine is not presently preferred over vasopressin as the angiographic treatment of choice for gastrointestinal bleeding, the preceding observation demonstrates the physiologic presence of adrenergic receptors in the intestinal vasculature and the potential use of beta-blockade as part of a vasoconstrictive regimen.

Lebrec et al. studied the effect of oral propranolol on portal hypertension and recurrent gastrointestinal bleeding in cirrhotic patients. In this group of patients, doses of propranolol that reduced heart rate by 25 percent produced a sustained decrease in portal venous pressure.[56]

This latter observation was then extended by the same investigators in a controlled study evaluating the role of oral propranolol in the prevention of recurrent bleeding from varices or gastric erosions in patients with cirrhosis and relatively good liver function. In their most recently published experience, which included 74 adult patients, among 38 patients who received propranolol only 1 patient rebled whereas among the 36 patients in the placebo group 16 rebled. Undesirable effects were not observed in any of the patients receiving propranolol. Thus, continuous oral administration of propranolol at doses reducing the heart rate by 25 percent was found to be useful for the prevention of recurrent gastrointestinal bleeding from varices or gastritis in patients with cirrhosis.[57]

MUCOSAL PROLIFERATION

The relationship of adrenoreceptor activity to cell proliferation was first examined by Von Naam and Cappel using fibroblasts,[58] although, subsequently, influence of adrenoreceptor activity on cell proliferation has been studied using a variety of systems. Epifanova and Tchoumak showed that following the intraperitoneal injection of epinephrine in the mouse, there was a diminution in the number of mitoses seen in the duodenal crypts of Leiberkuhn.[59] After the demonstration that the intestinal crypts had a rich adrenergic innervation, Tutton and Helme examined the influence of adrenoreceptor activity on crypt cell proliferation in the rat jejunum.[60,61] α- And β-adrenergic agonists were shown to have opposing effects on crypt cell proliferation, the α-system accelerating crypt cell proliferation and the β-system inhibiting proliferation.[62] These investigators also studied the effect of β-adrenergic blockade on crypt cell proliferation under conditions of stress felt to inhibit crypt cell proliferation possibly by increasing the adrenal output of epinephrine. In one study they showed that propranolol treatment of stressed rats significantly accelerated crypt cell proliferation when compared to a similar group of rats not treated with β-blockers.[63] Further characterization of the relationship of mucosal proliferation and stress ulceration are needed, although it is exciting to consider β-blockers as potentially useful agents in the prevention and treatment of stress ulcers.

ADVERSE GASTROINTESTINAL EFFECTS OF β-ADRENERGIC THERAPY

In four major reports, mild gastrointestinal disturbances (anorexia, nausea, vomiting, diarrhea, abdominal pain) have been seen to complicate the use of propranolol and other β-blockers. Stephen summarized the adverse reactions to oral propranolol based on reports to the manufacturer from 130 investigators.[64] Of 1500 patients estimated to have been treated with the drug, nausea occurred in 1 percent and diarrhea in 0.5 percent. Greenblatt and Koch-Weser surveyed 23 published studies in which a total of 797 patients were treated with oral propranolol for periods ranging from a few weeks to 6 years.[65] Gastrointestinal disturbances were the most common adverse reactions in these 797 patients, and were reported in 89 (11.2 percent). Zacharias reviewed the side effects of propranolol in 400 patients observed over a 10-year period and found only one patient requiring withdrawal of the drug because of diarrhea.[66] In the Boston Collaborative Drug Surveillance Program involving 268 hospitalized patients on propranolol, Greenblatt and Koch-Weser reported no incidence of diarrhea.[67] Gastrointestinal side effects observed with the eight β-blockers approved or about to be approved for use in the United States (propranolol, metoprolol, nadolol, atenolol, timolol, pindolol, labetalol, oxprenolol) are shown in Table 2. There are no significant differences between drugs with regard to gastrointestinal side effects and rarely is treatment discontinued for these reasons. In our extensive experience of more than 700 patients treated with various β-blockers, the incidence of gastrointestinal side effects was less than 1 percent (unpublished).

SCLEROSING PERITONITIS RELATED TO THE USE OF BETA-ADRENERGIC BLOCKING AGENTS

Practolol, one of the first generation of selective β_1-adrenergic blockers, was reported to induce an oculomucocutaneous syndrome[68] and sclerosing peritonitis.[69] Subsequent to those reports, approximately 40 cases of sclerosing peritonitis associated with the use of β-blockers have been reported in the English literature.[70–74] Sclerosing peritonitis has been observed almost exclusively in patients who have received practolol either

TABLE 2. GASTROINTESTINAL SIDE EFFECTS ASSOCIATED WITH BETA-ADRENERGIC BLOCKING THERAPY IN CARDIOVASCULAR DISEASE (IN ORDER OF FREQUENCY)

Diarrhea
Dyspepsia
Nausea
Flatulence
Abdominal pain
Constipation

alone or with other β-blockers such as propranolol or oxprenolol; in two patients, use of propranolol alone was associated with sclerosing peritonitis.[73,74] In three major series comprising 25 patients with sclerosing peritonitis associated with β-blocker therapy, the major symptoms reported were abdominal pain, vomiting, and weight loss. One important feature of this association is that symptoms of peritonitis may have their onset months after the cessation of β-blocker therapy. On physical examination, 76 percent of patients had an abdominal mass representing multiple loops of matted bowel. Abdominal distention was observed in 36 percent of patients. Ascites has only been reported once in this entity and the cell count of that fluid contained 8000 cells/cm^3, most of which were lymphocytes. Skin or eye involvement commonly marked the onset of the syndrome. In almost all patients with this syndrome, however, other organs are involved in addition to the peritoneum. These include the eye (xeropthalmia with or without corneal ulceration), skin (rash), lung (parenchymal lung involvement), and pleura (pleuritis accompanied by pleural effusion).

Roentgenologic examination of these patients showed evidence of an adhesive peritonitis, with fixation, separation, and dilatation of small bowel loops. Intestinal dilatation was quite marked and was usually extensive, with from one-third to all the small bowel affected. Most patients had evidence of incomplete small bowel obstruction, with profound delay in transit through the small bowel; complete obstruction to the flow of barium has uncommonly been demonstrated.[72] Because of progressive small bowel obstruction, laparotomy was necessitated in almost all cases. At laparotomy, gross thickening of the parietal and visceral peritoneum and dense adhesions with obliteration of the peritoneal cavity were noted. The peritoneum over the small bowel tended to be more involved than that over the large bowel and "cocooning" of the small bowel in saclike adhesions was commonly described. Retroperitoneal structures were usually normal in these cases when described.[68,69,71] Surgical therapy consisted of lysis of adhesions or peritoneal stripping with release of the underlying bowel. The short-term follow-up of patients surgically treated has shown remission of symptoms and some weight gain; however, the caliber of the small bowel and abnormal roentgenologic pattern persisted. Histologic examination of the fibrotic tissues removed at surgery shows fibrosis of the peritoneum with focal lymphocytic inflammatory infiltrates.

The mechanism by which practolol induces these changes is unknown. Of relevance are the studies by Smith and Butler on the long-term effects of propranolol in mice, in which intestinal abnormalities were demonstrated in 6 of 25 animals.[75] The earliest abnormality was observed in the serosal cells, the nuclei of which became hyperplastic and plump. A few macrophages became adherent to each other, and, in two animals, duodenal and colonic serosal granulomas developed. With practolol no longer being used, fibrosing peritonitis due to β-blockers has all but vanished. Whether the newer generation β-blockers have the potential to induce this side effect remains to be seen.

INTERACTION WITH GASTROINTESTINAL DRUGS

Recently, investigators have examined the pharmacologic interactions of propranolol with the widely used H$_2$ receptor antagonist, cimetidine.[76] Chronic cimetidine therapy (300 mg four times a day for 7 days) in normal subjects caused a reduction in liver blood flow as well as an inhibition of hepatic drug–metabolizing enzymes, thereby resulting in a reduction of the clearance of intravenously administered propranolol and a reduction in the elimination of oral propranolol. The physiologic relevance of these findings was demonstrated by the markedly lower resting pulse rates after propranolol plus cimetidine than after propranolol alone.

CONCLUSION

There is a growing experience emphasizing the importance of the sympathetic nervous system in gastrointestinal physiologic regulation, and β-adrenergic blocking drugs will undoubtedly play an important role in patient management and in our understanding of multiple gastrointestinal disorders. There are already specific entities for which β-blockers represent a potentially useful mode of therapy, e.g., variceal bleeding, and the future will certainly bring others. The exact therapeutic role for β-adrenergic blockade in gastrointestinal disorders will be better defined as laboratory and clinical experiences continue to accumulate.

REFERENCES

1. Frishman WH: β-Adrenoceptor antagonists—new drugs and new indications. N Engl J Med 305:500, 1981.
2. McMurphy DM, Boreus LO: Pharmacology of the human fetus: Adrenergic receptor function in the small intestine. Biol Neonate 13:325, 1968.
3. Hart SL, Mir MS: Adrenoreceptors in the human foetal small intestine. Br J Pharmacol 41:567, 1971.

4. Reddy V, Moran NC: An evaluation of the adrenergic receptor types in isolated segments of the small intestine of the rabbit. Arch Int Pharmacodyn Ther 1976:326, 1968.

5. Van Rossum JM, Mujic M: Classification of sympathomimetic drugs of the rabbit intestine. Arch Int Pharmacodyn Ther 155:418, 1965.

6. Norberg KA: Adrenergic innervation of the intestinal wall studied by fluorescence microscopy. Int J Neuropharmacol 3:379, 1964.

7. Diksnit BB: Acetylcholine formation by tissues. Q J Exp Physiol 28:243, 1938.

8. Blair MR, Clark BB: An evaluation of the action of substance P on the jejunum of the rabbit. J Pharmacol Exp Ther 117:467, 1956.

9. Innes IR, Kosterlitz HW, Robinson JA: The effects of lowering the bath temperature on the responses of the isolated guinea pig ileum. J Physiol (Lond) 137:396, 1957.

10. Day M, Vane JR: An analysis of the direct and indirect actions on the isolated guinea pig ileum. Br J Pharmacol 20:150, 1963.

11. Green JP, Carlini EA: The presence in sciatic nerve of material that releases acetylcholine. J Pharmacol Exp Ther 143:96, 1964.

12. Lum BKB, Kermani MH, Heilman RD: Intestinal relaxation produced by sympathomimetic amines in the isolated rabbit jejunum: Selective inhibition by adrenergic blocking agents and by cold storage. J Pharmacol Exp Ther 154:463, 1966.

13. Rosen OM, Erlichman J, Rosen SM: The structure activity relationships of adrenergic compounds that act on the adenyl cyclase of the frog erythrocyte. Mol Pharmacol 6:524, 1970.

14. Ruoff HJ: Rat gastric mucosal cAMP and cGMP after adrenergic stimulation and blockade. Eur J Pharmacol 44:349, 1977.

15. Burges RA, Blackburn KJ: Adenyl cyclase and the differentiation of β-adrenoreceptors. Nature 235:249, 1972.

16. Gagnon DJ, Belisle S: Stimulatory effects of catecholamines on the isolated rat colon after beta-adrenergic blockade with oxprenolol and propranolol. Eur J Pharmacol 12:303, 1970.

17. Gagnon DJ, Devboede G, Belisle S: Excitatory effects of adrenaline upon isolated preparations of human colon. Gut 13:654, 1972.

18. Hart SL, Mir MS: Adrenoreceptors in the human foetal colon. Br J Pharmacol 42:662P, 1971.

19. Smith J, Kelly KA, Weinshilboum RM: Pathophysiology of postoperative ileus. Arch Surg 112:203, 1977.

20. Stasiewicz J, Szalaj W, Chmielewski J, Gabryelewicz A: Effect of propranolol on the intestinal peristalsis in thyroxine treated mice. Endocrinol Exp 6:87, 1972.

21. Thomas FB, Caldwell JH: Steatorrhea in thyrotoxicosis: Relation to hypermotility and excessive dietary fat. Ann Intern Med 78:669, 1973.

22. Ligumsky M, Karmeli F, Rachmilewitz D: Pathogenesis of diarrhea in thyrotoxicosis: Effect of throxine on rat intestinal fluid transport, mucosal

PGE$_2$ content, Na-K-ATPase and adenyl cyclase activities. (Abstr). Gastroenterology 78:1208, 1980.

23. Thorpe JAC: Effect of propranolol on the lower oesophageal sphincter in man. Curr Med Res Opin 7:91, 1980.

24. Rees MR, Clark RA, Noldsworth CD, et al: The effect of β-adrenoreceptor agonists and antagonists on gastric emptying in man. Br J Clin Pharmacol 10:551, 1980.

25. Bass P, Patterson MA: Gastric secretory responses to drugs affecting adrenergic mechanisms in rats. J Pharmacol Exp Ther 156:142, 1967.

26. Misner A, Pendleton RG, Staples R: Effects of adrenergic drugs upon gastric secretion in rats. Gastroenterology 57:294, 1969.

27. Danhof IE, Geumei A: Effect of propranolol on gastric acid secretion in rats. Br J Pharmacol 46:170, 1972.

28. Curwain BP, Nolton P, Spencer J: Enhancement by propranolol of gastric acid secretion in response to pentagastrin in conscious dogs. Br J Pharmacol 48:341P, 1973.

29. Kronborg O, Pederson T, Stadil F, Rehfeld JF: The effect of β-adrenergic blockade upon gastric acid secretion and gastrin secretion during hypoglycemia before and after vagotomy. Scand J Gastroenterol 9:173, 1974.

30. Hayes JR, Ardill J, Kennedy TL, et al: Stimulation of gastrin release by catecholamines. Lancet 1:819, 1972.

31. Hayes JR, Ardill J, Shanks RG, Buchanan KD: Effect of catecholamines on gastrin release. Metabolism 27:385, 1978.

32. Stadil F, Rehfeld JF: Release of gastrin by epinephrine in man. Gastroenterology 65:210, 1973.

33. Brandsborg O, Brandsborg M, Christensen NJ: The role of the β-adrenergic receptor in the secretion of gastrin: studies in normal subjects and in patients with duodenal ulcers. Eur J Clin Invest 6:395, 1976.

34. Leichter SB, Permutt MA: Effect of adrenergic agents on post-gastrectomy hypoglycemia. Diabetes 24:1005, 1975.

35. Taub M, Bonorris GG, Chung A, et al: Effect of propranolol on bile acid cholera enterotoxin-stimulated cAMP and secretion in rabbit intestine. Gastroenterology 72:101, 1977.

36. Donowitz M, Charney AN, Hynes R: Propranolol prevention of cholera enterotoxin-induced intestinal secretion in the rat. Gastroenterology 76:482, 1979.

37. Binder JH, Filburn C, Volpe BT: Bile salt alteration of colonic electrolyte transport: Role of cyclic adenosine monophosphate. Gastroenterology 68:503, 1975.

38. Coyne MJ, Bonorris GG, Chung A, et al: Propanolol inhibits bile acid and fatty acid stimulation of cyclic AMP in human colon. Gastroenterology 73:971, 1977.

39. Coyne MJ, Bonorris GG, Chung A, et al: Inhibition by propranolol of bile acid stimulation of rabbit colonic adenylate cyclase in vitro. Gastoenterology 71:68, 1976.

40. Conley D, Coyne M, Chung A, et al: Propranolol inhibits adenylate cyclase and secretion stimulated by deoxycholic acid in the rabbit colon. Gastroenterology 71:72, 1976.

41. Kinzie JL, Grimme NL, Alpers DH: Cyclic AMP dependent amino acid uptake in intestine: the importance of β-adrenergic agonists. Biochem Pharmacol 25:2727, 1976.

42. Morris AI, Turnberg LA: Influence of isoproterenol and propranolol on human intestinal transport in vivo. Gastroenterology 81:1076, 1981.

43. Parsons RL, Trounce JR: Propranolol absorption in Crohn's disease and coeliac disease. Br Med J 1:103, 1977.

44. Schneider RE, Babb J, Bishop H, Mitchard M: Plasma levels of propranolol in treated patients with coeliac disease and patients with Crohn's disease. Br Med J 2:794, 1976.

45. Rudick J, Gonda M, Rosenberg R, et al: Effects of a beta-adrenergic receptor stimulant (isoproterenol) on pancreatic exocrine excretion. Surgery 74:338, 1973.

46. Kelly GA, Rose RC, Nahrwold DL: Characteristics of inhibition of pancreatic secretion by isoproterenol. Surgery 82:680, 1977.

47. Roze C, de la Tour C, Chariot J, et al: Isoproterenol induced pancreatic secretion in rats: a comparison with secretin. Biomedicine (Paris) 24:410, 1976.

48. Crema A, Benzi G, Frigo GM, Berte F: Occurrence of α and β receptors in the bile duct. Proc Soc Exp Biol Med 120:158, 1965.

49. Henrich H, Singbartl G, Biester J: Adrenergic induced vascular adjustments—initial and escape reactions. I. Influence of beta-adrenergic blocking agents on the intestinal circulation of the rat. Pfluegers Arch 346:1, 1974.

50. Ross G: Effects of epinephrine and norepinephrine on the mesenteric circulation of the cat. Am J Physiol 212:1037, 1967.

51. Swan KG, Reynolds DG: Effects of intra-arterial catecholamine infusions on blood flow in the canine gut. Gastroenterology 61:863, 1971.

52. Price HL, Cooperman LH, Warden JC: Control of the splanchnic circulation in man. Role of beta-adrenergic receptors. Circ Res 21:333, 1967.

53. Wilson SE, Bennet G, Winston MA, Jabour A: Potentiation of epinephrine-induced mesenteric vasoconstriction with β-blockade. J Surg Res 23:274, 1977.

54. Rosch J, Dotter CT, Rose RW: Selective arterial infusions of vasoconstrictors in acute gastrointestinal bleeding. Radiology 99:27, 1971.

55. Lee SP, Tasman-Jones C, Wattie WJ: Traumatic hemobilia: a complication of percutaneous liver biopsy. Gastroenterology 72:941, 1977.

56. Lebrec D, Bernau J, Rueff B, et al: Propranolol in prevention of recurrent gastrointestinal bleeding in cirrhotic patients. Lancet 1:920, 1981.

57. Lebrec D, Poynard T, Hillon P, Benhamou JP: Propranolol for prevention of recurrent gastrointestinal bleeding in patients with cirrhosis: a controlled study. N Engl J Med 305:1371, 1981.

58. Von Naam E, Cappel L: Effect of hormones upon cells grown. II. The ef-

fect of hormones from the thyroid, pancreas and adrenal gland. Am J Cancer 39:354, 1940.

59. Epifanova OI, Choumak M: On the action of adrenaline upon the mitotic cycle of intestinal epithelium in mice. Tsitologiia 5:45, 1963.

60. Gabella G, Costa M: Adrenergic fibers in the mucous membrane of guinea-pig alimentary tract. Experientia 24:706, 1968.

61. Tutton PJM, Helme RD: The influence of adrenoreceptor activity on crypt cell proliferation in the rat jejunum. Cell Tissue Kinet 7:125, 1974.

62. Tutton PJM, Helme RD: Stress induced inhibition of jejunal crypt cell proliferation. Virchows Arch Abt B Zellpath 15:23, 1973.

63. Tutton PJM, Helme RD: The role of catecholamines in the regulation of crypt cell proliferation. I. Adrenergic stimulation and blockade. J Anat 116:467, 1973.

64. Stephen SA: Unwanted effects of propranolol. Am J Cardiol 18:463, 1966.

65. Greenblatt DJ, Koch-Weser J: Adverse reactions to β-adrenergic receptor blocking drugs: A report from the Boston Collaborative Drug Surveillance Program. Drugs 7:118, 1974.

66. Zacharias FJ: Patient acceptability of propranolol and the occurrence of side effects. Postgrad Med J 52:87, 1976.

67. Greenblatt DJ, Koch-Weser J: Adverse reactions to propranolol in hospitalized medical patients: a report from the Boston Collaborative Drug Surveillance Program. Am Heart J 86:478, 1973.

68. Eltringham WK, Espinger HJ, Windsor CWO, et al: Sclerosing peritonitis due to practolol: A report on 9 cases and their surgical management. Br J Surg 64:229, 1977.

69. Brown P, Read AE, Baddeley H, et al: Sclerosing peritonitis an unusual reaction to a β-adrenergic blocking drug (practolol). Lancet 2:1477, 1974.

70. Cook AIM, Foy P: Sclerosing peritonitis and practolol therapy. Ann R Coll Surg Engl 58:473, 1976.

71. Marshall AJ, Baddeley H, Barritt DW, et al: Practolol peritonitis. Q J Med 46:135, 1977.

72. Lee REJ, Baddeley H, Marshall AJ, Read AE: Practolol peritonitis. Clin Radiol 28:119, 1977.

73. Harty RF: Sclerosing peritonitis and propranolol. Arch Intern Med 138:1424, 1978.

74. Ahmad S: Sclerosing peritonitis and propranolol. Chest 79:361, 1981.

75. Smith B, Butler M: The effects of long-term propranolol on the salivary glands and intestinal serosa of the mouse. J Pathol 124:185, 1978.

76. Feely J, Wilkinson GR, Wood AJJ: Reduction of liver blood flow and propranolol metabolism by cimetidine. N Engl J Med 304:692, 1981.

CHAPTER 17

β-Adrenoceptor Blockade in Anxiety States: A New Approach to Therapy?

William H. Frishman

Although the early workers in β-adrenergic pharmacology hypothesized that the drugs would be of use in patients with angina pectoris and arrhythmia, they may not have foreseen the wide spectrum of therapeutic indications for these drugs that is now being evaluated.[1] β-Adrenoceptor blocking agents have been found to be efficacious in many neuropsychiatric disorders, endocrine disorders, and in diseases of other organ systems.[1] As a result of the continued inventiveness of clinical investigators there is little doubt that the list of therapeutic applications for β-blockers will continue to grow.

The first psychiatric application of β-adrenergic blockade was reported in 1966 by Granville-Grossman and Turner,[2] who suggested that propranolol might be useful in treating anxiety. The multitude of studies appearing since then have tended to confirm this early suggestion.[3–9] Nevertheless, there are still many unresolved issues concerning the use of β-blockers in treating anxiety, and the U.S. Food and Drug Administration has not yet approved anxiety states as a therapeutic indication for β-blockade. In this chapter, the effects of β-adrenoceptor blockers in the treatment of anxiety will be assessed.

Based on an article which appeared in Cardiovascular Reviews and Reports, Volume 2, pp 447–459, May 1981, with permission.

WHAT IS ANXIETY?

We all have anxiety in our everyday life—work, social situations, family interactions, and even leisure activities may give rise to the vague emotion of anxiety. These anxieties of daily life can legitimately be called normal, and a certain amount of anxiety may be necessary to carry out certain daily functions. However, there may be extremes of this condition. Pathologic anxiety occurs when a person complains of anxiety that is frequent, more severe, and more persistent than he is accustomed to and can tolerate. Some patients describe anxiety symptoms as a change in their emotional status and a departure from their previous normal state. The pathologic state of anxiety constitutes an attack and may qualify as a medical illness. On the other hand, other patients admit to having always been more anxious than their peers. This pathologic high-trait anxiety may indicate an abnormal personality or may be just an extreme of the norm.[10]

The anxiety state refers to anxiety felt at a moment in time—"I feel anxious at this moment"—whereas the anxiety trait refers to a habitual tendency toward anxiety in general—"I often feel anxious." It has been suggested that anxiety, both as a trait and as a syndrome, is strongly influenced by genetic factors, evidence that encourages a biologic approach to the problem. Some properties of subjective anxiety are characteristics but not exclusive of it. Anxiety has an unpleasant quality that can be almost intolerable, and it is a perspective emotion directed toward the future.[10]

Anxiety is a component of many psychiatric states—depression, phobias, obsessive–compulsive disorders, schizophrenia, organic confusional states, epilepsy, and delirium tremens. When anxiety is the major feature of the clinical picture without any other disturbances, the term "anxiety state" is applied. The incidence of anxiety states is estimated to be 2 to 5 percent of the total population and 7 to 16 percent of all psychiatric patients. It appears to be most common in young adults and affects both sexes equally. Despite its prevalence, in recent years anxiety has generally not received the physiologic and biochemical attention in research that the affective disorders and functional phychoses have.[10]

Physiologic and biochemical changes are concomitant to all emotions but are particularly noticeable in anxiety and anger. Psychologic (somatic) symptoms of anxiety include tightness in the throat, difficulty in breathing, sense of constriction in the chest, epigastric discomfort or pain, palpitations, dizziness and weakness, and dryness of the mouth. Tremor, sudden micturition or defecation, vomiting, or sweating may also occur. Many objective measures of the physiologic changes under-lying these symptoms have been made. Pulse rate has been noted to be elevated, forearm blood flow increased, and finger-pulse volume de-creased; sweat gland activity is augmented, salivation is reduced, and muscle activity is markedly raised. Electoencephalograms of anxious patients show a generally increased voltage except in the α-wave band. Such changes are felt to reflect alterations in autonomic activity, mainly increases in sympathetic discharge, particularly of the α-adrenoceptor system. Another psychologic concept related to anxiety is arousal or ac-tivation. When there is a low level of activation or arousal, the subject is asleep or drowsy. On the other hand are extreme emotional stages such as terror and rage, with a high level of activation. Thus, anxiety may be conceived as a behavioral state dependent on, though not suffi-ciently defined by, underlying physiologic arousal.[10]

The extent to which the experience of the physical symptoms of anxiety is due to the direct result of autonomic discharge, particularly sympathetic discharge, has long been a matter of dispute. The James–Lange[11] theory proposed that "the feeling of bodily changes as they oc-cur is the emotion," whereas Cannon[12] considered that bodily changes and the emotion accompanying them both have a common origin in the brain. Sherrington[13] also demonstrated that the intactness of the periph-eral nervous system is not a necessary prerequisite for emotion. In 1964, after reexamining the literature, Breggin[14] concluded that there was evi-dence favoring both points of view. He suggested that sympathetic ac-tivity may generate mental disturbance, particularly if there has been a previously learned association between autonomic and subjective symp-toms. At this juncture, all current models of anxiety are largely specu-lative; the nature of the interaction between mind and body, which leads to the subjective clinical experience of anxiety, requires further study and clarification.

RATIONALE FOR USING β-ADRENOCEPTOR BLOCKING DRUGS IN ANXIETY

There are convincing arguments for the use of β-adrenoceptor blockade in anxiety states. Frohlich and associates[15] administered the β-adrener-gic stimulating drug isoproterenol to three groups of individuals, the first of which had been experiencing palpitations, chest discomfort, and anx-iety without evidence of any organic basis. The second group had had essential hypertension, and the third group consisted of normotensive volunteers. Isoproterenol had a much greater effect on the heart rate and chest discomfort of the first group than it had on the other two groups. Furthermore, about two-thirds of the first group developed severe anxiety. This occurred only when isoproterenol was given, whereas saline had no effect on any of these patients. These investigators concluded that isoproterenol-induced anxiety was secondary to the peripheral stimulation of hypersensitive β-adrenergic receptors. They described their first group as showing a hyperdynamic β-adrenergic circulatory state. And infusion of isoproterenol into anxious individuals without this syndrome failed to produce the dramatic emotional outburst seen in patients with increased β-adrenergic reactivity. Frohlich and his coworkers also demonstrated that β-adrenoceptor blockade with propranolol could control this hyperdynamic adrenergic state and the emotional outburst. This suggested an important role for β-adrenoceptor blocking compounds in treating anxiety syndromes in which heightened sympathetic tone is often seen.

SITES OF ACTION OF β-ADRENOCEPTOR BLOCKING DRUGS: CENTRAL VERSUS PERIPHERAL

It has been shown in animal models that propranolol has some direct actions on the central nervous system.[16] Sufficient dosage of propranolol has sedative, antitremor, and anticonvulsive action.[16] The drug potentiates barbiturate and chlorohydrate sedation and decreases alcohol narcosis.[16] When introduced directly into the brain of experimental animals, propranolol inhibits the central effects of catecholamines.[16] There is also evidence of β-adrenoceptor blocker enhancement of growth hormone secretion and an influence on brain neurotransmitter levels.[16] A limbic system site of action, particularly in the area of amygdala, has been suggested for these agents.[16]

     Various human studies also suggest some degree of direct central action of β-blockers, although the existence of a central β-receptor has not yet been established. Propranolol reportedly has both antipsychotic and psychotogenic effects and can cause toxic psychoses, nightmares, and hallucinations.[16,17] These hallucinations are often hypnagogic and usually visual.[16] Normal subjects receiving single 40 or 80 mg doses of oral d,l-propranolol may exhibit increases in reaction time and impairment in hand–eye coordination.[18] Impaired performance in pursuit–rotor testing, consistent with a central depressant action, has been reported after administration of intravenous oxprenolol. Although the β-blocker practolol does not exhibit selective uptake into the central nervous system, it reportedly can cause depression, vivid dreams, and fatigue.[16]

Clearly, the extent of cerebral uptake need not correlate with potency of central nervous system effects.[16] It has also been suggested that the impairment in reaction time with propranolol might be related to a peripheral effect on muscle motor coordination.[16]

More convincing experimental studies have indicated a primary peripheral rather than a central site of action of β-adrenergic receptor blockers. Sedative effects of propranolol in humans have not been consistently demonstrated.[16] A single 120-mg dose affects neither the sleep of EEG-monitored subjects nor the changes induced by dextroamphetamine and imipramine.[16] Using a wide range of psychomotor function tests, EEG auditory-evoked responses, and mood and bodily symptom ratings, Lader and Tyrer[19] found no consistent central effects of d,l-propranolol (120 mg) or d,l-sotalol (240 mg) in acute dosage in normal subjects.[19] However, a subjective sense of "drowsiness" was observed with sotalol. Both sotalol and propranolol caused subjects to feel more "troubled," suggesting a dysphoric effect.[16] In a double-blind crossover pilot study, d-propranolol (40 mg per day), which passes into the brain but lacks β-blocking activity, had no significant antianxiety effects compared with placebo, according to investigator ratings.[20] Other β-blockers with less brain uptake have antianxiety effects similar to those produced by propranolol. This suggests that peripheral β-adrenergic blockade is the primary mode of action of d,l-propranolol in decreasing anxiety. Most of these studies suffer from methodologic difficulties, since investigators tend to focus their ratings on the autonomically mediated symptoms of anxiety, not taking into consideration effects of mood. Tyrer and Lader[21,22] concluded that β-blockers have a place in the treatment of certain patients with anxiety, but as an adjunct rather than as the sole therapy.

Additional studies imply that propranolol, in contrast to diazepam, lacks central antianxiety actions. Normal subjects who were given a single dose of d,l-propranolol (120 mg), d-propranolol (120 mg), diazepam (6 mg), or placebo, and who were exposed to anxiety-provoking situations, were studied by performances tests, subjective mood scales, EEG- and auditory-evoked responses, finger tremor, and other physiologic measurements. Although adequate β-blockade was reportedly achieved, neither d,l- nor d-propranolol showed any beneficial effect on mood or evidence of sedation in contrast to diazepam.[23] Also, d,l-propranolol was not preferred to the d-isomer. Thus, in normal subjects, propranolol appears to lack significant central antianxiety effects at the dosage administered. The same investigators similarly studied chronically anxious patients, six with somatic manifestations of anxiety and six with psychic (experimental or subjective) anxiety, using d,l-propranolol, diazepam, and placebo, but now with a flexible dosage.[24] Again, findings confirmed that diazepam has a predominant central action and propranolol mainly a peripheral one.[24] Propranolol reduced pulse rate and finger tremor in cases in which it was beneficial. In a related report using patient and psychiatrist ratings of anxiety, these investigators found diazepam (a mean dose of 9.6 mg per day) more effective than propranolol (mean dose 120 mg per day) or placebo in relieving anxiety. Propranolol was more effective than placebo and was comparable to diazepam in patients with somatic manifestations of anxiety, but not in those with primarily psychic anxiety.[6] Patients with psychic anxiety preferred placebo to propranolol, perhaps because of undesirable peripheral or central effects of propranolol. These contrasts with diazepam are of interest since propranolol in a conflict experiment with rodents seemed similar to another benzodiazepine, chlordiazepoxide.[16] In another, double-blind crossover placebo-controlled trial of propranolol (160 mg per day) in patients with neurotic anxiety of thyrotoxicosis, Ramsay and colleagues[25] were unable to demonstrate any alterations in psychic anxiety using clinical ratings and psychologic testing.

Finally, Stone and coworkers[26] administered 60 mg of propranolol or placebo orally in divided doses to 24 healthy nonanxious male subjects during a 24-hour period prior to experimental stress procedures. Significantly lower initial anxiety levels were observed in the propranolol group as measured from speech samples and as correlated with plasma free–fatty acid levels. However, a stress interview increased anxiety scores to comparable levels in both groups. The investigators concluded that propranolol produces antianxiety effects in situations in which there is no acute stress. In another report, the same investigators elaborate on peripheral versus central mechanisms to account for their findings.[27]

In summary, it appears that although β-blockers may have central actions, it is likely that the antianxiety effects of β-adrenoceptor blockade are related to peripheral mechanisms. The relatively lipid-insoluble β-blockers, which enter the brain in relatively small concentrations, are effective against anxiety.[9,16] The effects of β-blockers on anxiety are probably unrelated to the membrane depressant properties that some of those agents manifest; the d-isomer of propranolol, which has membrane activity and no β-blocking properties, is ineffective in treating anxiety.[16] The β-blocker sotalol, which lacks membrane properties, has been shown to be effective in anxiety syndromes.[22] Practolol, which demonstrates β₁-selectivity, has been shown to affect the peripheral manifestations of anxiety comparably to propranolol.[9,16] The pharmacologic differences between those β-blocking drugs that have been shown to be useful in anxiety are illustrated in Table 1. It appears that

TABLE 1. PHARMACOLOGIC PROPERTIES OF β-ADRENOCEPTOR BLOCKING DRUGS USED IN ANXIETY

Drug	β_1-Selective	ISA*	Lipid Soluble
Alprenolol	−	+	+
Oxprenolol	−	+	+
Practolol	+	+	−
Propranolol	−	−	+
Sotalol	−	−	−

*Intrinsic sympathomimetic activity (partial agonist activity)

β_1-selective agents, nonselective agents, lipophilic agents, nonlipophilic agents, and drugs with and without intrinsic sympathomimetic activity are all equally effective in anxiety syndromes.

ANTIANXIETY EFFECTS OF β-ADRENOCEPTOR BLOCKADE: SOMATIC VERSUS PSYCHIC

Human studies using β-adrenoceptor blocking drugs in the treatment of anxiety cover a spectrum of disorders and states that include chronic anxiety, psychocardiac disorders, stress responses or situational anxiety, organic and addictive states, and schizophrenia.[16] A number of studies have demonstrated that propranolol can reduce somatic manifestations of anxiety in humans, such as tachycardia, palpitations, sweating, diarrhea, and tremor.[2,4,9,22,26] In contrast, studies indicating beneficial effects on psychic anxiety have been methodologically unsatisfactory.[16] It would appear that although propranolol improves some of the peripheral somatic manifestations of anxiety, there is no consistent evidence of its efficacy in relieving psychic anxiety.[16]

Suzman[4] studied 513 patients with "uncomplicated anxiety" using propranolol in flexible doses (40 to 300 mg per day) on a long-term single-blind basis and found overall improvement with propranolol and an 88 percent relapse rate with placebo.[4] Improvement occurred in muscular weakness and tremors, shakiness, fatigue, breathlessness, palpitations, tendency to hyperventilate and sigh, headache, and functional gastrointestinal and urologic symptoms. Effects on edema and excessive sweating were less constant, and vasospastic disturbances of the extremities tended to be aggravated. Improvement was also observed in nervousness, agitation, irritability, insomnia, weeping spells, nocturnal panic states, and depression and fear associated with somatic symptoms. There was little beneficial effect on phobic or obsessive–compulsive traits. Propranolol also prevented the appearance of symptoms and electrocardiographic changes during voluntary hyperventilation. Suzman[4] found that higher dosage could also control the more severe psychic symptoms.

In a general practice study, Wheatley[3] compared propranolol and an anxiolytic drug of proven efficacy, chlordiazepoxide. One hundred and five patients were treated for 6 weeks under full double-blind conditions, 51 with propranolol (30 mg three times daily) and 54 with chlordiazepoxide (10 mg three times daily). No difference was detected between the drugs except that chlordiazepoxide was found to be more effective in alleviating depression and sleep disturbance. The patients' ratings revealed that both drugs were beneficial after 1 week of treatment. After 6 weeks of treatment, proportional improvement was better with chlordiazepoxide, although this difference was not statistically significant. As noted by Whitlock and Price,[28] Wheatley's study suffers from the lack of a placebo group. In a 2-week double-blind crossover study of propranolol (up to 600 mg per day), Kellner and colleagues[24] found no significant "short-term" antianxiety effects of propranolol, although there was a trend toward a superiority over placebo.

It appears that β-adrenergic blockade will relieve many of the peripheral or somatic manifestations of anxiety.[29] Psychic manifestations may be indirectly relieved by alleviating the somatic symptoms, lending support to the James–Lange hypothesis.

USE OF β-ADRENERGIC BLOCKING DRUGS IN PSYCHOCARDIAC DISORDERS

β-Adrenergic blocking agents reportedly provide striking improvements in the group of autonomically mediated functional cardiovascular disorders or psychocardiac disorders known by various names, some of which may be distinguishable by physiologic and physical criteria.[16,30] These syndromes are listed in Table 2. The original syndrome, neurocirculatory asthenia, or irritable heart syndrome, is characterized by resting tachycardia, dyspnea, palpitations, exhaustion, marked reduction in work capacity, precordial pain, dizziness, nervousness, tremor, sweating, headache, syncope, sometimes elevated or variable blood pressure, and the absence of readily demonstrable organic disease. In some patients there are systolic ejection clicks noted on physical examination, nonspecific ST–T-wave electrocardiographic changes are seen, and increased cardiac output, increased left ventricular stroke volume, and altered peripheral vascular resistance are demonstrated.[16,30] Sensitivity to

TABLE 2. THE PSYCHOCARDIAC DISORDERS[16]

Da Costa syndrome
Hyperkinetic β-adrenergic circulatory state
Hyperkinetic circulatory state
Hyperkinetic heart syndrome
Neurocirculatory asthenia
Vasoregulatory asthenia
Neurovegetative tachycardia
Nervous heart syndrome
Mitral valve prolapse syndrome
Autonomic imbalance with tachycardia
Cardiac neurosis
Functional heart disorder
Hyperventilation syndrome
Irritable heart syndrome
Soldier's heart
Cardiophobia

isoproterenol is observed in some of these individuals.[15,16] Infusion of this drug produces a syndrome that resembles an acute anxiety attack, with reversal upon infusion of propranolol but not placebo. Although there are no unequivocal controlled studies for β blockers in the treatment of these heart disorders, several reports indicate that β-blocking agents provide an effective and specific treatment for the signs and symptoms of functional cardiac illness, including tachycardia, palpitations, tremor, and systolic hypertension.[15,16,31–39] It has also been shown that β-adrenoceptor blocking drugs will normalize resting and exercise-induced electrocardiographic changes that might be anxiety related, whereas electrocardiographic changes related to ischemic heart disease persist.[5,40] Some investigators have even suggested the use of β-blocker treatment for assessing nonspecific ST-segment and T-wave abnormalities to differentiate them from ischemic causes.[40]

It is of interest that in psychiatric studies in which the "anxiety state" was diagnosed, the reported symptoms were very similar to those seen in patients presenting with a psychocardiac disorder. Table 3 lists the nature and frequency of somatic complaints of patients presenting to the cardiac and psychiatric facilities of the Massachusetts General Hospital.[41,42] This table illustrates that groups of patients with functional cardiovascular complaints and those with nervous complaints are often indistinguishable from one another with respect to symptom patterns. It

TABLE 3. COMPARATIVE FREQUENCIES OF SOMATIC AND PSYCHOLOGIC
SYMPTOMS IN PATIENTS WITH CARDIAC AND PSYCHIATRIC DISEASE
(MASSACHUSETTS GENERAL HOSPITAL)[41,42]

Symptom	Cardiology Patients (% with symptoms)	Anxiety Neurotics (% with symptoms)
Palpitations	97	90
Tires easily	95	78
Breathlessness	90	75
Nervousness	88	99
Sighing	79	20
Dizziness	78	55
Faintness	70	20
Apprehension	61	80
Headache	58	65
Paresthesias	58	25
Weakness	56	65
Trembling	54	70
Breath unsatisfactory	53	73
Insomnia	53	48
Shakiness	47	70
Fatigued all the time	45	76
Sweating	45	62

further suggests that simple notions of somatic events "causing" anxiety, or vice versa, do not reflect the true complexity of human functioning.

OTHER NEUROPSYCHIATRIC APPLICATIONS OF β-ADRENOCEPTOR BLOCKING THERAPY

The effects of β-adrenoceptor blockers on stress responses have been described for public speaking and stress interviews, venipuncture, dental surgery, ski-jumping, exercise, race-car driving, concert performance, civil unrest, "exam-nerves," and stage fright.[16] There is a great deal of attention now being addressed in the lay literature about β-adrenoceptor blockers being "confidence medicines" that individuals can self-administer prior to stressful activities.

Taggart and Carruthers[43] studied normal subjects and patients with coronary artery disease in a double-blind crossover study with a placebo and a single 40-mg dose of oxprenolol and found that oxprenolol suppressed or eliminated the tachycardia, ECG changes, and plasma epinephrine– and plasma free–fatty acid elevations in response to public speaking in both groups. Propranolol in doses of 40 mg or less was shown to be remarkably effective in limiting the physical responses known collectively as stage fright.[44] However, the psychologic aspects of stage fright may still be disabling even after somatic manifestations are eliminated. β-Blockade with propranolol has only an indirect effect on the emotional aspects of stage fright. This facet of the problem is perhaps better treated by self-hypnosis training.

Imhof and Brunner[35] telemetrically studied ski-jumpers; Eliasch and colleagues[45] investigated fright-stimulation subjects, and Mechtens and Tetsch[46] examined patients undergoing dental surgery. These investigators found that β-adrenoceptor blockers reduced stress-induced tachycardia under their respective experimental situations.

Taggart and Carruthers[43] found that an oral dose of oxprenolol given 1 hour before race-car driving suppressed the tachycardia and the increased plasma free–fatty acids and blood glucose demonstrated in the same drivers without β-blockade. Taylor and Meeran[47] used a single dose of oxprenolol (40 mg) and placebo in a double-blind study of the tachycardias associated with motor-car driving, isoproterenol infusion, and walking. Tachycardias induced by driving or isoproterenol infusion were significantly reduced with oxprenolol, while the magnitude and duration of reduction in exercise tachycardia were substantially less. Thus, it appears that tachycardia due to emotional stress is mediated almost entirely by β-adrenergic receptors, whereas tachycardia due to exercise is only partially mediated by β-adrenergic receptors.

Because propranolol does not sedate, Brewer[48] considered it suitable for use in abnormally anxious students taking examinations. In a double-blind trial, propranolol was administered in doses sufficient to reduce resting pulse to 55 to 60 beats per mintue. The drug was compared with placebo, systematic desensitization, and no treatment. Propranolol caused no impairment of exam performance and may have improved performance in persons who would otherwise be handicapped by severe anxiety, especially those in whom cardiovascular manifestations were prominent. Conway[49,50] achieved successful results with propranolol up to 200 mg per day administered several weeks before examinations in students with a history of severe preexamination tension. He increased the dose, starting at 10 mg three times per day until the heart rate fell below 70 beats per minute. Eisdorfer and colleagues[51] administered propranolol (10 mg intravenously) or placebo to 28 male volunteers over 60 years of age and found significantly improved performance on a verbal learning task with propranolol.

Anecdotal reports suggest that propranolol reduces heroin-induced euphoria, ameliorates narcotic-withdrawal syndromes, and may be useful in treating narcotic addiction.[16,52] However, no adequate clinical trials have been conducted with propranolol or with the newer β-adrenoceptor blocking agents in treating narcotic addiction, and the effectiveness of these drugs in this condition is questionable.[52] Propranolol has been successfully used to manage patients undergoing acute alcohol withdrawal.[16,52,53] The drug's effects on alcohol-withdrawal symptoms are felt to be due to blockade of central nervous system β-adrenoceptors with a subsequent decrease in sympathetic outflow. However, one cannot rule out a peripheral β-blocking effect for treatment of this problem. Patients with mild to moderate symptoms of alcohol withdrawal responded to 40 to 160 mg of oral propranolol daily over 6 days of therapy. Agitation and tremors lessened, none of the patients developed delirium tremens or withdrawal seizures, and all tolerated the drug well. β-Blockers have also been suggested as a "hangover" remedy.[16]

The use of β-adrenoceptor blocking drugs in the treatment of psychosis is highly controversial.[18,28] Several studies have appeared that describe the use of propranolol (up to 5800 mg per day) in schizophrenic patients.[17] In general, favorable results have been claimed in patients with acute psychotic states, while chronically affected patients do not seem to respond. The beneficial response to β-blockade sometimes becomes apparent within hours.

Despite the initial excitement generated by β-blockers in the treatment of acute psychosis, none of the clinical trials with these drugs were based on a double-blind design. The possibility of spontaneous clinical remission and the concomitant use of other antipsychotic drugs were not taken into consideration.[54] The possible mechanism for a β-blocker response in patients with acute schizophrenia has also not yet been elucidated. If it relates to a central nervous system effect, those lipid-soluble drugs that rapidly cross the blood–brain barrier (metoprolol, propranolol) might prove to be more efficacious than β-adrenoceptor blocking agents that do not demonstrate this property.

There is some evidence that heightened adrenergic activity may play a role in some varieties of tremors, including essential, familial, and senile tremors, and familial essential myoclonus.[52] Most of the patients with benign action tremors noted clinical improvement with 60 to 240 mg of oral propranolol daily. A few patients showed virtually complete resolution of the tremor, while the majority of the patients reported mild improvement. The best responses were obtained in younger patients who had shorter histories of tremor. To date, there are no good clinical studies using the newer β-blocking drugs for treatment of tremor. Whether or not nonselective β-blockers will prove more efficacious than those with β_1-selectivity has yet to be determined.[52]

Potential use of β-blockers for stuttering, migraine, phantom limb, and fatty acid elevating effects of smoking have been suggested.[1] Linken[55] reported three cases of LSD-induced anxiety states that were rapidly relieved by oral propranolol (10 mg three times per day).[55] A recent report suggested the use of β-adrenoceptor blocking drugs in treatment of narcolepsy.[56]

RECOMMENDATIONS REGARDING THE USE OF β-ADRENOCEPTOR BLOCKERS FOR ANXIETY STATES OR PSYCHOCARDIAC DISORDERS

When does one treat the symptoms associated with anxiety or psychocardiac disorders? In general, nonanxious individuals infused with epinephrine are conscious of tachycardia but have little fear, whereas anxiety-prone individuals in the same situation report anxiety and panic as well as tachycardia. Tyrer[57,58] states that the anxious patients who benefit most from β-blockers are those with mainly somatic complaints mediated by sympathetic activity, i.e., palpitation, trembling, dizziness, shaking, or blushing. Sweating, muscle tension, headache, dry mouth, nausea, frequency of micturition, and diarrhea are less affected by β-blockade. These last symptoms are not readily connected with the physiologic activity of the β-receptors. Patients in whom the first group of symptoms are primary events associated with anxiety may do well on β-blockers alone. In contrast are those patients with primary psychic anxiety, marked by forebodings and dread. They too complain of somatic symptoms, but the correlation between bodily symptoms and psychologic changes seem to be low; in other words, somatic symptoms may not reflect true psychologic changes in this group. Patients with primary psychic anxiety are not helped much by β-blockers; indeed, the condition may be exacerbated by them. There is still no evidence that sympathetic activation is reduced by β-blockade in stress; therefore, it is not surprising that subjective psychic anxiety is little affected. In some of these patients the bodily symptoms of anxiety may have assurance value, and their abolition may make matters worse. Patients treated with beta-blockers need to be carefully selected, and they must be warned of the expected side effects (see below).[58]

In summary (Fig. 1), for patients who have primarily somatic anxiety, β-blockers are potential drugs of choice. In the usual therapeutic dose range, the drugs have few side effects, and there is little chance of drowsiness, tolerance, dependence, or abuse. β-Blockers may also be combined with centrally acting anxiolytic agents. However, in situations in which there is a great deal of psychic anxiety, such as severe phobia without much somatization of the anxiety, a centrally acting anxiolytic such as diazepam should be used in place of a β-blocking drug. When using β-blockers as antianxiety drugs, a small dose should be used initially since sympathetic tone varies between patients and one has to observe these patients quite closely for psychologic effects.

UNWANTED SIDE EFFECTS OF β-ADRENOCEPTOR BLOCKER THERAPY IN TREATMENT OF ANXIETY

Despite the fact that some members of the lay press are advising the widespread use of β-blocking drugs for children and adults to relieve anxiety, these drugs have definite side effects related to their basic pharmacologic properties, which are potentially serious (see Chapter 5).[59,60] Adverse cardiovascular effects include congestive heart failure, pulmonary edema, bradycardia, myocardial conduction disturbances, and hypotension. Most of these effects, however, occur in patients with organic heart disease whose cardiovascular stability is dependent on

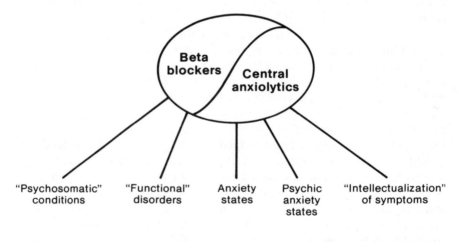

SOMATIC   PSYCHOLOGICAL

Figure 1. Possible relationship between anxiety symptom profile and anxiolytic treatment.

sympathetic stimulation. An incidence of hypertension as high as 33 percent has been reported during propranolol treatment of psychoses.[16] A rapid withdrawal of propranolol in treatment of anxiety syndromes may dispose patients with angina pectoris to myocardial infarction. Patients with bronchospasm should not be treated with β-adrenergic drugs.[59]

In a survey of approximately 1500 patients receiving oral propranolol therapy, Stephen[61] reported a number of unexpected neuropsychiatric side effects. Twenty-two patients reported lightheadedness or dizziness, 7 experienced insomnia, and 18 complained of fatigue. Five patients experienced visual blurring or hallucinations, and mental confusion was reported in one. Dornhorst, in his comment on Stephen's paper, stated that he had seen one case of hypnagogic hallucinations clearly related to propranolol therapy.[16] Hallucinations, nightmares, and insomnia have been mentioned by a number of authors.[16] These appear not to be spurious occurrences. There are also reports of acute toxic psychoses or confusional states attributable to propranolol. Changes in mood and affect caused by β-antagonists have also been described. Waal[62] claimed a high incidence of depression in 89 propranolol-treated patients. The incidence approached 50 percent after 3 months of treatment with doses greater than 120 mg a day and seemed to increase with both dose and duration of treatment. Two patients attempted suicide. Those patients with a history of depression associated with reserpine treatment seemed more likely to be depressed with propranolol. Sullivan[63] has noted behavioral evidence of "depression" in propranolol-treated rats similar to that induced with reserpine, apparently due to effects of both these drugs on tyrosine hydroxylase.

Fatigue, lassitude, and decreased exercise tolerance are not infrequent complaints of patients taking large doses of β-adrenergic blocking drugs, and it may be difficult to differentiate these responses from the manifestations of true depression. The exact incidence and significance of depression or confusion, hallucinations, and insomnia associated with propranolol and related drugs are not clear at present, but the β-antagonists clearly appear to have the potential to produce alterations in level of consciousness and affect in some individuals. Greenblatt and Koch-Weser[60] have recently examined reports of adverse psychic reactions to oral propranolol among 797 patients (Table 4).[60]

Neuropsychiatric side effects are of special significance if β-blockers are to be used in the treatment of anxiety states, since there can be difficulty in distinguishing these side effects from underlying anxiety symptoms. Many investigations of β-blockers in the treatment of anxiety either have not considered the important question of neuropsychiatric adverse reactions or have not reported any serious ones.[16] Lader

TABLE 4. CENTRAL NERVOUS SYSTEM SIDE EFFECTS OF ORAL PROPRANOLOL AMONG 797 PATIENTS[16,60]

Side Effects	Number of Patients	Percentage
Sleep disturbance	34	4.3
Dizziness	33	4.1
Fatigue	25	3.1
Mental depression	13	1.6
Hallucinations	4	0.8

and Tyrer[19] noted subjective feelings of "drowsiness and fuzziness" in some patients treated with sotalol and a sense of "being troubled" with sotalol and propranolol. They suggested that mood changes could be secondary to the perception of somatic effects of β-adrenergic blockers.[19,22] Wheatley found significantly fewer side effects with propranolol (30 mg three times daily) than with chlordiazepoxide.[3] The major untoward effect was drowsiness (propranolol 8 percent versus chlordiazepoxide 12 percent). Yet 12 percent of the patients omitted dosages because of side effects of propranolol versus 11 percent of patients receiving chlordiazepoxide. In the studies of Granville-Grossman and Turner,[2] and Bonn and colleagues,[9] more patients complained of side effects—usually tiredness, dizziness, nausea, or headache—with β-blockers than with placebo.

CLINICAL IMPLICATIONS

Studies of currently available β-adrenergic blocking drugs have contributed greatly to the development of anxiety theory. The importance of beta-adrenergic blockade to the understanding of anxiety derives from the fact that the sympathetic nervous system is activated in anxiety, and β-adrenoceptor blockade modifies some of the bodily responses to this activation. Studies of the pharmacologic effects of β-adrenoceptor blockers in anxiety must always be related back to the subjective reported experience of anxiety or fear. No matter how elaborate the measurements we use, in the end we have to ask the patient how he is feeling. Selective blockade of somatic effects of anxiety is useful primarily if the source of anxiety is also thereby affected. In other words, there should be interaction of a somatopsychic sequence of events whereby the somatic symptom is contributing to maintenance of anxiety. A useful effect in anxiety can be expected if there is clinical evidence that the inappropriate sympathetic activity is contributing to the stress and anxiety. For instance, a β-blocker might be of use in a public speaker who feels stressed by hand trembling. If the hand trembling is relieved by the β-blocker, and the speaker achieves an increased level of confidence, then the level of anxiety may be relieved. However, if hand trembling does not bother the speaker, treating him with a β-blocker will not affect him in any therapeutic way and may even reduce his performance level.

Peripheral β-blockade is a more likely mechanism for the action of these drugs on anxiety than any central effects that they might have. Also the presence or absence of cardioselectivity, intrinsic sympathomimetic activity, or lipophilicity in a β-blocker does not seem to influence the effects of a drug on anxiety. However, these differences may be significant in adverse reactions seen with these drugs.

The place of β-adrenoceptor blockade in the treatment of anxiety is still being evaluated. At the present time, none of the β-blockers would seem superior to conventional benzodiazepines for the treatment of chronic anticipatory and free-floating anxiety. β-Blockers have not yet been systematically compared with antidepressants to examine their role in spontaneous panic attacks and agoraphobia. Acute situational and anticipatory anxiety (e.g., public speaking), or at least the somatic manifestations of such anxieties, may be conditions in which β-blockers offer some advantage, but further research would be necessary to support this indication. There is a great danger also in a widespread use of these agents as "confidence" drugs. A certain degree of normal anxiety is necessary in many of our activities of daily living, and performance can be blunted with an inappropriate use of these agents.

How should β-blockers be used in anxiety states? Classification of anxiety states can help distinguish patients with predominantly central or psychic anxiety, in whom somatic complaints are of secondary importance, from those with somatic anxiety, with prominent somatic manifestations often in the cardiovascular system.[7,64] β-Adrenoceptor blockade would be expected to be particularly effective in the second group, as described by Tyrer and Lader.[6] However, the majority of patients with anxiety cannot easily be classified as belonging definitively to one of these two groups, as they have both central and somatic symptoms. Lader[7] has suggested that a combination of a centrally acting drug such as benzodiazepine, in small dosage with a β-adrenoceptor blocking drug, should therefore produce some maximum therapeutic advantage.

We have, of course, not yet mentioned the role of nonpharmacologic interventions (psychotherapy, behavior therapy, biofeedback) in anxiety. Although we cannot extensively review here the comparative efficacy of all these interventions, the following points are worth noting: (1) There are no studies definitively comparing psychotherapy, pharmacotherapy, and combined therapy. (2) Available evidence suggests that for nonpsychotic anxiety, combined psychotherapy and pharmacotherapy is more effective than either therapy alone.[65] (3) Behavior therapy and biofeedback must be considered as quite viable treatments (preferable to psychotherapy), though not clearly preferable to pharmacotherapy for clearly somatic or focused (phobic) anxiety. (4) Supportive or exploratory psychodynamic psychotherapy is probably the treatment of choice for psychic anxiety. The addition of pharmacologic treatment to psychologic intervention may well increase efficacy, as we have just suggested, but individual patient differences must of course be considered by the clinician. Thus, the meaning to the patient of being on one, another, or both types of treatment, the patient's preference (which will affect compliance), and the chronic (characterologic) or acute (situational) nature of the psychic anxiety must all be considered in choosing a therapeutic modality.

In closing, a completely new era of β-adrenoceptor research has been launched, one that may not only provide insights into therapy, but more important, may give new insights into the mind and neuropsychiatric illness.

SUMMARY AND CONCLUSIONS

1. β-Adrenoceptor drugs have contributed to the development and understanding of anxiety theory.
2. The sympathetic nervous system is activated in anxiety, and β-blockade modifies some of the bodily responses to this activation.
3. β-Blockers do not directly affect the psychic component of anxiety, only some of the somatic consequences. In situations where the somatic consequences are aggravating the anxiety syndrome itself, then the drug may be useful.
4. The presence or absence of cardioselectivity, intrinsic sympathomimetic activity, and lipophilicity in a β-blocker does not seem to influence the effects in anxiety. However, these differences may be operative in adverse reactions seen with the drugs.
5. Benzodiazepines are still superior to β-blocking drugs in the treatment of chronic anticipatory and free-floating anxiety.
6. β-Blockers may be useful in acute situational or anticipatory anxiety (e.g., public speaking).

7. There is a danger of the use of these drugs as "confidence" drugs. β-Blocking drugs have definite side effects and may depress individuals who are dependent on a "normal level of anxiety" in their activities of daily life.

8. β-Blockers have been shown to be useful for anxiety syndromes manifested by primary somatic complaints (psychocardiac disorders) and should be avoided in patients with predominant psychic components in their anxiety syndrome. For the combination of both psychic and somatic symptoms, the combination of tranquilizer, β-blocker, and psychologic treatment might be useful. Where psychic symptoms predominate, psychologic interventions may be most useful.

REFERENCES

1. Frishman W: Clinical Pharmacology of the Beta-Adrenergic Blocking Drugs. New York, Appleton-Century-Crofts, 1980.
2. Granville-Grossman KL, Turner P: The effect of propranolol on anxiety. Lancet 1:788, 1966.
3. Wheatley B: Comparative effects of propranolol and chlordiazepoxide in anxiety states. Br J Psychiatry 115:1411, 1969.
4. Suzman MM: The use of beta-adrenergic blockade with propranolol in anxiety syndromes. Postgrad Med J 47 (Suppl):104, 1971.
5. Suzman MM: Propranolol in the treatment of anxiety. Postgrad Med J 52 (Suppl 4):168, 1976.
6. Tyrer PJ, Lader MH: Response to propranolol and diazepam in somatic and psychic anxiety. Br Med J 2:14, 1974.
7. Lader M: Somatic and psychic symptoms in anxiety. Adv Clin Pharmacol 12:21, 1976.
8. Tanna VT, Penningroth RP, Woolson RF: Propranolol in the treatment of anxiety neurosis. Compr Psychiatry 1:319, 1977.
9. Bonn JA, Turner P, Hicks DC: Beta-adrenergic blockade with practolol in treatment of anxiety. Lancet 1:814, 1972.
10. Lader MH: The peripheral and central role of the catecholamines in the mechanisms of anxiety. Int Pharmacopsychiatry 9:125, 1974.
11. Lange CG, James W: The Emotions. Baltimore, Williams and Wilkins, 1922.
12. Cannon WB: The James-Lange theory of emotions. A critical examination and an alternative theory. Am J Psychol 39:106, 1927.
13. Sherrington CS: Experiments on the value of vascular and visceral factors in the genesis of emotion. Proc Soc Med 66:390, 1900.
14. Breggin PR: The psychophysiology of anxiety. J Nerv Ment Dis 139:558, 1964.

15. Frohlich ED, Tarazi RC, Dustan HP: Hyperdynamic β-adrenergic circulatory state. Arch Intern Med 123:1, 1969.

16. Shader RI, Good MI, Greenblatt DJ: Anxiety states and beta-adrenergic blockade, in Klein DF, Gittleman-Klein (eds), Progress in Psychiatric Drug Treatment. New York, Brunner Mazel, 1976.

17. Yorkston NJ, Zaki SA, Malik MKU, et al: Propranolol in the control of schizophrenic symptoms. Br Med J 4:633, 1974.

18. Jefferson JW: Beta-adrenergic receptor blocking drugs in psychiatry. Arch Gen Psychiatry 31:681, 1974.

19. Lader MH, Tyrer PJ: Central and peripheral effects of propranolol and sotalol in normal human subjects. Br J Pharmacol 45:557, 1971.

20. Bonn JA, Turner P: d-Propranolol and anxiety. Lancet 1:1355, 1971.

21. Tyrer PJ, Lader MH: Beta-adrenergic receptor blockade in the treatment of anxiety. Lancet 2:542, 1972.

22. Tyrer PJ, Lader MH: Effects of beta-adrenergic blockade with sotalol in chronic anxiety. Clin Pharmacol Ther 14:413, 1976.

23. Tyrer PJ, Lader MH: Physiological and psychological effects of ± propranolol, + propranolol and diazepam in induced anxiety. Br J Clin Pharmacol 1:379, 1974.

24. Tyrer PJ, Lader MH: Physiological responses to propranolol and diazepam in chronic anxiety. Br J Clin Pharmacol 1:387, 1974.

25. Ramsay I, Greer S, Bagley C: Propranolol in neurotic and thyrotoxic anxiety. Br J Psychiatry 122:555, 1973.

26. Stone WN, Gleser GC, Gottschalk LA: Anxiety and β-adrenergic blockade. Arch Gen Psychiatry 24:620, 1973.

27. Gottschalk LA, Stone WN, Gleser GC: Peripheral versus central mechanisms for antianxiety effects of propranolol. Psychosom Med 36:47, 1974.

28. Whitlock FA, Price J: Use of β-adrenergic blocking drugs in psychiatry. Drugs 8:109, 1974.

29. Kellner R, Wilson RM, Muldawer MD, et al: Anxiety in schizophrenia. The response to chlordiazepoxide in an intensive drug study. Arch Gen Psychiatry 32:1246, 1973.

30. Frohlich ED: Beta-adrenergic blockade in the circulatory regulation of hyperkinetic states. Am J Cardiol 27:195, 1971.

31. Besterman EMM, Friedlander DH: Clinical experience with propranolol. Postgrad Med J 4:526, 1965.

32. Bollinger A, Ganger M, Pylkkanen PO, et al: Treatment of the hyperkinetic heart syndrome with propranolol. Cardiology 49 (Suppl 2):68, 1966.

33. Furberg C: Adrenergic β-blockade and physical working capacity. Acta Med Scand 182:119, 1967.

34. Furberg C, Morsing C: Adrenergic beta-receptor blockade in neurocirculatory asthenia. Pharmacol Clin 1:168, 1969.

35. Imhof P, Brunner H: The treatment of functional heart disorders with beta-adrenergic blocking agents. Postgrad Med J 46:96, 1970.

36. Marsden CW: Propranolol in neurocirculatory asthenia and anxiety. Postgrad Med J 47 (Suppl):100, 1971.

37. Nordenfelt I, Persson S, Redfors A: Effect of a new adrenergic β-blocking agent H56/28 on nervous heart complaints. Acta Med Scand 184:465, 1968.
38. Thulsesius O, Hansson R, List E: Cardiospecific beta-adrenergic blockade in the treatment of nervous heart symptoms. Curr Ther Res 15:805, 1973.
39. Bourne HR, Thomson PD, Melmon KL: Diagnosis and treatment of beta-adrenergic receptor hyperresponsiveness. Arch Intern Med 125:1063, 1970.
40. Taggart P, Carruthers M, Somerville W: Emotions, catecholamines an the electrocardiogram, in Yu PN, Goodwin JF (eds), Progess in Cardiology (7). Philadelphia, Lea and Febiger, 1978, 103–124.
41. Wheeler EO, White PD, Reed EW, et al: Neurocirculatory asthenia (anxiety neurosis, effort syndrome, neurasthenia). JAMA 142:878, 1950.
42. Miles HWM, Barabee EL, Finesinger JE: Evaluation of psychotherapy with a follow up study of 62 cases of anxiety neurosis. Psychosom Med 13:83, 1951.
43. Taggart P, Carruthers M, Somerville W: Electrocardiogram, plasma catecholamines and lipids and their modification by oxprenolol when speaking before an audience. Lancet 2:341, 1973.
44. Brantigan CO, Brantigan TA, Joseph N: Effect of beta-blockade and beta-stimulation on stage fright. Am J Med 72:88, 1982.
45. Eliasch H, Rosen A, Scott H: Systemic circulatory response to stress of simulated flight and to physical exercise before and after propranolol blockade. Br Heart J 29:671, 1967.
46. Mechtens E, Tesch P: Die injizierbare kombination eines lokalanesthetikums mit einem beta rezeptorenblocker. Dtsch Zahnaerztl Z 23:581, 1968.
47. Taylor SH, Meeran MK: Different effects of adrenergic beta-receptor blockade on heart rate response to mental stress, catecholamines and exercise. Br Med J 4:257, 1973.
48. Brewer C: Beneficial effect of beta-adrenergic blockade on "exam nerves. Lancet 2:435, 1972.
49. Conway M: Final examinations. Practitioner 296:795, 1971.
50. Conway M: Response to propranolol and diazepam in somatic and psychic anxiety. Br Med J 2:671, 1974.
51. Eisdorfer C, Nowlin J, Wilke F: Improvement of learning in the aged by modification of autonomic nervous system activity. Science 170:1327, 1970.
52. Frishman W, Silverman R: Clinical pharmacology of the new beta-adrenergic blocking drugs. Part 3: Comparative clinical experience and new therapeutic applications. Am Heart J 98:1191, 1979.
53. Sellers EM, Deyani NC, Silm et al: Propranolol decreased noradrenaline secretion and alcohol withdrawal. Lancet 1:94, 1976.
54. New drugs for schizophrenia. (Editorial). Br Med J 4:614, 1975.
55. Linken A: Propranolol for LSD-induced anxiety states. (Letter). Lancet 2:1039, 1971.
56. Kales A, Soldatos CR, Cadieux R: Propranolol in the treatment of narcolepsy. Ann Intern Med 93:741, 1979.
57. Tyrer P: The Role of Bodily Feelings in Anxiety. London, Maudsley Monograph, No. 23, 1976.

58. Beta-adrenergic blockade and anxiety. (Editorial). Lancet 2:611, 1976.
59. Frishman W, Silverman R, Strom J, et al: Clinical pharmacology of the new beta-adrenergic blocking drugs. Part 4: Adverse effects. Choosing a β-adrenoceptor blocker. Am Heart J 98:256, 1979.
60. Greenblatt D, Koch-Weser J: Adverse reactions to beta-adrenergic receptor blocking drugs: A report from the Boston Collaborative Drug Surveillance Program. Drugs 7:118, 1974.
61. Stephen SA: Unwanted effects of propranolol. Am J Cardiol 18:463, 1966.
62. Waal HJ: Propranolol-induced depression. Br Med J 2:50, 1967.
63. Sullivan JL, Segal DS, Kuczenski RT, et al: Propranolol-induced rapid activation of rat striatal tyrosine hydroxylase concomitant with behavioral depression. Biol Psychiatry 4:193, 1972.
64. Turner P: Beta-adrenoceptor blockade in hyperthyroidism and anxiety. Proc Roy Soc Med 69:375, 1976.
65. Luborsky L, Singer B, Luborsky L: Comparative studies of psychotherapies. Arch Gen Psychiatry 32:495, 1975.

Index